Practical Manual of
OBSTETRICS

Practical Manual of OBSTETRICS

SECOND EDITION

Amitava Pal
MBBS (Hons) DGO MS DNBE (Obs Gyn) FICMCH
Professor
Department of Obstetrics and Gynecology
Burdwan Medical College
Burdwan, West Bengal, India

Rupali Modak
MBBS (Hons) MD (Gold Medalist)
Assistant Professor
Department of Obstetrics and Gynecology
RG Kar Medical College
Kolkata, West Bengal, India

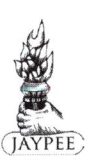 *The Health Sciences Publisher*

New Delhi | London | Panama

Jaypee Brothers Medical Publishers (P) Ltd

Headquarters

Jaypee Brothers Medical Publishers (P) Ltd
4838/24, Ansari Road, Daryaganj
New Delhi 110 002, India
Phone: +91-11-43574357
Fax: +91-11-43574314
Email: jaypee@jaypeebrothers.com

Overseas Offices

J.P. Medical Ltd
83 Victoria Street, London
SW1H 0HW (UK)
Phone: +44 20 3170 8910
Fax: +44 (0)20 3008 6180
Email: info@jpmedpub.com

Jaypee-Highlights Medical Publishers Inc
City of Knowledge, Bld. 235, 2nd Floor, Clayton
Panama City, Panama
Phone: +1 507-301-0496
Fax: +1 507-301-0499
Email: cservice@jphmedical.com

Jaypee Brothers Medical Publishers (P) Ltd
17/1-B Babar Road, Block-B, Shaymali
Mohammadpur, Dhaka-1207
Bangladesh
Mobile: +08801912003485
Email: jaypeedhaka@gmail.com

Jaypee Brothers Medical Publishers (P) Ltd
Bhotahity, Kathmandu, Nepal
Phone: +977-9741283608
Email: kathmandu@jaypeebrothers.com

Website: www.jaypeebrothers.com
Website: www.jaypeedigital.com

© 2017, Jaypee Brothers Medical Publishers

The views and opinions expressed in this book are solely those of the original contributor(s)/author(s) and do not necessarily represent those of editor(s) of the book.

All rights reserved. No part of this publication may be reproduced, stored or transmitted in any form or by any means, electronic, mechanical, photocopying, recording or otherwise, without the prior permission in writing of the publishers.

All brand names and product names used in this book are trade names, service marks, trademarks or registered trademarks of their respective owners. The publisher is not associated with any product or vendor mentioned in this book.

Medical knowledge and practice change constantly. This book is designed to provide accurate, authoritative information about the subject matter in question. However, readers are advised to check the most current information available on procedures included and check information from the manufacturer of each product to be administered, to verify the recommended dose, formula, method and duration of administration, adverse effects and contraindications. It is the responsibility of the practitioner to take all appropriate safety precautions. Neither the publisher nor the author(s)/editor(s) assume any liability for any injury and/or damage to persons or property arising from or related to use of material in this book.

This book is sold on the understanding that the publisher is not engaged in providing professional medical services. If such advice or services are required, the services of a competent medical professional should be sought.

Every effort has been made where necessary to contact holders of copyright to obtain permission to reproduce copyright material. If any have been inadvertently overlooked, the publisher will be pleased to make the necessary arrangements at the first opportunity.

Inquiries for bulk sales may be solicited at: jaypee@jaypeebrothers.com

Practical Manual of Obstetrics

First Edition: 2013

Second Edition: **2017**

ISBN: 978-93-86150-92-9

Printed at Sanat Printers

Dedicated to

*Our Parents,
Teachers and Students*

PREFACE TO THE SECOND EDITION

The acceptance of first edition by students and doctors has encouraged us to bring out the earlier second edition. All the chapters are thoroughly revised and special attention is paid for correction of spelling mistakes. The formats of some questions are changed and answers are simplified in many areas. A few new questions relevant to examination purpose are also added in different chapters. Emphasis has been paid on some important topics, such as specimens of hydrocephalus, conjoined twin and anencephaly, drugs in obstetrics, role of Doppler in pregnancy, and hyperemesis gravidarum. One important postgraduate topic *Nonimmune Hydrops Fetalis* and fetal anemia is included in this edition. Contents have been revised to incorporate evidence-based approach.

We are very much thankful to Dr Santanu Bar, MS, RMO-cum-clinical tutor, Burdwan Medical College, Burdwan, West Bengal, India, for his contribution on *Role of Doppler in Pregnancy*. We are also grateful to all our colleagues and seniors of our departments for planning and execution of this edition.

We hope, this edition will also be helpful for students and doctors in this fraternity.

We thank Shri Jitendar P Vij (Group Chairman) and Mr Ankit Vij (Group President) of M/s Jaypee Brothers Medical Publishers (P) Ltd, New Delhi, India, for their interest to bring out this edition expeditiously despite many problems.

Feedback is always welcome for further edition.

Amitava Pal
Rupali Modak

PREFACE TO THE FIRST EDITION

This book is written to meet the long-standing demand of the students. It is not a textbook. All the readers are requested to go through a textbook before reading this book. This book is very much helpful for undergraduate and postgraduate students of medical fraternity, students of nursing and also for clinicians who practice in the field of obstetrics. Much emphasis is paid on four essential attributes like knowledge, skill, experience and judgment to tackle the different obstetrical problems in day-to-day practice.

This book mainly deals with the practical aspects of obstetrics including specimen, instruments, operations and to identify, investigate, diagnose and manage more common clinical problems in the field of obstetrics. Essential diagrams, photographs, tables and flowcharts have been judiciously selected. The interventions described are based on latest scientific evidence. Majority of the chapters are written in questions and answers form which are commonly asked in examinations. The questions have also been divided into different categories.

So, this book is very much helpful for the students for a quick revision purpose before any practical examinations of India and abroad. It may also be used as a bedside guide.

The readers will determine the strength and weakness of this edition. Feedback is always welcome for further revised edition.

Amitava Pal
Rupali Modak

CONTENTS

1. **Specimens**   1–36
   - Ectopic Pregnancy 1
   - Rupture of Uterus 11
   - Hydatidiform Mole 16
   - Placenta with Umbilical Cord 24
   - Anencephaly 32
2. **Instruments and Drugs**   37
   - Sponge-holding Forceps 37
   - Kocher's Artery Forceps or Clamps 38
   - Allis Tissue Forceps 39
   - Green-Armytage Hemostatic Forceps 40
   - Simple Rubber Catheter and Foley's Catheter 41
   - Drew Smythe Catheter 44
   - Sim's Double-bladed Posterior Vaginal Speculum 44
   - Vulsellum 47
   - Uterine Sound 48
   - Cervical Dilators 50
   - Hegar's Dilators 51
   - Hawkins-Ambler's Dilators 51
   - Uterine Curette (Flushing) 52
   - Ovum Forceps 54
   - Karman's Plastic Cannula 55
   - Abdominal Retractors 55
   - Pinard's Metal Fetoscope 56
   - Mucus Sucker 58
   - Umbilical Cord Scissors with Disposable Umbilical Cord Clips 61
   - Blunt Hook and Crochet 62
   - Lumbar Puncture Needle 62
   - Drugs in Obstetrics 65
   - Antihypertensives 67
   - Labetalol 67
   - Hydralazine Hydrochloride (Drangeen) 68
   - Other Drugs 74
   - Corticosteroids 76
3. **Obstetric Operations and Interventions**   78
   - Cesarean Section 78
   - Episiotomy 86
   - Dilatation and Evacuation/Suction and Evacuation 92
   - Destructive Operations 95
   - Instruments for Decapitation 99
   - Surgical Management of PPH 101
   - Obstetric Forceps 108
   - Ventouse 118
   - Version 123
   - Other Operations 126
4. **Maternal Pelvis and Fetal Skull**   142

- Pelvis 142
- Fetal Skull 149

5. **Normal Labor and Labor in Malposition and Presentation** 158
   - Flying Questions on Normal Labor 162
   - Programmed Labor 167
   - Labor in Abnormal Presentation: Face 174
   - Brow Presentation 176
   - Breech Presentation 177
   - Cord Prolapse 189
   - Compound Presentation 190

6. **Assessment of Fetal Well-being** 194
   - Daily Fetal Movement Count 194
   - Fetal Heart Rate Monitoring 194
   - Fetal Distress and Monitor 195
   - Classification, Causes and Mechanism of Fetal Heart Rate Pattern 196
   - Antepartum Fetal Surveillance 205
   - Examples of Some Abnormal Fetal Heart Rate Baseline 207
   - Fetal Heart Rate Deceleration 209
   - Fetal ECG Waveform Analysis (ST Analyzer—STAN) 211

7. **Partograph** 213

8. **Ultrasonography in Obstetrics** 223
   - First Trimester Pregnancy Problems 226
   - Pregnancy of Unknown Location 229
   - USG in Second and Third Trimester 231
   - Ultrasonography Doppler 240
   - Questions on Doppler in Fetal Hypoxia 241
   - Role of Doppler in Pregnancy 243

9. **X-ray in Obstetrics** 247
   - Breech Presentation 247
   - Hydrocephalus 250
   - Transverse Lie 252
   - Anencephaly 255
   - Multiple Pregnancy 257
   - Conjoined Twins 262
   - Intrauterine Fetal Death 263

10. **Obstetric Cases** 267
    - History Taking 267
    - Chief Complaints in Chronological Order 267
    - Normal Pregnancy at Term 278
    - Case Discussion on Rh-negative Mother 291
    - Primigravida with Floating Head 303
    - A Case of Multiple Pregnancy 311
    - Postdated Pregnancy 323
    - Puerperium 329
    - A Case of Anemia in Pregnancy 343
    - Post-cesarean Section Pregnancy 352
    - Antepartum Hemorrhage 359
    - Abruptio Placentae 367
    - A Case of Pre-eclampsia 374
    - A Case of HIV in Pregnancy 397
    - Intrauterine Growth Restriction 412
    - A Case of Pregnancy with Diabetes 420

- A Case of Heart Disease in Pregnancy   432
- Jaundice in Pregnancy   444
- Recurrent Pregnancy Loss   453
- Epilepsy in Pregnancy   462
- Thyroid Disorder in Pregnancy   467
- Hypothyroidism   468
- Hyperthyroidism in Pregnancy   472
- Obesity and Pregnancy   475
- A Case of Beta Thalassemia and Pregnancy   479

11. Flying Questions   **484**
- Liquor Amnii, Hydramnios and Oligohydramnios   484
- Hydramnios   485
- Oligohydramnios or Oligoamnios   487
- Preterm Labor   489
- Chorioamnionitis   493
- Shoulder Dystocia   494
- Induction of Labor   497
- Complications of Third Stage of Labor   505
- Inversion of Uterus   510
- Abortion Problem   512
- Gynecological Disorder in Pregnancy   519
- Hyperemesis Gravidarum   523
- Nonimmune Hydrops Fetalis and Fetal Anemia   525
- Maternal Death   531
- Perinatal Mortality Rate   533

Appendices   *535*
- *Appendix 1: Nutrition in Pregnancy   535*
- *Appendix 2: Physiological Changes in Pregnancy and Diagnosis of Pregnancy   542*
- *Appendix 3: Fetal Circulation   550*
- *Appendix 4: Different Types of Female Pelvis 553*

Index   *555*

Tips of Oral–Practical Examination in Obstetrics

A. GENERAL

- *Appearance of the student*: Dress should be simple, light colored, hair style should not irritate others, clean shave of beard (if religiously permissible), neat and clean ironed apron with roll number tag in front and covered shoes should be used.
- *Confidence*: Student must have self-confidence; knowledge of the subject may be optimum, but the candidate should not be nervous during examination.
- *Alertness*: Listen the questions of examiner carefully, do not be casual, if one does not understand the question, he or she can say politely 'pardon me sir or madam' or 'please repeat the question'.
- *Presentation*: Answer should be concise and relevant to the questions. Avoid unnecessary gesture, posture and mannerism during communication. Do not give wrong answer or argue with the examiners as you are not the master of the subject, or quote any name of the book in support of your answer.
- *Problem during examination*: Attract the attention of coordinator.
- *Equipments*: Students should be well-equipped with their own instruments necessary for examination of the patient (Blood pressure measuring instrument, stethoscope, hammer, measuring tape, skin marking pencil, etc).

B. SPECIAL POINTS

Each and every moment from the time of entry to exit of the Obstetrics table are countable and if examiner does not greet you with the word 'sit down'; you will welcome him politely with the words 'Good morning sir/madam—may I take seat'.

- *Specimen:* Do not lift the specimen from the table. Look the specimen jar on both sides by turning it on the table an handle it carefully because any spillage of formalin may irritate the examiner. Diagnose the specimen of tissue origin carefully before answering question.
- *Instrument:* Take the instrument as directed by examiner. See the instrument carefully and student is expected to know their points of identification and use in obstetrics. If examiner is liberal and allows one to take any instrument from the table, take the instrument on which he has the best confidence. Students must know the details of different drugs which are commonly used in obstetrics.
- *Maternal and fetal skull:* A lot of practice at home may help you in examination.

- *Radiological and, USG plate or partographic and CTG tracing if given in examination:* Scrutinize once before answering questions. Repeated examination during the process of questioning and answering creates a bad impression unless indicated by examiners.
- *Long case:* Read the full text several times before presentation as the examiner will take the history sheet. If the examiner asks you 'tell me the summary'—you will briefly summarize the case history with emphasis on relative positive and negative findings, but if the examiner sticks on 'diagnosis'—say only the 'diagnosis'.
- *Identification of slides if any:* Identify the pathological slides under microscope and write the diagnosis and 3-5 salient points in favor of diagnosis.

C. TO INCREASE THE SELF-CONFIDENCE AND SKILL FOR EXAMINATION

- Attend the classes (lecture, demonstration and ward clinic) regularly as the experienced teachers are the best guide
- Start group discussion on a topic with the fellow students or questioning and answering among themselves
- Teach the fellow students and juniors after preparation of a case or a topic
- Communication skill can be improved by practice and effort
- Speak in front of mirror for self-correction

So, regular practice with specimen, instruments, pelvis and fetal skull, X-ray and USG or tracing of partograph and cardiotocography personally, and in groups; regular group discussion with fellow students; prompt and clear answer with confidence in examination may allow a good score of the candidate in oral- practical examination.

PLATE 1

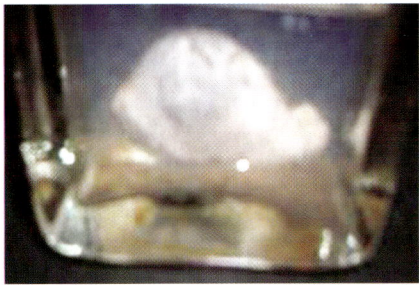

Figure 1.1A: Unruptured tubal ectopic pregnancy

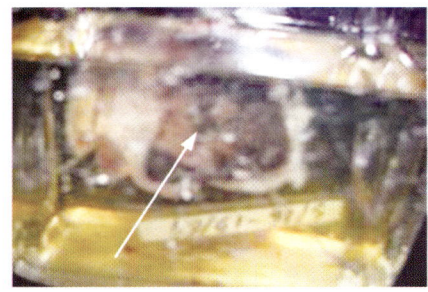

Figure 1.1B: Tubal mole (Black spot marked by arrow) on cut section

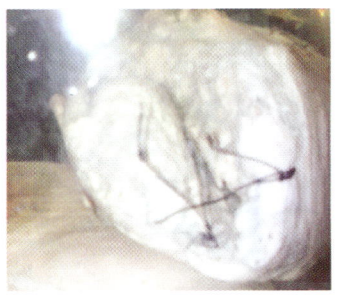

Figure 1.2: Rupture of uterus (Subtotal hysterectomy done)

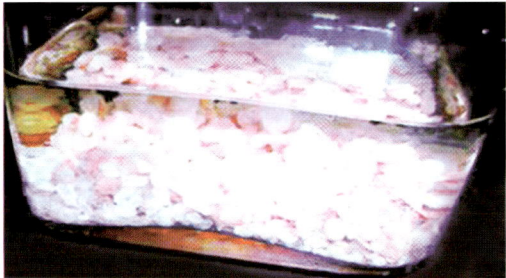

Figure 1.3: Specimen of hydatidiform mole

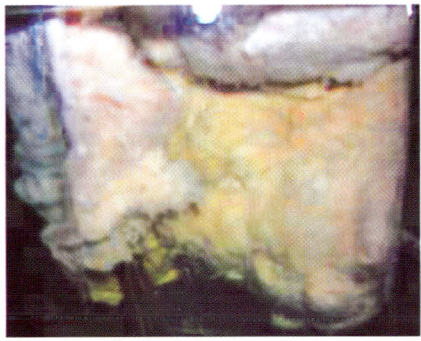

Figure 1.7A: Maternal surface of placenta (rough due to cotyledons)

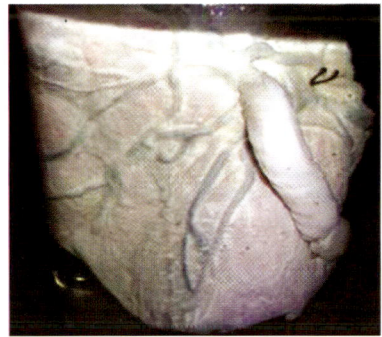

Figure 1.7B: Placenta—Fetal surface (umbilical cord and umbilical blood vessels)

PLATE 2

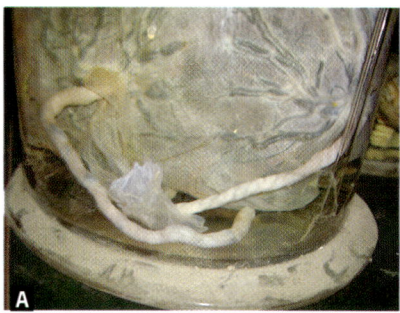 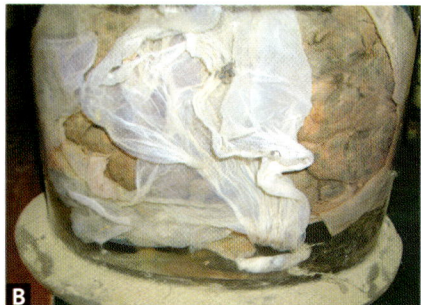

Figures 1.8A and B: (A) Placenta of uniovular twin pregnancy (fetal surface); (B) Placenta of twin pregnancy (maternal surface) (single placenta with 2-cords and no vessel anastomosis on fetal surface)

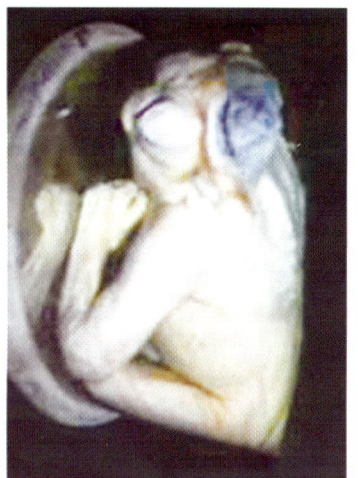 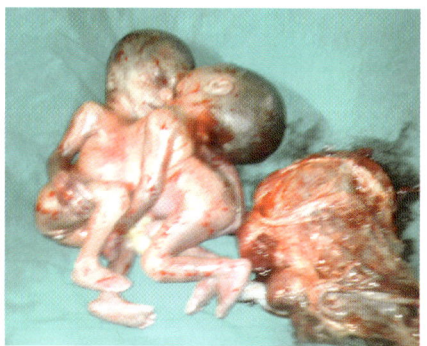

Figure 1.10: Anencephaly

Figure 1.12: Conjoined twin with placenta (Thoracopagus)

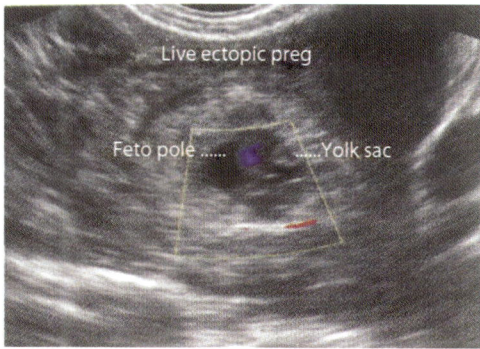

Figure 8.8: EVS—shows a live ectopic pregnancy

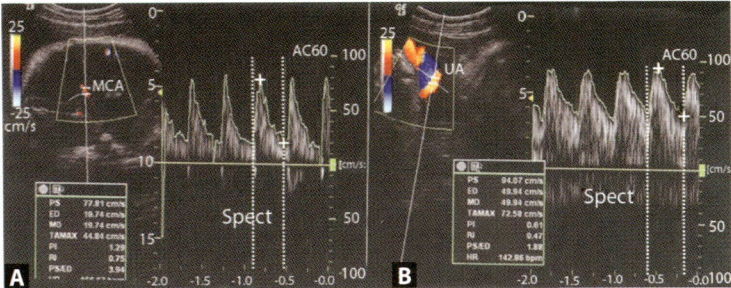

Figures 8.17A and B: (A) Blood flow in MCA (MCA-PI = 1.29, RI = 0.75); (B) Blood flow in umbilical artery (UmA-PI = 0.61, RI = 0.47)

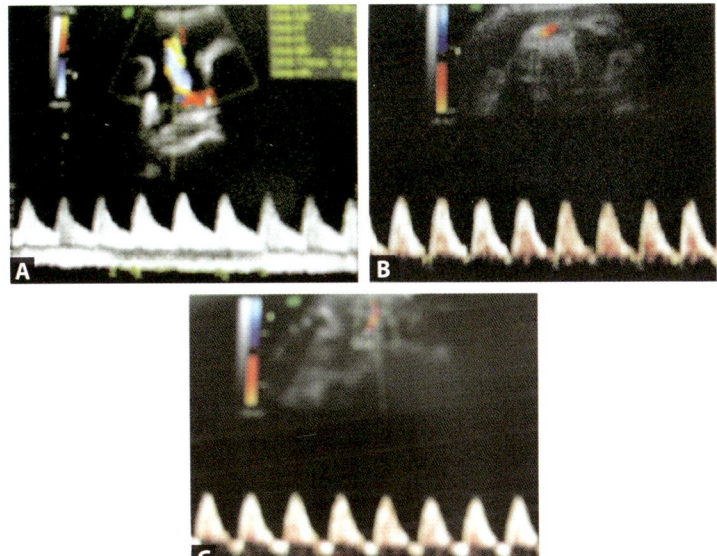

Figures 8.19A to C: (A) Normal umbilical artery Doppler, (B) Absent end-diastolic flow in UmA, (C) Reversed end-diastolic flow in UmA

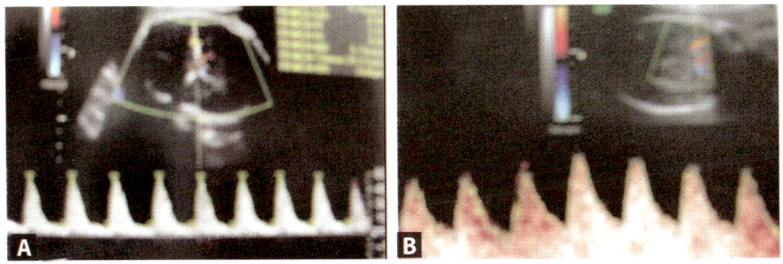

Figures 8.20 A and B: Middle cerebral artery. (A) Normal middle cerebral artery wave form, (B) Redistribution of MCA in a case of severe IUGR (brain-sparing effect)

PLATE 4

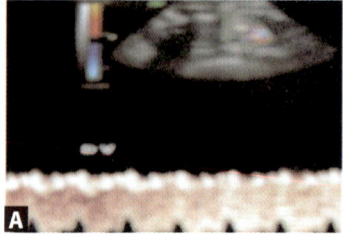 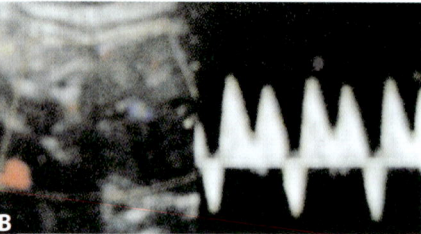

Figures 8.21 A and B: (A) Normal ductus venosus with Doppler waveform, (B) DV waveform with reversed a-wave

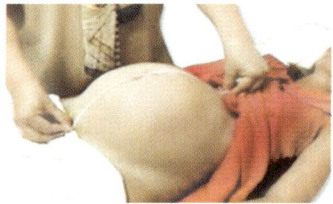 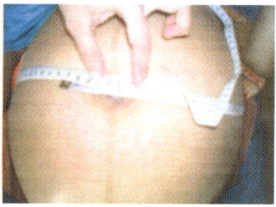

Figure 10.1A: Symphysis fundal height measurement

Figure 10.1B: Measurement of abdominal girth at the level of umbilicus

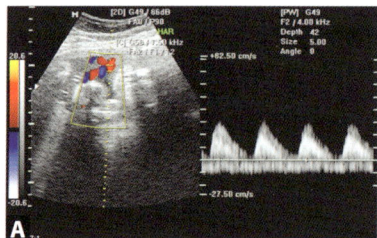 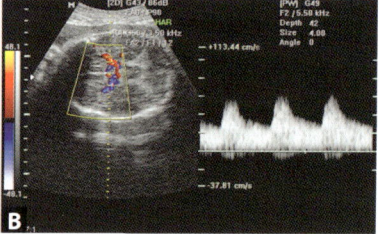

Figures 10.23 A to B: (A) UmA—Absent end diastolic flow (IUGR), (B) MCA increased diastolic flow (IUGR)

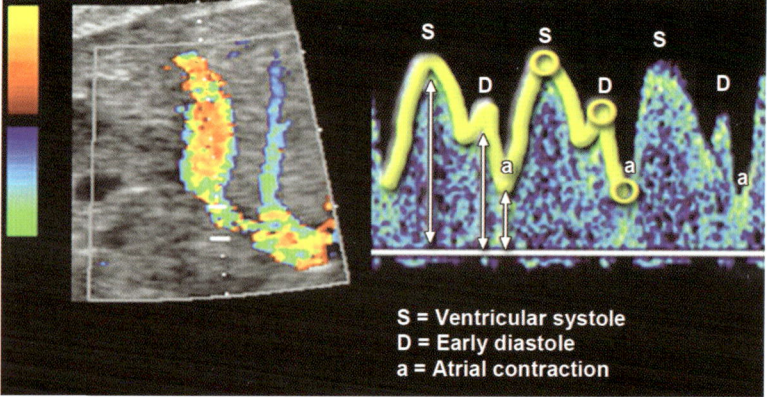

Figure 10.24: Normal Doppler study in ductus venosus (DV)

Chapter 1

Specimens

ECTOPIC PREGNANCY

Specimen of Tubal Pregnancy

Q. How do you identify the tubal ectopic pregnancy?

Ans. Identify the fallopian tube and confirm it by fimbrial end and look carefully, whether ovary is attached with it or not and the ectopic pregnancy is in tube, so this specimen is unruptured tubal ectopic pregnancy (Figure 1.1A).

Q. Which operation is performed here?

Ans. Salpingectomy of the affected tube.

Q. Do you know any other management of unruptured tubal ectopic pregnancy?

Ans. a. Medical management (discussed later).
b. Conservative surgery by salpingotomy/salpingostomy or laparoscopic aspiration.

Q. What is ectopic pregnancy?

Ans. Any pregnancy, where the fertilized ovum is implanted in any site other than normal uterine cavity is called ectopic pregnancy.

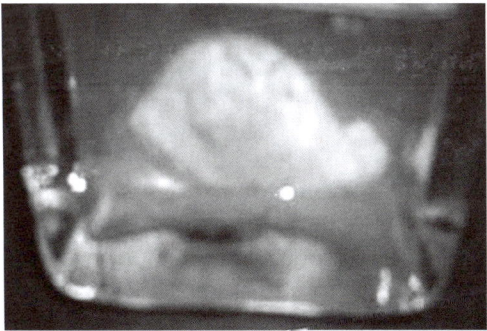

Figure 1.1A: Unruptured tubal ectopic pregnancy
(For color version, see Plate 1)

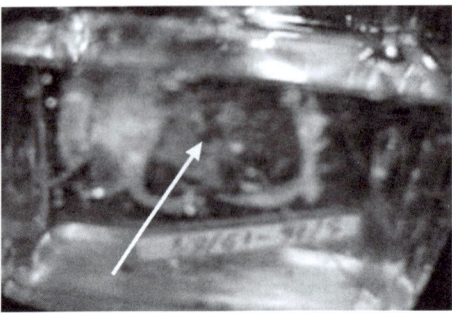

Figure 1.1B: Tubal mole (Black spot marked by arrow) on cut section *(For color version, see Plate 1)*

Q. What is the incidence of ectopic pregnancy in fallopian tube?
Ans. 95% to 99%.

Q. What is the most common site of tubal ectopic pregnancy?
Ans. Ampulla (70%) as it is the normal site of fertilization.

Q. What is the incidence of ectopic pregnancy in other part of the tube?
Ans. Fimbrial—11%; Isthmic—12%; Interstitial—2% to 3%.

> **Note**
> *Other sites: Ovarian–2%; Cervical–<1%; Abdominal –1%. After one ectopic pregnancy chances of recurrence is 10%.*

Q. What are the causes of ectopic pregnancy?
Ans. 1. **Acquired causes:**
   a. Pelvic inflammatory disease (PID).
   b. *Surgical:*
      – Surgical reconstruction of tube (Tuboplasty)
      – Spontaneous recanalization occurs after ligation
   c. Intrauterine contraceptive device (IUCD).
   d. Endometriosis.
   e. Broad ligament tumor and ovarian tumor—kinking of the tube.
   f. *In vitro* fertilization (IVF) and gamete intrafallopian transfer (GIFT).
   2. **Congenital causes:**
   Hypoplasia, undue tortuosity of the tube and accessory lumina.

Q. What is the outcome of ectopic pregnancy?
Ans. a. *Tubal abortion:* Complete or incomplete.
   b. *Tubal mole:* The dead ovum remains in the tube and subjected to repeated small choriodecidual hemorrhage, which converts it to carneous mole. If pregnancy is small, then mole absorbed partially and give rise to a small and often symptomless hematosalpinx (Figure 1.1B).
   c. *Tubal rupture:* Intraperitoneal/extraperitoneal (Common in isthmic ectopic pregnancy).
   d. Secondary/abdominal pregnancy.

Specimens

Q. What are the clinical types of ectopic pregnancy?

Ans. Chronic (common) and acute type.

Q. How do you diagnose chronic ectopic pregnancy?

Ans. History
1. The patient has a short period of amenorrhea.
2. Symptoms of early pregnancy—nausea, breast tenderness.
3. Abdominal pain due to:
   - Distension of the tube
   - Choriodecidual hemorrhage
   - Escape of blood in the peritoneal cavity (associated with syncope).
   (Combination of abdominal pain and syncopal attack is the most important symptom of ectopic pregnancy).
4. Vaginal bleeding—mild, following pain. This is uterine in origin due to separation of decidua.
5. Shoulder tip pain may occur in heavy peritoneal collection of blood and when the patient is lying down.
6. A large pelvic hematocele may cause retention of urine.

On examination (O/E)
1. Pallor+, pulse rate (PR) is high, intermittent pyrexia.
2. Early pregnancy change of breast.
3. Tenderness and muscle guard over lower abdomen.
4. Intestinal distention by peritoneal fluid.
5. Hemoperitoneum of 2 to 3 weeks causes bruising around umbilicus (Cullen's sign)—not so common.

Per vaginal (P/V)
1. Irregular tender mass on the affected side felt through the fornix.
2. Ill-defined tender semisolid swelling in pouch of Douglas (POD).
3. Arterial pulsation through the fornix (occasionally).

Investigations: UPT(+ve), Serum β-hCG level, laparoscopy, laparotomy D&E
1. *Hemoglobin percent (Hb%)*: Lower, leukocyte count is high, pregnancy test is positive in 50% of cases.
2. *Ultrasonography (USG)*: Bagel's sign—on endovaginal sonography (EVS) hyperechoic ring around the gestational sac in the adnexal region, but more often they are seen as a small inconglomerate mass near the ovary with no evidence of sac or embryo—blob sign. Hemoperitoneum may also be found. Transvaginal sonography (TVS) can diagnose 80% of ectopic pregnancy.
3. *Laparoscopy* is helpful for diagnosis of ectopic pregnancy (EP) and for definitive surgery as well in the same setting.
4. *Culdocentesis*:
   - +ve inference—0.5 mL of unclotted blood
   - –ve inference—0.5 mL of serous blood
   - Indeterminate—no fluid.
5. Final diagnosis—by laparotomy/laparoscopy.
6. Important finding: If beta-human chorionic gonadotropin (β-hCG) is not detected in serum, the diagnosis of ectopic pregnancy is ruled out. In 90% of ectopic pregnancy, β-hCG level is less than 6,500 m IU/mL.

It has also shown that if increase in β-hCG level over 2 days period (48 hours) is less than 66%, the chance of ectopic pregnancy is high in absence of intrauterine gestational sac on repeat TVS.
7. **D and E:** No products of conception, only small amount of endometrial tissue.

Q. How do you diagnose a case of ruptured ectopic pregnancy?

Ans. History
1. Short period of amenorrhea.
2. Excruciating pain in the hypogastrium.
3. Features of shock (pallor, low blood pressure (BP), PR increased, cold clammy skin, oliguria).

O/E
1. Features of shock.
2. Presence of free fluid may cause dullness of lower abdomen.

P/S
Vagina is pale.

P/V
1. Acute tenderness and pain due to movement of cervix by vaginal examination is the leading sign.
2. POD is often felt soft, fluctuant, full and tender due to pelvic hematocele.

Investigations
1. UPT may be positive, complete blood count (CBC), Hb%—low.
2. USG—empty cavity with fluid in POD/abdomen.
3. Culdocentesis—Aspiration contains blood.

Q. How do you manage a case of ectopic pregnancy?

Ans. Resuscitation and operation will go side by side. Resuscitation is done by moist oxygen, intravenous (IV) fluid (by ringer lactate [RL], normal saline [NS] or plasma expander, blood) operation—Laparotomy is followed by:
   a. *Salpingostomy:* A linear incision over ectopic pregnancy along <2 cm on the antimesosalpinx border provided the pregnancy is in ampullary part and size is less than 5 cm. It is not suitable in the isthmic pregnancy. Small bleeding sites are cauterized, no sutures are used on incision line. Serum β-hCG level >6000 mIU/L are associated with high risk of implantation into the muscularis having more tubal damage.
   b. Segmental excision and end-to-end anastomosis for isthmic pregnancy.
   c. Milking of the tube—in ampullary pregnancy, where pregnancy can be easily dislodged.
   d. Salpingotomy: A longitudinal incision is made on the antimesenteric border of the fallopian tube, the products are removed with forceps or gentle suction and one layer closure of the incision with 7-0 interrupted vicryl suture.

> **Note**
> After operation Beta-hCG level falls quickly and is approximately 10% of preoperative values by day 12. Persistent trophoblastic risk (pre after conservative surgery requires prophylactic methotrexate with a dose of 1 mg/m² body surface area (BSA).

e. *Salpingectomy:* Removal of the affected tube is the usual procedure—radical surgical procedure

> **Note**
> See gynecological part for details of operation on ectopic pregnancy, a-d are conservative surgical treatment. Expectant management of ectopic pregnancy may be done, if there is serial decrease of β-hCG level (or if β-hCG level <1500 mIU/mL), diameter of ectopic mass ≤3.5 cm and no evidence of intra-abdominal bleeding or rupture by EVS (endovaginal sonography).

Q. Do you remove ovary during salpingectomy operation?

Ans. No, it is always preserved for future pregnancy, but it is removed, if it is pathological.

Q. How do you diagnose early unruptured ectopic pregnancy and how do you manage it?

Ans. The likelihood of EP is suspected in woman who has just missed period and experience abdominal pain or vaginal bleeding, especially when a patient has a past history of PID/infertility/tubal surgery/medical termination of pregnancy (MTP) or using IUCD.

Diagnosis
a. Urine for pregnancy test (UPT)
b. By USG (EVS)—empty uterine cavity and adnexal mass is seen.
c. β-hCG—in normal pregnancy, this hormone level doubles over 2 days; in abnormal gestation, the rate is much lower or absent.
d. Color flow Doppler—see USG in obstetrics.

> **Note**
> Vaginal USG of indeterminate type can detect EP/ or complete abortion at 5 to 6 weeks when β-hCG value is lower than 2,000 IU/mL. Rapidly falling of hCG level (50% over 48 hours) occurs with complete abortion, whereas with ectopic pregnancy level rises or plateau.

Q. What are the criteria for medical treatment?

Ans. The criteria for the medical treatment are as follows:
a. Patient is of good health, hemodynamically stable and able to return for follow-up examination
b. Unruptured EP
c. No evidence of intrauterine pregnancy
d. Ectopic mass is less than 3.5 cm
e. hCG less than 5,000 IU/L

f. No yolk sac seen
g. No fetal heart tone.

Q. What are the agents used for medical management of EP?

Ans. Methotrexate, mifepristone, potassium chloride, actinomycin, prostaglandins (PGs), hyperosmolar glucose, anti-hCG antibodies.

Q. How methotrexate is used?

(For post graduates)

Ans. a. Intra sac methotrexate by EVS/laparoscopic guidance, where reduced dose is required.

b. *Systemic methotrexate:*
1. *Single dose*: Systemic injection of methotrexate is used, 50 mg/m² is administered on day 1. Up to 13% of cases required second dose, if the hCG level does not reduce by 15% between 4 to 7 days.

   If β-hCG level declines 15% or more between days 4–7 the treatment is successful and β-hCG is followed up weekly until it is undetectable. The Beta-hCG level is somewhat increased between day 1 and 4, over baseline due to lysis of trophoblast. The observation is normal and does not indicate failed treatment. Any subsequent increase in β-hCG level or a decrease of less than 15% between days 4 and 7 is an indication of second dose on day 7, using the same criteria for judging response (on day 11). If required, a third dose can be administered on day 11 and the response is evaluated by measuring β-hCG again on day 14. Although, a fourth dose can be administered on day 14.

   Surgical treatment is recommended after 2 weeks of failed medical treatment.

2. In two dose regimen methotrexate is used on Day 1 and day 4 in the dose of 50 mg /m². If serum β-hCG declines 15% or more between days 4 to 7 levels are monitored weekly until the level becomes undetectable. If the β-hCG concentration decreases by less than 15% between day 4 and 7, a third dose is administered on day 7 and using the same criteria for judging response (on day 11), a fourth dose may be necessary on day 11 and serum β-hCG concentration is again measured on day 14.

3. *Another regime (Multiple dose):* Injection methotrexate IM, 1 mg/kg body weight (BW) should be given on day 1, 3, 5,7 (four doses) with folinic acid (0.1 mg/kg IM) on day 2, 4, 6, 8 until the serum β-hCG declines by 15% from the previous value. Thereafter, β-hCG levels are monitored on a weekly basis until the level becomes undetectable. After methotrexate treatment more of ectopic mass enlarges due to hematoma formation but such observation do not predict treatment failure. In severe pain, USG should be done promptly to detect copious peritoneal fluid which suggest rupture of tubal pregnancy. Surgical treatment is needed when ruptured ectopic is suspected or diagnosed or when the patient refuses medical treatment.

> **Note**
> - *Repeat dosing may be required, if β-hCG level increase or plateau*
> - *Transient increase in pain is common in days to weeks after methotrexate administration. This is caused by separation of trophoblastic tissues from the tubal wall with varying amount of intraperitoneal bleeding. This separation pain may be managed on outpatient basis but severe pain may require hospitalization for observation to rule out rupture and intraperitoneal hemorrhage.*

Q. How methotrexate act?

Ans. Methotrexate is a folic acid antagonist and folate is essential for deoxyribonucleic acid (DNA) synthesis and effective against rapidly dividing cells.

Q. What are the contraindications of methotrexate therapy?

Ans. Intrauterine pregnancy, severe anemia, leukopenia (< 3×10^9/L), thrombocytopenia, active infection, human immunodeficiency virus (HIV)/acquired immunodeficiency syndrome (AIDS), renal and liver disease, peptic ulcer and ulcerative colitis, breastfeeding. Other relative contraindications—gestational sac >3.5 cm, embryonic cardiac activity present.

Q. What will you do in case of failure of methotrexate therapy?

Ans. Repeat the dose; if fails to resolute, go for surgery.

Q. When do you choose the procedure for laparoscopic surgery?

Ans. The adnexal mass must be 3–5 cm in diameter or free fluid in POD.

> **Note**
> *It is easily approachable for any kind of tubal operation (see operation in Gyne part).*

Q. What are the indications of hysterectomy in case of disturbed ectopic pregnancy?

Ans. Patient's age greater than 40 years when associated with:
 a. Ectopic pregnancy due to widespread pelvic adhesion.
 b. Uterus is diseased.
 c. When the patient is in a good condition.
 d. Interstitial pregnancy.

Q. What is interstitial pregnancy?

Ans. When the implantation occurs in the interstitial portion of the tube.

Q. When does it rupture?

Ans. It ruptures around 16–20 weeks.

Q. How do you diagnose this condition?

Ans. Diagnosis is very difficult and confused with pregnancy in bicornuate uterus, pregnancy with fibroid uterus, pregnancy in a rudimentary horn. There may be asymmetrical enlargement of one cornu.

Q. How do you treat this case?

Ans. Surgical: Hemodynamically unstable patient generally requires laparotomy:
   a. *If the uterine wall is severely damaged:* Total abdominal hysterectomy (TAH) and unilateral salpingo-oophorectomy to control hemorrhage.
   b. *If patient wishes for further pregnancy:* Partial hysterosalpingectomy, but there is a risk of rupture of the uterus in future pregnancy.
   c. Cornual resection and repair of the defects or cornuostomy.

> **Note**
> Administration of methotrexate (systemic or laparoscopy or hysteroscopy) has been demonstrated as a viable option in the patient without evidence of uterine rupture and overall success rate is 83% in unruptured interstitial hemodynamically stable pregnancy.

Q. What is the incidence of ovarian pregnancy?

Ans. One percent of all EP.

Q. What are the types of ovarian pregnancy?

Ans. Intrafollicular, extrafollicular or combined.

Q. Can you diagnose ovarian pregnancy preoperatively?

Ans. It is very difficult to diagnose preoperatively with certainty.

Q. What are Spiegelberg's criteria for ovarian ectopic pregnancy?

Ans.
   a. The tube on the affected side must be intact
   b. The fetal sac must occupy the position of ovary
   c. The ovary and the sac must be connected with the uterus by ovarian ligament
   d. Definite ovarian tissue must be present in the wall of the sac.

Q. What is the treatment of ovarian pregnancy?

Ans. At operation, the affected ovary usually has to be sacrificed.

Q. What is cornual pregnancy?

Ans. Implantation occurs in the rudimentary horn of the uterus. This horn does not always communicate with the rest of the uterine cavity. Spermatozoa ascends through the normal part of uterus and tube and fertilize in the peritoneal cavity, this then enter the tube of rudimentary horn.

Q. What is the fate of cornual pregnancy?

Ans. Rupture of the horn occurs at 12–20 weeks of pregnancy with intraperitoneal hemorrhage and shock.

Q. What is the differential diagnosis of cornual pregnancy?

Ans. Uterine fibroid, ovarian tumor, interstitial type of tubal pregnancy.

Specimens

Q. How can you differentiate it from interstitial pregnancy?

Ans. Position of the round ligament, which is attached lateral to the sac and the long pedicle by which rudimentary horn is attached to the uterus—cornual pregnancy.

Q. What is the treatment?

Ans. a. Remove the rudimentary horn.
b. If the pedicle is short and attachment is wide, hysterectomy is the treatment of choice.

Q. Which abdominal pregnancy is common?

Ans. Secondary due to rupture of tubal pregnancy (1 in 15,000 births) and subsequent intra-abdominal reimplantation of conception and it also may occur after tubal abortion.

Q. How primary abdominal pregnancy is diagnosed?

Ans. *Studdiford's criteria*:
a. Presence of normal tubes and ovaries with no evidence of recent or past pregnancy
b. No evidence of uteroplacental fistula
c. The presence of a pregnancy, related exclusively to the peritoneal surface and early enough to eliminate the possibility of secondary implantation after primary tubal nidation.

Q. How do you diagnose secondary abdominal pregnancy?

Ans. a. Braxton Hicks contraction is absent clinically
b. *USG of abdomen*: The uterus may be seen as a separate mass in relation to the gestational sac
c. *X-ray of abdomen*:
- Absence of uterine outline and placental shadow
- Intermingling of maternal gas shadow with the fetal parts (Bishop's sign)
- An abnormal high position of fetus
- Fetal parts overlapping maternal spine in the lateral view (Weinberg's sign).

> **Note**
> It commonly occurs after tubal abortion or less often after uterine rupture.

Q. How do you treat such patient?

Ans. As soon as diagnosis is made laparotomy should be done as the delay may lead to spontaneous intraperitoneal hemorrhage.
- Removal of the placenta, if it is not adherent to any vital organ.
- If adherent to broad ligament and uterus, go for hysterectomy.
- If placenta is adherent to bowel then cut the cord, close to the placenta and leave it. It usually gets absorbed or occasionally forms abscess.
- The place of methotrexate is doubtful in this case.

Q. What are nontubal ectopic pregnancies?

Ans. They are cervical pregnancy, abdominal pregnancy, ovarian pregnancy, cesarean section scar pregnancy (rare) and it may also occur on omentum, liver spleen and retroperitoneal.

FOR POSTGRADUATES

Q. What is cesarean section scar pregnancy (CSP)?

Ans. Implantation of embryo within the myometrium of prior cesarean delivery scar (incidence 1 in 2000 normal pregnancies).

Q. How do you diagnose CSP?

Ans.
a. Pain and bleeding are common symptoms
b. 40% of women are asymptomatic
c. Diagnosis is made on routine sonography in early pregnancy

USG (TVS): Cervico-isthmic pregnancy and CSP are very difficult to diagnose by USG

USG Features in CSP:
 i. Bright hyperechoic endometrial stripe
 ii. The uterine cavity is empty
 iii. An empty cervical canal
 iv. An intrauterine mass is seen in the anterior part of uterine isthmus
MRI is useful when sonography is inconclusive.

Q. How do you treat CSP?

Ans. There is no standard treatment:
 i. Hysterectomy is an acceptable initial choice for uncontrolled bleeding and patient wants sterilization
 ii. Fertility preserving options are:
  a. Local injection of methotrexate
  b. Conservative surgery like suction curettage, or transvaginal aspiration, hysteroscopic removal or isthmic excision and uterine artery embolization.

> **Note**
> *These procedures are done solely or adjunctive with methotrexate.*

Q. What is cervical pregnancy?

Ans. Cervical pregnancy is one that implants entirely within the cervical canal.

Q. What is the incidence of cervical pregnancy?

Ans. 1:250 to 1:18000 deliveries (0.2% of ectopic pregnancies).

Q. What are the predisposing factors of cervical pregnancy?

Ans.
a. Therapeutic abortion previously
b. Previous cesarean section
c. Asherman's syndrome
d. IUI and IVF.

Specimens

Q. What are the clinical criteria of diagnosis of cervical pregnancy?

Ans.
a. The distended cervix is smaller on P/V examination
b. On curettage, no evidence of trophoblastic tissue
c. The product of conception is confined within the cervix
d. The internal os is closed.

> **Note**
> Cervical pregnancy is associated with profuse vaginal bleeding without abdominal pain.

Q. What is the USG criteria for diagnosis of cervical pregnancy?

Ans.
a. Ballooning of cervical canal
b. Gestational sac is within the endocervix
c. Internal os is closed
d. No evidence of intrauterine pregnancy.

Q. What is Rubin's criterion for diagnosis of cervical pregnancy?

Ans.
a. There must be cervical gland opposite to placental attachment
b. The placental attachment to the cervix must be intimate
c. The whole or a portion of the placenta must be situated below the entrance of uterine vessels or below the peritoneal reflection of the anterior and posterior surface of the uterus
d. No fetal element should be present in the corpus uteri
e. Cervix is enlarged and soft equal in size or bigger than fundus.

Q. Management of cervical ectopic pregnancy?

Ans.
a. Hysterectomy is the only treatment of choice
b. Other surgical alternatives less radical to hysterectomy are sometime helpful
  1. D and C operation
  2. To control bleeding
     i. Packing of the uterus and cervix
     ii. Intracervical 30 mL Foley's catheter and inflate the bulb
     iii. Deep lateral cervical stitches or placement of cervical circlage
     iv. In some cases bilateral internal iliac artery ligation
     v. Uterine artery embolization
c. *Medical*: Some patients may be treated with methotrexate either intra-amniotically or systematically. Therapeutic success has been reported with the use of etoposide or combination chemotherapy.

RUPTURE OF UTERUS

The specimen is of uterus (subtotal hysterectomy) where tubes and ovaries are absent, cervix is also absent (Figure 1.2).

Q. Why this operation was done?

Ans. This was done for rupture of uterus.

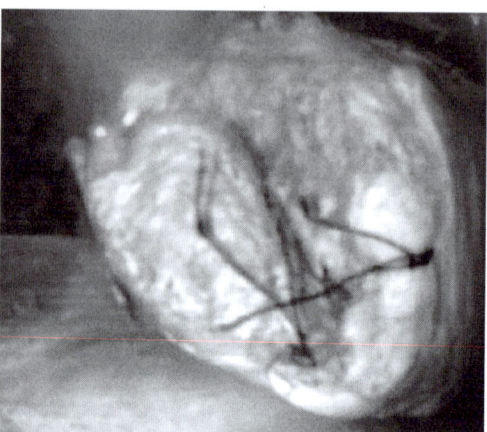

Figure 1.2: Rupture of uterus (Subtotal hysterectomy done)
(For color version, see Plate 1)

Q. What are the causes of uterine rupture during pregnancy?

Ans. Spontaneous rupture (rare)
  a. Congenital maldevelopment of uterus—rupture most common at mid trimester.
  b. Spontaneous rupture at last trimester
   • Previous operation [myomectomy or classical cesarean section (CS)]—common
   • Old perforation (MTP)
  Others—trauma of myometrium by endometrial ablation and hysteroscopy

Traumatic (rarest)
Fall, crushing accident or blow on abdomen.

Q. How do you diagnose rupture of uterus during pregnancy?

Ans. a. Acute abdominal pain with features of shock.
  b. Contracted uterus is felt as a suprapubic mass.
  c. Easily palpable fetus.
  d. Fetal heart sound (FHS)—absent.

Q. What are the causes of rupture of uterus during labor?

Ans. Spontaneous
  a. Obstructed labor: Malpresentation, malposition, cephalopelvic disproportion (CPD), hydrocephalus.
  b. Multiparity causes more fibrous tissue and malnutrition produces certain changes in myometrium and susceptible to rupture, CPD due to big baby is also an important factor.
  c. The cesarean or hysterotomy scar rupture (very common).
  d. Injudicious use of oxytocics.

Traumatic
  a. Internal version, or external cephalic version.
  b. Extraction of fetus through the incomplete dilated cervix.
  c. Operative delivery like difficult forceps, craniotomy, decapitation.

Specimens

Q. What are the different types of rupture pathologically?

Ans. a. *Complete:* When all the coats of the uterus are involved including peritoneum. Here hemorrhage is intraperitoneal.
It usually results in death of fetus.
b. *Incomplete:* When peritoneum is not involved and fetus usually lies in the uterine cavity
- Spontaneous rupture is more often complete than incomplete
- Traumatic rupture is more often incomplete than complete.

Q. What are the complications of ruptured uterus?

Ans. a. Hemorrhage
b. Shock
c. Sepsis
d. Peritonitis
e. Renal failure
f. Paralytic ileus
g. Maternal mortality and morbidity
h. High fetal mortality.

Q. Is rupture of lateral wall of uterus complete or incomplete?

Ans. Lateral wall of pregnant uterus is uncovered by peritoneum. Rupture of this site may include whole thickness of muscular wall of uterus and still be incomplete, as it only opens up the broad ligament, but does not tear the peritoneum.

Q. Why incomplete rupture and broad ligament hematoma is more common on left side of the uterus?

Ans. a. Dextrorotation of the uterus exposes lateral wall to increased stress of labor.
b. Passive venous congestion in the left broad ligament due to left ovarian vein draining into the left renal vein at right angle.

Q. Rupture is more common in classical CS than LSCS, why?

Ans. Rupture of classical CS is 2% and half of these cases occur before the onset of labor. Rupture in lower segment cesarean section (LSCS) is rare (0.4% or less).

> **Note**
> Two previous sections carry 3- to 5-folds increased risk over one previous section.

Rupture occurs due to the following reasons in classical CS:
a. Defective healing of classical scar due to contraction and relaxation in uterine involution.
b. Difficulty in approximation of edges.
c. Incomplete hemostasis and infection.
d. Placenta on the scar makes the scar tissue weak.

Q. What are the signs and symptoms of rupture uterus in labor?

Ans.
a. Signs of prolonged and difficult labor.
b. Acute pain on lower abdomen, unexplained sudden maternal tachycardia.
c. Previous labor pain stops when rupture occurs.
d. Pallor and shock appears due to intra-abdominal hemorrhage.
e. The uterine outline is completely lost and fetus is felt most superficially when palpating the patient's tender abdomen.
f. FHS is absent.

Vaginal examination
a. Hemorrhage through the cervical orifice (os).
b. The presenting part often goes up.
c. Hematuria on catheterization, if bladder is involved.
d. Cervix hangs like a curtain.

In an atypical case
a. General condition is satisfactory.
b. The uterine outline is intact, if rupture is incomplete.
c. Tenderness and fullness in suprapubic and iliac region.
d. The FHS is absent or irregular.
e. An unexplained collapse during the late first and early second stage of labor with tender inert uterus with slight bleeding should suggest rupture of uterus and not accidental hemorrhage.
f. When a patient collapse after difficult vaginal delivery, it is advisable to explore the uterus after manual removal of placenta (MRP).

Q. How do you manage the case?

Ans. General:
a. Stop oxytocin, if running.
b. Moist oxygen inhalation.
c. Start IV fluid (NS/RL) with wide bore needle.
d. Continuous bladder drainage.
e. Blood transfusion in severe hemorrhage.
f. Continuous maternal monitoring.
g. Emergency laparotomy with rapid operative delivery.

Definitive repair of the tear:
a. If the tear is small.
b. There must be strong reason to preserve the uterine function.
c. Clean wound and edges are not ragged as in rupture of LSCS scar.
d. If patient does not want issue perform tubal ligation with repair.

> **Note**
> *If patient have pregnancy after repair of uterine rupture, go for elective CS as soon as fetus is mature or at 36–37 weeks of gestation before the onset of labor.*

Hysterectomy (Subtotal or supracervical):
- When the tear is irregular, irreparable and edges are friable.
- In colporrhexis (Total hysterectomy may be needed).
- Lateral tears with broad ligament hematoma.
- When the uterus is infected.

If bladder is involved—*repair of bladder in two layers followed by hysterectomy and Foley catheter is kept in bladder for 10 days (for details see the case discussion of post cesarean section pregnancy—chapter 10).*

Q. What are the postoperative complications?

Ans. Hemorrhage, shock, peritonitis, rarely pulmonary embolism.

> **Note**
>
> If the site of ruptured scar is on the lower uterine segment (LUS) the rate of repeat rupture or dehiscence in labor is 6%, and if the scar includes upper segment of uterus the repeat rupture rate is 32%.

Q. Outline the procedure of subtotal hysterectomy?

Ans. *Principles of the procedure*: Supracervical part of uterus is removed.
Procedure:
- Clamp, cut and transfix the round ligament of both sides
- Clamp, cut and transfix the tube and ovarian ligament of both sides to preserve ovaries as the patient is young
- Clamp, cut and ligate the both-sided uterine arteries
- Cut the uterus above the level where uterine arteries are ligated
- Close the cervical stump with interrupted sutures
- Secure hemostasis and close the abdomen with a drain if required.

Q. How do you manage rupture with broad-ligament hematoma?

Ans. Features of shock is more than p/v bleeding
Management: Correction of shock and definitive treatment by following steps:
1. If rupture creates broad-ligament hematoma, clamp, cut and tie the round ligament on the affected side.
2. Open the anterior leaf of broad ligament.
3. Drain the hematoma.
4. Inspect the area carefully for injury of uterine artery or its branches and ligate the bleeding vessels.
5. In complicated cases subtotal hysterectomy.

Q. How do you administer postoperative care after subtotal hysterectomy?

Ans.
- IV drip with NS/RL for 24-48 hours (prolonged infusion may alter electrolyte balance)—so sodium and potassium level should be noted every alternate days
- Ensure the level of consciousness by supervision of vital signs (BP, pulse, respiratory rate and urine output) and temperature every 15 minutes during the first hour, then every 30 minutes for the next hours.
- Transfuse blood, if necessary.
- If vital signs become unstable, relaparotomy as internal bleeding may be the cause.
- If there are signs of infection (fever) give combination antibiotics (Ampicillin —2 g every 6 hours, plus gentamicin 5 mg/kg IV every 24 hours plus.
  Metronidazole 500 mg IV 8 hourly, until she is fever free for 48 hours.

6. Give analgesic.
7. Remove the abdominal drain after 48 hours, if there are no signs of infection or minimum collection in the drain bag.
8. Remove abdominal sutures 5 days after surgery.
9. Ensure that the patient is eating regular diet before discharge from hospital.

HYDATIDIFORM MOLE (SYNONYMS VESICULAR MOLE GESTATIONAL TROPHOBLASTIC DISEASE/NEOPLASIA)

Q. What is this specimen?

Ans. This is the specimen of hydatidiform mole (Figure 1.3). (Description of the specimen—cystic grape-like structures from pin-head to large size).

Q. What is the histology? What is the histological classification?

Ans.
a. Trophoblastic proliferation of cytotrophoblast and syncytiotrophoblast.
b. Hydropic changes in the stroma with cistern formation.
c. Absence of fetal blood vessels.

Histological: Classification
a. Hydatidiform mole (complete and partial).
b. Invasive mole (chorioadenoma destruens).
c. Choriocarcinoma.
d. Placental site trophoblastic tumor (PSTT).

Q. What are the risk factors of H mole?

Ans.
a. Maternal age greater than 40 years.
b. Teen age less than 19 years.
c. Asian woman.
d. Malnutrition.
e. Immunologic and genetic factors are also responsible.

Q. What is the complete mole?

Ans. Complete mole (without embryo fetal remnants) has 90% of 46 XX karyotype (Figure 1.4).

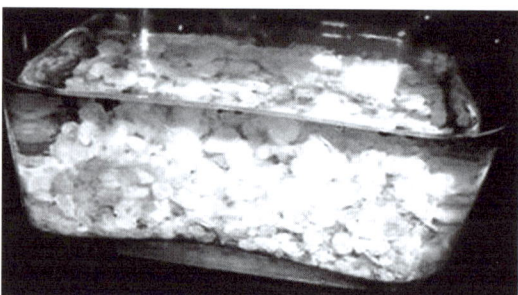

Figure 1.3: Specimen of hydatidiform mole *(For color version, see Plate 1)*

Specimens

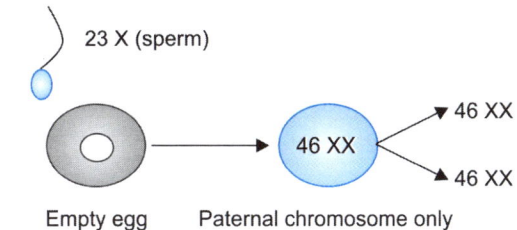

Figure 1.4: Complete mole

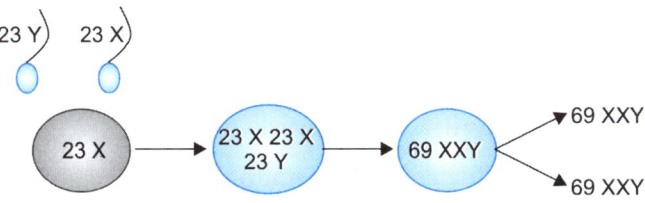

Figure 1.5: Partial mole

In 10% of cases, 46 XY are present. Chances of malignancy are high in 20% of complete mole.

Q. What is partial mole (with embryo-fetus)?

Ans. Karyotype is 69XXY. Fertilization by two sperms, one with 23X and another with 23Y (dispermy) with normal ovum containing 23X.
Fetal tissue is present (Figure 1.5).
Less likely to develop malignant change (5%).

Q. How do you differentiate partial and complete hydatidiform mole?

Ans. See difference of partial and complete hydatidiform mole below:

Features	Partial mole	Complete mole
Fetal tissue	Present	Absent
Swelling of villi	Focal	Diffuse
Trophoblastic hyperplasia	Focal	Diffuse
Stromal inclusions	Présent	Absent
Scalloping of villous	Present	Absent
Karyotype	69XXY, 69XYY	46XX (90%) 46XY (10%)
Trophoblastic neoplasia	~5%	~20%
USG	Cystic spaces at placental site, ratio of transverse and anteroposterior diameter of gestational sac is more than 1.5 along with fetus or fetal tissue	Snowstorm appearance

Q. Define H mole.
Ans. It is a noninvasive abnormal placenta characterized by enlarged, edematous chorionic villi with variable amounts of proliferative trophoblast. It is a benign neoplasm with malignant potential.

Q. Why H mole is formed?
Ans.
a. Primary death of fetus results in failure in villus circulation and consequence edema and liquefaction of stroma.
b. Primary error in the development of the vessels in the core causing villus to become overloaded with fluid and food staffs, the later then provide epithelial cells with excessive growth stimulus for proliferation.
c. Anoxia causes active fluid secretion into the core of the villus, as well as cellular hyperplasia.

Q. How does the patient present?
Ans.
a. Period of amenorrhea—8 to 12 weeks or more.
b. Vaginal bleeding.
c. Pain abdomen.
d. Passage of grape-like vesicles.
e. Excessive vomiting, hypertension.
f. Fetal movement is absent, if gestational age (GA) is greater than 20 weeks.

Q. How will you diagnose H mole?
Ans.
a. History
b. General survey—pallor, BP (may increase), hyperthyroidism in 7% of cases due to increased level of hCG in H mole.

P/A
a. Uterine size is enlarged than period of amenorrhea in 50% of cases, in some cases, size correspond or even less, due to discharge of moles per vagina.
b. Doughy feeling, i.e. no fetal part is felt.
c. FHS—absent.

P/V
a. Os—closed, internal ballottement is absent.
b. Bilateral cystic enlarged ovary in 25–50% of cases (Lutein cyst).
c. Bloody discharge.
d. Discharge of vesicles (50%).

Investigations
a. β-hCG level is very high, both in urine and blood—urinary hCG level, of 3,50,000 to 5 million IU/L above 100 days, is strongly indicative. Biweekly rising titer is helpful.
b. Sonography—'snowstorm appearance' in complete mole (Figure 1.6)
   - Sonolucent area due to blood clot
   - Absence of gestational sac at 5–7 weeks
   - Repeat scan a week later.

   (Differential diagnosis of snowstorm appearance—missed abortion, degenerated fibroid).
c. Others—Renal, hepatic and thyroid function test, chest radiography.

Specimens

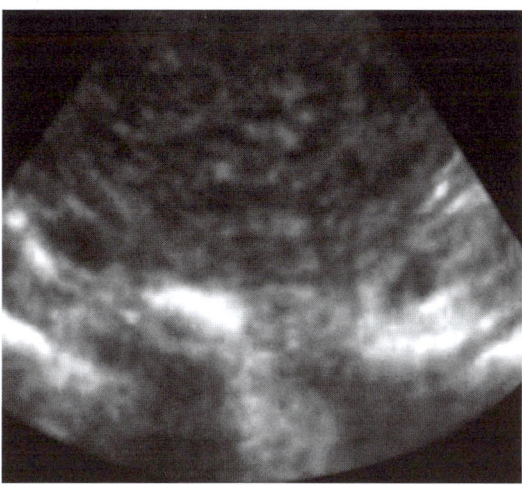

Figure 1.6: USG—H mole

Q. What are the complications of H mole?

Ans.
a. Hemorrhage (severe uterine hemorrhage is treated by traditional hysterectomy).
b. Shock.
c. Sepsis.
d. Perforation (may need emergency hysterectomy in cases of invasive mole associated with uterine rupture and intraperitoneal hemorrhage).
e. Preeclamsia (in 25% of cases below 20 weeks)
f. Hyperthyroid/Thyroid storm (propylthiouracil, methimazole, Lugol's iodine, β-adrenergic blocker and steroids may be needed).
g. Theca leutin cyst rupture/torsion (This infrequent situation is managed by laparoscopy/laparotomy).
h. Acute respiratory distress syndrome (ARDS)—may be seen after evacuation of mole due to embolization of trophoblastic cells after evacuation.
i. Malignant change (5%).

Q. What are the high-risk factors for malignancy in H mole?

Ans.
a. Complete mole.
b. Bilateral theca lutein cyst (> 6 cm).
c. Age above 40 years.
d. Serum hCG—1 million U/L before starting treatment.
e. Uterine size is large for gestational age.
f. Slow decline of β-hCG level.

Q. How do you treat a case of H mole?

Ans.
a. Start IV drip with RL. Oxytocin is administered only after dilatation of cervix and partial evacuation to aid hemostasis.
b. Grouping and cross-matching for blood
c. Antibiotic by IV route
d. Early evaluation

e. **Partial expulsion:**
   - Os open—suction evacuation by cannula (no. 10–12 according to size of the uterus) with 10 units of syntocinon
   - Os closed—slow dilatation by—laminaria tent and cerviprime (intracervical) gel or misoprostol per vagina and then suction evacuation followed by gentle curettage.

   At the end of first week, repeat curettage for complete evacuation of uterus and sending the material for history and physical (H/P) examination is not mandatory. It is done only in presence of persisting trophoblast in the uterine cavity. Repeated evacuation may cause high chance of requiring chemotherapy and may increase rate of complications.

f. **Follow-up:**
   Total hysterectomy (surgical extirpation of adenexa even for benign indication)
   - If patient's age is greater than 35 years
   - Elderly with completed family
   - Perforating mole and placental site trophoblastic tumor
   - Patient not responding to chemotherapy
   - Uncontrolled vaginal bleeding.

> **Note**
>
> Hysterectomy reduces the incidence of malignancy than suction D and C (<5% versus 20%), but follow-up is necessary.

Hysterotomy
Seldom done nowadays, done in case of excessive bleeding, vomiting, oliguria, but tightly closed cervix.
Patient should be followed up for 2 years.
Theca lutein cysts: It disappears after several weeks of molar evacuation. Enlarged cyst may undergo torsion, infarction or rupture, and oophorectomy should be considered in these conditions, otherwise aspiration of fluid under aseptic precaution may be required in big-sized cysts by USG or laparoscopy.

Q. What is the incidence of recurrence in H mole?
Ans. About 0.8–2.9% risk of recurrence after one mole and 15–18% after two moles.

Q. When will you start chemotherapy?
Ans.
a. In high-risk groups (as mentioned above).
b. When the patient cannot be followed up properly.
c. High level of hCG persisting for 2 months after evacuation.
d. Any detectable hCG in the serum after 9 weeks.
e. Persistent uterine bleeding, even if trophoblastic tissues are not available by curettage. This is the indication of myometrial invasion.
f. Evidence of metastasis in brain and lungs.

Q. Which drug is used in prophylactic chemotherapy?
Ans. Oral methotrexate 5 mg TDS × 5 days. A total of 3 courses are given at a gap of 5–7 days.

Specimens

Q. How do you follow-up a case of H mole?

Ans. Protocol: Weekly for 8 weeks, monthly for 10 months and patient should not conceive for 1 year.

> **Note**
>
> *After evacuation, patient is monitored weekly for serum β-hCG level until it becomes normal for 3 consecutive weeks, followed by monthly determination until the levels are normal for 6 consecutive months. The hCG level becomes normal after 9 weeks of evacuation. Contraception is required for hormonal follow up (see below).*

Procedure

At each visit, history relevant to:
1. Irregular bleeding P/V
2. Central nervous system (CNS) disturbances such as headache, vomiting
3. Hemoptysis and breathlessness.

A. Full general survey (pallor, jaundice, thyroid gland's condition) and abdominal and pelvic examination for:
1. Sub-involution of uterus
2. Theca lutein cyst
3. Vaginal secondaries

A chest X-ray is advised routinely on diagnosis of mole, if it is normal, it is repeated monthly, until hCG becomes normal.

Serum β-hCG assay at each visit—becomes negative after 9 weeks in majority of cases; in a few cases, the titre becomes high, even after normal level of β-hCG. When it is high, exclude:
  a. Pregnancy.
  b. Choriocarcinoma.
  c. Enlarged ovary.

Q. What are the criteria for repeat curettage?

Ans. a. Irregular bleeding P/V
  b. The uterus does not involute satisfactorily
  c. If β-hCG level is still positive, 6 weeks after evacuation.

Q. What is the contraceptive practice in H mole?

Ans.
- Patient should not be allowed to become pregnant for 1 year
- IUCD—no, for irregular bleeding
- Condom—preferable
- Low-dose oral contraceptive pill (OCP)—use, after β-hCG level becomes normal.

FOR POSTGRADUATES

> **Note**
>
> *Prevalence of choriocarcinoma is 5% of gestational trophoblastic diseases (GTDs). Choriocarcinoma is preceded by mnemonic "MEAN" M: Mole in 50%; E: Ectopic pregnancy- 2.5%; A: Abortion (spontaneous) in 25%; N: Normal pregnancy in 22.5%.*

Q. What are the different types of gestational trophoblastic neoplasia?

Ans. a. *Non-metastatic:* No evidence of disease outside the uterus.
[*Treatment*: Single agent chemotherapy—methotrexate—0.4 mg/kg day IV or intramuscularly (IM) for 5 days course, and repeat the same dose after 7 to 10 days]. [Day 1, 3, 5, 7 with methotrexate Injection with folinic acid 0.1 mg/kg per day on 2, 4, 6, 8th day].
b. *Metastatic:* Any disease outside the uterus.

Good prognosis of metastatic disease (Treat by single agent chemotherapy initially)
1. Short duration less than 4 months.
2. Urinary hCG less than 1,00,000 IU/24 hours or serum β-hCG less than 40,000 IU/mL.
3. No metastasis to brain or liver.
4. No significant prior chemotherapy.

Metastatic poor prognosis
1. Long duration greater than 4 months.
2. Urinary hCG greater than 1, 00,000 IU/24 hours or serum.
2. β-hCG greater than 40,000 IU/mL.
3. Metastasis to brain and liver.
4. Unsuccessful prior chemotherapy.
5. Gestational trophoblastic tumor following term pregnancy.

Q. What is the protocol of MAC regime?

Ans. Chemotherapy of poor-prognostic disease (multidrug therapy)
  I. Methotrexate—10 to 15 mg/day IV or IM
   Dactinomycin—10 to 12 µg/kg/day IV
   Chlorambucil—8 to 10 mg/day per mouth or Cyclophosphamide—3 to 5 mg/kg/day IV
   1. Give the course for 5 days
   2. Repeat the cycle with minimum interval of 10–14 days as toxicity allows.
  II. Continue repetitive chemotherapy until:
   1. Three courses after negative serum β-hCG titers.
   2. Remission is defined as three consecutive normal weekly β–hCG titer.

Switch on to alternative chemotherapy if
a. Titer rise (10 fold or more)
b. The plateau after two courses of MAC regime
c. New metastasis appear
   - Do not begin or continue a course of chemotherapy, if white blood cell (WBC) count less than 3,000/µL
   - Granulocytes less than 1,500/µL
   - Platelet count less than 1, 00,000/µL
   - Blood urea nitrogen (BUN), serum glutamic oxaloacetic transaminase (SGOT), serum glutamic pyruvic transaminase (SGPT) serum bilirubin significantly elevated, laboratory values obtain daily during treatment cycle.

Specimens

Q. What is alternative chemotherapy for poor prognosis patient of choriocarcinoma?

Ans. EMA-CO (E—etoposide, M—methotrexate, A—dactinomycin, C—cyclophosphamide, O—vincristine).

Q. What is invasive mole?

Ans. It is a type of invasive mole that penetrates the uterine wall and causes internal hemorrhage.

Q. Differences between invasive mole and choriocarcinoma.

Ans. *Invasive mole*
  a. Villus structure is present. Trophoblastic invasion of uterine wall and not the blood vessels.
  b. Locally malignant and does not kill the patient by distant metastasis.

  Choriocarcinoma
  Villus structure is absent. Invasion of myometrium, blood vessels, tissue necrosis and hemorrhage, kills the patient by distant metastasis to lungs (over 75%), brain, and vagina (50%).

Q. What is the treatment of choriocarcinoma?

Ans. a. Correction of anemia, multiparity—total hysterectomy/ chemotherapy.
  b. Conservative chemotherapy till the lesion regresses and vaginal or pulmonary deposits disappear spontaneously.
  c. Vaginal deposits are removed sometimes by wide excision and pulmonary deposit disappears spontaneously, but in drug resistant cases pulmonary segmental resection is to be done.
  d. Irradiation is often as an adjunct to chemotherapy for brain and liver metastasis.

Q. What is the partial molar degeneration of placenta?

Ans. In this case, only a part of the placenta undergoes molar changes, the rest of it remains normal. So, a fetus is usually present. This condition may occur in singleton pregnancy, but more common in multiple pregnancies. USG helps to diagnose the condition.

Q. What will you do if complete hydatidiform mole coexists with two fetuses?

Ans. In the past, it was terminated immediately following the diagnosis. The circumstances have been changed in recent years.
  The absolute indication of immediate evacuation of pregnancy includes:
  a. Development of pre-eclampsia (severe, not managed by medical treatment)
  b. Intractable vaginal bleeding
  c. Severe hyperemesis gravidarum
  d. Hyperthyroidism
  e. Evidence of trophoblastic embolism.
  Some authors have also been suggested that, in the absence of fetal anomalies, the pregnancy can be allowed to continue upto term

irrespective of the development of persistent gestational trophoblastic disease (PGTD) provided there are no other complications as mentioned above. Postpartum dangers may be high that may require chemotherapy.

> **Note**
> Chances of miscarriage and preterm delivery is high in such cases.

Q. What is the incidence of H mole with a coexistent fetus?
Ans. The incidence is very rare; 1 in 22,000 to 1,00,000 pregnancies.

Q. What is placental site trophoblastic tumor (PSTT)?
Ans. This is an uncommon trophoblastic tumor composed principally of cytotrophoblast cells and the lesion is microscopic to follow a soft, brown, partly hemorrhagic mass, which protrude in the uterine cavity and infiltrate the uterine musculature. In addition to vaginal bleeding, cytotrophoblast cells produce hPL resulting hyperprolactinemia which can result amenorrhea and galactorrhea.

Q. How does PSTT differ from choriocarcinoma?
Ans. This produces relatively little hCG than choriocarcinoma in relation to the size of tumor. There is typical myometrial invasion with rare systemic metastasis. High proportion of β-hCG (>30%) is considered diagnostic.

Q. How do you treat placental site trophoblastic tumor?
Ans. Curettage is not generally done as it causes perforation due to uterine muscle infiltration. Treatment of choice is hysterectomy as this is resistant to chemotherapy.

Q. What is the fate of placental site trophoblastic tumor?
Ans. a. It may be benign with a capacity for spontaneous regression.
b. It may be highly malignant with resistance to cytotoxic drugs.

Q. Is there any requirement of anti-D globulin in Rh -ve mother with molar pregnancy?
Ans. Anti-D globulin should be given to the mother, if she is Rh -ve for all practical purpose, irrespective of complete or partial mole.

> **Note**
> See also the specimen of choriocarcinoma in gynecological part.

PLACENTA WITH UMBILICAL CORD

Q. What is this specimen?
Ans. This is the specimen of placenta with umbilical cord.

Q. What is its weight?
Ans. About 500 gram or in relation to fetal body weight is 1/6th to 1/7th of the weight of fetus.

Q. In which condition the size of the placenta increases?
Ans. Syphilis, diabetes and erythroblastosis (placental weight—2,000 gram).

Specimens

Q. What is its shape?

Ans. It is disc-shaped (15 to 20 cm in diameter). It is thickest in the center, with maximum thickness of about 25 mm, and then diminished towards periphery.

Q. What is the type of human placenta?

Ans. Hemochorial, because of direct contact of human blood and chorion.

Q. How does it develop?

Ans. Chorionic frondosum and decidua basalis form the discrete placenta. Chorion leave disappears. Placenta begins to develop at 6th week and is completed by 12th week.

Q. What are the surfaces and how do you identify it?

Ans. a. Maternal surface—spongy, 15 to 20 lobes or cotyledons, which are limited by fissures. Each fissure is occupied by decidual septum. Only the decidua basalis and the blood in the intervillus space are of maternal origin (Figure 1.7A).

b. Fetal surface is glistened with the umbilical cord attached near the center. At term, 4/5th of placenta is of fetal origin (Figure 1.7B).

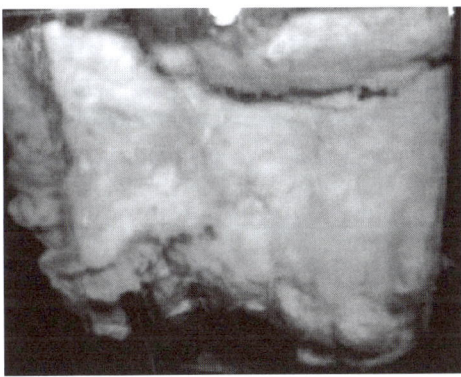

Figure 1.7A: Maternal surface of placenta (rough due to cotyledons) *(For color version, see Plate 1)*

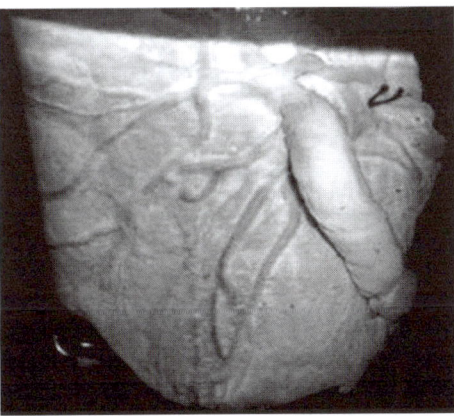

Figure 1.7B: Placenta—Fetal surface (umbilical cord and umbilical blood vessels) *(For color version, see Plate 1)*

Q. What are the structures of placenta?

Ans. From fetal side to maternal side:
  a. Amniotic membrane
  b. Chorionic plate
  c. Choriodecidual space—contains stem villi with their branches, the space is filled with maternal blood.
  d. Basal plate—from outside inward
      i. Part of compact and spongy layer of deciduas basalis
      ii. Nitabuch's layer of fibrinoid degeneration of the outer syncytiotrophoblast at the junction of cytotrophoblastic shells and deciduas
      iii. Cytotrophoblastic shell
      iv. Syncytiotrophoblast.

Q. What is choriodecidual space?

Ans. It is bounded on inner side by chorionic plate, outside by basal plate, limited on the periphery by fusion of two plates. It is lined internally on all sides by syncytiotrophoblasts and is filled with maternal blood. Numerous branching villi arising from stem villi enter into the space and contribute the chief content of choriodecidual space.

Q. What are primary, secondary and tertiary villi?

Ans.
- Primary villi contain only the syncytiotrophoblast and cytotrophoblast cells.
- Secondary villi contain outer syncytiotrophoblast and cytotrophoblast cells with mesoderm.
- Tertiary villi contain: (from outside inward)
    i. Outer syncytiotrophoblast
    ii. Cytotrophoblast
    iii. Basement membrane
    iv. Central stroma contains fetal capillaries, primitive mesenchymal cells and Hofbauer (phagocytic cells) (Figures 1.8A and B).

Q. What is placental grading by USG?

Ans. See Grannum's Classification in USG (Chapter-8)

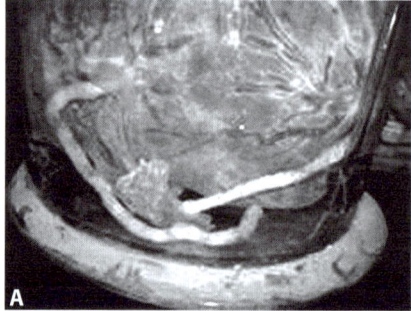
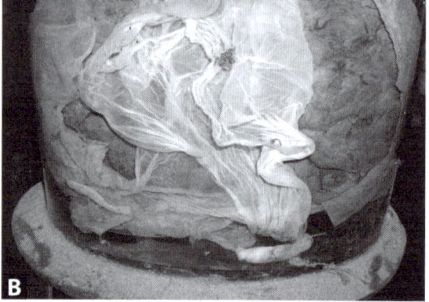

Figures 1.8A and B: (A) Placenta of uniovular twin pregnancy (fetal surface); (B) Placenta of twin pregnancy (maternal surface) (single placenta with 2-cords and vessel anastomosis on fetal surface) *(For color version, see Plate 2)*

Specimens

Q. How many spiral arteries are in normal placenta?
Ans. 200.

Q. What is the rate of blood flow through uteroplacental unit?
Ans. 500 mL/min at term.

Q. What is the rate of fetal blood flow through the placenta?
Ans. 400 mL/min.

Q. What is placental barrier?
Ans. In the villi, maternal and fetal blood flow are separated by a barrier (0.025 mm thick) and consist of:
  a. Syncytiotrophoblast
  b. Cytotrophoblast
  c. Basal membrane
  d. Stromal tissue
  e. Endothelium of fetal capillaries with basement membrane.

Q. What is α-zone and β-zone of the placental membrane?
Ans. The thin zone of terminal villi (0.002 mm) 'α-zone' for fetomaternal exchange and the thick zone of terminal villi, i.e. β-zone are for hormone synthesis.

Q. What is Nitabuch's membrane?
Ans. It is a fibrinoid deposit in the outer syncytiotrophoblast adjacent to the decidua. This membrane limits further invasion of decidua by trophoblasts.

Q. When this membrane is absent?
Ans. It is absent in placenta accreta.

Q. What are the functions of placenta?
Ans. 1. **Transport:**
  a. Oxygen is transported by diffusion
  b. Water, glucose, sodium ions (Na^+), potassium ions (K^+), calcium ions (Ca^{2+}) and phosphorus pass from maternal to fetal side by passive diffusion
  c. Amino acid is transported by active process
  d. Iron and water soluble vitamin are transported by active mechanism to the fetus.
 2. **Synthesis:**
  a. Enzyme—heat stable alkaline phosphatase, cysteine aminopeptidase (CAP)
  b. Protein hormone—hCG and human placental lactogen (HPL)
  c. Steroid hormone—estrogen and progesterone
  d. Pregnancy-associated placental protein—pregnancy associated plasma protein A (PAPP-A), pregnancy associated plasma protein-B (PAPP-B), etc.
 3. **Respiratory**
 4. **Nutritive**
 5. **Excretory**
 6. **Barrier and immunological function.**

Q. What are the abnormalities of placenta?

Ans. a. Placenta succenturiate (Figure 1.9A):
An accessory lobe, which remains at a distance from main placenta and is connected to the main placenta by membrane containing umbilical blood vessels.
Significance: It causes postpartum hemorrhage (PPH), shock, sepsis and placental polyp.

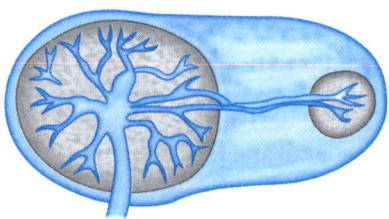

Figure 1.9A: Placenta succenturiata

b. Placenta bipartia or tripartia (Figure 1.9B):
Placenta is divided incompletely at the periphery into two or three lobes and this has no obstetrical significance.

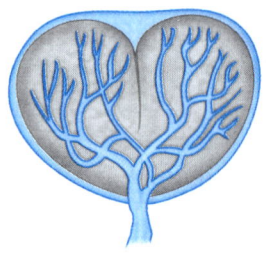

Figure 1.9B: Placenta bipartia

c. Placenta duplex or triplex (Figure 1.9C):
Here, the placenta is completely divided into two or more lobules. The small lobules are attached with the main placenta by membrane or blood vessels.
Significance: Antepartum hemorrhage (APH), PPH, retained bits.

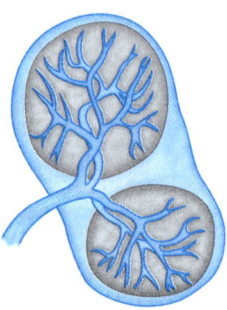

Figure 1.9C: Placenta duplex

d. **Placenta membranacea**—Large, 15 inch in diameter. Here, the placenta develops from chorion laeve and from chorion frondosum.

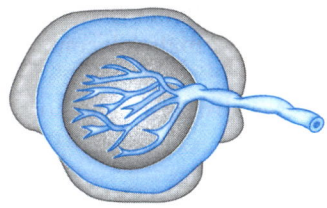

Figure 1.9D: Placenta circumvallate

e. **Placenta circumvallate:** Partial or complete ring divide the fetal surface into the distinct central and peripheral portion (Figures 1.9D and E).

The rim is raised yellowish-white in color and ½ inch broad and is composed of double layer of chorion, which undergoes infarction when the ring coincide with the placental margin. The condition is called placenta marginata.

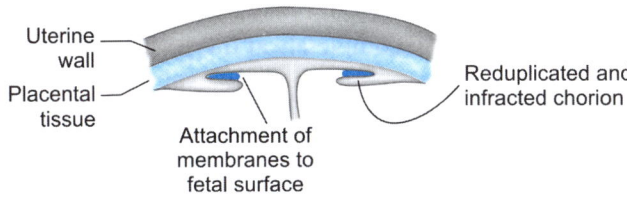

Figure 1.9E: Circumvallate placenta (Schematic diagram)

Central zone is slightly depressed and normal appearance, but peripheral zone may be 5 to 7.5 cm in breadth. Placental tissue is thicker over peripheral zone. Vessels radiate from the cord up to the ring and then disappear. The probable explanation is that during early development, the chorionic frondosum is too restricted for nutrition of the fetus, to compensate for this the peripheral villi grow outwards splitting the decidua basalis into two layers.

Significance: Abortion, APH, Preterm labor, intrauterine growth restriction (IUGR), intrauterine fetal death (IUFD), hydrorrhea gravidarum.

f. **Battledore placenta (Figure 1.9F):**
Cord is attached to the margin of the placenta.
Significance: Cord presentation and cord prolapse.

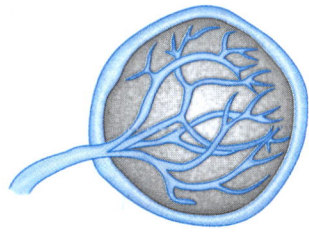

Figure 1.9F: Battledore placenta

g. **Velamentous insertion of the cord (Figure 1.9G):**
Cord is inserted in the membrane and cord vessels traverse some distance along the membrane to reach the placenta.
Significance: Vasa previa is associated with placenta previa (here, the fetal blood loss is significant). Here intrapartum bleeding is common rather than antepartum bleeding.

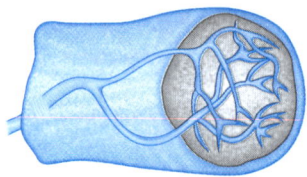

Figure 1.9G: Velamentous insertion of the cord

Q. What are the diseases of placenta?

Ans. Placental polyp, cyst, hydatidiform degeneration, edema and infarction and placental tumor (hemangioma—rare).

Q. How do you examine the placenta?

Ans. Maternal surface
  a. Lobules of the placenta.
  b. The lobules should fit together.
  c. The margins should be regular.
  d. If there is missing of lobules, they do not fit together.

Fetal surface
  a. Attachment to umbilical cord to placenta.
  b. The umbilical vessels passing from the cord and fades into the margin.
  c. Look for free ending vessels, which may indicate succenturiate lobe has been left behind in uterus.

Membrane
  a. The chorion is the layer in contact with the uterus—rough and thick.
  b. The amnion is the inner layer—thin and shiny.
  c. The amnion can be peeled up to the insertion of the cord.
  d. If the membrane is ragged, place them together and ascertain their completeness.

Umbilical cord
Look for artery and vein (normal A2, V1). If only one artery is found, look for congenital defect of the baby.

Q. What is normal length of the cord?

Ans. 50 to 60 cm and diameter is 12 mm.

Q. What are the structures of the cord?

Ans. 1. Amnion
  2. Wharton's jelly (a hydrated glycoprotein matrix accumulates around the large vessels in the umbilical cord following enclosure of ectoderm)

3. Umbilical artery (2) and umbilical vein (1) [A2V$_1$]
4. Remnant of umbilical vesicle (yolk sac and its vitelline duct
5. Allantois
6. Obliterated extraembryonic coelom.

Q. What are the complications of long cord?

Ans. a. May lead to cord knots
 b. Nuchal cord
 c. Cord prolapse
 d. Cord entanglement
 e. Fetal distress
 f. Fetal death.

Q. What is short cord and mention its clinical significance?

Ans. Short cord, length— 35 to 46 cm.
 a. Malpresentation (breech).
 b. Temporary arrest of descent.
 c. Separation of placenta (accidental hemorrhage).
 d. Inversion of uterus.
 e. Fetoplacental hematoma.
 f. Tearing of the cord.
 g. May be associated with congenital anomalies and trisomy-21.
 h. FGR, or Fetal death.

Q. Why there is twisting of the cord?

Ans. Due to the embryonic/fetal movement.

> **Note**
> Two vessels cord is associated with aplasia or atrophy, 30% with single umbilical artery may have congenital defect of fetus.

Q. How umbilical cord develops?

Ans. The umbilical cord begins to develop in the 5th postmenstrual week, when a bridge of mesenchymal tissue condensed between ventral surface of the embryo-forming connecting stalk. The connective tissue of the cord is Wharton's jelly, a ground substance made up of predominantly mucopolysaccharide.

Q. Which types of major fetal anomalies are associated with SUA (single umbilical artery)?

Ans. a. Fetal heart anomaly.
 b. CNS defect.
 c. Kidney problem.
 d. Chromosomal anomalies such as trisomy 13 and 18, but no such association with trisomy-21.

> **Note**
> SUA on USG should thoroughly search fetal anomalies, and if anomaly is found the risk of aneuploidy also increases, amniocentesis may be needed later on.

ANENCEPHALY

Q. What is this specimen?

Ans. This is the specimen of anencephaly.

Q. What is anencephaly?

Ans. Absence of cranial vault and much of the forebrain of fetus, eye balls are bigger and sometime protrude, neck is short (Figure 1.10).

> **Note**
>
> *Female baby is at increased risk (70%), aneuploidy and folic acid deficiency may be the underlying etiology. It is an open type of neural tube defect, other is open spina bifida where fetal spinal column does not close completely (normally neural tube fuses at 24–28 days post conception). Anencephaly is also caused by the drugs like valproic acid and clomiphene citrate.*

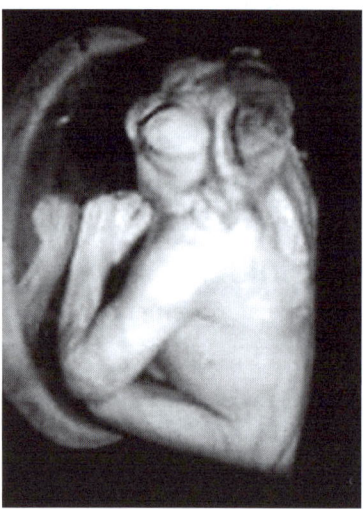

Figure 1.10: Anencephaly *(For color version, see Plate 2)*

Q. How can you diagnose anencephaly?

Ans. By USG (10–12 weeks), X-ray (not preferable now-a-day) and increased level of MSAFP or amniotic fluid alpha fetoprotein.
USG: Inability to get a view of BPD (biparital diameter), cranial vault and brain tissue.

Q. How can you reduce the incidence of open neural tube defect (NTDs)?

Ans. By administration of folic acid (500 μg), 2 months before conception and continue for at least 12 weeks of pregnancy. To prevent the recurrence of NTDS higher dose (5 mg) of folic acid is required in high risk cases having previous history of open neural tube defects.

Q. What are the complications?

Ans. Polyhydramnios (50%), preterm labor, post-dated pregnancy, mal-presentation, obstructed labor and shoulder dystocia.

Specimens

Q. What are the associated anomalies with anencephaly?

Ans. Spinabifida (26%), cleft lip (26%), omphalocele (6%) and cardiac anomalies (5%).

> **Note**
>
> *For other questions and answers see the chapter of X-ray, USG and flying oral questions on anencephaly.*

Hydrocephalus (Figure 1.11)
[Hydro= water (CSF), Cephalus = Head]

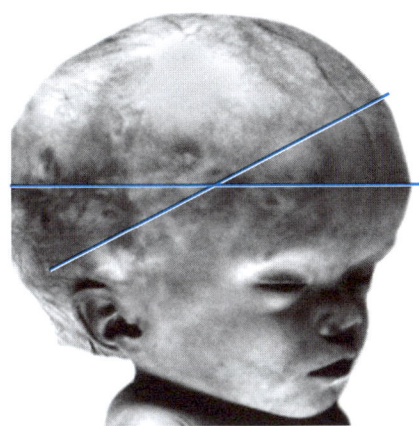

Figure 1.11: Hydrocephalus

Q. What is this specimen?

Ans. This is the specimen of fetus showing enlarged head (head circumference >50 cm) which is suggestive of hydrocephalus due to increased CSF volume (0.5L–1.5L).

Q. What are the pathophysiology/causes of hydrocephalus?

Ans. a. *Pathophysiology*: Obstructive and nonobstructive variety
b. *Causes*: Congenital or acquired by TORCH infection.

> **Note**
>
> *Aqueductal stenosis is caused by Fetal-TORCH infection.*

Q. How do you diagnose hydrocephalus clinically?

Ans. a. Minor cases are very difficult to diagnose.

In moderate-to-severe cases:
b. The head is felt larger, softer than normal head
c. The head is high up and impossible to push into the pelvis
d. *P/V findings in labor*: The sutures are wide apart, anterior fontanel is wider and the skull bones are thin and feels like the sensation of a ping-pong ball.

Q. What is the USG finding?

Ans. *USG findings:* Dilation of ventricles (more than 10 mm), dangling choroid plexus, thinning out of cerebral cortex (see Chapter 8 of USG in Obstetrics).

> **Note**
> Lateral ventricle consists of anterior (frontal) horn, posterior (occipital) horn, atrium containing glomus of choroid plexus and inferior (temporal) horn. As the fetus grows the ventricular size decreases and inferior horn is obliterated by 18 weeks. In second trimester, the lateral ventricles are present as anterior and posterior horn and atrium which is studded with choroid plexus. Dilatation of only posterior horn seen in agenesis of corpus callosum, which is known as colpocephaly.

Q. What is the mode of delivery?

Ans. There is no conclusive evidence regarding the mode of delivery. Cesarean section should be considered for maternal indications, maternal request after counseling hydrocephalus where vaginal delivery is not possible, breech and large fetal lesions for advancement of intrauterine and pediatric surgery. Previously craniocentesis and vaginal delivery was the only option.

Q. What are the obstetric complications?

Ans. Obstructed labor and rupture of uterus.

Q. What are the different sites for shunt operation in utero in hydrocephalic baby?

Ans. Ventricle-peritoneal cavity/ventricle-pericardial cavity shunt.

Q. What malformations are generally associated with hydrocephalus?

Ans. Most common malformations associated are spina bifida, Arnold-Chiari malformation (a group of anomalies with herniation of cerebellar tonsil through the foramen magnum and downward displacement of pons and medulla oblongata and cerebellar hypogenesis), and Dandy-Walker malformation (see Chapter 8, USG in Obstetrics).

Que. What is the mode of delivery?

Ans. There is no conclusive evidence regarding the mode of delivery. Cesarean section should be considered for maternal indications, maternal request after counseling hydrocephalus where vaginal delivery is not possible, breech and large fetal lesions for advancement of intrauterine and pediatric surgery. Previously craniocentesis and vaginal delivery was the only option.

> **Note**
> Breech presentation occurs in 25% of cases and recurrence rate is 5%.

Conjoined twin (Siamese twins) (Figure 1.12)

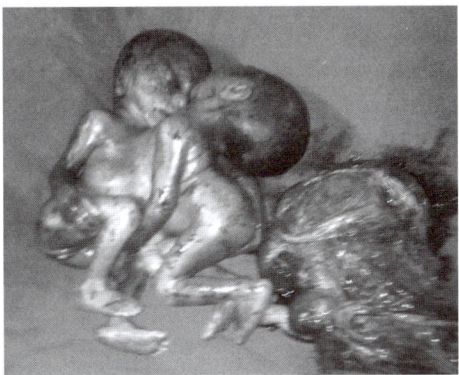

Figure 1.12: Conjoined twin with placenta (Thoracopagus)
(For color version, see Plate 2)

Q. What is this variety?

Ans. This is thoracopagus:
  a. 73% are connected at mid-torso (at the chest wall or upper abdomen)
  b. 23% at lower torso (sharing hips, legs, or genitalia)
  c. 4% at upper torso (connected at the head).

> **Note**
> Other types are omphalopagus, pyopagus, ischiopagus, craniopagus and Janiceps rarest type of conjoined twin: 2 faces are attached but oriented in opposite direction.

Q. What is the cause of conjoined twin?

Ans. Imperfect division of zygote after development of embryonic disc, i.e. after 13 days of fertilization.

Q. How do you diagnose it?

Ans. By targeted USG at mid-pregnancy and X-ray.

Q. What are the diagnostic criteria on X-ray?

Ans. a. The two heads are at the same level
  b. Convex aspects of the vertebral column of the two fetuses is generally apposed to each other.

Que. How do you diagnose conjoined twin by USG?

Ans. a. Apparent fusion
  b. No separating membrane
  c. Anomalies in a twin pair
  d. More than three vessels in umbilical cord
  e. Both fetal heads persistently at the same level
  f. Backward flexion of cervical and thoracic spine
  g. No change in relative position of the fetus.

Q. How do you deliver the conjoined twin?

Ans. Majority advocates LSCS to avoid traumatic and difficult vaginal delivery.

Iniencephaly: This is a lethal anatomy with defect in occiput, involving foramen magnum, retroflexion of entire spine and open spinal canal defects of variable degrees. Associated abnormalities like hydrocephaly, microcephaly, ventricular atresia and holoprosencephaly (the abnormality is complete or partial deficiency of falx leading to alobar, semi-lobar or lobar type of holoprosencephaly) are known.

Chapter 2

Instruments and Drugs

SPONGE-HOLDING FORCEPS

Q. Describe the instrument.

Ans. This is a long instrument with oblong serrated and fenestrated rings at the anterior end and catches at the other end (Figure 2.1).

Q. What are the uses of sponge-holding forceps in obstetrics and gynecology?

Ans. Obstetrics
  a. Holding the swab for antiseptic dressing before any operative procedure.
  b. For removal of membranes after delivery of placenta.
  c. To catch hold the cervix to see the tear of the cervix and to repair it.
  d. As an alternative of ovum forceps to remove the products of conceptions.
  e. Cervical encirclage operation in cervical incompetence.

Gynecology
  a. A golley may be used to push the bladder after incising the peritoneum of anterior pouch in abdominal hysterectomy.
  b. To catch hold the swab to see the bleeding points in the deeper pelvic tissue.
  c. To remove the fibroid polyp with thin pedicle.
  d. Temporary clamping of infundibulopelvic ligament in myomectomy operation.

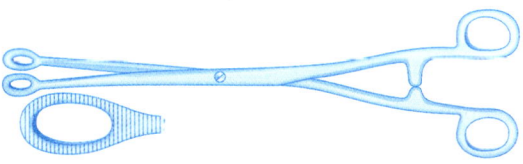

Figure 2.1: Sponge-holding forceps

KOCHER'S ARTERY FORCEPS OR CLAMPS

Q. How will you identify the instrument?

Ans. It is an instrument with transversely serrated blades and teeth (2×1) at the tip and catch at the handle (Figure 2.2).

Q. What are the uses of this instrument in obstetrics?

Ans.
a. To clamp the umbilical cord after delivery of the baby at least 6 cm away from its naval attachment.
b. For artificial low rupture of membrane (ARM) in case of surgical induction of labor.
c. To clamp the pedicles in obstetrical hysterectomy.

> **Note**
> Two Kocher's clamps are necessary for cord clamping—one at baby side and other at the mother side (see cutting of the cord, chapter-5).

Q. What are the indications of low ARM? What are the complications?

Ans. In postdated pregnancy, pregnancy induced hypertension (PIH), eclampsia, abruptio placentae.

Complication— see induction of labor (chapter 11).

Q. In which conditions you will not perform low ARM?

Ans. In case of intrauterine death (IUD) of fetus, central placenta previa, free floating head and hydramnios to prevent cord prolapse and accidental hemorrhage, ARM is not generally done in HIV, hepatitis B and C infected mothers.

> **Note**
> In hydramnios if low rupture of membrane is done, allow slow release of liquor by pressing the vulva by both palms to prevent the complications of accidental hemorrhage and cord prolapse. Alternatively if vertex is not well applied to the lower uterine segment, membrane is ruptured in several places with 26-gauze needle held with ring forceps under direct visualization by Sim's speculum for slow release of amniotic fluid if membrane bulges.

Q. What are the uses of Kocher's artery forceps in gynecology?

Ans. It can be used as a hysterectomy clamp for abdominal and vaginal hysterectomies for clamping of uterine vessels for better gripping of the instruments.

Q. What do you note following ARM?

Ans.
a. Color of liquor
b. Cord prolapse
c. Bleeding per vagina
d. FHS.

Instruments and Drugs

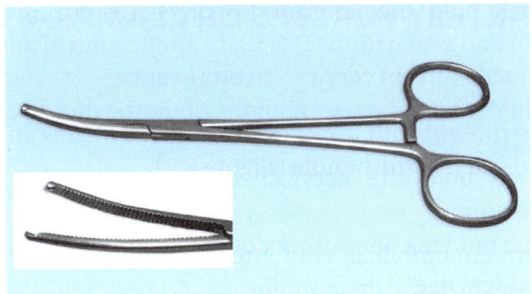

Figure 2.2: Kocher's artery forceps
(see transversely serrated blades with 2 × 1 teeth at the tip)

Q. What is the use of small artery forceps?
Ans. To catch hold of the bleeding points during operation, holding ends of suture materials, to hold parietal and visceral peritoneum and to crush the tube before tubectomy operation.

ALLIS TISSUE FORCEPS

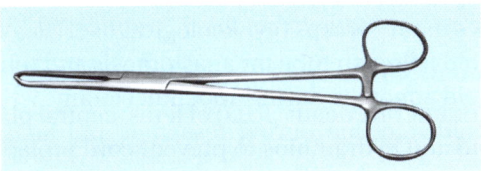

Figure 2.3A: Allis tissue forceps

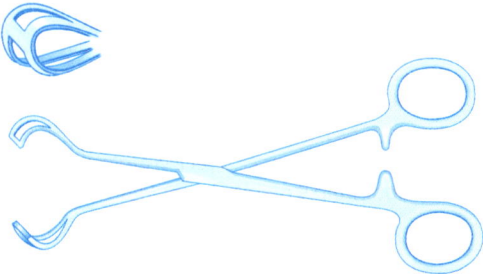

Figure 2.3B: Babcock's tissue forceps

Q. How will you identify this instrument (Allis)?
Ans. This is a pair of forceps with fine teeth (3–4) at one end and catch at the handle (Figure 2.3A).

Q. What are the uses of Allis tissue forceps?
Ans. Obstetrical use
    a. To hold the tissues like peritoneum, sheath, vaginal mucosae and skin.

b. To catch hold the anterior lip of cervix during operations like dilation and evacuation (D & E); in application of Shirodkar stitch or McDonald stitch in cervical incompetence.
c. To hold the angles of cut margins of uterus during cesarean section (2 pairs).
d. To catch hold the cervical stump for its closure in subtotal hysterectomy.
e. To catch hold the apex of episiotomy while suturing.

Gynecological use
a. To hold the skin, peritoneum, sheath in different gynecological abdominal operations or anterior lip of the cervix in D and C operation.
b. To catch hold the small myoma during enucleation operation.
c. To catch hold the vaginal vault after abdominal/radical hysterectomy operation, to pick up the vagina in Fothergill's operation, in anterior colporrhaphy, posterior colpoperineorrhaphy, in repair of VVF and RVF.
d. To pick-up the loop of fallopian tube during tubectomy operation.

Q. Name the other type of tissue forceps.

Ans. a. Lane's tissue forceps for holding tough tissues and bulk of tissues like skin and parietal tissues, etc.
b. Babcock's tissue forceps (gynecological use) (Figure 2.3B):
  i. To hold fallopian tube for anastomosis and tubectomy operation
  ii. To hold appendix during appendicectomy.
  iii. To hold intestine during resection and anastomosis in bowel injury
  iv. To remove the lymph glands and to hold the ureter in Wertheim's operation
  v. To hold the ovary in ovarian cystectomy operation
  vi. Dissection of vascular sheath in ligation of anterior division of internal iliac artery.

GREEN-ARMYTAGE HEMOSTATIC FORCEPS

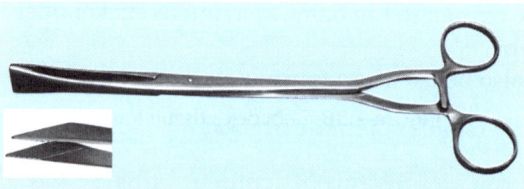

Figure 2.4: Green-Armytage hemostatic forceps

Q. How will you identify this instrument?

Ans. The instrument consists of triangular blades with fine serrations at one end and catch on the other end (Figure 2.4).

Q. What are the uses of this forceps?
Ans.   a. It is used to hold the angles of the cut margins of the uterus during cesarean section, the broad tip with fine serrations cause proper hemostasis with least tissue damage.
b. To trace cervical tear after vaginal delivery
c. As an alternative of sponge holding forceps.

Q. Have you seen this instrument to use now a days?
Ans. No.

Q. What is the disadvantage of this instrument?
Ans. It holds the wide area of the uterine tissue.

Q. Which instrument is used instead of it?
Ans. Two pairs of Allis tissue forceps for angles of the incision commonly.

> **Note**
> It can be used for holding swab and antiseptic dressing.

SIMPLE RUBBER CATHETER AND FOLEY'S CATHETER

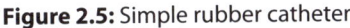

Figure 2.5: Simple rubber catheter

Q. Have you seen to use a rubber catheter in obstetrics practice?
Ans. Yes, for evacuation of bladder.

Q. In which conditions have you seen to use it?
Ans.   a. Evacuation of bladder in second stage of labor
b. Before or after any obstetric operations—forceps, destructive operations
c. In postpartum hemorrhage (PPH), retained placenta before manual removal.

Q. What are the other uses of a rubber catheter in obstetrics?
Ans.   a. To give oxygen to the baby, as a mucus sucker after delivery of head of a baby.
b. It can also be used as a tourniquet.

Q. What is the length of female urethra?
Ans. 4 cm.

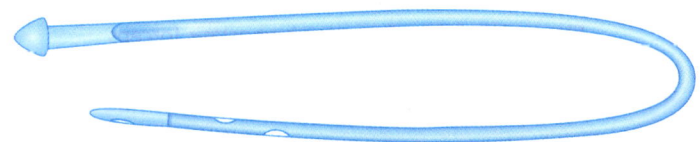

Figure 2.6: Disposable plastic catheter

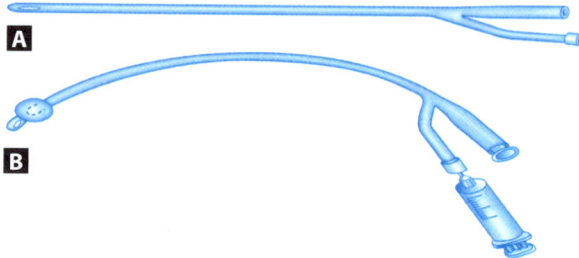

Figures 2.7A and B: Foley's catheter

Q. What is Foley's Catheter?

Ans. It is a self-retaining catheter of different sizes (Figure 2.7 A) and look the inflated bulb adjacent to the tip when water is introduced through side channel (Figure 2.7 B). The maximum capacity of the bulb is written on the wall of the catheter. The catheter should be deflated before removal from bladder.

Q. What are the uses of Foley's catheter in obstetrics?

Ans.
a. In early retroverted gravid uterus, where retention of urine is the complaint.
b. In suspected cases of bladder injury like after difficult forceps delivery, after destructive operations, in case of obstructed labor, in unconscious patient as in eclampsia and in septic cases or patients with obstetric shock and in postpartum hemorrhage (PPH) cases to measure urine output.
c. For introduction of ethacridine lactate extra-amniotically in the uterine cavity for midtrimester abortion.

Q. What are the uses of Foley's catheter in gynecology?

Ans.
a. In acute and chronic retention of urine by central cervical fibroid and ovarian tumor impacted in pouch of Douglas (POD).
b. Preoperative—before many gynecological operations like abdominal and radical hysterectomy and is maintained following operation for continuous bladder drainage.
c. Postoperative—after vaginal hysterectomy, Fothergill's operations in prolapse uterus and even after repair of vesicovaginal fistula (VVF), current procedural terminology (CPT), stress urinary incontinence (SUI). Other uses are:
   i. For hysterosalpingography and sono hysterography to investigate female infertility
   ii. As a part of treatment of Asherman's syndrome
   iii. To achieve hemostasis in myomectomy operation.

> **Note**
> *In chronic retention of urine slow release of urinary catheter for prevention of bladder hemorrhage.*

Instruments and Drugs

Q. Have you seen to use a metal female catheter in obstetrics and what will be the harm?

Ans. No, there may be more chances of urethral damage.

Q. In suspected cases of bladder injury, for how many days the self-retaining catheter is kept?

Ans. Ten days with strict monitoring of urine output to exclude the catheter blockage. Ensure that the urine is clear before removing the catheter.

Q. How will you sterilize the catheter?

Ans. A simple rubber catheter is sterilized by simple boiling, a Foley's catheter or disposable catheter are available in a sterilized pack (sterilized by gamma radiation).

Q. How will you introduce female catheter?

Ans. The bladder should be catheterized in aseptic precautions to avoid infection, in the following way:
  i. Highly disinfected gloves should be worn on both hands
  ii. Then left index finger and thumb is used to open the introitus to identify the urethral opening.
  iii. Take a sterile cotton swab soaked with savlon and clean the introitus with single stroke from above downwards (not from below upwards to avoid contamination of organism from perianal region).
  iv. Take the sterile rubber catheter and hold it 4 cm away from the tip and introduce through the opening of urethra and clear urine identifies that the catheter is in bladder.
  v. In case of self-retaining catheter, it should be introduced 5-7 cm in bladder and when clear urine is seen the bulb of the catheter is insufflated with sterile water of 10 to 20 mL by a sterilized syringe through the side tube of the catheter (or according to its capacity written on the catheter).

Q. In which condition will you keep catheter for a prolonged period?

Ans. For 10–12 days

Obstetrical conditions:
  a. After repair of bladder injury (due to rupture of uterus, or during cesarean section or laparotomy).
  b. After destructive operation.
  c. Following surgery of uterine rupture and prolonged or obstructed labor.
  d. Conditions like puerperal sepsis with pelvic peritonitis
  e. Massive perineal edema.

Gynecological conditions:
  a. After surgical repair of VVF, CPT, SUI.
  b. After radical hysterectomy in cancer cervix
  c. After posterior colpoperineorrhaphy (3–5 days).

Q. What is the important complication of catheterization?

Ans. Cystitis, urinary tract infection (UTI) (see also catheter in gynecological instruments in gynecology part).

DREW SMYTHE CATHETER

Q. How do you identify the instrument?

Ans. It is a long metal catheter with two curvatures with a stillete inside which projects beyond the catheter. The catheter has an opening at the side of the tip (Figure 2.8).

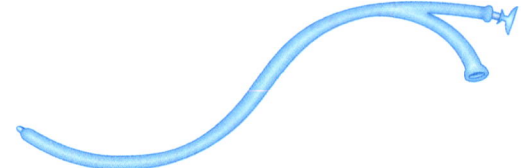

Figure 2.8: Drew Smythe catheter

Q. What are its uses?

Ans. a. For high rupture of membrane in case of hydramnios.
  b. In case of hydrocephalus with breech presentation, the cerebrospinal fluid (CSF) is drained through the spinal cord after delivery of the trunk especially when associated with spina bifida.

Q. What do you mean by high rupture of membrane?

Ans. The rupture of membrane above the presenting part for drainage of liquor.

Q. What are the advantages of high rupture of membrane?

Ans. a. Measured amount of liquor is drained.
  b. Chances of accidental hemorrhage and dry labor are less.
  c. Smooth dilation of cervix due to the presence of fore water.

Q. What are the disadvantages of high rupture of membrane?

Ans. a. Injury of placenta, fetus and uterine wall may occur as it is a blind procedure.
  b. Increased risk of infection.
  c. Low rupture of membrane may occur during the procedure.

SIM'S DOUBLE-BLADED POSTERIOR VAGINAL SPECULUM

Q. Describe Sim's speculum.

Ans. It is a double-bladed speculum. The narrow blade is for nulliparous vagina and the other side for multiparous vagina (Figure 2.9).

Q. Where is it used most frequently? Other obstetrical uses?

Ans. In the labor room for visualization of cervix, in repair of cervical tear, D and E operation. Other uses in obstetrics are S/E of vesicular mole, in evaluation of antepartum hemorrhage (APH), and cervical circlage operation.

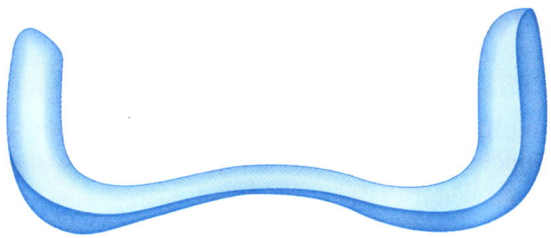

Figure 2.9: Sim's speculum

Q. What are its uses in gynecology?

Ans. a. To retract the posterior vaginal wall.
b. To visualize the anterior vaginal wall to detect the fistula keeping the patient in left lateral and sim's position.
c. To inspect the cystocele and urethrocele or cyst on anterior vaginal wall.
d. To visualize cervix along with anterior vaginal wall retractor.
e. To collect urine in case of vesicovaginal fistula (VVF).
f. It is used in certain operations, like D and C, repair of cystocele.
g. To see enterocele by double speculum examination.
h. For culdocentesis.

Q. Which instrument is used along with Sim's speculum to see the anterior wall of vagina/cervix?

Ans. Sim's anterior vaginal wall retractor (Figure 2.10).

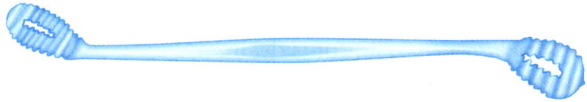

Figure 2.10: Sim's anterior vaginal wall retractor

Q. What are the disadvantages of Sim's speculum?

Ans. a. It is not self-retaining, assistant is required for holding it.
b. In cystocele, cervix cannot be visualized well only with this instrument.

Q. Where it is not used in gynecology?

Ans. Any operations on perineum like:
a. Posterior colpoperineorrhaphy
b. Repair of complete perineal tear (CPT)
c. Cyst on posterior vaginal wall.

Q. How do you introduce this instrument in vagina?

Ans. a. Ask the patient to evacuate the bladder.
b. Patient should be in lithotomy/dorsal position at the edge of the table.
c. Lubricate the instrument with savlon.
d. Separate the introitus by gloved left thumb and index finger and ask the patient to relax the perineum.

e. The instrument is held by right hand and introduced gently along the lateral wall of vagina in aseptic way and then rotate through 90° to bring it in the midline (not a good method). In patient, it will be introduced directly as the instrument is designed for direct application and vagina is wider from side-to-side than from front to back.

Q. What is Sim's triad?

Ans. a. Sim's position.
b. Sim's speculum.
c. Sim's-silver wire used for repair of VVF.

Q. What is Sim's position?

Ans. The female should lie on left lateral position with chest prone to bed, left thigh is semi-flexed and right lower limb is carried over the left.

Q. Advantage of Sim's position?

Ans. Better visualization of anterior vaginal wall due to ballooning of vagina.

Q. Have you seen to use other speculum? Where is it used mostly? What is the name of that instrument?

Ans. Yes, the name of the instrument is Cusco's bivalve self-retaining vaginal speculum, it is mostly used in gynecological outpatient department (OPD).

Q. How do you introduce the instrument in the vagina?

Ans. The closed valve should be introduced directly in the vagina as like Sim's speculum.

Q. What is the advantage of this instrument?

Ans. It has self-retaining device and no assistant is required (Figure 2.11).

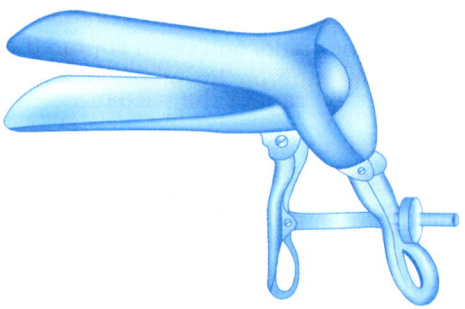

Figure 2.11: Cusco's speculum

Q. What are the uses in gynecology?

Ans. a. To inspect the cervix for ulcer, cancer, growth (polyp) and discharge and vaginal vault.
b. To take cervical cytology, cautery of cervix and intrauterine contraceptive device (IUCD) insertion in gynecology OPD.
c. To take cervical swab for bacteriology.

VULSELLUM

i. Multiple teeth vulsellum (Figure 2.12A)
ii. Single tooth vulsellum (Figure 2.12B)

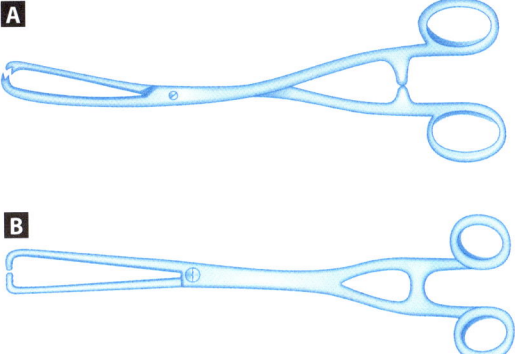

Figures 2.12A and B: (A) Multiple teeth vulsellum; (B) Single tooth vulsellum

Q. Name the different parts of multiple teeth vulsellum?

Ans. Multiple teeth at one end and catch at the other end.

Q. What are the uses of multiple teeth vulsellum?

Ans. Obstetrical use

To hold the anterior lip of cervix in D and E and suction evacuation operation, destructive operation to hold the fetal parts.

Gynecological use
a. To hold the anterior lip of the cervix in the operations like D & C, vaginal hysterectomy, cervical cautery and taking biopsy from cervix.
b. To hold the posterior lip of cervix—(i) for opening of pouch of Douglas in vaginal hysterectomy operation, (ii) during colpotomy for drainage of pelvic abscess (iii) if there is a friable growth on anterior lip of cervix, (iv) for culdocentesis in ruptured ectopic pregnancy, (v) for biopsy from anterior lip of cervix, (vi) vaginal ligation by posterior colpotomy.
c. To hold and pull the fundus during abdominal hysterectomy (exception: do not hold the fundus during TAH + BSO (Total abdominal hysterectomy with bilateral salpingo-oophorectomy), if the indication is endometrial carcinoma).
d. To hold the myoma during myomectomy operation, to grasp the fibroid polyp for polypectomy.

Q. What are the uses of single tooth vulsellum?

Ans. a. To hold the cervix after amputation in Fothergill's operation.
b. To hold the nulliparous cervix

Disadvantages of single tooth over multiple teeth vulsellum
a. The grip is weak
b. This can cut easily through the cervix, if it is soft.

Disadvantages of multiple teeth vulsellum—cervical injury and bleeding.

UTERINE SOUND

Figure 2.13: Uterine sound

Q. Describe the instrument.

Ans. Graduated, olive pointed, malleable, metallic uterine sound. It is angulated at a distance of 2½ inch from the tip (Figure 2.13).

Q. What are the uses of uterine sound in gynecology?

Ans. a. To measure the length of the uterine cavity.
b. To confirm, whether the uterus is anteverted (AV)/retroverted (RV).
c. It acts as a first dilator of cervix.
d. To find out, whether the IUCD is inside the uterus or not along with X-ray when the thread of the device is missing.
e. To distinguish between uterine inversion and pedunculated polyp.

Q. Why is it called sound?

Ans. Formerly, it was used to detect stone of urinary bladder.

Q. When this instrument is not used?

Ans. In pregnancy and hydatidiform mole for fear of perforation.

Q. What is the length of uterine cavity?

Ans. 2½ inch (uterocervical length).

Q. How do you introduce this instrument?

Ans. First do bimanual examination to have an idea about the size of uterus and, whether the uterus is AV/RV. The cervix is pulled down and steadied by Allis' tissue forceps or vulsellum. If the uterus is RV, the tip of the instrument should be directed downwards or if AV, the tip should be kept in upward direction.

Q. What are the common causes of increased uterine length?

Ans. Pregnancy and sub-involution of uterus (obstetric cause).
Gynecological causes:
a. Uterine fibroid/adenomyosis
b. Uterine prolapse
c. Congenital hypertrophic elongation of cervix
d. Metropathia hemorrhagica
e. Perforation of uterus.

Q. What are the common causes of decreased uterine length?

Ans. a. Congenital hypoplastic uterus (Uterus: cervix = 1:1)
b. Submucous fibroid
c. Inversion of uterus
d. Menopausal uterus.

Instruments and Drugs

Q. Complications/disadvantages?

Ans. Infection, perforation, hemorrhage, broad ligament hematoma.

Q. Contraindications?

Ans.
  a. When pregnancy is suspected
  b. Acute infection of uterus and cervix
  c. Hydatidiform mole.

Q. What are the common instruments causing perforation?

Ans.
  a. Uterine sound
  b. Cervical dilators
  c. Cannula
  d. Curette (commonest)
  e. Ovum forceps.

Q. What are the common sites of perforation?

Ans. Fundus of uterus, cornu, lateral wall of uterus causing broad ligament hematoma, coils of intestine.

Q. Which uterus is more prone to perforation?

Ans. Gynecology
  a. Acutely anteverted and retroverted uterus
  b. Cervical stenosis
  c. Distorted uterine cavity by fibromyoma and intrauterine adhesion
  d. Small menopausal uterus,
  e. Acute infection of uterus and cervix,
  f. Endometrial and cervical cancer
  g. Endometrial tuberculosis
  h. Congenital anomaly of uterus
  i. Distorted anatomy due to previous surgery.

Obstetrics
  a. Pregnant uterus
  b. Puerperal uterus
  c. Molar pregnancy
  d. Hyper involuted uterus due to prolonged lactation
  e. Advanced gestational age
  f. Uterine sepsis
  g. Nulliparity
  h. Cervical stenosis.

Q. How will you diagnose perforation?

Ans.
  a. Sudden loss of resistance
  b. Apparent lengthening of uterine cavity
  c. Unusual position and movement of the instrument
  d. Bleeding per vagina (PV)
  e. Features of shock may be present.

Q. How do you manage perforation by this instrument or by cervical dilators?

Ans.
  a. Stop the operative procedure transiently and assess bleeding and hemodynamic stability.

b. Intravenous infusion with ringer lactate and cross match blood and observe the patient if she is hemodynamically unstable.
c. Laparoscopy for location of site of perforation and intraperitoneal hemorrhage if the patient is stable/and intra abdominal injury.
d. If laparoscope is not available and P/V bleeding is more or features of shock is present, go for laparotomy immediately.
e. In majority of the cases perforation by uterine sound is small and close observation is to be done and the perforation tends to heal spontaneously.
f. Hysterectomy for big broad ligament hematoma. Other intra-abdominal organs like intestine, colon and omentum should be looked for any damage and managed accordingly after laparotomy. In younger patient open the broad ligament and repair of bleeding vessels or internal iliac artery ligation of both sides.

> **Note**
> Cervical dilators or uterine curette causes big size perforation.

g. If large perforation occurs on fundus, anterior or posterior wall of uterus, products are to be removed through the rent after laparotomy and later repair of the rent with absorbable suture.
h. If laparoscope is available evacuation under laparoscopic guidance from below and repair of the rent by suturing under laparoscopic guidance.
i. If patient is multigravida and does not want further pregnancy, concomitant bilateral tubectomy operation should be undertaken if the patient is in clinically stable condition.

> **Note**
> Chances of rupture uterus is more in future pregnancy if ligation is not done. Lateral perforation near the uterine vessels is more likely to result in hemorrhage than midline lacerations.

CERVICAL DILATORS

Q. Name the different types of dilators.

Ans. Hegar's dilators (Figure 2.14)

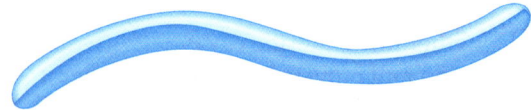

Figure 2.14: Hegar's dilator

Hawkins—Ambler's dilators (Figure 2.15)
Das's dilators—These are similar to Hawkin-Ambler's dilators, but the bases of these dilator are flat.

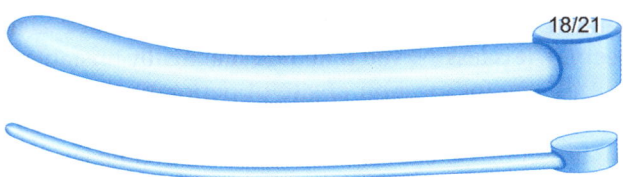

Figure 2.15: Hawkins' Ambler's dilators

HEGAR'S DILATORS

Q. What is the description of the instrument?
Ans. Each dilator is double-ended, curved in opposite direction.

Q. How many dilators are there in a set?
Ans. Twelve dilators.

Q. What is the lowest size and highest size?
Ans. Lowest is 1/2 and highest is 23/24. The number represents diameter in millimeter. With 1/2 Hegar's dilator, the cervical canal with internal os is dilated up to 1 mm with one end and the other end dilates the canal up to 2 mm. Keep the instrument in situ for 2–3 seconds for the purpose of dilatation.

Q. What is the advantage of this instrument?
Ans. Both the ends can be used.

Q. Uses in gynecology?
Ans. a. As a part of D&C
   b. Before hysteroscopy.
   c. Diagnosis of incompetent os—passage of no 8 Hegar's dilator in cervix up to internal os without resistance or pain or discomfort.
   d. Drainage of pyometra and hematometra.
   e. In Fothergill's operation before amputation of cervix.
   f. Therapeutic in cervical stenosis.

Q. Uses in obstetrics?
Ans. Before curettage, evacuation of products of conception, and for MTP.

> **Note**
> For suction and evacuation, ideally one size less than the diameter of suction cannula is used. The size of the suction cannula corresponds to the size of the uterus in weeks of gestational age.

Q. What are the complications of cervical dilatation?
Ans. Cervical tear, broad ligament hematoma, hemorrhage, infection, perforation.

HAWKINS-AMBLER'S DILATORS

- Lower size 3/6 mm; highest size 18/21 mm

- Single-ended with tapering tip, slightly curved and circular thumb rest at the other end. It is less curved than Hegar's dilator.

Q. One set contains how many dilators?
Ans. 16.

Q. What is the use of Hawkins Ambler's dilator?
Ans. For gradual dilation of external os, cervix including internal os.

Q. What do you mean by 18/21?
Ans. The tip of the dilator is 18 mm and the thickest diameter behind [3.75 cm (1½ inch)] the tip is 21 mm.

Q. What are the different sizes?
Ans. 3/6; 4/7; 5/8; 6/9; 7/10; 8/11; 9/12; 10/13; 11/14; 12/15; 13/16;14/17; 15/18; 16/19; 17/20;18/21. The first 7 sizes (3/6 to 9/12), are used in gynecology and for MTP.

Q. What are the indications of dilatation only?
Ans. a. For drainage of lochiometra, pyometra and hematometra
 b. Tubal insufflation (not popular in present days)
 c. Before introduction of intrauterine contraceptive device (IUCD)
 d. Before doing amputation of cervix
 e. After cervical cautery
 f. Before hysteroscopy
 g. Endometrial ablation
 h. Spasmodic dysmenorrhea.

Q. What are the indications of curettage only?
Ans. a. To diagnose hormonal status of uterine endometrium by Sharman's curette.
 b. Fractional curettage for diagnosis of endometrial carcinoma.

Q. How do you manage a uterine perforation by cervical dilator?
Ans. See the management of perforation by uterine sound. Perforation by cervical dilator is bigger in size than uterine sound. So operative correction is required.

> **Note**
>
> For cervical dilatation, Hawkins-Ambler's dilator is the best in comparison to Hagar, as single end is used for much more cervical dilatation than two ends of Hagar's dilator, but Hegar's dilators are used commonly for cervical dilatation in clinical practice.

UTERINE CURETTE (FLUSHING)

Q. Describe the instrument (flushing curette).
Ans. One side is blunt and hollow inside and opened at other end. Antiseptic solution was introduced through other end to flush the uterine cavity, but is not widely used nowadays in obstetrics (Figure 2.16).

Instruments and Drugs

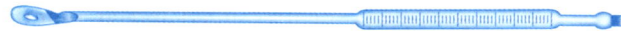

Figure 2.16: Flushing curette

Q. Describe the other type of curette.

Ans. A long slender instrument with two fenestrated ends, one side sharp and other side is blunt (See D & E or S & E operation).

Q. What are the uses of uterine curette?

Ans. For curetting of endometrial cavity in obstetrical operations like D & E or S & E for MTP, incomplete abortions, missed abortions. For D & C operation in gynecology, to detect endometrial pathology like TB, endometrial cancer, proliferative or secretory endometrium, detection of luteal phase defect (LPD).

Q. What are the indications of D & C operation?

Ans. Diagnostic (Gynecology)
    a. Infertility due to luteal phase defect (2nd half of cycle)
    b. Dysfunctional uterine bleeding (DUB)
    c. Tuberculous endometritis
    d. Carcinoma of body of uterus
    e. Choriocarcinoma uterus
    f. Placental polyp.

Therapeutic
    a. DUB (not significant)
    b. Placental polyp (significant).

Prior to some operation
    a. Fothergill's operation.

Q. Contraindications of D & C.

Ans. a. When pregnancy is suspected
    b. Sepsis of uterus until sepsis is controlled as it may cause breakdown of leukocyte barrier, which causes dissemination of infection.

Q. How long uterine curettage should be done?

Ans. It is done until the uterine cavity is empty and sufficient material is obtained.

Q. When do you say the uterine cavity is empty in obstetrics?

Ans. When the gritty sensation is felt in all the walls of the uterus during curettage.

Q. What is the most vulnerable complication of dilation and curette?

Ans. Perforation of the uterus.

Q. What are the indications of laparotomy in perforation of uterus?

Ans. a. Lateral uterine wall perforation
    b. Perforation of pregnant uterus by dilators
    c. Suspected injury to the bowel and omentum
    d. Lowering of vital signs.

Q. What are the dangers of excessive uterine curettage?

Ans. a. The basal layer may be off to expose the underlying myometrium and the walls of uterus may get adherent resulting uterine synechiae
b. Morbid adhesion of placenta in later pregnancy.

Q. What is the complaint and treatment of uterine synechiae?

Ans. Scanty period or amenorrhea.
Treatment: Treatment is dilation and separation of uterine wall adhesion by curettage, followed by insertion of IUCD inside the uterine cavity or hysteroscopic separation of uterine adhesion and insertion of loop.

Q. What is the use of blunt curette?

Ans. It is used mainly in obstetrics, hydatidiform mole, incomplete abortion or in any case of D & E operation or suction evacuation.

OVUM FORCEPS

Q. Describe the instrument.

Ans. It is a long forceps with a fenestrated end at one end (differentiating point from sponge holding forceps, i.e. no serrations on the fenestrated blade, and no catch on the other end) (Figure 2.17).

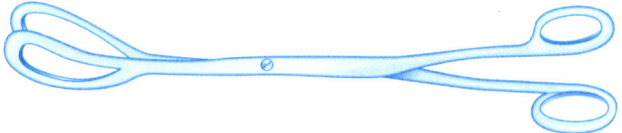

Figure 2.17: Ovum forceps

Q. Why there is no catch in this instrument?

Ans. Application of catch will break the products of conception and removal will be difficult. If uterine wall is caught by mistake it slips due to lack of catch and no injury occurs in the uterus.

Q. What are the indications of its use?

Ans. Obstetrical use
a. Remove the products of conception in D & E operation, during MTP, incomplete and missed abortion.
b. To remove moles in hydatidiform mole, placental beats from gravid uterus.

Gynecological use
a. To take out uterine polyp.

> **Note**
>
> *If there is any small perforation of small intestine during D & E operation repair the rent quickly in two layers by delayed absorbable suture after laparotomy and if part of the intestine is devitalized due to pull of intestine by ovum forceps inside the uterine cavity, it should be released and resection anastomosis should be done and in case of rectal or colon injury, colostomy may be required primarily followed by permanent repair in collaboration with surgeon.*

KARMAN'S PLASTIC CANNULA

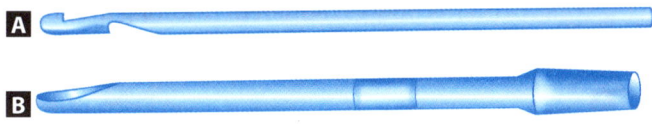

Figures 2.18A and B: (A) Plastic Karman's cannula; (B) Suction cannula

Q. Describe the Karman's cannula.

Ans. It is a hollow, transparent, flexible tube (7-9 inch) made of plastic. The uterine distal end is closed and rounded and the other end is opened. Below the distal tip two triangular shaped opening exists on opposite side (Figure 2.18A).

Q. What is the other type of suction cannula?

Ans. Other type (Berkeley's) of suction cannula is made of plastic and is thicker (6, 8, and 10 mm) in diameter with a single lateral opening below the closed end (Figure 2.18 B).

Q. What are the different sizes?

Ans. 5 sizes—4 mm, 6 mm, 8 mm, 10 mm and 12 mm.

Q. What is its use?

Ans. It is mainly used in obstetrical suction operation like D & E for MTP, incomplete, abortion and hydatidiform mole. The convex hood which over hangs each opening acts as a curette when the canula is drawn on the uterine endometrium.

Q. Why the sizes are different?

Ans. Different sizes indicate diameters of cannula in 'mm'. 6 mm cannula is used for 6 weeks size uterus, 8 mm cannula is used for 8 weeks size uterus and so on. 12 mm cannula (wide bore) is used to evacuate the uterus in hydatidiform mole.

Q. How will you sterilize the instrument?

Ans. It is sterilized by keeping it in savlon solution for half an hour to one hour.

> **Note**
>
> In suspected cases of perforation stop suction procedure immediately because if the cannula enters into the abdomen through the uterine rent, the abdominal contents like greater omentum and loop of intestine may come out side during the suction procedure. (See suction and evacuation operation).

ABDOMINAL RETRACTORS

Q. What is the use of Doyen's retractor? Disadvantages.

Ans. It is used as an abdominal wall retractor for obstetrical operation like cesarean section delivery, ectopic pregnancy and gynecological

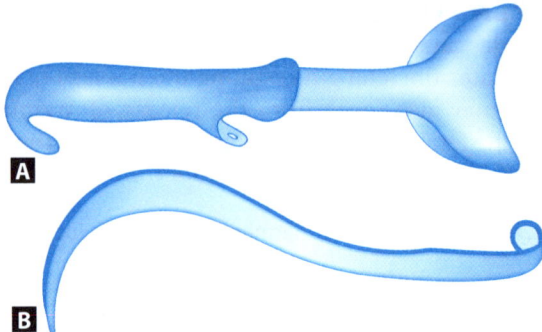

Figures 2.19A and B: (A) Doyen's retractor; (B) Deaver's retractor

operations like hysterectomy, myomectomy and ovariotomy (Figure 2.19A).

Disadvantages:
Does not retract bladder wall, space occupying when large size is used.

Q. What is the use of Deaver's retractor?
Ans. Mainly used in gynecological operation like Wertheim's operation to retract the dissected bladder from vagina or as lateral retractor in gland dissection of pelvis. It is also used to retract bladder in abdominal hysterectomy operation (Figure 2.19B).

PINARD'S METAL FETOSCOPE

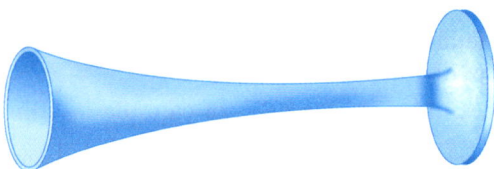

Figure 2.20: Fetoscopre

Q. What is the use of Pinard's metal fetoscope?
Ans. To auscultate fetal heart sound (FHS) at 17 weeks to 20 weeks of pregnancy. The broad open end is placed on mother's abdomen vertically and ear is placed on the other end (Figure 2.20).

Q. What is normal fetal heart rate (FHR)?
Ans. It varies from 110 to 160 beats/minute in at term baby.

Q. What are the different methods of recording fetal heart sound?
Ans. Stethoscope (18–20 weeks), fetal Doptone (10 weeks), FHR monitoring by cardiotocography (CTG) and USG (6th weeks, endovaginal sonography–5th week).

Q. How do you monitor fetal condition in antepartum period?
Ans. By assessment of amniotic fluid index (AFI), NST, biophysical profile (BPP) and ultrasound Doppler of umbilical blood vessels.

Instruments and Drugs

Q. Why meconium comes in fetal distress?

Ans. Fetal hypoxia causes increase impulse of para sympathetic nerve which stimulates the fetal gut resulting the passage of meconium. The mechanism may also result from the release of Arginine-vasopressin (AVP) from the fetal pituitary secondary to hypoxia. The AVP stimulates the smooth muscles of colon to contract and release meconium in amniotic fluid.

Q. What is meconium?

Ans. Meconium is a viscous substance from the intestinal tract consisting of water, lanugo, desquamated fetal intestinal cells, skin cells, vernix, amniotic fluid, pancreatic enzyme and bile pigment. Meconium aspiration causes injury of fetal lung.

Q. What are the signs of fetal distress in labor and how do you manage it?

Ans.
a. Persistent fetal tachycardia (FHR >160 beats/minute)
b. Bradycardia (FHR <110 beats/minute)
c. Bradycardia with irregular FHR—most vulnerable
d. Excessive fetal movement
e. Passage of meconium stained liquor in cephalic presentation when membrane is ruptured.

Management: Turn the patient in left lateral position, oxygen inhalation, rapid infusion of IV fluid (NS or RL), stop syntocinon if induction is going on and expedite delivery by forceps or cesarean section (CS) according to clinical findings.

Q. Why fetal blood pH falls in fetal distress?

Ans. Prolonged fetal anoxia causes metabolic acidosis and leads to fall in fetal blood pH.

Q. How do you collect fetal scalp blood for assessment of pH?

Ans. A plastic cone is inserted transvaginally in the fetal vertex. A cervix needs to be at least 4–5 cm dilated and the vertex is at or below -1 cm station and membrane should be ruptured. Ethyl chloride is spread to produce hyperaemia. Scalp is re-cleansed with silicon grease and then using a lancet, the scalp is pricked and blood is collected in a heparinized tube. Scalp blood pH of ≤7.20 is consistent with fetal acidosis, and a pH of 7.20–7.25 is borderline, and should be repeated immediately. A pH of ≥7.25 is reassuring and repeated every 20–30 minutes as long as the pattern persists, and the fetus is not acidotic.

Q. Questions on different sites of FHS in different presentations/positions of fetus *in utero*.

Ans. Fetal heart sound (FHS) is best heard through the back in cephalic and breech presentation but in face presentation it is best audible through the chest

Occiput:
a. In OA position—FHS is located in the middle of the spinoumbilical line of the same side

b. In Occipito lateral position—It is heard more laterally
c. In OP—FHS is heard on mother's flank.

Breech:
a. In Complete breech—FHS is usually located at a higher level of umbilicus.
b. In Frank breech—FHS is heard at a lower level in the mid line due to early engagement.

Face:
a. Mento-anterior—FHS is distinctly audible on the midline of anterior abdominal wall.
b. Mento-posterior—FHS is audible on the flank of the maternal abdomen.

Transverse:
a. Dorso-anterior—Below the umbilicus.
b. Dorso-posterior—At a higher level of umbilicus and often indistinct.

Q. In which conditions FHS is difficult to locate?

Ans. Obese mother, polyhydramnios, occiput posterior position, IUFD.

Q. When do you auscultate FHS in labor?

Ans. In the first stage of labor, FHS should be checked every 30 minutes and every 15 minutes in second stage of labor. For women with pregnancies at risk, fetal heart rate auscultation is performed at least every 15 minutes in first stage and every 5 minutes during the second stage of labor. Continuous fetal monitoring may be used with evaluation of the tracing every 15 minutes during the first stage of labor and every 5 minutes during the second stage. Auscultation should be done at the height of uterine contraction and after the contraction until the fetal heart rate comes back to the base line (see the Assessment of Fetal Well-being- Chapter 6)

MUCUS SUCKER

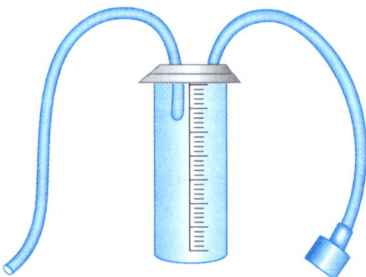

Figure 2.21: Disposable mucus sucker

Q. What is the use of mucus sucker?

Ans. For clearing the air way of the newborn (mouth, oropharynx and nostrils orderly). The narrow end is introduced into baby's mouth and the broader end is placed on operator's mouth for creation of negative suction (Figure 2.21).

Instruments and Drugs

> **Note**
>
> It is an evidenced based fact that routine suction is not mandatory in vigorous babies for newborn survival. On the contrary it may lead to complications including trauma, infection, desquamation, braycardia and increased incidence of pneumothorax.

Q. What is the advantage of this instrument?

Ans. The color and amount of the aspirated material can be visualized as it is made of transparent plastic (in metallic mucus sucker this can not be visualized until it is opened). The negative suction pressure should not be very high. It should be around 100 mm Hg. High pressure (around 200 mm Hg) can cause injury of mucous membrane of mouth and throat).

Q. What is asphyxia neonatorum?

Ans. Failure to initiate and sustain breathing at birth causing birth asphyxia.

> **Note**
>
> *Perinatal asphyxia according to American Academic of pediatrics is:*
> i. Cord umbilical pH <7.0 with base deficit >10 meq/L,
> ii. Neonatal neurologic manifestation is suggestive of hypoxic ischemic encephalopathy (HIE),
> iii. Evidence of multi organ dysfunction of cardiovascular system, renal, GIT system, hematologic or pulmonary.

Q. What are the causes of asphyxia?

Ans. **Antepartum**—Placental insufficiency and fetal anoxia, e.g. PIH, abruptio placentae
Intrapartum—Prolonged hypoxic labor, traumatic delivery, opiate drugs, anesthesia
Postpartum—Immaturity, cerebral trauma, congenital abnormalities, such as diaphragmatic hernia.

Q. What is vigorous baby?

Ans. 'Vigorous baby' is defined as strong respiratory efforts, good muscle tone, and heart beat greater than 100 bpm.

Q. How will you asses the condition of baby at birth?

Ans. By Apgar score – (she is an anesthetist).

Q. What is 'Apgar score'?

Ans. Apgar [appearance (1), pulse (4), grimace (5), activity (2), respiration (3)] score (see below)

Sign	0-point	1-point	2-point
1. Skin color (appearance)	Cyanosis pallor	Peripheral cyanosis	Pink
2. Muscle tone (activity)	Flaccid	Moves limbs	Good
3. Respiratory effort (respiration)	None	Grasp	Good
4. Heart rate (HR)[pulse]	None	<100	>100
5. Response to stimulation on nasal catheter (grimaces)	None	Slight grimace	Good

Q. Practical value of Apgar score.

Ans. 7 to 10—good
4 to 7—slightly asphyxiated and baby needs treatment
Less than 4—bad case, require treatment.

Q. How do you resuscitate an asphyxiated baby?

Ans. Principle of management is A, B, C, D, E

A—Airway is open and clear;
B—Breathing spontaneous or assisted
C—Circulation of oxygenated blood
D—Drugs
E—Evaluation

Procedure

a. Place the baby in a warm, clear and firm surface
b. Remove the wet towel and wrap the baby with second dry towel excluding first
c. Clear the airway by suction first the mouth and then nose when needed
d. Dry the baby thoroughly with a clean, warm towel.

The above steps should be completed within 30 seconds, then assess breathing

e. If regular breathing and crying—give the baby to mother
f. If still not breathing or has gasping respiration;
   - Select appropriate mask—no. '1' for normal weight or no. '0' for small babies
   - Reposition the neck in neutral or slightly extended position
   - Place the mask on the baby's face to cover chin, mouth and nose to obtain seal
   - Squeeze the bag at the rate of 30 to 60/minute

   After 1 minute, assess breathing
   - Regular breathing or cry—give the baby to mother
   - Breathing slow less than 30/minute or gasping or apnoeic—conduct ventilation, once breathing is regular provide on going care.
   - If no breathing in 20 minute of ventilation if only gasping and no spontaneous breathing after 30 minutes of ventilation-stop ventilation and reassure mother and family.

Advanced resuscitation (Figure 2.22):

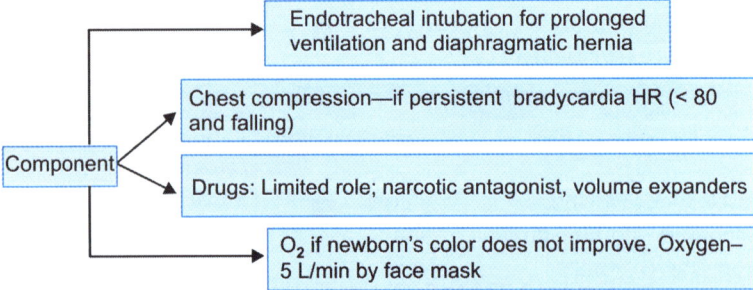

Figure 2.22: Advanced resuscitation of newborn

Instruments and Drugs

> **Note**
> If the baby does not cry in 30 seconds take steps to resuscitate the baby.

> **Note**
> Meconium should be passed by 24 hours and urine is passed by 48 hours in a newborn baby. Suction of oropharynx of fetus is not recommended even in the face of meconium stained liquor (updated NRP 2010 guideline). The baby is allowed to cry on its own if the infant is vigorous. However in meconium stained liquor, if the infant is not vigorous, tracheal suction should be performed under direct laryngoscope immediately after delivery as antepartum suctioning of oro-pharynx upon delivery of head before delivery of shoulders which is used commonly in obstetric practice cannot prevent meconium aspiration with the first breath of baby. There is also no evidence-based support for routine suction of stomach contents when meconium is noted in amniotic fluid.

UMBILICAL CORD SCISSORS WITH DISPOSABLE UMBILICAL CORD CLIPS

Q. What is the use of umbilical cord scissors?

Ans. The umbilical cord scissors is used for cutting the cord (Figure 2.23A).

Q. What is its advantage over normal scissors?

Ans. The umbilical cord contains Wharton's gelly and is covered by amniotic membrane. So, when ordinary scissors are used to cut the cord it tends to slip. Here the blades are so curved that they meet at the tip leaving a gap for cord when closed. So it avoids the slipping of the cord.

Q. How does umbilical clip acts?

Ans. The clip has two arms with a hinge and a spring action. When it is applied around the cord the tips are locked around the cord [See Figure 2.23 B (open clip) and Figure 2.23 C (closed clip)].

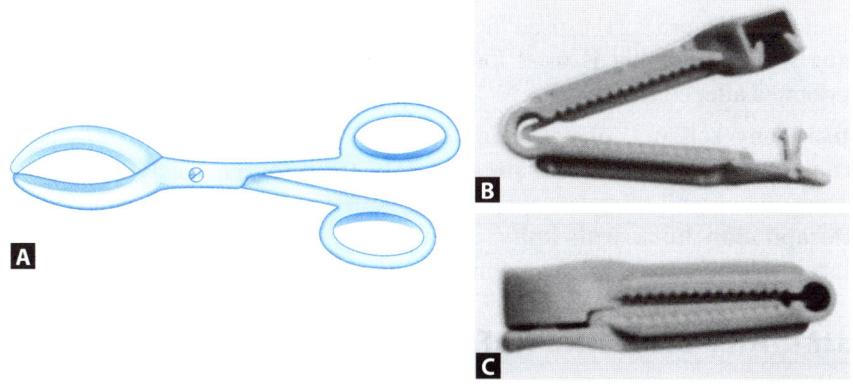

Figures 2.23A to C: (A) Umbilical cord scissors,
(B and C) Disposable umbilical cord clips (open and closed)

> **Note**
>
> Diabetes in pregnancy, cord round the neck, IUGR Rh-isoimmunization, HIV infected mother, fetal distress where early cord clamping (<1 minute) is necessary. Late cord clamping (1–3 minutes) is required for all births in developing countries who does not need resuscitation to allow extra, amount of blood from mother to baby for preservation of iron store and prevention of fetal anemia. Early cord clamping is not recommended unless the neonates need immediate resuscitation for asphyxia. It should not be performed even in preterm baby due to risk of overloading or cardiac failure.

Q. When milking of the cord before clamping is hazardous?

Ans.
a. CVS anomalies
b. Asphyxia with circulatory failure
c. Intracranial hemorrhage (ICH)
d. Maternal feto blood group incompatibility.

> **Note**
>
> - Early or immediate cord clamping is associated with intraventricular hemorrhage (IVH), respiratory distress syndrome (RDS), late onset sepsis, anemia and elevated lead levels.
> - Delayed cord clamping beyond 1 minute, the infant is at an increased risk of developing polycythemia, transient tachypnea, jaundice, elevated blood pressure, and patent ductus arteriosus.

BLUNT HOOK AND CROCHET

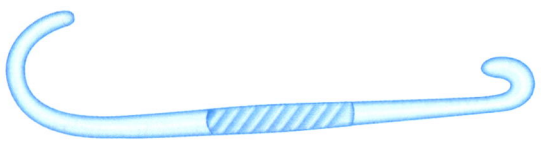

Figure 2.24: Blunt hook and crochet

Blunt hook (Figure 2.24) is used for breech traction in impacted breech, where fetus is dead. Crochet is used for hooking down the decapitating head or perforated after coming head.

Episiotomy scissors, obstetric forceps, cup of ventouse, instruments of craniotomy operations (Oldham's cranial perforator, cranioclast, cephalotribe and bone nibbling forceps) and instruments of decapitation operation (Decapitation hook with knife, embryotomy scissors)—All discussed in obstetrical operations and interventions (*see Chapter 3*).

LUMBAR PUNCTURE NEEDLE

Q. What are the uses of lumbar puncture (LP) needle in obstetrics?

Ans. a. To collect amniotic fluid for biochemical, cytological and cytogenetic study (see amniocentesis).

b. Spectrophotometric analysis of amniotic fluid bilirubin in Rh isoimmunized mother.
c. For drainage of CSF in hydrocephalus when cervix is < 4 cm dilated.
d. For drainage of liquor in acute hydramnios.
e. To introduce hypertonic saline in amniotic cavity for midtrimester abortion (not a very popular method now a day for some severe complications like cardiovascular accident, renal failure and coagulation defect).

Shirodkar's Needle

Q. What is this instrument?

Ans. This is shirodker's needle (determine right or left).

Q. How will you identify this instrument?

Ans. The needles are made of stainless steel having 5 cm, half circle blunt tipped needle with an eye at the tip and the other end has stout handle (Figure 2.25).

Q. How many needles are needed for operations?

Ans. Two.
The needle is for right side (Figure 2.25A)
The needle is for left side (Figure 2.25B).

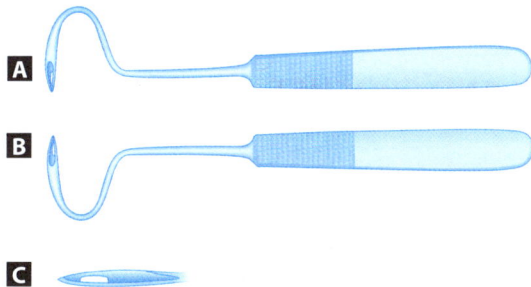

Figure 2.25: Shirodkar's needle: (A) Right, (B) Left, (C) Tip of the needle

Q. Use?

Ans. It is used for Shirodkar's cervical circlage operation to treat cervical incompetence.

Q. How do you introduce right and left needle during operation?

Ans. a. Anteriorly 1.5 cm transverse incision is made on the cervical mucosa and lift the bladder.
b. 1 cm longitudinal incision is made on the posterior aspect on the mucosae at the junction of cervix and vagina.
c. Cervical cerclage suture is passed through the needle.
d. The needle is passed through the right angle of the anterior incision and then through submucosal substance on the right side of the cervix, finally emerge through the posterior incision. The suture material is removed.
e. The other end is threaded in the left needle which is passed through the left angle of anterior incision and then through submucous

substance of left side of the cervix to the posterior incision. The suture comes out.

f. The suture is fixed on the posterior aspect of cervix.
g. Vaginal mucosal incision on anterior and posterior aspect are sutured by catgut suture.

Q. What are the complications?

Ans. a. Peroperative—hemorrhage, rupture of membrane, and bladder injury
b. Immediate postoperative—threatened abortion, preterm labor and sepsis
c. Delayed postoperative—cervical dystocia, bucket handle tear, uterine rupture if labor is allowed with encirclage suture.

Q. What is the other method of cervical encirclage operation?

Ans. McDonald operation (simpler and currently practised).

> **Note**
> For other questions on cervical incompetence, see the long case of recurrent pregnancy loss (Chapter 10)

Willets' Scalp Traction Forceps

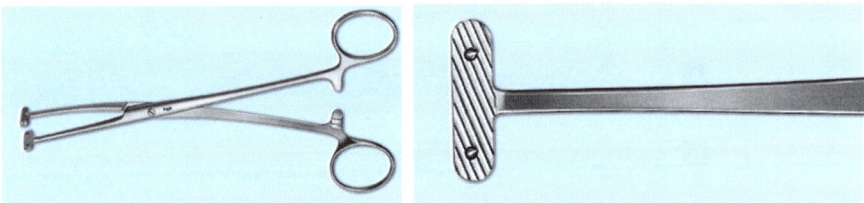

Figure 2.26: Willets' scalp traction forceps

Q. Describe the instrument.

Ans. The ends of the blades are T-shaped with oblique serrations and made of stainless steel. One of the blades has two tiny teeth side by side which fit in the whole of other blade to achieve a firm grip on the scalp of fetus. A ratchet lock is found on the handle (Figure 2.26).

Q. What are the different sizes?

Ans. It is available in two sizes: 18.7 cm and 30 cm in length.

Q. Use?

Ans. Not generally used at present.
1. To control bleeding in type I and II anterior placenta previa with vertex presentation. The fetal scalp is grasped by forceps after rupture of membrane and continuous traction is applied.
2. To administer traction on the fetal head after craniotomy to facilitate the head delivery.
3. During head delivery in LSCS (not used in modern obstetrics for trauma to fetal head).

4. In case of cord prolapse scalp traction is used after replacement of the prolapsed cord above the level of fetal head to prevent recurrence of cord prolapse (not used in modern obstetrics).

Q. What are the complications?

Ans. a. Injury to the fetal scalp.
   b. Scalp hematoma and infection.
   c. Injury to maternal soft tissue.

DRUGS IN OBSTETRICS

Magnesium Sulfate

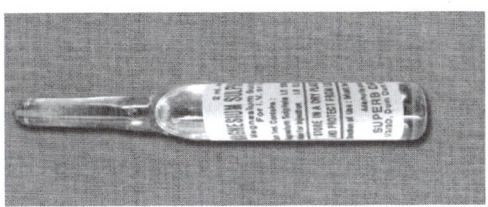

Figure 2.27: Ampoule of injection magnesium sulfate

Preparation
a. Inj $MgSO_4$ (50% w/v), 1 ampoule = 2 mL = 1 g, $MgSO_4$ used for both IM and IV (Figure 2.27).
b. Inj $MgSO_4$ (25% w/v), 1 ampoule = 2 mL = 0.5 g, 2 ampoule = 4 mL = 1g, $MgSO_4$ used only for IV route (not usually available).

Use: Anticonvulsant.

Mechanism of action:
1. Reduces end plate sensitivity to acetyl choline
2. Reduces acetyl choline release
3. Blocks Ca^{++} influx into the neurones of brain (magnesium blocks the N-methyl-D aspartate (NMDA) receptors in the brain, which is activated by asphyxia leading to calcium influx into the neurons which causes cell injury. Magnesium blocks these receptors and reduces Ca^{++} influx and protects the neurone from damage).
4. Causes vasodilatation with subsequent reduction of cerebral ischemia
5. Direct depressant action on utérine muscle.

Indications:
Parenteral: Ideal drug in prevention and treatment of convulsion in pre-eclampsia and eclampsia, tocolytic in preterm labor.

Contraindications: Myasthenia gravis, impaired renal function.

Side effects
Maternal: Respiratory depression, muscular paresis, flushing, perspiration, headache, rarely pulmonary edema.
Fetal: Lethargy, hypotonic, rarely respiratory depression.

Antidote: 10 mL 10% calcium gluconate over 10 minutes (Rule of 10)

Different regimes of injection Magnesium sulfate used in eclampsia:
a. Pritchard
b. Zuspan
c. Low dose regime.

a. **Pritchard:**
Loading dose:
- Magnesium sulfate of 20% solution, 4 g (= 8 mL +12 mL NS = 20 mL) IV over 5 minutes
- Then 10 g 50% $MgSO_4$ solution, 5 g in each buttock as deep IM injection with 1 mL 2% lignocaine in the same syringe aseptically
- If convulsion recurs after 15 minutes, give 2 g $MgSO_4$ (20% solution IV (i.e. 4 mL 50% magnesium sulfate + 6 ml of normal saline) over 5 minutes.

Maintenance dose:
- 5 g $MgSO_4$ (50% solution) + 1 mL lignocaine 2%, IM every 4 hours into alternate buttock
- Continue treatment with $MgSO_4$ for 24 hours after delivery or the last convulsion, which ever occurs last].

Disadvantage: Pain and infection at the IM injection site.

b. **Zuspan:** Loading dose 4 g IV infusion (20%) over 15–20 minutes; Maintenance dose: 1 g/hour IV infusion [Inj $MgSO_4$ (5 g) in 500 mL NS IV infusion, if rate of infusion is 1 g/hour infuse 100 mL/hour].

c. **Low dose:** Loading dose: 4 g IV over 3–5 minutes; maintenance dose: 2 g IM/IV diluted 3 hourly.

Recurrent convulsion- inj $MgSO_4$ 2 g IV over 5 minutes.

Monitoring of magnesium sulfate
a. Urine output should be at least 30 mL/hour
b. Deep tendon reflex (patellar reflex) should be present
c. Respiration rate (RR) should be more than 16 breaths/minute
d. Pulse oxymetry should be >96% of oxygen saturation.

> **Note**
> The oxygen saturation starts to drop even before respiratory depression. In the therapeutic range magnesium sulfate slows neuromuscular conduction and depresses central nervous system irritability. For this reason deep tendon reflex, maternal respiratory rate and state of consciousness must be frequently monitored to detect magnesium toxicity. The drug should not be given if serum creatinine level is >1 mg%.

Withhold or delay the drug if:
- Respiratory rate falls below 16/minute
- Patellar reflex is absent
- Urinary output falls below 30 mL/hour over preceding 4 hours.

Magnesium toxicity
1. Stop magnesium injection
2. In case of respiratory arrest—assist ventilation by (mask and bag or intubation)
3. Calcium gluconate (rule of 10) 10 mL 10% over 10 minutes, repeated dosage may be required until respiration begins to antagonize the effects of magnesium sulfate.

4. Use second line anticonvulsant drug if required (Phenytoin sodium)
(For other questions—see long case of pre-eclampsia)

ANTIHYPERTENSIVES

NICE Guideline (2011)

If SBP is ≥150 mm Hg and diastolic BP (DBP) in pregnancy is >100 mm Hg, antihypertensive drugs are used.

Goal to maintain BP:
Systolic (SBP): at 130–150 mm Hg
Diastolic (DBP) 90–100 mm Hg, but not below 80 mm Hg to prevent cerebral hemorrhage hypertensive encephalopathy, CCF, placental abruption and HELLP. The drug of choice is Labetalol.
Antihypertensive treatment in mild pre-eclampsia is harmful to the fetus as it may cause:
a. Fetal growth restriction (FGR)
b. Impaired neurodevelopment
c. Iatrogenic premature intervention.

LABETALOL

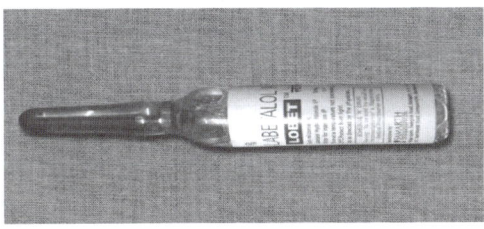

Figure 2.28: Injection Labetalol (1 ampoule=10 mg)

Preparation

Injection: Intravenous (IV) (Figure 2.28)
Oral: 100 mg tablet
Use—Antihypertensive
Mechanism of action—Combined α-and β-blocker (Flowchart 2.1).

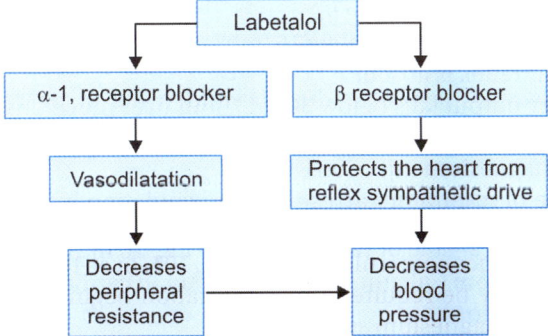

Flowchart 2.1: Mechanism of action of labetalol

Indications: Antihypertensive in pregnancy and hypertensive crisis.
Contraindications: CCF, hepatic disorders, asthma, COPD, heart block.
Side effects: Rash and liver damage, fetal hypoglycemia.
Dose:
a. *Oral:* Initial dose—100 mg twice daily, may be increased at weekly intervals by 100 mg thrice daily
Further dose titration may be required to 100–400 mg tds in second and third trimester. Maximum of dose up to 2400 mg daily.
b. *Intravenous bolus dose*: Start with 10–20 mg by slow IV over 2 min period, if no response in 10 minutes 40 mg (4 ampoules) IV bolus then 80 mg (8 ampoules) every 10 minutes with maximum total dose of 300 mg (30 ampoules) per episode. Onset of action 5 minute, peak effect 10-20 minute; duration of action 45 minutes to 6 hours.
c. *Intravenous infusion*:

Dilution:
Add 40 mL of labetalol in 250 mL of IV fluid
Resultant solution contain 200 mg of labetalol (5 mg/mL) in 290 (250 +40) mL ≈300 mL of solution, i.e. = 2 mg/3 mL

IV infusion:
- Start at the rate of 20 mg/hour (20 mg = 30 mL/60 min; 450 drops /60 min as 1ml is 15 drops; so the drip rate =7- 8 drops/minute)
- Double the dose every 30 minutes until a satisfactory response is obtained or a dose of 60 mg /hr is reached.

(For other questions see case discussion of pre-eclampsia; Chapter—10).

HYDRALAZINE HYDROCHLORIDE (DRANGEEN)

Preparation

Injection: Intravenous (IV)—20 mg
Mechanism of action: It causes direct relaxation of vascular smooth muscles especially on arterioles than veins.
Indications: Anti-hypertensive in pregnancy and hypertensive crisis
Dose:
Intravenous bolus dose: Initial 5–10 mg in 3–4 minutes then 10 mg every 20–30 minutes to a maximum dose of 30 mg. Repeat in several hours as necessary. Onset of action is 10–20 minutes.

Advantage: It reduces BP quickly even when hypertension is severe.

Disadvantage:

Mother: Tachycardia, nausea and vomiting, headache, muscle tremor.
Fetal: Fetal distress may occur due to sudden fall of BP reducing utero-placental blood flow.

Nifedipine

Preparation: Oral capsule or tablet (5 mg/10 mg/20 mg) (Figure 2.29).
Mechanism of action: Calcium channel blocker in cardiac muscle and blood vessels (vasodilatation).

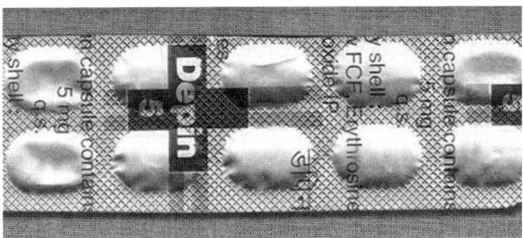

Figure 2.29: Oral preparation

Uses: Hypertension, prevention of preterm labor.
Side effects: Flushing, hypotension, tachycardia, and headache (may confuse the picture of pre-eclampsia).
Routes: Oral, intranasal, sublingual (better not to use).
Dosages
Hypertension: 5–20 mg bd/tds; max dose 200 mg
Prevention of preterm labor: 20–30 mg stat orally followed by and 10–20 mg tds/day.
Precaution: 1. Use with $MgSO_4$ may be hazardous as nifedipine may cause a dangerous fall in BP, so the BP should be monitored carefully, 2. Sublingual use should be prohibited as it can precipitate acute myocardial infarction.

Oxytocics

Oxytocin
This is a hormone secreted by posterior pituitary. It is synthesized in supraoptic and paraventricular nucleus of hypothalamus. Increases frequency and force of myometrial contraction.

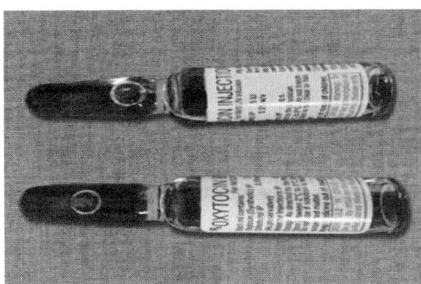

Figure 2.30: Syntocinon ampoule

Preparation: Injection (ampoule 5U or 10 U); storage temperature is $\leq 30°C$ (Figure 2.30).
Mechanism of action: Uterine stimulant by action on myometrial receptors:
1. Direct stimulatory effect on myometrium by mobilization of intracellular calcium ion.
2. Stimulates decidual PG production and causes contraction of uterus.

Uses:
1. Induction and augmentation of labor.
2. Prevention and treatment postpartum hemorrhage (PPM).
3. In breast engorgement.

Contraindications:
1. Cephalopelvic disproportion (CPD)
2. Malpresentation
3. Previous two CS
4. Grand multipara
5. Incoordinate uterine action
6. Fetal distres
7. Cardiac disease.

Side effects:
Maternal: uterine hyperstimulation, uterine rupture, water intoxication, hypotension in large doses and in improper monitoring.
Fetal: Fetal distress.

Plasma half life: 10–12 minutes.

Protocol: a. Low-dose protocol (2–5 U/L), b. High-dose protocol (10 U/L)
The proposed infusion rate in recent studies are) 0.5 to 1mU/min, instead of 3 mU/min. According to recent reports, the proposed interval for oxytocin increments ranged between15 and 60 minutes, without significant differences in rates of failed induction.

It should not be given by IV bolus for fear of sudden hypotension and marked increase in cardiac output, myocardial ischemia and chest pain.

(For other questions see induction of labor and complications of 3rd stage of labor in Chapter 11).

Methylergometrine

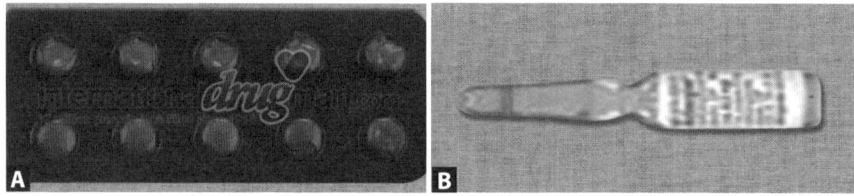

Figures 2.31A and B: (A) Methylergometrine tablet; (B) Injection of methergin

Preparation: Ergometrine is available 0.25 mg or 0.5 mg ampoules (Figure 2.31B) while methylergometrine is available as 0.2 mg ampoule and 0.2 mg tablets (Figure 2.31A).

Nature: Uterine stimulant (retraction of uterine muscle fibers).

Storage temperature of injection: 2°C to 8°C, otherwise potency is lost.

Onset of action: Oral: 10 min, IM: 4–7 min, IV: 40 sec.

Mechanism of action: Vasoconstrictor and uterine smooth muscle agonist and causes uterine retraction.

Uses
Routine management after delivery of the placenta; in management of PPH; following S/E, in MTP and incomplete abortion.

Side effects
Nausea, vomiting, diarrhea, pulmonary hypertension, coronary artery vasoconstriction, severe systemic hypertension (especially in patients with preeclampsia), convulsions.

Contraindications: Hypertension, PIH, hypersensitivity, before second twin is born, heart disease, vascular disease, Rh-negative mother after birth of anterior shoulder of baby.

Half life: 1-2 hours.

Dosage
Parenteral: 1 mL (0.2 mg) after delivery of the anterior shoulder or after delivery of the placenta, or during the puerperium. May be repeated as required, at intervals of 2-4 hours in the management of PPH.

Oral: Adults—0.2 mg 3 or 4 times daily in the puerperium for a maximum dose of 1 week.

Dinoprostone (Prostaglandin Gel)

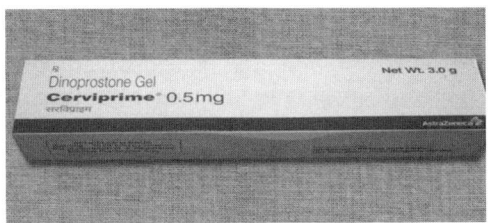

Figure 2.32: Cerviprime gel

Preparation: Prostaglandin E2 gel [0.5 mg (2.5 mL) in a prefilled plastic device with a specially designed nozzle for proper placement in the cervical canal (Figure 2.32)].

Uses: Induction of labor.

Mechanism of action:
- Binds to myometrial cells to cause myometrial contractions.
- Cervical ripening with softening and dilatation of cervix in labor induction, prior to late first trimester of pregnancy and for second trimester MTP.

Contraindications
Not to use in labor of women with:
a. Scarred uterus (previous CS or uterine surgery)
b. Grand multipara
c. Hypersensitivity
d. Asthma
e. Glaucoma
f. Active cardiac, pulmonary, renal or other hepatic diseases, and manufacturers' recommendation caution with ruptured membrane.

Side effects: nausea, vomiting, diarrhea, vaginal irritation, hyperstimulation of uterus.

Dosage : 0.5 mg (2.5 mL) over 6-12 hrs with 3 doses in 24 hrs intracervically.

Disadvantage: Intracervical administration is difficult than intravaginal insert.

Advantage:
a. More significant intracervical softening in intracervical insertion,
b. Low-risk of hyperstimulation.

Vaginal route: PGE2 application in vagina (posterior fornix) is easy and most practical. The commonly used doses are 3–5 mg and the dose of PGE2 be varied according to the patient's cervical score, permitting a lower dose of PGE2 to be used in many cases. A commonly used approach of cervical ripening and labor induction with PGE2 is to administer 3 mg at 4–6 hours intervals for two doses, followed by oxytocin induction or augmentation in 12–18 hours if necessary.

Monitoring: Check regularly the woman's pulse, BP, uterine contraction, FHR during induction of labor by prostaglandins.

Carboprost or Prostodin

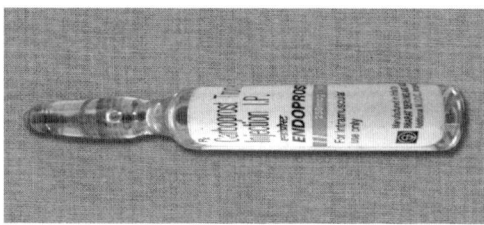

Figure 2.33: Injection prostodin ampoule

Preparation: Injection prostaglandin (15-methyl PGF2α) for IM uses only (no IV use). The injection is stored at the temperature of 2°C–8°C
1 amp contains 125 or 250 µg prostaglandin (Figure 2.33).

Uses:
a. Prophylaxis and treatment of PPH
b. Medical termination of pregnancy (MTP) for softening of cervix in first trimester
c. MTP in second trimester of pregnancy.

Mechanism of action:
a. Myometrial contractions by binding with myometrial cells
b. Cervical ripening with softening and dilatation of cervix.

Contraindications: See the contraindications of dinoprostone.

Side effects: Nausea, vomiting, diarrhea, vaginal irritation, rupture of uterus

Dosage:
a. Active management of third stage of labor 125 µg IM after delivery of baby.
b. For management of PPH–250 µg in every 15–90 minutes interval, not exceeding 8 doses (Total dose 2 mg).

Misoprostol

Preparation: Prostaglandin E1 tablet—25 µg, 50 µg, 100 µg, 200 µg, 600 µg (stable at room temperature) (Figure 2.34).

Uses
1. (a) MTP in first trimester, (b) abortion, (c) induction and augmentation of labor, (d) prevention of PPH (600 µg).

Instruments and Drugs

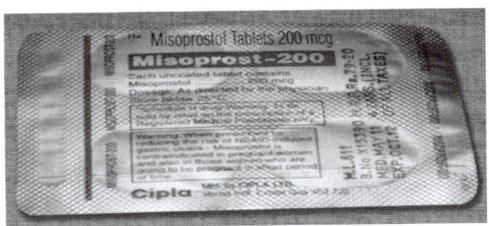

Figure 2.34: Misoprostol tablets

2. Cervical priming before D and E, or other gynaecological procedures like D&C or hysteroscopy.

Advantage: Inexpensive, long half life (4 hours) can be given in hypertension and asthma.

Mechanism of action
a. Binds to myometrial cells to cause strong myometrial contractions.
b. Cervical ripening with softening and dilatation of cervix.

Routes of administration (Table 2.1)
a. *Oral*: Action is rapid and short duration (100 µg oral dose is as effective as a 25 µg intravaginal dose).
b. *Vaginal*: Action is slow and sustained (bioavailability of vaginally administered misoprostol is three times higher than that of orally administered). Do not use > 50 µg at a time and do not exceed 4 doses (200 µg) for induction of normal labor at term.
c. *Sublingual*.
d. *Per rectal* (action is not good, onset of action is delayed).

> **Note**
> Close monitoring at 1 hour interval is necessary for early detection of fetal distress.

Table 2.1: Pharmacokinetic parameters of 4 routes of administration of misoprostol

Route	Onset of action[a] (minutes)	Peak action[b] (minutes)	Duration of action[c] (minutes)
Oral	8	60	120
Sublingual	11	60	180
Vaginal	20	120	240
Rectal	100	120–180	240

[a] Time to increase uterine tonus; [b] Time to peak uterine tonus; [c] Duration of regular uterine contraction

Complications
Uterine hyperstimulation, tachysystole, uterine rupture, fetal heart rate abnormalities, amniotic fluid embolism, meconium passage, meconium aspiration syndrome (MAS).

Dose of misoprostol for induction of labor, for PPH and MTP (see induction of labor —chapter 11).

Discontinuation of PGs and beginning of oxytocin infusion, if
a. Membrane is ruptured
b. Cervical ripening is achieved
c. Goal of labor has been achieved.

> **Note**
> Do not use oxytocin within 6–8 hours of using misoprostol management of first trimester pregnancy loss—(a) PGE1, 600 μg orally or 600 μg orally initially or at 4 hours, or (b) 800 μg vaginally; concomitant vacuum aspiration may be required for greater success rate (97%).

OTHER DRUGS

Tranexamic Acid

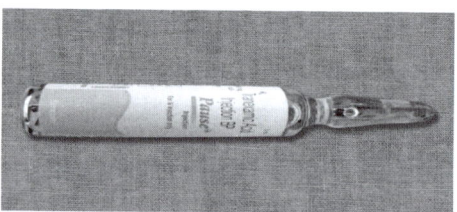

Figure 2.35: Ampoule of tranexamic acid injection

Nature: Anti-fibrinolytic (Injectable, and oral form is available)
Uses: (a) Traumatic PPH, (b) DUB, (c) Menorrhagia for Cu-T
Mechanism of action: Binds to lysine binding site on plasminogen and prevent its combination with fibrin.
Side effects: Nausea, diarrhea, headache, giddiness, thrombophlebitis.
Contraindications: Severe renal insufficiency, hematuria.
Dose: 10–15 mg/kg 2–3 times a day.
In apprehension of PPH injection may be given within 1 hour of cesarean section (Figure 2.35).

> **Note**
> Better not to use in very old age with menorrhagia and in severe hypertension.

Iron Sucrose

Nature: Injectable iron (Figure 2.36)
Different preparations of injectable iron:
Iron dextran (inferon), iron sorbitol citrate (jectofer), iron sucrose, ferric carboxy maltose (500 mg/10 mL).

Composition: Iron sucrose—100 mg/5 mL
Indications:
a. Iron deficiency
    i. Poor compliance to oral iron
    ii. Inadequate absorption of oral iron
    iii. Lack of response to oral iron
b. Anemia of those patients suffering from chronic hemodialysis.

Instruments and Drugs

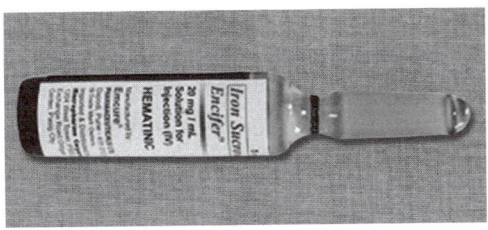

Figure 2.36: Ampoule of iron sucrose injection

Contraindications: Hypersensitivity, iron overload.

Adverse effects: Hypotension, anaphylactoid reactions, musculoskeletal pain, diarrhea, nausea vomiting, abdominal pain, pruritus, elevated liver enzymes, pain at injection site, chill and rigor.

Dosage
- 100 mg (5 mL) one ampoule by IV route weekly—4 such
- The infusion must be at 100 mg is diluted in 100 mL of normal saline and infuse at a rate of 100 mg/15 minute, three times weekly (Day 1, Day 3, Day 5).
- Expected rise in Hb 0.7–1 g %/week.

> **Note**
> Ferric carboxy maltose is not widely used in pregnancy anemia but may be used safely in puerperium.

For other questions see case discussion on anemia in pregnancy (Chapter 10).

Injection Anti-D Globulin

Nature: Injectable preparation (monoclonal and polyclonal) by IM route.
Mechanism of action: Hide the Rh-D antigen in the maternal system on fetal RBCs after fetomaternal bleed, hence prevents maternal antibody formation by immune system.
Uses: Prevention and prophylaxis of postabortal or postdelivery Rh is immunization.

Recommended dose of Anti-D:

Pregnancy complications	Dose of RhIG
a. First trimester abortion	50 µg
b. Ectopic pregnancy <13 weeks	50 µg
c. Second trimester abortion	300 µg
d. Ectopic pregnancy >13 weeks	300 µg
e. Invasive procedure, e.g. amniocentesis	300 µg

Prevention
a. 300 µg of anti-D postdelivery
b. During pregnancy two doses of 500 IU (100 µg) anti-D at 28 and 34 weeks can reduce the incidence of sensitization to 0.1%. Alternatively, a single dose of 300 µg at 28 weeks provides protection up to 40 weeks, but 300 µg of anti-D postdelivery (within 72 hours) is mandatory. If it is not administered within 3 days of delivery, a dose within up to 9–10 days may provide protection.

c. Rh D immunoglobulin should be given slowly by deep IM route in deltoid muscle. If large dose (>5 mL) is required, it is advisable to administer it in divided doses at different sites.
d. Additional anti-D should be given where the FMH is estimated to be more than usual. Tests such as K-B test or flow cytometry can be used for estimation of FMH where the clinical situation is suggestive of abruption placentae, or the clinical situation like manual removal of placenta.
e. For every 15 mL of fetal RBCs (30 mL of fetal blood) exposed to maternal circulation, 300 µg of RhIgG should be administered
f. 10 µg additional anti-D should be given for every additional 0.5 mL of fetal RBCs in maternal circulation.

(If mother is sensitized previously, as determined by elevated level of maternal Rh antibodies, administration of RhIgG is of no value).
Contraindications: Hypersensitivity
(For other questions see case discussion on Rh negative mother)

CORTICOSTEROIDS

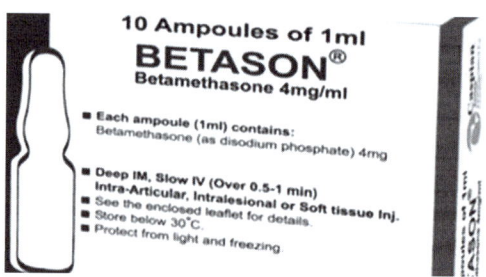

Figure 2.37: Ampoule of betamethasone

Antenatal corticosteroids are used to reduce the incidence and severity of respiratory distress syndrome (RDS) and other neonatal morbidity including IVH (intraventricular hemorrhage), necrotizing enterocolitis, patent ductus arteriosus and periventricular leukomalacia. It is also used in HELLP syndrome.

Two **glucocorticoids regimes** are found to be effective
1. Injection betamethasone 12 mg intramuscularly every 24 hours apart for 2 doses.
2. Injection dexamethasone 6 mg IM every 12 hours total 4 doses. The oral preparation of dexamethasone should not be used.

Repeat or booster dose is not needed after 48 hours as no safety data is available. Weekly repeated dose may be reduce the head circumference of fetus or may cause low birth weight of baby and may be also impair neuropsychological development of child later in life. These effects may be more marked with dexamethasone therapy, hence betamethasone is preferred. So *rescue therapy* (repeated corticosteroid dose when delivery becomes imminent and more than 7 days have passed since the initial dose) is not preferable.

Mechanism of fetal lung maturity: It induces the Type -II pneumocytes of lung alveoli to produce surfactant in adequate amount (lecithin and sphyngomyelin ratio :: 2:1).

> **Note**
> The doses of corticosteroid are same for multiple pregnancy as for singleton pregnancy.

Relative contraindications:
- May be used with caution in severe pre-eclampsia
- Impaired glucose tolerance test (GTT).

Indications: Preterm labor, PROM, preeclampsia, APH, FGR:
Indicated between 28 and 34 weeks of pregnancy, but may be used in usual doses before elective cesarean section in advanced gestational age too.

Contraindications:
1. Diabetic mother (can be used with strict maintenance of blood glucose level).
2. Chorioamnionitis.

Risks of antenatal corticosteroid treatment
a. In insulin dependant diabetes mellitus steroid treatment always results in 48–96 hours of increased blood glucose which is very much difficult to control with standard insulin regime and sometime IV infusion of insulin is necessary.

   An algorithm to guide glycemic management during systemic betamethasone therapy:
   - Day 0: (1st dose betamethasone at 16:00 hours) 30% increase in bed time insulin
   - Day 1: (2nd dose betamethasone 24 hours later) 50% increase in all (presteroid) insulin doses
   - Day 2: 50% increase in all (presteroid) insulin doses
   - Day 3: 30% increase in all (presteroid) insulin doses
   - Day 4: 20% increase in all (presteroid) insulin doses
   - Day 5: Gradual reduction of presteroid insulin doses

b. Maternal treatment with betamethasone but not dexamethasone has been associated with transient reduction of fetal heart rate variability and body and breathing movement in several studies. When it occurs, typically between 48 and 72 hours after the first dose, the alteration of fetal biophysical profile (BPP) is striking. Both short-and long-term heart rate variability is reduced. The effects resolve spontaneously by the 4th day.

c. Antenatal steroids enhance cell differentiation and maturation rather than cell growth.

d. Flare up of infection in chorioamnionitis occurs.

> **Note**
> In India, one components of betamethasone, i.e betamethasone sodium phosphate is available, which does not have betamethasone sodium acetate, hence may not be effective in fetal lung maturity. So, dexamethasone is a very useful drug for fetal lung maturity and also economical in India.

Chapter 3

Obstetric Operations and Interventions

CESAREAN SECTION

Q. What is cesarean section (CS)?

Ans. The delivery of fetus placenta and membrane through an incision in the abdominal and uterine wall after 28 weeks of pregnancy.

Q. What is primary CS?

Ans. The first CS performed on a pregnant mother is known as primary CS.

Q. What is elective CS?

Ans. An elective CS is one, which is performed on a patient before the onset of labor or before the occurrence of any complications.

Q. What are the indications of CS?

Ans. **A. General**
  a. Fetal distress in pregnancy and labor
  b. Cephalopelvic disproportion (CPD)
  c. Post CS pregnancy with non-engaged head
  d. Delay in the first stage of labor due to disorder of uterine activity (Uterine dystocia) or non-progress of labor
  e. Cord prolapse
  f. Severe pre-eclampsia, eclampsia
  g. Abruptio placentae where baby is living
  h. Failed induction.

> **Note**
> *Never forget 3Ds: Fetal distress, CPD, uterine dystocia.*

B. Elective indications

Placenta previa, previous two CS, intrauterine growth restriction (IUGR), BOH, maternal diabetes, and breech (preterm), post-dated pregnancy, and transverse lie, pregnancy following repair of VVF, oligohydramnios (liquor pocket <1 cm).

Q. What are the different types of anesthesia used for CS?

Ans. Spinal, general anesthesia (GA), epidural (Spinal is the most common in our institution).

Obstetric Operations and Interventions

Q. What are the complications of spinal anesthesia and how do you manage it?

Ans.
a. Hypotension (due to spinal blockade and obstructed venous return due to uterine compression by great vessels);
Treatment: Uterine displacement by left lateral position, intravenous crystalloid hydration, and intravenous injection of ephedrine or phenylephrine
b. High spinal blockade (due to excessive dose of local anesthesia);
Treatment: as before along with effective ventilation by tracheal intubation
c. Spinal headache (due to leakage of CSF);
Treatment: Use of caffeine, which is a cerebral vasoconstrictor for pain relief, and with severe headache an epidural blood patch (10–20 ml of autologeus blood without anticoagulant) in the epidural space at the site of dural puncture is effective
d. Convulsion (due to CSF hypotension);
Treatment as like spinal headache
e. Bladder dysfunction—*treatment* is by catheterization
f. Meningitis/or arachnoiditis—Supportive and antibiotics and physician's opinion.

Q. What are the contraindications to spinal anesthesia?

Ans.
a. Refractory maternal hypotension
b. Maternal coagulopathy
c. Thrombocytopenia
d. Patient-getting heparin
e. Untreated maternal bacteremia
f. Skin infection at the site of spinal needle puncture
g. Increased intracranial pressure by mass lesion.

Q. Epidural block is best, why?

Ans.
a. Avoids danger of GA
b. Improves uterine retraction
c. Patient is conscious—can see her child
d. Rapid postoperative recovery.

Q. What are the disadvantages of epidural block?

Ans. Time taken—prolonged, total spinal blockade, ineffective analgesia, hypotension, maternal fever and back pain.

Q. When GA is required?

Ans. *Antepartum hemorrhage (APH)*: In placenta previa to avoid hypotension.

Q. What are the different types of CS?

Ans.
a. Lower segment cesarean section (LSCS)
b. Classical cesarean section.

Q. What do you mean by lower segment of uterus?

Ans. See preterm labor (Chapter 11).

Q. How do you perform lower segment cesarean section (LSCS)?

Ans. It can be performed either by:
  a. Midline subumbilical abdominal incision (Figure 3.1a).
  b. Paramedian (right or left) (Figure 3.1b)
  c. Transverse suprapubic incision (Pfannenstiel incision) (Figure 3.1c).

Q. What are the steps of LSCS?

Ans.
  a. Bladder is empty, confirm fetal heart sound (FHS) and take informed consent for operation.
  b. Anesthesia—Spinal/epidural/general anesthesia.
  c. Dressing with antiseptic lotion and draping.
  d. Skin incision (Figure 3.1c)—pfannenstiel incision—3 cm above symphysis pubis in supine position at 15° tilt on left side to prevent supine hypotensive syndrome. The incision should be of adequate width to accommodate delivery (12–15 cm is typical).
  e. Incision on rectus sheath, split the muscle in midline and then separate, parietal peritoneum is opened and enter into the abdominal cavity.
  f. Introduce Doyen's retractor.
  g. Identify the round ligament of uterus on both sides (important) and correct dextrorotation first if required.
  h. *Technique*:
   i. The loose uterovesical fold of peritoneum is picked up, cut and pushed down with bladder (not more than 5cm caudally) to expose the lower segment (Figure 3.2A). The bladder is then retracted by Doyen's retractor which was introduced beforehand.

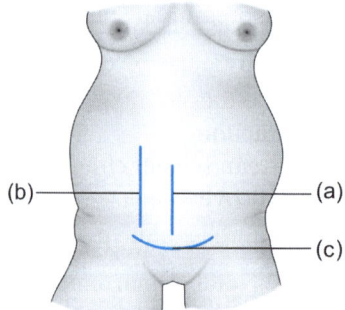

Figure 3.1: Abdominal incisions during cesarean section: (a) midline subumbilical; (b) right paramedian; (c) Pfannenstiel

   ii. A small nick is made (1–2 cm) through the midline of the lower uterine segment and deepens until membrane protrudes, it should be below the level where the vesicouterine serosa was incised to bring the bladder down (Figure 3.2B).
   iii. The uterine incision is widened with index fingers or make it at least 10 cm by cutting with scissors and then rupture of

Obstetric Operations and Interventions

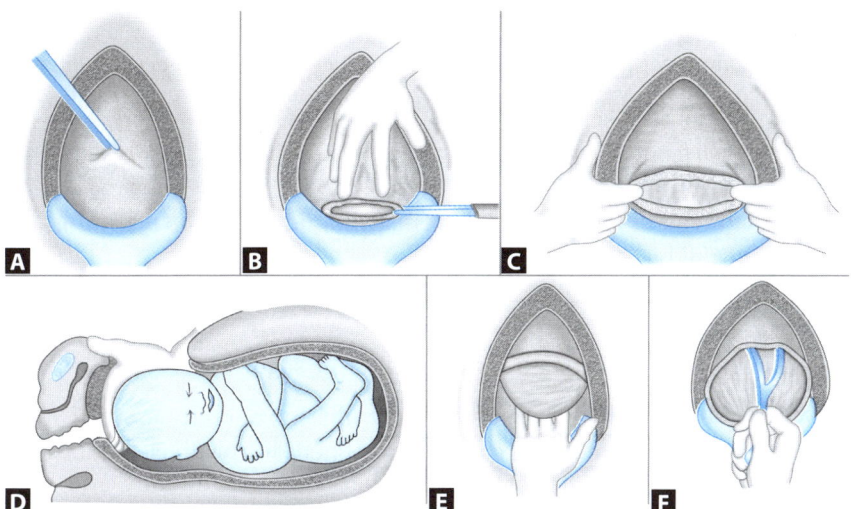

Figures 3.2A to F: Steps of lower segment: (A) Loose peritoneum is picked up and cut; (B) Lower segment of uterus is cut; (C) Uterine incision is widened; (D and E) Delivery of head by hand method; (F) Delivery of head by forceps

      membrane (Figure 3.2C) is done, to allow delivery of head and trunk of fetus without tearing the lateral uterine margins.

iv. The operator's right hand is passed into the uterine cavity through the incision to lift the baby's head, and Doyen's retractor is taken out while the assistant gives the fundal pressure to push the baby out and suck the baby's mouth and nostrils when it is delivered (Figures 3.2D and E).

v. Sometimes, it is necessary to extract the head by low forceps (Figure 3.2F).

vi. Uterine oxytocics are used after delivery of the baby (confirm no other baby is inside) clamp the cord, cut it in between the clamp and hand over the baby to the pediatrician.

vii. Give a single dose of prophylactic antibiotic after the cord is clamped and cut and keep the gentle traction on the cord and massage the uterus and deliver the placenta and membrane (wait for natural separation of placenta for reduction of bleeding and do not mop vigorously in the uterine cavity, rather examine the placenta to see any missing of cotyledons or membrane).

viii. Uterine incision is repaired in two layers by 1-0 vicryl or catgut by continuous suture excluding the visceral peritoneum.

ix. Peritoneal toileting done.

x. All the bleeding points should be secured meticulously.

xi. Counting of mops and instruments before abdominal closure is essential.

xii. Abdomen is closed in layers.

xiii. Vaginal toileting is done to see the amount of bleeding.

> **Note**
>
> Misgav-Ladach technique is the technique where incision to delivery interval of baby is reduced considerably with minimal use of instruments. Here a Joel-Cohen abdominal incision is made. It is a straight transverse incision (10 cm) through the abdominal skin 3 cm below the level of anterior superior iliac spine. The abdomen is opened by finger separation and stretching. Neither visceral nor parietal peritoneum is closed. Uterus is closed in a single layer by locking continuous suture followed by rectus sheath and skin in the Misgav-Ladach technique.

Classical CS

Longitudinal incision on the upper uterine segment.

Q. What are the indications of classical CS?

Ans.
a. Lower segment is not easily approached due to dense adhesion of bladder or presence of fibroid
b. Lower segment is highly vascular due to placenta previa
c. Lower segment is infiltrated with carcinoma cervix
d. Impacted shoulder presentation with drained liquor/back down in transverse lie
e. Conjoined twin
f. Postmortem CS
g. Successful repair of high vesicovaginal fistula (VVF).

Q. What are the techniques of Classical CS?

Ans.
a. A midline incision is made through the anterior wall of uterus—the uterine fundus lies above and the reflection of uterovesical fold below
b. As soon as membrane is encountered, it is ruptured
c. The fetal foot is grasped and baby is delivered after version as a breech delivery
d. This is followed by delivery of placenta
e. The wound is closed in three layers:
   i. Close the first layer of deeper uterine muscle excluding decidua by chromic '1-0' catgut or polyglycolic suture material (1-0) continuously.
   ii. Close the second layer of uterine muscle using interrupted 1 chromic catgut (or polyglycolic suture material).
   iii. Close the superficial muscle fibers and serosa using a continuous '0' chromic catgut (or polyglycolic acid suture material) with atraumatic needle.

Problems during Surgery

1. Deeply Engaged Head

a. A deeply engaged head may require to be pushed by an assistant with fingers in the vagina aseptically. The Trendelenberg position of mother is of real help in this case.

b. *Patwardhan's method*: First, one upper limb is delivered followed by opposite upper limb then back is delivered followed by fetal abdomen and lower limbs. The fetal head is lastly delivered. It is possible only when fetal back is anterior and amount of liquor is adequate.

2. Floating Head

Floating head is delivered by forceps, vectis or vacuum. During forceps application, slight fundal pressure helps to push the head towards incision, sagittal suture is placed transversely with the concavity of pelvic curve towards the fetal occiput. Lower blade (left blade) is applied first followed by anterior (right) and fetal head is delivered by controlled extension. The handles of forceps are elevated and mild traction is applied and head is then lifted out of the lower segment of uterus.

3. Baby Breech

- Wide uterine incision is made
- Grasp the foot and deliver it through the incision
- Deliver the legs and body up to the shoulders and then deliver the arms
- *Difficulties in head delivery*: Fetal head is delivered by Mauriceau-Smellie-Veit maneuver or forceps or in further difficulty GA may be required for uterine relaxation; though the operation was started by spinal anesthesia.

4. Lower Uterine Segment is not Well-formed

Cesarean section at 34 weeks (not in labor) or lower uterine segment is very narrow, may need undesirable variations of uterine incisions like:
a. Low vertical cesarean section or Kronig incision (LVCS).
b. J-shaped incision (a transverse low uterine incision passing upwards through one side of the uterus).

Advantage
Apposition is good.

Disadvantage of vertical incision
Low vertical incision may go upwards as in classical CS or may extend downwards involving bladder.

5. Baby Transverse

Baby's back up (near the top of the fundus)—usually, does not need classic incision for delivery
- Introduce the right hand through the uterine incision line and reach up to the fundus and find ankle of the fetus
- Grasp the ankle and gently pull through the incision to deliver the legs and complete the delivery as in breech.

Baby's backdown
- A high vertical uterine incision is the incision of choice
- After the incision, reach into the uterus and find the feet, pull these through the incision and complete the delivery as in breech
- The repair is as in classical CS.

6. Placenta Previa

Anterior placenta previa: Try to incise uterine wall above its margin, but if placenta is on the line of incision cut through it and deliver the fetus and quick cord clamping to prevent unnecessary blood loss from fetus.

a. After delivery, if the placenta cannot be separated manually, the diagnosis is placenta accreta, which is commonly found in previous cesarean section scar, needs cesarean hysterectomy in many cases (Here total hysterectomy is needed as the placenta is low down). Other methods of management of adherent placenta with previous scar are discussed in the case discussion of placenta previa.
b. High risk of postpartum hemorrhage (PPH), so vertical or horizontal compression suture in the lower uterine segment or separate placental bed sutures, tight-packing of lower segment is important before hysterectomy.
c. Classical section may be needed when lower segment is very vascular.

7. Bleeding is not Controlled after Delivery of Baby and Placenta

Take the uterus out of the abdominal cavity and see the bleeding points clearly. Assistant will give temporary pressure on abdominal aorta for reduction of bleeding and suction is used to keep the operative field clear

a. *Extension of incision angle*: Repair it properly, but if fails a subtotal or total hysterectomy is carried out as cervix is not easy to identify. Mobilize the bladder 2 cm below the tear. If possible place a suture 1 cm below the upper end of cervical tear and keep traction on the suture to bring the lower end of the tear into views as the repair continues.
b. *Atonic uterus*:
   i. IV Ringer lactate, oxytocics, blood transfusion
   ii. If fails—B-Lynch suture/uterine and ovarian artery ligation/internal iliac artery ligation of both sides in a step wise manner.
   iii. If all the measure fail—subtotal hysterectomy.

Q. What are the complications of CS?

Ans. Preoperative
   a. Anesthetic complications such as hypotension, adult respiratory distress syndrome (ARDS), pulmonary edema.
   b. *Hemorrhage*:
      i. Atonic hemorrhage.
      ii. Injury to uterine vessels due to extension of the angles.
      iii. Broad ligament hematoma.
   c. Injury to the bladder
   d. Injury to the intestine.

Postoperative
   a. PPH
   b. Paralytic ileus
   c. Infection and wound dehiscence.

Obstetric Operations and Interventions

Q. Advantages of lower transverse or Kerr incision in LSCS.

Ans. a. Less hemorrhage during operation.
b. Easy suturing.
c. Better union as it takes little part in uterine involution.
d. Incidence of scar rupture is less (if it occurs, it will occur during labor).
e. Incidence of placental implantation is less on the lower segment scar when compared to classical CS.
f. Trial of labor may be acceptable.

> **Note**
> Tubal ligation (Pomeroy method) may be added to LSCS, if family is completed otherwise insert Cu-T during operation after placental delivery and before closure of uterine incision as a temporary method of contraception. In both the cases prior informed consent of the patient/husband is necessary.

Q. What are the indications of peripartum hysterectomy?

Ans. Peripartum hysterectomy means removal of uterus after vaginal delivery or cesarean section. It may be total or subtotal hysterectomy
a. *Emergency indications:*
  i. Uterine rupture
  ii. Uncontrolled uterine hemorrhage
  iii. Placenta accreta
  iv. Uterine infection
  v. Persistent uterine atony
  vi. Uterine trauma after varieties of obstetric manipulations
  vii. Lateral trauma extension of the lower uterine segment into the uterine artery
b. *Non-emergency indications*: Significant uterine pathology such as
  i. Cervical carcinoma *in situ*
  ii. Uterine leiomyoma.

Q. Which factors increase the risk of cesarean section?

Ans. a. Medical diseases associated with pregnancy such as diabetes, heart disease, severe anemia, jaundice, etc.
b. Pregnancy-associated diseases such as placenta previa, pre-eclampsia, eclampsia.
c. Indications of cesarean section such as obstructed labor, prolonged labor, and prolonged rupture of membrane which increases maternal exhaustion, dehydration, operative morbidity, atonicity of uterus and sepsis.
d. Anesthesia in full stomach just before operation causes aspiration in lung.
e. Hypotension due to spinal/epidural anesthesia, if proper preloading is not performed.

Q. What are the causes of maternal death after cesarean section?

Ans.
a. Hemorrhage due to operation (normal blood loss on an average during LSCS is 1000 mL), PPH and rectus sheath hematoma, if remains undetected
b. Shock
c. Sepsis
d. Amniotic fluid embolism
e. Severe reaction due to blood transfusion
f. Coagulation failure
g. Renal failure.

Q. How do you prevent maternal mortality from cesarean section?

Ans.
a. Avoid unnecessary cesarean section.
b. Proper selection of patient for elective and emergency operation.
c. Skill of operating surgeon and anesthetist.
d. Detection of high-risk factors in antenatal period and prevention of anemia by prophylactic iron and folic acid.
e. Prevention of postoperative shock—by oxygenation, IV infusion of colloid, crystalloid, blood and blood products.
f. Prevention of infection by prophylactic antibiotics after clamping the cord of baby, because sepsis after cesarean section is very difficult to manage.
g. Judicious blood transfusion after cross matching and proper monitoring during transfusion.
h. Preloading by normal saline before spinal anesthesia to prevent hypotension and its complications such as acute renal failure.
i. Watch of vitals (pulse, respiration rate, temperature, BP, per vaginal or intra-abdominal bleeding, and urine output) every 4 hours for 48 hours after operation.

Q. How do you reduce higher cesarean section rate in practice?

Ans.
a. Vaginal birth after cesarean section in non-recurrent indication.
b. Maintenance of partographic chart during active phase of labor.
c. Amnioinfusion in selected cases of PROM.
d. External cephalic version or breech extraction according to the condition during breech delivery.
e. Option of destructive operation in some cases.
f. Liberal use of scalp blood pH when fetal distress is diagnosed by CTG can reduce the cesarean rate.

EPISIOTOMY

Q. What is episiotomy?

Ans. A planned surgical incision on the perineum and posterior vaginal wall in the second stage of labor just prior to crowning of the presenting part to facilitate delivery (Epision= pubic region; tomy= to cut).

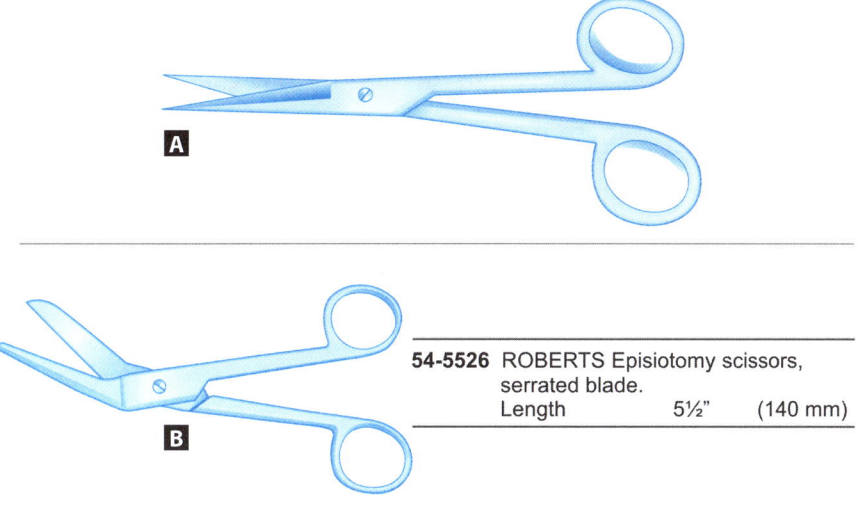

Figures 3.3A and B: (A) Sharp end scissors; (B) Episiotomy scissors

Q. What are the uses of episiotomy scissors (Figures 3.3A and B)?
Ans. a. For episiotomy/perineotomy
b. For cutting the umbilical cord (most common operation in labor room).

> **Note**
> Blunt ended scissors are usually used in episiotomy to avoid injury on rectum.

Q. What are the indications of episiotomy?
Ans. a. Rigid perineum, but not in all cases of primigravida
b. Complicated vaginal delivery (breech, shoulder dystocia, face to pubis delivery)
c. Fetal distress
d. Delivery following repair of CPT
e. In any instrumental delivery.

> **Note**
> Episiotomy may cause anal sphincteric dysfunction and incontinence may be due to decreased anal squeeze pressure.

Q. What are the types of incision?
Ans. a. Median—in the middle of the introitus (Start from the mid-point of fourchette/or 6 o'clock position for about 2.5 cm in the midline)
b. Lateral—episiotomy is made at an angle of 90° to the midpoint of fourchette
c. Mediolateral—episiotomy is made at an angle of 45° to the midpoint of fourchette. Scissors are positioned at 5 O'clock or 7 O'clock and incision is extended for 3-5 cm towards ipsilateral ischial tuberocity. This type is most commonly preferred
d. J-shaped—first start from midline and then tilts lateral ward.

Q. What are the advantages and disadvantages of median episiotomy?

Ans. **Advantage:** It heals well, scar tissue formation is less.
Disadvantage: If it extends downwards, then it causes complete perineal tear.

Q. When do you perform episiotomy?

Ans. a. Perineum is thinned out
b. Just before crowning of the head—head does not recede back in between contractions (3–4 cm of head is visible during contraction).

Q. What structures are cut during mediolateral episiotomy?

Ans. a. Posterior vaginal mucosa
b. Superficial and deep perineal muscles
c. A few fibers of levator ani when it is deep
d. Blood vessels and some cutaneous nerves on perineum
e. Fascia and skin.

> **Note**
>
> *Muscles attached to perineal body: Paired—Transverse perinea superficialis, Transverse perinea profundus, Levator ani; unpaired—Bulbospongiosus, sphincter ani externus (few fibers). Sphincter urethra membranace.*

Obstetrical perineum: It is the space between the vagina and anal canal (size 4 cm × 4 cm).

Q. What is the nerve supply of vulva?

Ans. a. Branches of the pudendal nerve
b. Branches of the posterior femoral cutaneous nerve of thigh
c. Genital branch of genitofemoral nerve
d. Ilioinguinal nerve
e. Inferior hemorrhoidal nerve
f. Perforating cutaneous nerves.

> **Note**
>
> *The pudendal nerve (S2, 3, 4) has three branches: the clitorial perineal, and inferior hemorrhoidal that innervate clitoris, perineal muscles, inner perineal skin and external anal sphincter (EAS).*

Q. What are the steps of episiotomy?

Ans. Anesthesia
a. Infiltration of local anesthesia (10 mL, 1% lignocaine) along the proposed line of incision. Care should be taken that needle should not be in the vein. Never inject, if blood is aspirated otherwise convulsion and coma of the individual may occur (Figure 3.4).
b. Minimum 2 minutes of time should be allowed.
c. *Technique*:
  i. Place the fingers between the baby's head and perineum
  ii. Use a pair of scissors to cut the perineum 3 to 4 cm in the mediolateral direction (Figure 3.5)
  iii. Incision is made just before crowning, if it is made too early it causes more bleeding

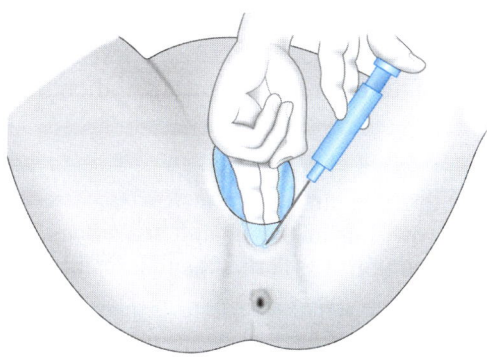

Figure 3.4: Infiltration of perineal tissue with local anesthetic

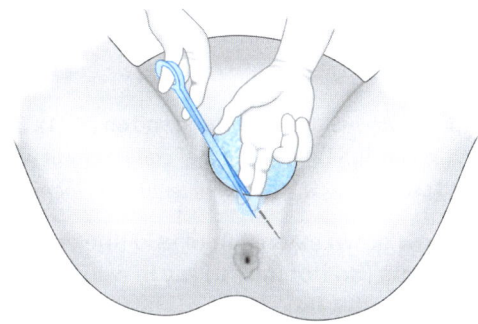

Figure 3.5: Technique of left mediolateral episiotomy

    iv. Control the baby's head and shoulders as they deliver ensuring that the shoulders have rotated to the midline to prevent extension of episiotomy.
- d. *Repair (Figure 3.6)*:
  - i. Close the vagina with 1-0 catgut suture
  - ii. Start the repair at about 1 cm above the apex of episiotomy wound because some blood vessels may retract upwards
  - iii. Vaginal mucosae—continuous suture up to the level of vaginal opening bringing the points 2a and 2b (Figure 3.6)
  - iv. Muscles—close the perineal muscles by interrupted sutures
  - v. Perineal skin—closes the skin by interrupted 2-0 absorbable sutures.

Q. Postoperative care of episiotomy wound.

Ans.
- a. Dressing with antiseptic solution or antibiotic ointment
- b. Pain killer orally (NSAID) and local magnesium sulfate compress
- c. Ambulation–Allow to move after 12 hours
- d. Removal of stitch is not necessary when catgut is used as a suture material.

Q. What are the complications?

Ans.
- a. Extension of the wound—upwards, downwards leading to hemorrhage

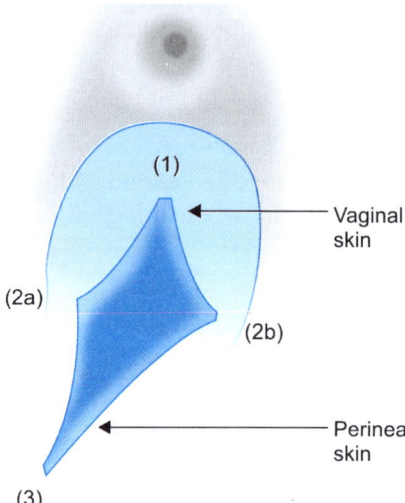

Figure 3.6: Repair of episiotomy—Start from (1) and end on (3): (1). Extent of episiotomy in vaginal mucosa (apex), (2a and 2b)–Lateral extent of episiotomy of wound; (3). Extension in the perineal muscles and skin

    b. CPT (due to low down extension of mid line episiotomy)
    c. Vulval hematoma (do not miss to say in examination)
    d. Retention of urine
    e. Infection, secondary hemorrhage, non-union
    f. Rectovaginal fistula (RVF)
    g. Perineal scar, dyspareunia and scar endometriosis (rare).

Q. Common causes of vulval hematoma.
Ans. *Obstetrical causes:*
    a. Improper hemostasis during repair of episiotomy wound—most common.
    b. Trauma to the small artery adjacent to the vaginal wall during later stage of delivery.
    c. Precipitate labor—Expulsion of fetus in < 3 hours due to vigorous uterine and abdominal contraction.
Gynecological causes:
    a. Rape.
    b. Accidental fall on a sharp object.

Q. How do you diagnose vulval hematoma?
Ans. a. Complain of pain on perineum and retention of urine
    b. On examination, general condition: poor, pulse—tachycardia, blood pressure (BP) is low, swelling of the vulva is present.

Q. How do you treat vulval hematoma?
Ans. a. Start IV drip with Ringer lactate (RL)
    b. Arrange for blood transfusion by grouping and cross-matching
    c. Antibiotics— By IV route
    d. Send the patient to the operation theater

Obstetric Operations and Interventions

  e. Incise hematoma under GA and evacuate the blood clot and after proper hemostasis close the wound with a drain which should be removed after 48 hours.
  f. Continuous catheter drainage by self-retaining catheter for 24–48 hours.

Q. What will you do if CPT occurs?

Ans. Immediate repair, if it is identified within 24 hours otherwise it should be repaired after 3 months when infection is controlled and tissue involution is complete.

Q. Why immediate repair is good?

Ans.
  a. Union is good for high vascularity
  b. Less chance of infection
  c. Identification of each structure is very easy.

Q. Which suture material is preferable?

Ans. Polyglycolic suture material over catgut is preferred for more tensile strength, non-allergic and lower probabilities of infection.

Q. What will be the line of treatment, if infection of episiotomy wound occurs?

Ans.
  1. Mild—no antibiotics, only local dressing with betadine solution.
  2. Severe but does not involve deep tissue—ampicillin 500 mg orally qds plus metronidazole 400 mg thrice daily for 5 days.
  3. If the infection is deep and involves muscles—injection ampicillin 1 g IV after skin test plus injection gentamicin 60 mg IM plus metrogyl infusion 400 mg IV stat and continued for 3 days according to the severity of infection then switch on oral preparation for another 4 days. Resuturing is done after 2 to 4 weeks, if there is gaping of the wound.

Q. What are the different degrees of perineal tears?

Ans.
- 1st degree—vaginal and perineal skin are torn
- 2nd degree—perineal body (perineal muscles) is involved, not the anal sphincter
- 3rd degree—sphincters of anal canal
  - 3a: <50% thickness of external anal sphincter (EAS) torn
  - 3b: >50% thickness of EAS torn
  - 3c: Internal anal sphincter (IAS) torn
- 4th degree—a third degree tears with involvement of anal mucosa.

Q. How can you prevent perineal injury?

Ans.
  a. Delivery of head by modified Ritgen maneuver (giving pressure on the fetal chin through the perineum by right hand covered with a sterile towel while suboccipital region of fetal head is held against symphysis pubis).
  b. Judicious episiotomy.
  c. Judicious use of forceps (forceps causes more perineal trauma than ventouse).
  d. Elective cesarean section prevents perineal damage.

DILATATION AND EVACUATION (D/E)/SUCTION AND EVACUATION (S/E)

Q. Pick up the instruments for D/E or S/E operation.

Ans.
a. Sponge-holding forceps
b. Catheter (rubber/plastic)
c. Posterior vaginal speculum
d. Multiple-teeth vulsellum/Allis' tissue forceps
e. Cervical dilators
f. Ovum forceps for (D/E); Karman's cannula for S/E
g. Curette.

Q. What are the indications of S/E operation?

Ans.
a. Medical termination of pregnancy (MTP) in first trimester of pregnancy.
b. Evacuation of hydatidiform mole by wide bore Karman's Cannula.
c. Missed abortion, incomplete abortion or inevitable abortion.

Q. Have you seen S/E operation?

Ans. Yes.

Q. In which condition have you seen this operation?

Ans. In incomplete abortion, MTP in first trimester.

Q. What are the steps of D/E or S/E operation?

Ans.
a. Informed consent before operation
b. Ask the patient to evacuate the bladder
c. Position of the patient—lithotomy
d. Anesthesia—GA/paracervical block
e. Antiseptic dressing and draping
f. If bladder is full catheterization in aseptic precaution
g. P/V examination to see the size and direction of uterus (A/V or R/V)
h. Introduce the posterior vaginal speculum
i. Anterior lip of the cervix is hold by multiple-teeth vulsellum/Allis' tissue forceps (the later is preferable for least tissue trauma)
j. The Hegar/Hawkins-Ambler's dilators should be passed gradually from lower to higher size (6 mm for 6 weeks; 8 mm for 8 weeks; 10 mm for 10 weeks of uterine size) to dilate the cervix and internal os (up to 9/12 Hawkins-Ambler's dilator) (Figure 3.7).

> **Note**
> *The uterus is very soft in pregnancy. Passage of uterine sound through the cervix to assess the length and direction of the uterus may cause injury of uterus.*

k. Material is taken out by ovum forceps (in D & E operation) or by Karman suction cannula (S & E operation), which is attached to the suction apparatus and suction is carried out at an optimal pressure of 450 mm of Hg.
l. Suction is carried out by rotating the cannula and as the cavity empties, gripping sensation is felt over the cannula by the operator.

Obstetric Operations and Interventions

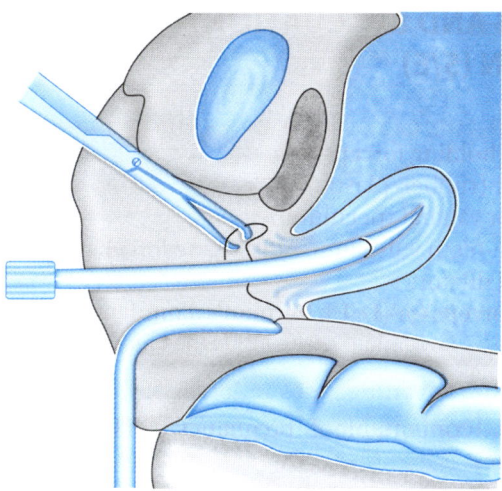

Figure 3.7: Introduction of cervical dilators

    m. Curettage is done gently until the gritty sensation is felt or the uterine cavity is empty (Procedure of curettage—see later). Examine the evacuated material and send the material for H/P examination.
    n. Perform bimanual examination to confirm the size and firmness of uterus.
    o. Swab the vagina to clear and look on the external os to see the amount of bleeding.
    p. Injection of oxytocics are given before curettage.

Q. What is the instrument?

Ans. Uterine curette (having blunt and sharp end) is made of stainless steel and 25 cm long. It is of three sizes (large, medium and small according to the diameter of sharp loop 8, 6, 4 mm respectively) (Figure 3.8).

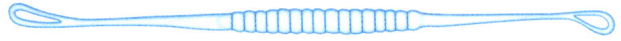

Figure 3.8: Uterine curette

Q. How do you proceed for uterine curettage?

Ans. Procedure: The curette is held by index finger and thumb. The cervix is steadied by vulsellum and curette is passed through the dilated cervical canal into the uterine cavity till the fundus is reached. The concave surface of sharp or blunt end is applied on the endometrial surface and stroke under gentle and firm pressure to draw the curette from fundus up to the internal os by clockwise or anticlockwise direction till the whole uterine surface is scrapped. The uterus is empty when gritty sensation is felt on all uterine surfaces during curettage, fetal tissue is absent and air bubble through blood comes out through the cervical os (Figures 3.9A and B).

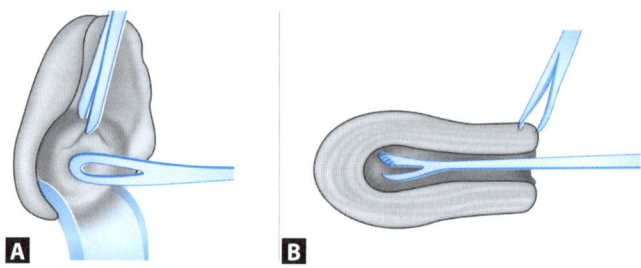

Figures 3.9A and B: (A) Introduction of uterine curette; (B) Uterine curette inside the uterine cavity

Q. What are the advantages of suction procedure?

Ans. a. Easy and comfortable to the patient
b. Blood loss is less
c. Can be done as an outpatient procedure
d. Hospital stay is less
e. Curettage may be done with cannula.

Q. What are the dangers of S/E operation or curettage?

Ans. *Immediate*
a. Uterine perforation (stop the suction procedure immediately as gut or omentum may come out through the rent due to suction procedure)
b. Tear of the cervix
c. Hemorrhage, shock and sepsis
d. Incomplete evacuation in suction procedure
e. Tip of the flexible plastic cannula may break inside the uterus which is removed by D and C or by operative hysteroscope.
Remote: Pelvic inflammatory disease (PID), tubal blockage (infertility), T-O mass, cervical incompetence, menstrual irregularities, cervical stenosis, Asherman's syndrome (uterine synechiae).

Q. Uterine forceps (the instrument is not widely used nowadays).

Ans. The forceps are slightly curved. It is introduced with the tip directed forwards and backwards as per direction of the uterus (Figure 3.10).

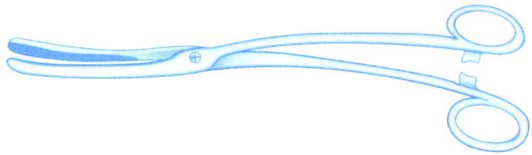

Figure 3.10: Uterine forceps (Bozeman)

Q. What are the uses of this instrument?

Ans. a. To dress the uterine cavity with sterile gauze and antiseptic solution following dilatation and evacuation (D and E) operations of obstetric indications, but not done in gynecological D and C operation.
b. To pack the uterine cavity with roller gauze in secondary hemorrhage under GA.
c. To grasp the tube for ligation.

FOR POSTGRADUATE STUDENTS

DESTRUCTIVE OPERATIONS

A. Craniotomy operation or decompression of hydrocephalic head
B. Decapitation
C. Evisceration
D. Cleidotomy.

Craniotomy Operation

Oldham's Cranial Perforator (Figure 3.11)

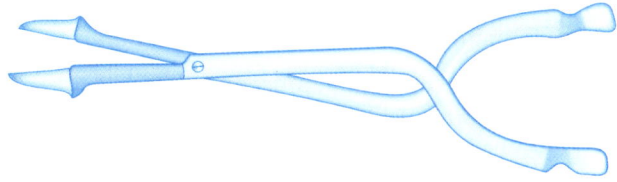

Figure 3.11: Opened Oldham's cranial perforator

Q. What is the use of this instrument?

Ans. For craniotomy operation.

Q. What are the indications of craniotomy?

Ans. a. Hydrocephalus (baby is living) [craniocentesis is preferable].
b. If fetus is dead and mother is unable to expel the baby—persistent occipitoposterior (POP), persistent mentoposterior, brow and after coming head of breech.
c. CPD (mild) with obstructed labor and the baby is dead.

> **Note**
> *Hydrocephalic head should be punctured by lumbar puncture needle when cervical os is more than 4 cm dilated to avoid rupture of uterus.*

Q. What are the conditions that must be fulfilled for craniotomy operation?

Ans. a. Dead or hydrocephalic baby
b. Cervix is almost fully dilated
c. Membrane must be ruptured
d. Pelvis is adequate
e. Head is engaged except in hydrocephalic baby
f. Bladder is empty.

Q. What are the steps of destructive operations?

Ans. a. History, examination of the patient and IV line with antibiotics
b. At least two units of blood are kept ready, compatible with patient's own blood.

c. Anesthesia under GA.
d. Position lithotomy, antiseptic dressing and draping.
e. Evacuation of bladder by self-retaining catheter, which should be kept in site after operation.
f. PV examination to confirm the previous finding, i.e. dilatation of cervix, membrane ruptured, presentation and position.

Perforation of fetal skull

g. Site of perforation:
   i. Vertex—through parietal bone
   ii. Face—through orbit or hard palate
   iii. Brow—through frontal bone.
h. The head is fixed by suprapubic pressure (first pelvic grip) and pressure is maintained throughout the procedure.
i. The selection site should be away from fontanelles and suture lines.
j. The left two fingers are placed at the selected site and the scalp tissue over it is cut slightly by a pair of scissors—this prevents perforator from slipping.
k. The closed perforator is introduced into the opening along with the palm and fingers of left hand at right angle to the presenting part.
l. The skull is perforated by a rotating movement on the scalp to establish a firm grip and then a strong steady push is given through the skull bone keeping the direction of perforator perpendicular to the skull.
m. The blades of the perforator are pushed in as far as the shoulder and then the handles are apposed—this causes separation of the blades at the tip for about an inch, thereby cutting through the skull bones. The instrument is then rotated through 90° and repeats the same procedure.
n. Thus, a '+' shaped incision is made for proper drainage of the brain matter.
o. The closed instrument is then introduced further in the cranial cavity and the brain matter is churned.
p. The instrument is then taken out under the guidance of left palm and fingers.
q. It is not necessary to wash out the content of the cranial cavity by Budin's cannula as was recommended in the past Budin's cannula (Figure 3.12): Double channelled catheter to washout the brain matter after craniotomy operation.
r. The perforated head may be collapsed sufficiently to permit the vaginal delivery.

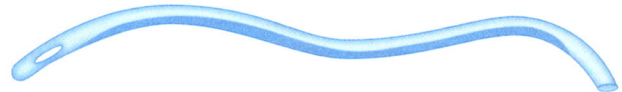

Figure 3.12: Budin's cannula

Cranioclast (Figure 3.13)

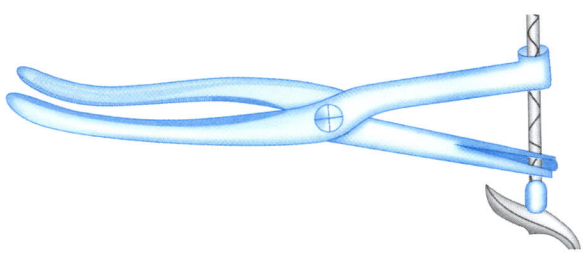

Figure 3.13: Crainoclast

Delivery of Perforated Head

s. The solid blade (male blade) of cranioclast is introduced through the perforation under guidance of left palm and fingers. An assistant is asked to hold it.
t. The position of the internal hand is now changed and placed in the sacral hollow. The fenestrated blade is now introduced from above, otherwise it will be difficult in locking of the blades. It is applied on any part of the skull lying posteriorly.
u. Blades are locked and screw is tightened.
v. Left hand is taken out.
w. PV examination is done to note any inclusion of maternal soft tissue or any bony projection from the fetal skull. Bone projections are removed, if present.
x. A tentative pull is applied for confirmation of good grip.
y. Direction of pull is just like forceps—downward, forward and then upward.
z. The placenta is removed manually. The syntocinon is given after delivery of baby.
- Inspection of maternal soft tissue like cervix, vagina and vulva for any tear or laceration, which are to be repaired and patient should be observed for 1 hour. Continuous catheter is maintained.

Q. In case of contracted pelvis how will you deliver the dead baby?

Ans. In case of contracted pelvis, the perforated head requires further diminution of size by three-bladed cephalotribe and the operation is called cephalotrypsy (Figure 3.14).

Q. What are the dangers of the operation?

Ans.
a. Hemorrhage
b. Shock
c. Sepsis
d. Injury of maternal soft tissues—cervix, vagina, uterus
e. Rectum—RVF
f. Bladder—VVF.

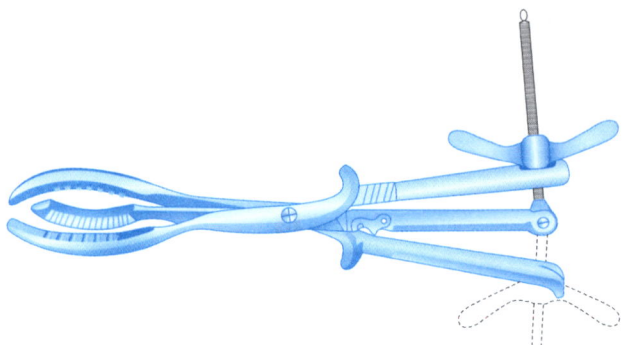

Figure 3.14: Cephalotribe

Q. How do you treat VVF, if it occurs during operation?

Ans. a. Continuous bladder drainage for 10 to 14 days
b. Antibiotics
c. Small fistula heals, but large fistula is reduced in size
d. The patient is discharged, if fistula persists and advise her to come after 3 months for repair as by that time involution of the scar and infection is controlled.

Q. How can you perform craniotomy in after coming head of hydrocephalus baby in breech presentation?

Ans. Discussed in details in X-ray (under hydrocephalic baby).

Bone-nibbling Forceps

Q. What is the use of Bone-nibbling forceps?

Ans. To remove the spicules of bone during craniotomy (Figure 3.15).

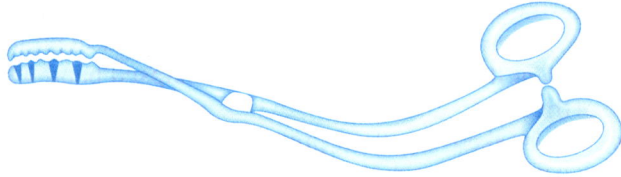

Figure 3.15: Bone-nibbling forceps

Q. Why nibbling of bone is necessary?

Ans. To avoid the trauma of the bladder, rectum and soft tissue of birth canal of mother.

Q. What are the contraindications of craniotomy operation?

Ans. a. Free floating head or > 3/5th head palpable per abdomen
b. Cervix is not fully dilated
c. Baby is living (except hydrocephalus)
d. Gross CPD when obstetrical conjugate <7.5 cm as the bimastoid diameter 7.5 cm is incompressible.

INSTRUMENTS FOR DECAPITATION (FIGURES 3.16A TO C)

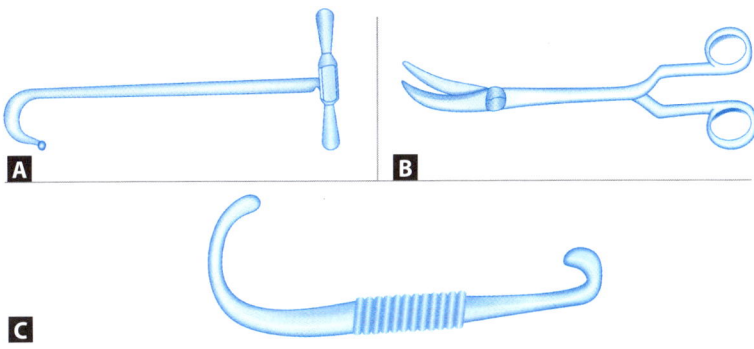

Figures 3.16A to C: Decapitation instruments; (A) Decapitation hook with knife; (B) Embryotomy scissors; (C) Breech hook with crochet

Q. What are the main instruments required for decapitation?

Ans. a. Decapitation hook with knife
b. Embryotomy scissors
c. Breech hook with crochet.

Q. What is the indication of decapitation?

Ans. A dead fetus in transverse lie without any signs and symptoms of threatened uterine rupture.

Q. Describe the procedure of decapitation.

Ans. a. General anesthesia
b. Lithotomy position
c. Antiseptic dressing and draping
d. Evacuation of bladder
e. Vaginal examination (Cervix fully dilated, fetal neck is within easy access), if there is no arm prolapsed, make one arm prolapsed.
f. Direction of the thumb in supinated prolapsed hand will point the side of the head
g. Assistant is asked to pull the prolapsed arm away from the head
h. This will make the neck stretched and accessible
i. The fingers of left hand are placed over the neck and the instrument (i.e. the knob) is introduced under the guidance of palm and fingers up to the level slightly over the neck. The tip of the instrument (i.e. the knob) is kept directed towards the fetal head and the hook of the instrument lies parallel to the floor.
j. The instrument is then rotated through 90° till the curve of the instrument encircles the neck and the tip of the hook is directed backwards and below the neck.
k. Fingers are now placed underneath the neck to guard the tip of the instrument against any injury of maternal soft tissue
l. By sea-saw movement, the neck is divided up to the cervical column. The instrument is pushed up, rotated through 90°. The internal

fingers are now placed over the neck and the instrument is then taken out under the guidance of palm and fingers.
m. The remaining soft tissue is divided by embryotomy scissors, which are introduced and taken out under guidance of palm and fingers.
n. By traction on the arm the trunk is easily delivered.
o. Delivery of the head (Give uterine fundal pressure to fix the head) (Figure 3.17).

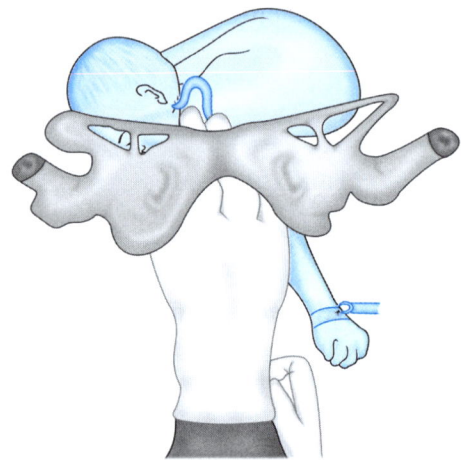

Figure 3.17: Introduction of decapitation hook with knife

- By putting right index finger into the mouth, if fails
- Traction by crochet and hook introduced into the mouth, if fails
- Application of forceps: an assistant fixes the head at the brim by abdominal grip
- *Double fixation of head*: Per abdomen by an assistant and PV by forceps and head is delivered by craniotomy

p. Placenta is removed manually
q. Uterine walls are palpated for any rupture
r. Uterine oxytocics
s. Cervix, vagina, bladder are inspected for any injury and care should be taken to protect the birth canal from injury by any projecting spicules of bones from the cut edge of the neck.

Q. What are the dangers of decapitation operation?
Ans. Hemorrhage (PPH), shock, sepsis, ruptured uterus, injury of the bladder (VVF) and soft tissue of mother like vagina, cervix and vulva.

Q. What is the postoperative care?
Ans. Antibiotics and catheter (self-retaining) is to be kept *in situ* for 7–10 days.

Q. Which instruments are kept in decapitation operation set?
Ans. a. Catheter
b. Decapitation hook with knife
c. Embryotomy scissors

d. Bone-nibbling forceps
e. Breech hook with crochet
f. Obstetric forceps
g. Cranioclast.

Decapitation Shaw

Use: Same as decapitation hook with knife.
Disadvantage: Blade is wider—more chances of injury to the uterus—more force are required.

Embryotomy Scissors

Q. **What are the uses of embryotomy scissors?**

Ans. a. Evisceration (fetal abdomen and thorax) is opened and viscera are removed in piecemeal.
b. Cleidotomy (cutting of the clavicle) in dead fetus especially in shoulder dystocia (common in anencephaly).
c. Spondylectomy—cutting of the fetal vertebral column.
d. Cutting of the soft tissue of neck after decapitation (Figure 3.18).

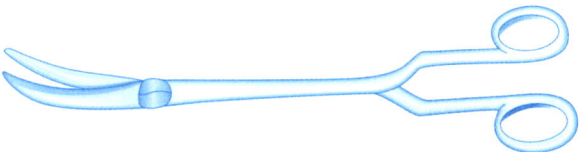

Figure 3.18: Embryotomy scissors

Q. **What is evisceration?**

Ans. It is the procedure of removing the viscera of a dead fetus in uterus. This facilitates delivery of the dead fetus due to the collapse of the chest and abdomen. Evisceration is indicated in cases of transverse lie with dead fetus, where the neck of the fetus is not easily accessible vaginally and fetal ascites. A prolapsed hand facilitates evisceration.

Q. **How do you reduce maternal morbidity or mortality by destructive operation?**

Ans. a. Vigorous preoperative resuscitation by IV fluid (NS/RL).
b. Correction of acidosis
c. Prophylactic antibiotics
d. Blood for grouping and cross-matching
e. Continuous catheterization.

SURGICAL MANAGEMENT OF PPH

Bimanual Uterine Compression (Figure 3.19A)

Form a fist and place in the anterior fornix and pressure against anterior wall and the other hand press deeply into the abdominal wall behind the uterus applying pressure on the posterior wall of the uterus. Maintain compression until the bleeding is controlled.

Aortic Compression per Abdomen (Figure 3.19B)

Apply downward pressure with a closed fist over the abdominal aorta directly through the abdominal wall:
- The point of compression is just above the umbilicus and slightly to the left
- Aortic pulsation can be felt through the anterior abdominal wall in the immediate postpartum period

With the other hand, palpate the femoral pulse to check the adequacy of compression:

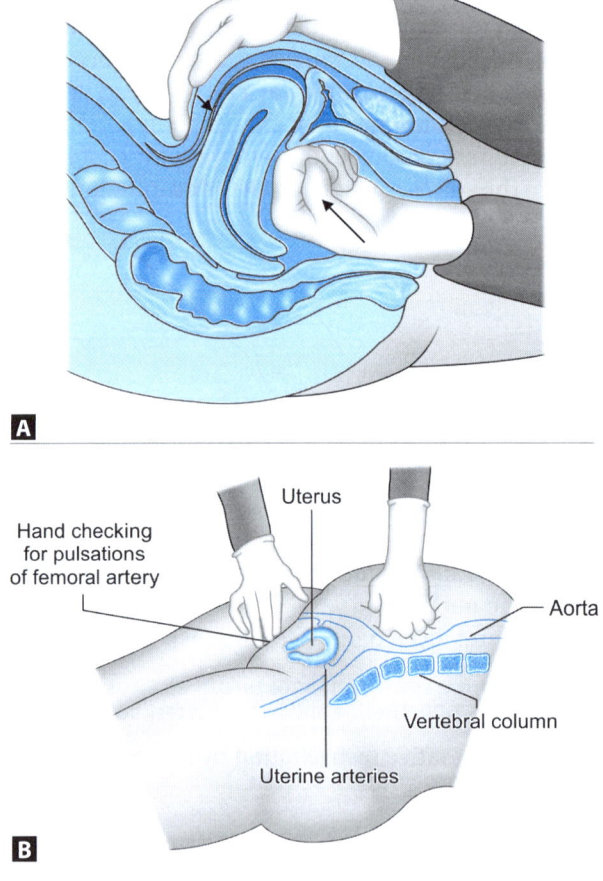

Figures 3.19A and B: (A) Bimanual uterine compression; (B) Aortic compression of abdominal aorta

- If the pulse is palpable during compression, the pressure exerted by the fist is inadequate
- If the femoral pulse is not palpable the pressure exerted is adequate.

Maintain compression until bleeding is controlled.

Uterine and Ovarian Artery Ligation (Figure 3.20)

1. See the site of uterine artery ligation
2. See the site of ovarian artery ligation adjacent to ovarian ligament.

Procedure:
a. Open the abdomen in layers to expose the uterus and broad ligament and retract the bladder.
b. Feel the pulsation of the uterine artery at the junction of uterus and cervix.
c. Using an absorbable suture, a large needle is passed through 2–3 cm of myometrium around the artery near the proposed site of lower uterine segment incision and tie it and secure the knot.
d. Suture is to be placed as close to the uterus as possible as the ureter lies 1 cm lateral to the uterine artery.
e. Repeat the same procedure on the other side.
f. Ligate the utero-ovarian artery just below the point where the ovarian ligament joins the uterus and repeats the same procedure on the other side.
g. Close the abdomen in layers.

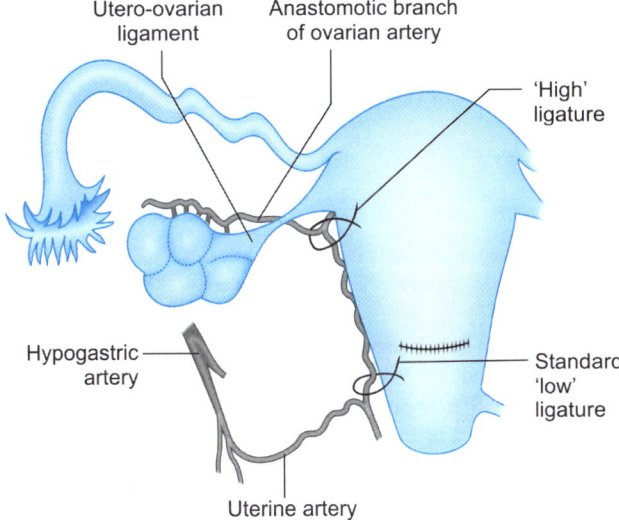

Figure 3.20: Uterine and ovarian artery ligation

Brace Suture (Figures 3.21 A to C)

1. B-Lynch suture.

Procedure

1. Start from right side, 3 cm below the incision and threaded through the uterine cavity to emerge 3 cm above the incision and 4 cm from the lateral border of uterus. Then, it passes over the fundus and goes to the posterior surface of the uterus. From the posterior surface, it comes again into the uterine cavity and from uterine cavity, again go out to the posterior surface a little distance away from the former and make a loop on the left side of the fundus and pierce 3 cm above and 3 cm below the incision line

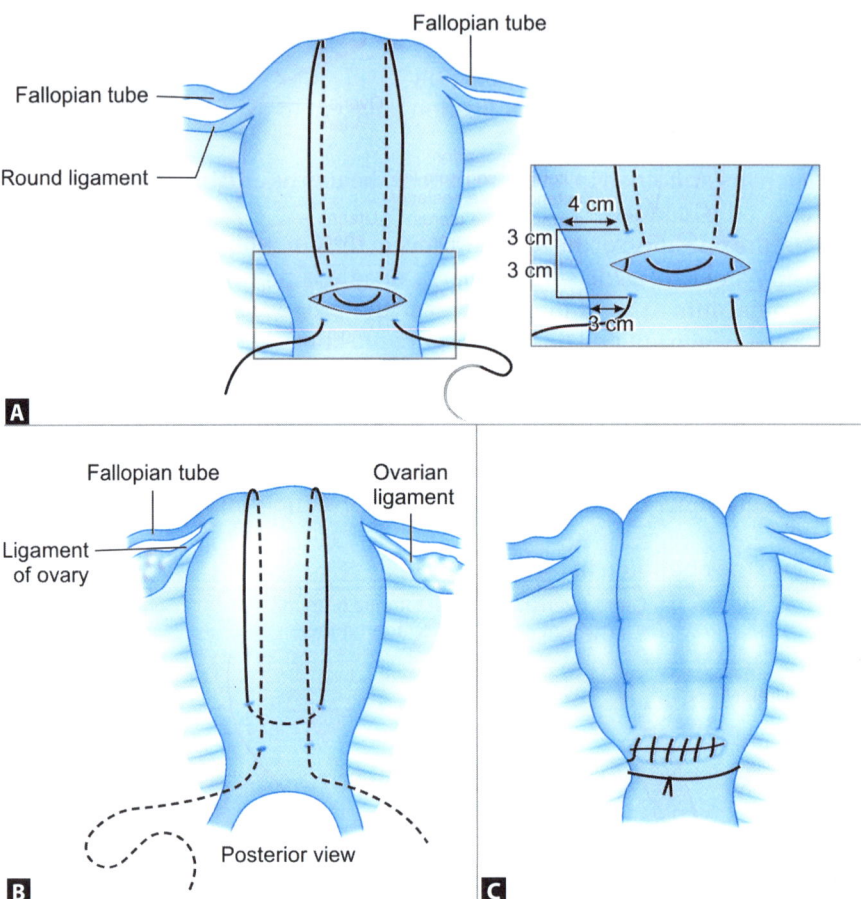

Figures 3.21A to C: B-Lynch procedure: (A) Front view; (B) Back view; (C) Knot

as on the right side. The suture is finally tied below the incision line of CS anteriorly.

2. Hayman uterine compression sutures are placed on two sides of uterus without opening the uterine cavity and uterovesical fold of peritoneum. The Cho multiple square sutures compress anterior and posterior wall of uterus at different sites. Blood may be inspissated in multiple square sutures of Cho (Figures 3.22A and B).

Bilateral Internal Iliac Artery Ligation (BIL) (Figure 3.23)

Q. What is the procedure?

Ans. This is the operative ligation of anterior division of the internal artery to achieve hemostasis in the operative field. It was first done by Kelly in 1894.

Q. What are the obstetric indications of internal iliac artery ligation?

Ans. a. Uterine rupture
b. Placenta accreta
c. Atonic PPH

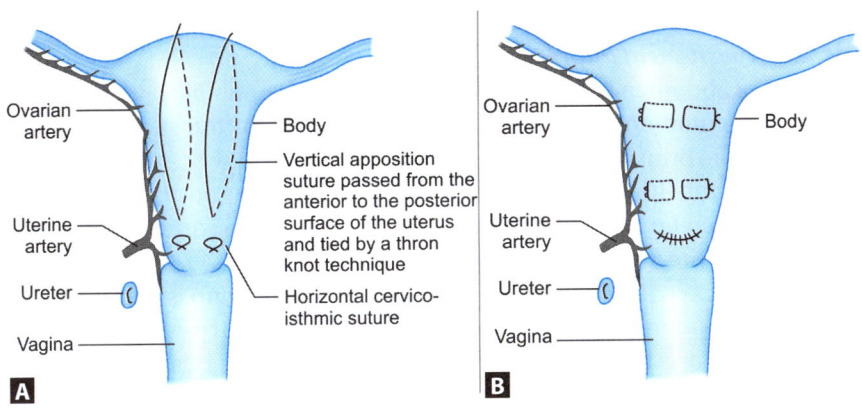

Figures 3.22A and B: (A) Hayman uterine compression suture; (B) Cho multiple square sutures at different sites of uterus

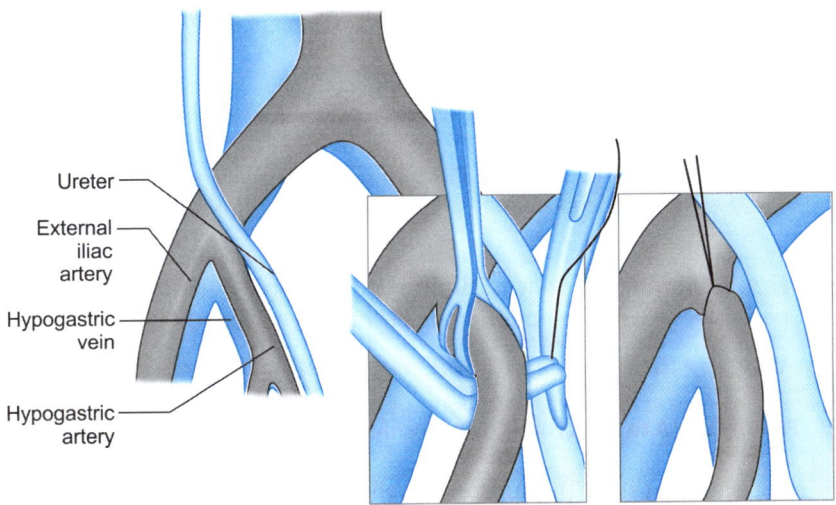

Figure 3.23: Internal iliac artery ligation

    d. Laceration of cervix
    e. Post-CS hemorrhage
    f. Broad-ligament hematoma.

Q. What are the branches of internal iliac artery?
Ans. Posterior division:
    1. Iliolumbar
    2. Superior gluteal
    3. Lateral sacral.
    Anterior division:
    a. *Visceral*—Superior vesicle, inferior vesicle, uterine, vaginal, middle rectal
    b. *Parietal*—Internal pudendal, inferior gluteal and obturator.

Q. What is the technique?

Ans. *Intraperitoneal approach:*
1. The abdomen is opened by paramedian infraumbilical incision.
2. The common iliac artery bifurcates in front of the sacroiliac joint (Pelvic brim).
3. The longitudinal incision is made on the posterior parietal peritoneum lateral to bifurcation of common iliac artery. The ureter lies in the medial flap of peritoneum.
4. The internal iliac artery is next lifted and bifurcation is reidentified.
5. The ligation is to be done distal to the branching of posterior division and close to the uterine artery to avoid collaterals from inferior mesenteric artery to feed the bleeding uterine artery.
6. The vessel is ligated with two free ties of number 1 black silk, 5 mm apart without ever cutting the major vessels.
7. It is important to work within the capsule of artery to avoid damaging vein, which may be closely associated of the artery capsule.
8. Do the same procedure on the other side.
9. The posterior peritoneum is closed.

> **Note**
> When external iliac artery is efficiently pressed in between thumb and index finger femoral arterial pulsation is absent. It is not true in case of internal iliac artery.

Extraperitoneal approach: Internal iliac artery is exposed extraperitoneally without opening the peritoneal cavity.

Q. What are the hemodynamic changes after ligation of artery?

Ans. After ligation of anterior division of internal iliac artery, there is a drop in the pulse pressure, a drop in mean BP and rate of blood flow through the collateral circulation. It transforms to a venous like system by eliminating the trip hammer effect. Collateral circulations develop in 45 to 60 minutes after the ligation, which are smaller in diameter than the internal iliac artery.

> **Note**
> Complications: 1. Immediate—injury of ureter, iliac veins, and accidental ligation of external iliac artery, 2. Late—bladder necrosis, peripheral nerve ischemia.

Manual Removal of Placenta (MROP) (Figures 3.24A and B)

1. IV drip with RL.
2. Informed consent is to be taken.
3. Anesthesia—GA (preferable for good uterine relaxation)/Regional anesthesia may be used.
4. Two units of blood must be kept ready at hand.
5. Aseptic technique is to be followed.
6. Lithotomy position of the patient.
7. Cleaning, draping and catheterization of the patient.

Obstetric Operations and Interventions

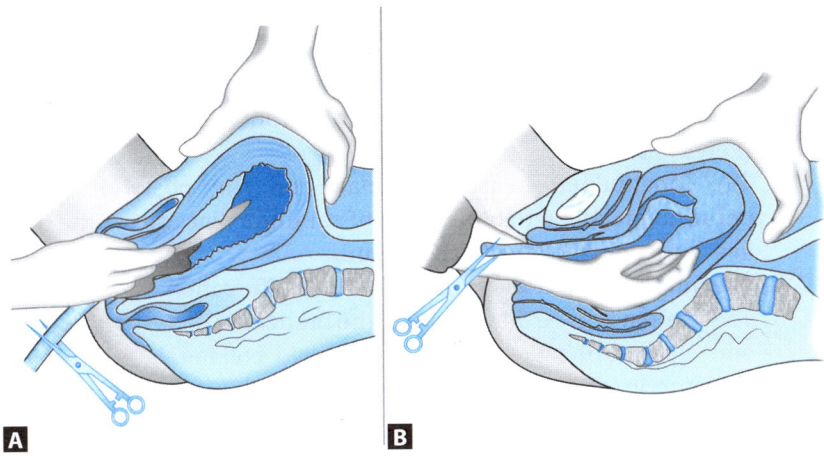

Figures 3.24A and B: Manual removal of placenta (MROP): (A) Introduction of hand for MROP; (B) Detaching the placenta

8. Follow the umbilical cord till the internal hand (right) reaches the cervical canal.
9. Keep the other hand (left) on the mother's abdomen to steady the uterus and internal fingers of right hand are introduced in the uterine cavity.
10. Locate the edge of the placenta and insinuate the ulnar border of the right hand in between the placenta and uterine wall. By alternate side-to-side movement (abduction and adduction movement) of hand the placenta is gently separated from the inner wall of the uterus.
11. If the placenta does not separate from the uterine surface by gentle lateral movement of the finger tips at the line of cleavage, suspect placenta accreta and proceed to laparotomy and possible subtotal hysterectomy.
12. When entire placenta is separated and remains in the palm of the operator's hand, bring out the placenta and membrane.
13. With the other hand (left) continue to provide counter-traction to the fundus by pushing it in the opposite direction of the hand (right) that is being withdrawn.
14. Palpate the inside of the uterine cavity carefully to ensure that all placental tissue has been removed.
15. Continue oxytocin drip (20 units in 1 L of NS or RL at 60 drops/minute)
16. Examine the placenta carefully.
17. Watch P (pulse)/R (respiration rate)/T (temperature)/BP (Blood pressure)/ PV (Per vaginal) bleeding and uterine contraction.
18. Prophylactic antibiotics should be given for intrauterine manipulation
19. Check the birth canal for tear.

Q. What are the complications?

Ans. Hemorrhage, infection and perforation, shock, and acute inversion of uterus when placenta is adherent to the uterine wall.

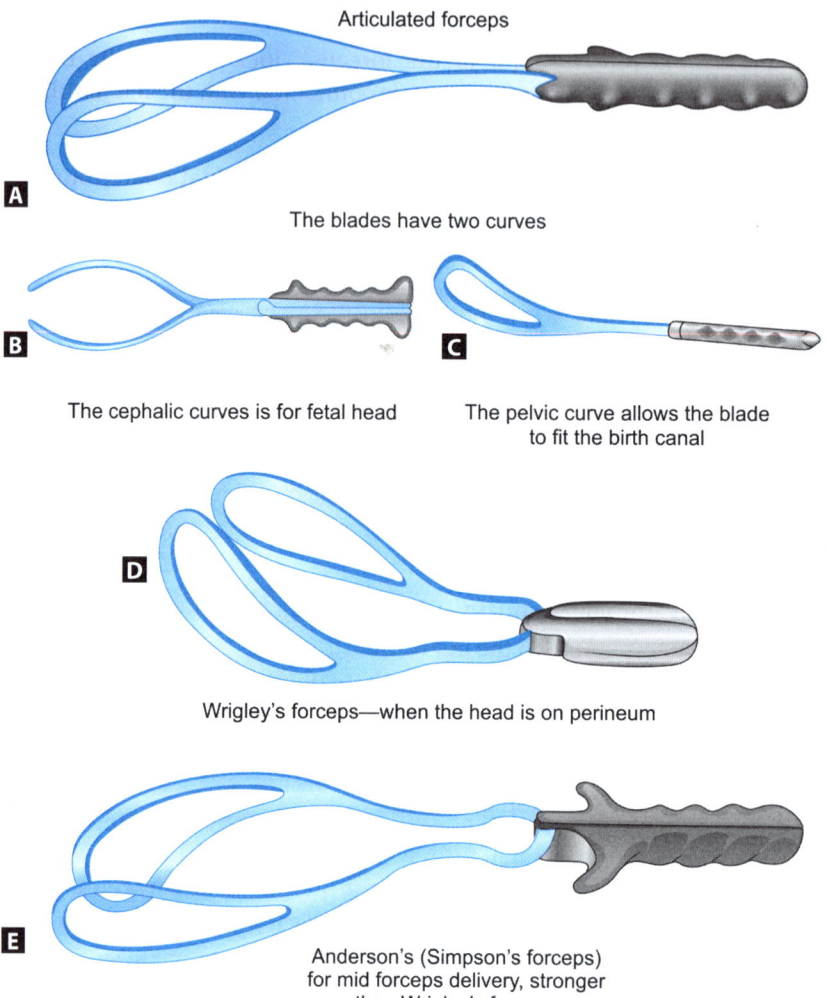

Figures 3.25A to E: Forceps: (A) Articulated forceps; (B) The cephalic curve is for fetal head; (C) The pelvic curve allows the blade to fit in the birth canal; (D) Wrigley's forceps: When the head is on perineum; (E) Anderson's (Simpson's forceps): For midforceps delivery, stronger than Wrigley's forceps

OBSTETRIC FORCEPS (FIGURES 3.25A TO E)

Q. What is this instrument?

Ans. Long-curved obstetric forceps/short-curved obstetric forceps according to the size of forceps.

Q. Who used forceps first?

Ans. A family doctor called Chamberlain.

Q. Have you seen the short-curved forceps?

Ans. Yes, that is the Wrigley's forceps.

Obstetric Operations and Interventions

Q. What are the different parts of forceps?

Ans. Blade, shank (gives length to the forceps), lock and handle but in midforceps (Das's forceps), a screw is connected with the left handle.

Q. Show me the curves of the blades and what is the length of the blade?

Ans. Cephalic curve: A curve, which fits well with the fetal head (four and half inch or 11.25 cm in radius) when articulated the curve allows the maximum space in the center (9.0 cm) for fetal head and at the tip 2.5 cm for fetal week.

Pelvic curve: A curve on the edge to fit in the cavity in the sacrum (7 inch or 17.5 cm in radius).

The length of the blade is 16 cm (Das's forceps).

Q. Why the blades are fenestrated?

Ans. a. To make the instrument lighter
b. Firm gripping of the head
c. Lesser compression of the head (0.5 cm).

Q. What is shank?

Ans. Metallic bar connecting the blade with the handle (L = 6.25 cm in Das's forceps; it gives length to the instrument).

Q. What are the different types of lock?

Ans. a. English—slot on each blade
b. French—pivot system
c. German—combination of the two.

Q. What is the length of the handle?

Ans. Length = 12.5 (Das's forceps).

Q. What is the length of the forceps?

Ans. Length is 37.5 cm or 15 inch (Das's forceps).

Q. How will you determine the right or left blade of forceps?

Ans. The cephalic curve faces medially, the pelvic curve faces upwards, the right and left blades of an obstetric forceps is are relation to the right and left side of maternal pelvis. In Das's forceps, the screw is placed on the left branch.

Q. What are the axis-traction devices?

Ans. a. Axis-traction rod (2) fitted with the notch at the lower part of fenestrated blade of long-curved forceps
b. Traction handle.

Q. Advantages of axis-traction mechanism.

Ans. Pulls the head along the axis of birth canal, so
a. Wastage of force is minimum
b. Advantage for beginners (pull is very easy)
c. A little unrotation of head is corrected automatically.

Q. Describe the axis-traction handle and points for identification of the side.

Ans. Each axis-traction handle has three curvatures (i.e. two vertical and one horizontal). The horizontal curve is in the middle. There are two knobs, upper knobs faces medially and fits into the notch at the lower part of fenestrated blade, while the lower knob faces forward and attaches with the traction handle and a groove lies laterally. During the process of traction the horizontal part of each axis traction rod should remain parallel with the shank of the forceps.

Q. Is axis traction rod necessary for forceps delivery?

Ans. When the head is high in the pelvis delivery is easier by axis traction rod as the pull is in the axis of the pelvis and a minimum of force is lost against the pubes. But high operation is replaced by cesarean section. True axis traction becomes progressively less important when the head is lower in the pelvis or nearer to the pelvic floor.

Q. What is the history of forceps?

Ans. Chamberlain brothers (Peter I and Peter II) invented the obstetric forceps in 1569. This was a family secret for 200 years. The original forceps had only cephalic curve. Levert (1747) introduced the pelvic curve. Smellie introduced English lock on the forceps blade. The axis traction device was introduced by Tarnier (1877).

Q. What are the types of forceps delivery?

Ans. According to American College of Obstetricians and Gynecologists (ACOG) Society:

Outlet forceps: The fetal skull reaches the perineal floor, the scalp is visible in between contraction, the sagittal suture is in the anteroposterior (AP) diameter or in the right or left occiput anterior (OA) or occiput posterior (OP), but not more than 45° from midline.

Low forceps: The leading edge of the skull is at +2 (in cm) or more. Rotation is divided in < 45° or > 45°.

Midforceps: The head is engaged, but the leading edge of the skull is above +2 (in cm) station.

High forceps: Not included in this classification.

Q. What are the common indications of forceps delivery?

Ans.
a. Fetal distress in second stage of labor
b. Maternal distress in second stage of labor
c. To cut short the second stage of labor as in eclampsia, pregnancy-induced hypertension (PIH), post-CS pregnancy, postmaturity, prematurity, patient under epidural analgesia, heart disease
d. After coming head of breech, face, POP position.

> **Note**
> For nulliparous the prolonged second stage is defined as >3 hours with or >2 hours without regional anesthesia; in parous women, it is defined as >2 hours with and >1 hour without regional anesthesia.

Obstetric Operations and Interventions

Q. What is 'prophylactic' forceps?

Ans. Forceps delivery to shorten the second stage of labor when maternal and fetal complications are anticipated. It prevents the mother from straining of bear down effect.

Indications—see the answer of the above question under "c".

Q. Have you seen to apply forceps in labor room?

Ans. Yes.

Q. In which condition have you seen?

Ans. Fetal distress in second stage of labor.

> **Note**
> *Prepare for any questions on fetal distress.*

Q. Conditions that must be fulfilled for forceps application.

Ans. There must be legitimate indication of forceps delivery in perspective of mother and fetus.
 a. Bladder should be empty*.
 b. Full dilatation of cervical os.
 c. Cervix must be fully taken up.
 d. Head must be engaged
 e. Membrane is ruptured.
 f. Sagittal suture must be on AP diameter of pelvis.
 g. Presence of normal uterine contraction and relaxation.
 h. Pelvis should be adequate.
 i. FHS +.

Remember the word FORCEPS (+): F—Full dilatation of cervical os and fully taken up of cervix, O—Occiput should be anterior and engaged, R—Rupture of membrane, C— Contraction of uterus should be normal, E—Evacuation of the bladder, P—Pelvis should be adequate, S—Sagittal suture must be on AP diameter of Pelvis, FHS +.

Q. How will you apply forceps?

Ans.
 a. Informed consent for forceps delivery is to be taken
 b. Assemble the forceps and take the left blade first and lubricate it (Figure 3.26A)
 c. Catheterization of bladder must be done
 d. Episiotomy after pudendal block/local infiltration anesthesia (2% Xylocaine) is to be made

Two methods of applying forceps:
 a. *Cephalic method*: The blades are applied on either side of BPD for better grip.
 The ear lies at the center of fenestra of the forceps and causes least compression on BPD.
 b. *Pelvic method*: Here the forceps blades are applied with reference to the maternal pelvis on either side and it may cause trauma to the fetal head. Not popular nowadays.

---

* Low or mid forceps do not generally cause bladder injury, but it should be evacuated before application of forceps for prevention of PPH following delivery, as full bladder may aggravate atonic PPH and empty bladder causes uterine contraction and prevents PPH.

Application of blades:
   i. Put on a pair of high-level disinfected sterile gloves and insert two fingers of right hand in the vagina on the side of fetal head. The handle of left blade is taken lightly by left index, middle and thumb in a pen-holding manner and is held vertically almost parallel to the right inguinal ligament. Now, slide the left blade gently between the head and fingers inside the vagina manipulated by thumb to the left lateral wall of pelvis so that it rests on the side of fetal head in front of left ear of the fetus (Figure 3.26B).
   ii. Repeat the same procedure on the other side by sliding the operator's left hand into the pelvis and using right blade of forceps (Figure 3.26C).

Q. How do you know the blades are correctly applied (Figures 3.28)?

Ans. i. The blade should be overparietal eminence
   ii. The shank must be in contact with the perineum
   iii. Superior surface of the handle should be directed upwards.

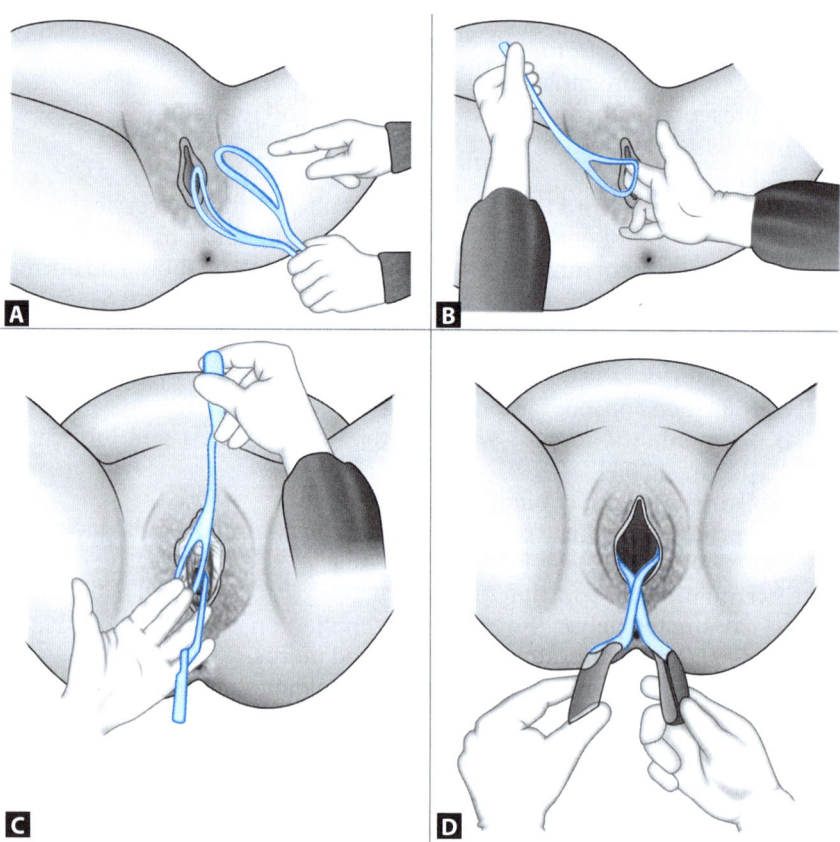

Figures 3.26A to D: (A) Assembling of forceps before application; (B) Introduction of left blade; (C) Application of right blade; (D) Locking of the blades

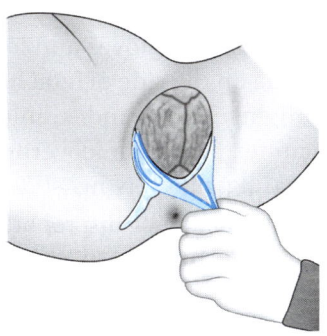

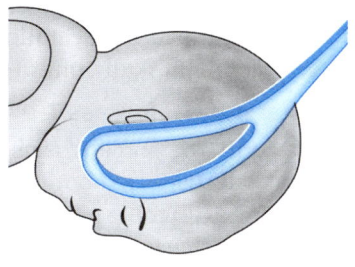

Figure 3.27: Gentle traction with an episiotomy

Figure 3.28: Correct application of forceps (mentovertical line)

Locking of the blade (Figure 3.26D):
  i. Depress the handle and lock the blades
  ii. Difficulty in locking usually indicates that the application is incorrect. Remove the forceps; recheck the position and reapply, only if rotation is confirmed.

Traction and removal of blades (Figure 3.27):
  The traction is given by gripping the handle with the middle finger in between shank and ring and index finger on either side. The low forceps or midforceps operation (2–3 pulls):
  i. The direction of pull downwards and backwards until the head comes to the perineum.
  ii. Pull is then directed downwards (horizontally) straight to the operator till the head is crowned.
  iii. Then pull 'upwards and forwards' towards mother's abdomen to deliver the head by extension.
  iv. In outlet forceps operation, the direction of pull is straight horizontal and then upwards and forwards towards the mother's abdomen.
  v. The blades are removed one after another, right blade is removed first.

Q. What are the complications of forceps delivery?

Ans. *Maternal*
  a. *Injury*: Soft tissue injury like vaginal/cervical tears, laceration, extension of episiotomy wound and third degree perineal tear, in rare cases, separation of pubic symphysis occurs, if it is applied in contracted pelvis.
  b. *PPH*: Traumatic, atonic and ruptured uterus.
  c. *Shock*: Blood loss, pelvic hematoma, prolonged labor and dehydration.
  d. Anesthetic complications.
  e. *Remote*: Chronic backache, genital prolapse and stress urinary.
  Incontinence (SUI) or anal incontinence.
  Fetal
  a. Birth asphyxia or death
  b. Intracranial hemorrhage
  c. Cephalhematoma

d. Facial palsy
e. Laceration of the face and scalp tissues or bruising
f. Scalp and facial lacerations
g. Fracture of skull bones.

Q. What is 'Trial forceps'?

Ans. The term 'trial forceps' is used when the forceps delivery is attempted in a case of suspected borderline mid pelvic contraction or disproportion keeping everything ready for LSCS. If moderate traction fails to overcome the resistance for descent forceps, blades are removed and go for CS.

Q. What is 'failed forceps'? How do you manage this condition?

Ans. Unsuccessful attempts to deliver the baby vaginally by forceps operation.
Forceps failed, if:
- If fetal head does not advance with each pull
- Fetus is undelivered after three pulls with no descent or after 30 minutes.

Causes
1. *Failure in application:* The criteria of forceps delivery is not fulfilled properly
2. *Failure in traction and delivery:* Wrongly directed traction, CPD, absence of uterine contraction, undiagnosed brow, hydrocephalus, fetal ascites, constriction ring.
3. *Wrong Choice of Forceps*

Prevention
- Proper selection of case and forceps
- No forcible traction.

Management
The patient should be managed in a well-equipped hospital.
a. Senior person is called to manage the case
b. Start IV line
c. Injection antibiotics
d. Formulate plan of delivery:
   1. LSCS, if baby is living
   2. Craniotomy, if baby is dead
   3. Ruptured uterus—laparotomy.

Q. How do you apply forceps in after coming head of breech (Figure 3.29)?

Ans. The forceps can be applied to the head once the head enters the pelvis and hair line at the nape of the neck is visible at the introitus. The trunk of the baby is lifted upwards and held by an assistant, the long-curved forceps are applied from below. The left blade is held in the left hand and is placed to the left side of maternal pelvis by the guidance of right thumb in between head and fingers. The right blade is placed on the opposite side and the blades are locked so that it occupies occipitomental diameter, one over each ear. The direction of pull is downward then forward and finally upward along the curve of Carus. This rolls the face over perineum, while occiput remains beneath the symphysis pubis until brow delivers, then the forceps, body and legs of fetus are raised together to complete the delivery of head. Forceps prevents the extension of head on neck.

Obstetric Operations and Interventions

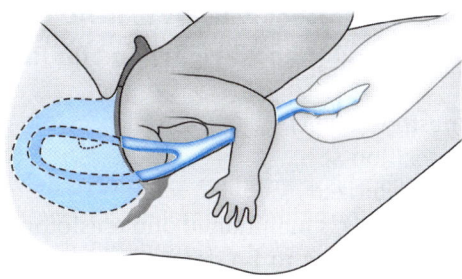

Figure 3.29: Forceps in after coming head of breech

Q. How do you apply forceps in a case of face presentation?

Ans. In face presentation (mentoanterior), the forceps may be applied direct. The pull is directed downwards, till the submentum hinges under the symphysis pubis, then the pull is directed upwards and forwards till the occiput is delivered (Figures 3.30).

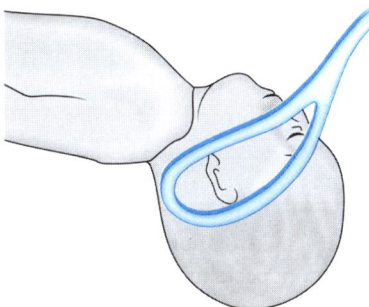

Figure 3.30: Forceps in mentoanterior (face)

Q. How will you deliver the head in a case of POP position?

Ans. The head is directed in the occiput posterior position and the head is low in the pelvis. Following a wide episiotomy (mandatory), the forceps is applied and first pull the head directly downwards until the bridge of nose hinges under the symphysis pubis, then the pull should be upward and forward to deliver the occiput and lastly downwards to deliver the face (Figure 3.31).

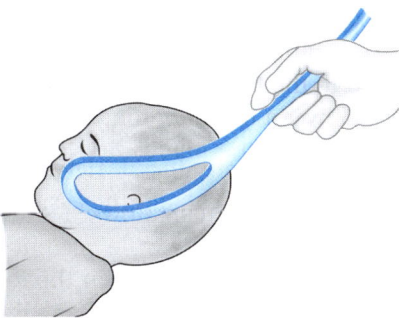

Figure 3.31: Forceps in persistent occipitoposterior position (POP)

Q. Manual rotation and forceps delivery in ROP.

Ans. I. Whole Hand Method (Choose right hand for ROP) (Figure 3.32)

Steps:
a. General anesthesia (GA)
b. Lithotomy position
c. Bladder is catheterized
d. Full surgical asepsis is maintained and episiotomy is made
e. Vaginal examination is to be done to find out occiput, if caput is formed the direction of unfolded pinna points towards occiput.

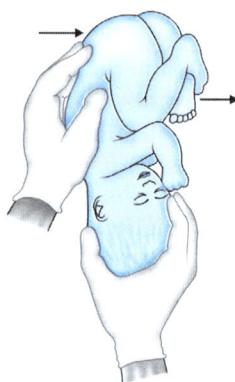

Figure 3.32: Manual rotation by whole hand method in right occipitoposterior (ROP)

Gripping of the Head
The fingers should be introduced in a cone-shaped manner. Four fingers of the pronated right hand are kept over the sinciput and thumb on the occiput. The hand is to be rotated by supination.

Rotation of the Head
a. Slight disimpaction for sufficient grip
b. Maintain flexion of the head
c. By movement of supination the right hand is rotated to bring the occiput anterior along the shortest route
d. Simultaneously, the back of the fetus is rotated by external hand from flank to the midline
e. A slight overcorrection is desirable.

Application of Forceps
After rotation, the right hand is placed on the left side of the pelvis and left blade of forceps is introduced, right blade is used in a usual manner. While introducing the blades the assistant will fix the head by suprapubic pressure.

Difficulties
a. Failure to grip the head
b. Failure to dislodge the head.

Obstetric Operations and Interventions

Dangers
During disimpaction, the fetal head may go above pelvic brim and cord may be prolapsed. Cesarean section is then the answer.

II. Half Hand Method
In this method, 4 fingers are into the vagina excepting the thumb. In ROP and ROT, the fingers are placed anterior to the head and pressure is applied by ulnar border of right hand on the side of parietal eminence tangentially (In LOT, the fingers are placed posterior and pressure is applied on the parietal bone by radial border of the hand).

Advantages:
a. Less chance of disimpaction
b. Can be manipulated by small hand

Disadvantage: Where disimpaction is needed discard the half hand method.

Q. How will you go for manual rotation and forceps delivery in LOP?

Ans. Fingers of the left hand are introduced in the same fashion (like manual rotation in ROP) and after rotation of the head, the left hand remains on the right side of the pelvis. So right blade of the forceps is introduced first and left blade is negotiated below the right blade otherwise locking of forceps will be difficult.

Q. What is Scanzoni-Smellie maneuver?

Ans. The double application of forceps, which is not used commonly for forceps rotation and forceps delivery in occipitoposterior position.

Principle
a. First application of the blades of forceps are to the sides of the head with the pelvic curve towards the face of the fetus.
b. In second application of pelvic curve is directed towards the occiput.

For first application:
 i. The right hand is passed into the vagina posteriorly to feel the rearear.
 ii. The left blade is applied over the ear held in position by assistant.
 iii. The operator's left hand is pushed in the right side of vagina to control the introduction of right blade.
 iv. It then rotated anteriorly until it lies over the left ear and opposite to the first blade.
 v. The forceps are then locked and handle elevated to flex the fetal head, dislodge the head very slightly upward and rotation in clockwise direction. This serves to rotate the head about occipitomental diameter.
 vi. Once the occiput is rotated anteriorly it is necessary to remove and reapply the forceps as described for OA delivery.

For second application:
 i. The forceps are then unlocked and the branch now on the left side of pelvis right branch is removed by pulling the handle downwards and inwards.
 ii. Other branch is held in position during the maneuver to stabilize the head in OA position.

iii. The right branch is now inserted immediately after the remaining branch has been removed. During this time, the occiput typically move to right occiput anterior (ROA). The left blade should be introduced below the right blade for easy locking.

Q. What is the function of forceps?

Ans.
a. Traction (most important)
b. Compression
c. Rotation of head
d. Protection of head from pressure of parturient canal
e. Delivery of head.

> **Note**
> In multigravida, the pull required in 13 kg and in primigravida is in 18 kg.

VENTOUSE

Vacuum is a method of delivery of fetal head using a traction device by creating a vacuum between it and the scalp (Figure 3.33).

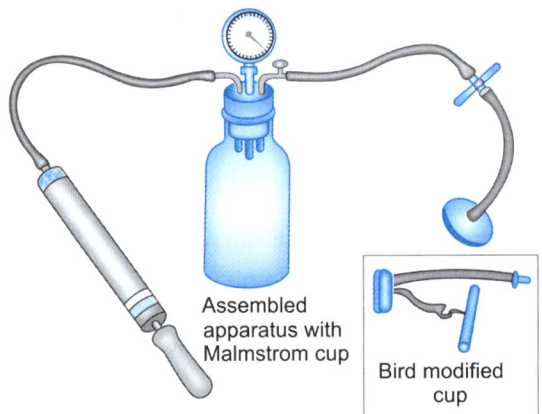

Figure 3.33: Essential components of ventouse

Q. What are the different parts of this instrument?

Ans.
a. Metallic cup (6 cm, 5 cm, 3 cm)—edges of the cup are inverted for firmer grip and artificial caput (chignon) formation and diameter varies from 40–60 mm.
b. Vacuum pump
c. Traction device.

Q. Character of silastic cup.

Ans. Soft cup is made of silastic material. The edges are soft and everted (no 'chignon' effect). The suction and traction ports are integrated into one port at the centre of the cup and this induces higher incidence of 'pop off' (disengagement of fetal head) due to lateral traction. Two sizes— 6 cm, 5 cm.

> **Note**
> Soft cup—Fewer neonatal scalp injury and higher failure rate.

Q. What are the indications of ventouse operation?
Ans.
a. Maternal exhaustion
b. Lack of advancement of head after 8 cm dilatation of cervix in a nulliparous woman
c. Prolonged second stage of labor
d. Deep transverse arrest (DTA) or OP (output posterior)
e. After an epidural analgesia
f. Delivery of head of second twin.

> **Note**
> Do not use in fetal distress as it takes a long time to build up the vacuum and delivery of the baby.

Q. What are contraindications?
Ans.
a. Fetal distress—as it takes more time to build up the vacuum
b. Face presentation/non-vertex presentation
c. Fetal coagulopathy
d. Premature baby.

Q. What are the conditions to be fulfilled?
Ans.
a. Cephalic presentation
b. Fetus in full term
c. Cervix is fully or at least more than 8 cm dilated
d. Unrotated fetal head at the perineum or at least at '0' station or no more than 2/5th above the symphysis pubis
e. Bladder must be empty
f. No bony resistance below the head.

Q. How do you operate ventouse?
Ans. *Pre-requisites:*
a. There should be legitimate indication of ventouse delivery
b. Check all connections and test the formation of vacuum on gloved hand
c. Provide encouragement to the patient
d. Episiotomy—after perineal infiltration of local anesthesia
e. Good uterine contraction and effective bearing down effort is required
f. Largest cup is used (for lesser chances of cup pop-off).

Application of cup (Figures 3.34 and 3.35A to F.)
a. Put the patient in lithotomy position
b. Aseptic P/V examination to assess the position of fetal head by filling sagittal suture and fontanelle
c. Identify posterior fontanelle

d. Separate the labia with left thumb and index finger and insert cup in transverse manner
e. Apply the largest cup, with the center of the cup over the sagittal suture, 3 cm in front of posterior fontanelle. This placement promotes flexion, descent and autorotation with traction
f. In case of metallic cup, the knob will face towards the occiput.

> **Note**
> *Anterior placement near the anterior fontanelle will aggravate deflexion and asymmetrical placement relative to sagittal suture will aggravate asynclitism.*

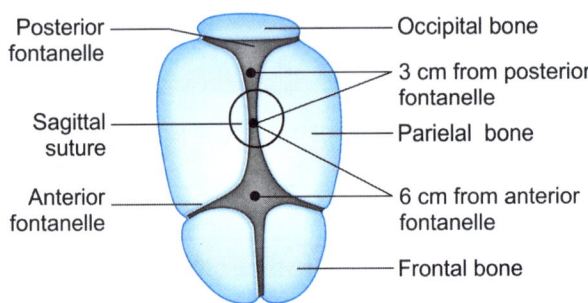

Figure 3.34: Landmark of fetal skull and suture lines and pivot point

g. Cranial flexion or pivot point—Imaginary spot on sagittal suture of fetal skull, located approximately 6 cm posterior to the centre of anterior fontanels or 3 cm anterior to posterior fontanels. Because the cup diameter is 5–6 cm when properly placed, the cup rim lies 3 cm from anterior fontanel. The centre of vacuum is positioned in cranial flexion or pivot point.
h. Check the application and ensure that no soft tissue (cervix/vagina) is entrapped between the cup and fetal head.

Creation of vacuum
- Connect the cup to the suction machine
- An initial vacuum of 0.1 kg/cm^2 negative pressure is made
- In case of metallic cup—a vacuum of 0.2 kg/cm^2 is induced by hand pump slowly taking at least 2 minute then the negative pressure gradually raised at the rate of 0.1 kg/cm^2 until it reaches to 0.8 kg/cm^2 in about 10 minutes (to give time for chignon formation and expand into the cup) **(Figure 3.35A)**.

Traction (Figures 3.35C to E):
a. After achieving maximum negative pressure, traction is given at right angle to the cup initially downwards and then extended upwards as the head emerges.
b. Traction should be synchronous with the uterine contraction and maternal expulsive efforts.
c. The cup is held on the hand with the left hand as traction is applied with right hand.
d. If there is no advancement during four successive uterine contractions, it is to be abnormal.
e. Duration of traction should never exceed over 30 minutes.

Obstetric Operations and Interventions

> **Note**
> *If the fetal head is tilted to one side or not flexed well, traction should be directed in a line that will help in correcting the tilt or deflexion of head (i.e. to one side or to other, not necessarily in midline).*

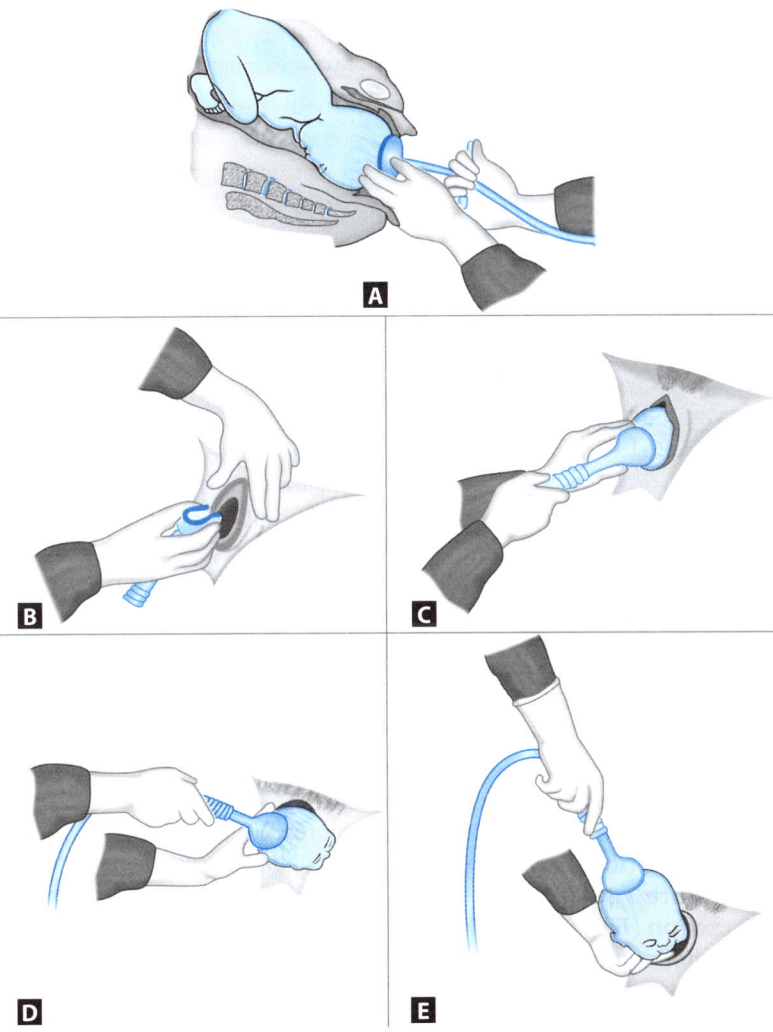

Figures 3.35A to E: (A) Applying traction by metallic cup; Silastic cup: (B) After application of antiseptic solution to the cup, the edges of the cup are carefully folded in to diminish the diameter and then inserted into the vagina; (C) Traction is given in the axis of the birth canal during uterine contraction, resulting the descent of fetal head; (D) By placing the thumb on the cup and index finger on the fetal scalp, traction force is monitored; (E) Delivery of the head

f. Between contraction check:
    i. Fetal heart rate (FHR)
    ii. Position of cup
g. If the cup slips more than twice, do not apply again.
h. Once head is extracted cup is removed by relieving vacuum pressure and complete vaginal delivery.

Q. When will you call the vacuum extraction has failed?

Ans. Vacuum extraction fails, if:
a. The head does not descend with each pull.
b. The head is undelivered after 3 pull with no descent or after 30 minutes of operation.
c. If the cup slips off the head twice with maximum negative pressure and proper direction of pull.

Q. If vacuum extraction fails what will you do?

Ans. Perform CS.

Q. What are the complications of delivery procedures?

Ans. *Mother:*
a. Avulsion of cervix/vaginal tissue, if such is entrapped in cup and fetal head
b. Vaginal, cervix or perineal tear
c. Vaginal hematoma.

Fetus:
a. Localized scalp edema (or chignon formed by metallic cup)—disappear in a few hours without treatment.
b. Injury of the scalp—abrasion, laceration, necrosis (rare).
c. Cephalhematoma—only observation requires 3 to 4 weeks to clear.
d. Intracranial hemorrhage.
e. Retinal hemorrhage.

> **Note**
> *Scalp injury and cephalhematoma are more common in metallic cup.*

Q. What are the advantages of vacuum over forceps?

Ans.
a. It is used when rotation of vertex is not proper
b. Can be applied in incompletely dilated cervix (smaller cup)
c. Less traction (10 kg)
d. Can be used safely when head of second twin is high up
e. Can be used safely in a cardiac patient in lateral position
f. Requires less technical skill.

Q. Advantage of forceps over ventouse.

Ans.
a. Forceps is safer in premature baby
b. It can be applied in face and after coming head of breech presentations
c. It can be used in acute fetal distress
d. Less costly and handy.

Obstetric Operations and Interventions

Q. What are the contraindications of instrumental delivery?

Ans. a. Fetal bone demineralization disorder
  b. Fetal bleeding disorders
  c. Unengaged fetal head (forceps is contraindicated)
  d. Vacuum delivery—pregnancy of <34 weeks of gestation.

Q. How do you deliver the head by silastic ventouse cup?

Ans. See Figures 3.35B to E.

VERSION

External Version

Q. What is external cephalic version (ECV)?

Ans. Manipulation is to be done usually before the onset of labor to convert a transverse or oblique lie or breech into cephalic presentation by abdominal route.

Q. Indications of ECV.

Ans. a. Breech is turned to cephalic
  b. Transverse lies to cephalic or podalic.

Q. What is the time of ECV?

Ans. Do not perform the procedure in less than 37 weeks as at or about 37 weeks of GA, the survival rate of baby is better after delivery and likely-hood of spontaneous version is low.

Q. (a) Can ECV be performed at 32 to 34 weeks? (b) What are the complications of ECV?

Ans. a. No, because baby may revert to breech position again
  b. Maternal and fetal complications such as premature rupture of membranes (PROM), Preterm labor, antepartum hemorrhage (APH), cord entanglement, umbilical cord prolapse, fetomaternal hemorrhage and rupture of uterus, may occur and baby is preterm to survive.

Q. What are the pre-requisites of ECV?

Ans. a. Single live fetus at 37 weeks or later
  b. Baby is of moderate size
  c. No IUGR, malformed baby, placenta previa, uterine anomalies
  d. Adequate amount of liquor or normal AFI
  e. No evidence of contracted pelvis
  f. Fetal presenting part is not deeply engaged
  g. Reactive nonstress test (NST) prior to attempt or after the procedure.

Q. What are the contraindications of ECV?

Ans. a. Maternal diseases like heart disease, diabetes
  b. Multiple pregnancy
  c. IUGR, oligohydramnios
  d. BOH, placenta previa

e. Post-CS pregnancy
f. Elderly primigravida
g. Hypertension, PIH
h. Rh-negative mother
i. Nonreactive NST or fetal heart rate tracing.

Q. Techniques of ECV.

Ans.
a. Informed consent must be taken
b. Woman should lie on back and foot end elevated
c. Note basal fetal heart rate (FHR)
d. Palpate abdomen to confirm presentation
e. Mobilization of breech—gently lift the lowest part from the pelvic inlet by grasping above the pubic bone (Figure 3.36A)

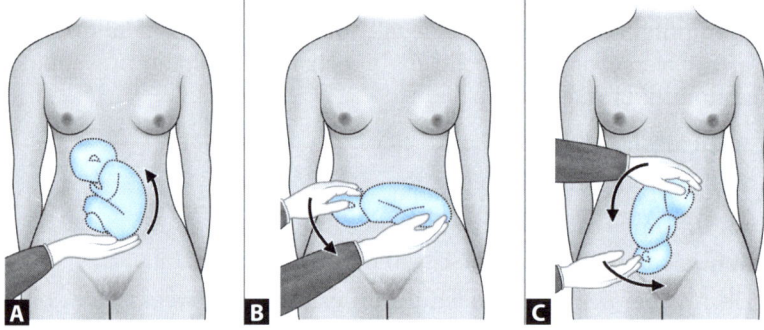

Figures 3.36A to C: External cephalic version (steps)

f. Move the breech to one iliac fossa towards the side of fetal back, the fetal head downwards towards the pelvic brim by maintaining flexion (Figure 3.36B).
g. After the fetus is brought to transverse position the hands are interchanged over the fetal poles and ECV is completed (Figure 3.36C).
h. Note the FHR, if an abnormality is detected:
  i. Turn the woman on left side.
  ii. Start oxygen 4 to 6 liter/minute by mask or nasal catheter
  iii. Reassess every 15 minutes
i. If procedure is successful:
  i. The woman should lie for another 15 minutes
  ii. Counsel her to return, if bleeding PV or pain occurs
j. If the procedure is still unsuccessful and FHR is good, version is tried under tocolytics (terbutaline 250 µg IV over 5 minutes or salbutamol 0.5 mg IV over 5 minutes)
k. If the procedure is still unsuccessful, attempt of the version after 1 week should be tried.

Q. If FHR abnormality persists, what will you do?

Ans.
a. Turn the woman on the left side
b. Reassess the FHR every 5 minutes
c. If FHR does not stabilize within next 30 minutes delivery by CS.

Internal Podalic Version (IPV) (Figure 3.37)

Q. What is IPV?

Ans. It is the procedure of conversion of fetal presentation from a transverse or cephalic presentation to the podalic presentation by intrauterine manipulation as well as abdominal maneuver.

Q. What is the indication?

Ans. In modern obstetrics, it has only one indication to deliver the second twin in a transverse lie when ECV fails. This is followed by breech extraction.

Other indications:
 i. Transverse lie with full dilatation of cervix and external cephalic version fails
 ii. Transverse lie with cord prolapse and fetal death in fully dilated cervix
 iii. Transverse lie with fetal malformation incompatible with life.

Q. What are the pre-requisites?

Ans. a. Cervix is almost fully dilated
 b. Presence of adequate amount of liquor
 c. Uterine relaxation persists in between contraction
 d. Membrane intact or just ruptured.

Q. What are the risks?

Ans. *Mother:*
 a. Injury to the cervix, vagina, perineum

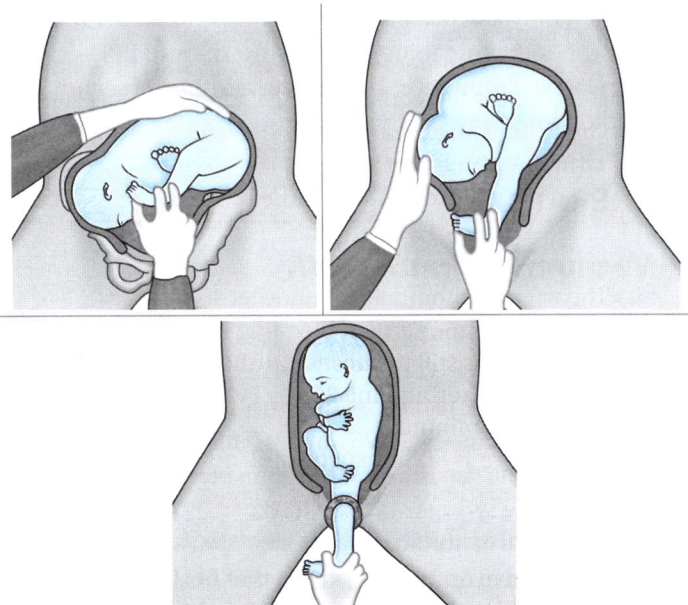

Figure 3.37: Internal podalic version (Different steps)

    b. Rupture of uterus
    c. PPH
    d. Hazards of emergency anesthesia.

Fetal: Fetal asphyxia, birth trauma, intracranial hemorrhage, fractures of limbs.

Q. What is the technique?

Ans.
a. IV infusion with Ringer lactate, blood grouping and cross-matching are necessary
b. Informed consent should be taken
c. Lithotomy position, antiseptic dressing and draping are required
d. Bladder should be evacuated by catheter
e. General anesthesia is preferable for uterine relaxation
f. Episiotomy is made
g. One hand is introduced in the uterine cavity and other hand steadies the uterine fundus (per abdomen)
h. The gloved hand is passed and identifies the fetal foot by moving along the back, buttock and thighs identify the ball of heel. Grasp the foot in between the index and forefingers and give gradual traction downward towards the pelvic inlet, and the other hand is kept on the fundus per abdomen for simultaneous assistance from above.
i. Pull the legs down the cervix and vagina and when knee is seen version is completed.
j. If cervix is fully dilated internal podalic version is followed by breech extraction and both the feet are brought down either simultaneously or one after other.
k. Manual removal of placenta is done and administer oxytocics.
l. Check the soft tissue injury, rupture uterus and PPH.
m. Prophylactic antibiotics should be administered for intrauterine manipulation.

OTHER OPERATIONS

Manual Vacuum Aspirator (MVA)

Q. Describe the instrument.

Ans. See the Figures 3.38A to C and 3.39.
1. It is a 60 cc syringe usually made with polyethylene with a capacity to hold a vacuum of 25–26 inches/600–650 mm of Hg which is equivalent to the vacuum created in an electric suction pump.
   The parts of the syringe are as follows:
   a. A barrel with calibrations
   b. A double valve or single valve set that fits to the tip of the barrel
   c. The tip of the syringe is fashioned to hold the cannula tight
   d. Plunger with arms that snap out when the plunger is pulled back

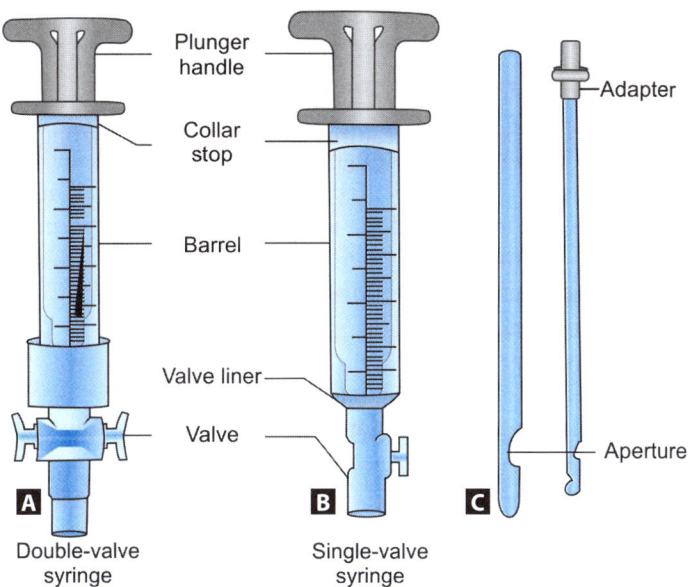

Figures 3.38A to C: (A) Double valve syringe; (B) Single valve syringe; (C) Cannula

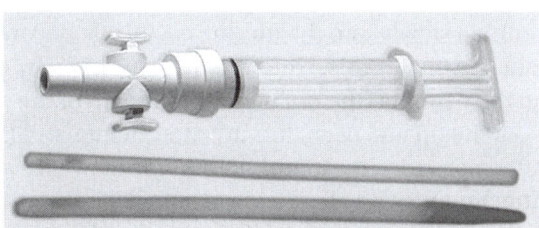

Figure 3.39: Equipment of MVA

    e. Collar-stop that hold and lock the plunger inside the syringe when fully pulled back out of the barrel
    f. Plunger O-ring
    g. Silicon for lubricating the O-ring.
2. Cannula—Flexible Karman's plastic cannula of sizes 4–12 mm (except 11) outside diameter corresponding to the period of gestation.

Each cannula has a closed-rounded tip with two opposing opening with an overlapping convex hood that acts as a curette.

Q. What are the indications of MVA?

Ans. MVA is recommended for termination of pregnancy up to 8 weeks of GA and also for management of incomplete abortion.

Q. Technique of MTP.

Ans. a. Counsel the client and ensure that the consent is obtained before the procedure

b. Ask the patient to evacuate the bladder
c. Give analgesia with pethidine (1 mg/kg BW but not more than 100 mg) IM or IV slowly or para cervical block
d. Preparation of MVA: (i) Assemble the syringe, (ii) Close the pinch valve, (iii) Pull back the plunger until its arms are locked
e. Preparation of the client: (i) Clean the perineum and vagina by antiseptic lotion or povidone iodine, (ii) Use clean perineal sheet, if available
f. Pelvic examination—To note size and position of uterus and condition of fornices.
g. *The procedure*:
   i. Insert the speculum gently in the vagina.
   ii. Clean the cervix with antiseptic solution starting with cervical os and then the surrounding area.
   iii. Hold the anterior lip of the cervix by Allis' tissue forceps and give steady traction.
   iv. Insertion of the cannula—Insert the cannula through the cervix into the uterine cavity just past the internal os by rotating the cannula while gently applying pressure. Start with cannula size 4 and gradually increase to the size that corresponds with the period of gestation.
   v. Measuring the uterine depth with cannula—Push the chosen cannula slowly into the uterine cavity just beyond the os until it touches the fundus. Note the uterine depth by the dots visible on the cannula (the dot nearest to the tip of the cannula is 6 cm from the tip and each dots are at 1 cm interval) (Figure 3.40).
   vi. After measuring the uterine depth withdraw the cannula slightly.
   vii. Attachment with the syringe—attach the prepared syringe to the cannula holding the Allis forceps and the end of the cannula

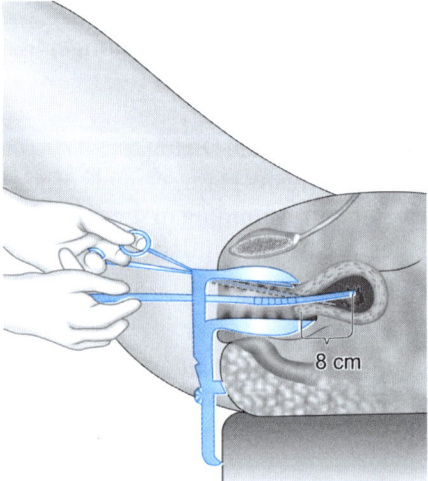

Figure 3.40: Measurement of uterine depth

Obstetric Operations and Interventions

in one hand and syringe in the other ensuring that the cannula does not move forward (Figure 3.41).

viii. Releasing the pinch valve—release the pinch valve on the syringe to release the vacuum into the uterine cavity. Bloody tissue and bubbles should begin to flow through the cannula into the syringe (Figure 3.42).

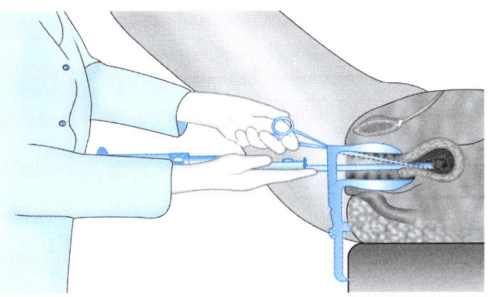

Figure 3.41: Attachment of cannula with syringe

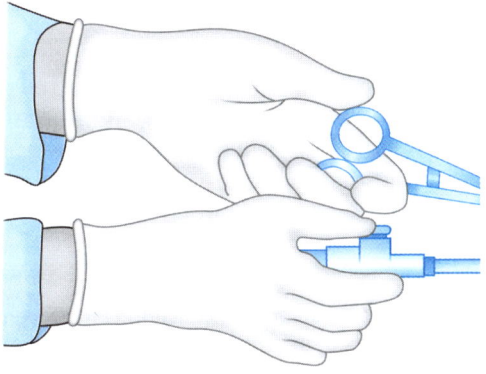

Figure 3.42: Releasing of pinch valve

ix. Evacuating the uterine contents—evacuate the remaining contents of the uterine cavity by gently rotating from side to side (10–12 o'clock) [do not rotate the cannula more than 180 degree) and then moving the cannula gently and slowly back and forth within the uterine cavity (Figure 3.43).

Ensure (i) The opening and openings on the cannula are not outside the cervical os, (ii) That the cannula is not pushed too much to avoid perforation, (iii) While the vacuum is well established and the cannula is in the uterus, ensure that the syringe is not grasped by plunger as it may cause the plunger arms to become unlocked and slide back into the syringe and push the contents into the uterus.

x. Check the signs of complete evacuation—(a) Red or pink foam and no more tissue seen in the cannula, (b) A gritty sensation is felt as the cannula passes over the surface of the evacuated

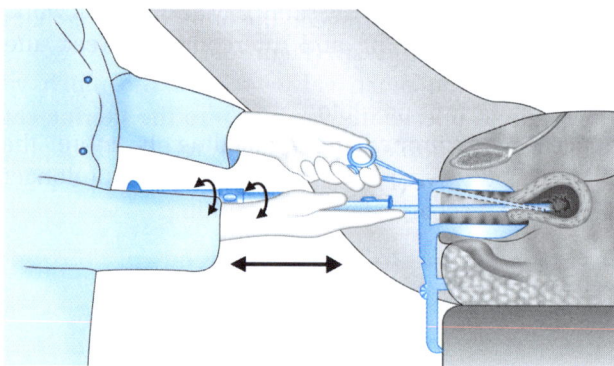

Figure 3.43: Evacuation of uterus

uterus, (c) The uterus contracts around the cannula (can feel the grip).

 xi. Withdraw the cannula and detach the syringe. Remove Allis forceps and speculum.

 xii. If evacuation is complete IUCD insertion as per national guideline.

Q. How do you confirm products of conception?

Ans. Strain and rinse the collected tissue to remove excess of blood clots, then place in a container of clean water, saline or weak acetic acid (vinegar) solution to examine. This will float like a tadpole. Tissue specimen will also be sent to pathology department, if indicated.

> **Note**
>
> *Absence of products of conception may indicate ectopic pregnancy.*

Q. What are the complications?

Ans. a. Complications of local anesthesia may be met.
  b. Complications of the procedure—excessive bleeding (due to cervical injury, incomplete emptying of uterus, uterine atony and perforation of uterus), and uterine perforation.
  c. Delayed complications—incomplete evacuation, continuation of pregnancy, infection.
  d. Remote complications—complications may occur during future pregnancy (adherent placenta, uterine rupture due to previous undiagnosed perforation), psychomotor symptoms, recurrent mid-pregnancy abortions, ectopic pregnancy, infertility, amenorrhea due to Ashermann's syndrome.

Q. Postoperative instructions.

Ans. a. Uterine cramps for a few days (T/T-NSAID)
  b. Some spotting or bleeding not more than usual period
  c. Natural menstruation will come back within 4–6 weeks

Obstetric Operations and Interventions

d. Resume—normal diet on the same day and normal work next day.
e. Avoid—vaginal douching and intercourse a week after bleeding stops.
f. Start OCP as early as possible.
g. Contact doctor immediately—bleeding is more than normal menstrual flow, severe lower abdominal pain, prolonged bleeding, foul-smelling discharge, fever, and fainting.

Q. Do you know first trimester (<7 weeks) medical abortion by drugs?

Ans. Yes.

Q. Which drugs are used and mention the dose schedule?

Ans. Standard dose is mifepristone 200 mg orally followed by 400 mcg misoprostol oral/vaginal.
First day (Day 1): Tablet mifepristone 200 mg orally.
Second day (Day 2–3): Two tablets of misoprostol (2 × 200 µg = 400 µg) orally/vaginally.
Third visit (Day 15): To ensure that the abortion is complete.

> **Note**
> Miferine kit contains one tablet of mifepristone 200 mg and 4 tablets of misoprostol [200 µg each, four tablets (800 µg) either oral or sublingual or per vaginal use at the same sitting].
> Chances of incomplete abortion are low (2%), Success rate 90–98%; failure rate 1–3%.
> Misoprostol is teratogenic. So there must be commitment to complete the abortion once the drug has been used.

Q. What are the contraindications of medical abortion?

Ans.
a. Anemia (Hb < 8 g%)
b. Suspected/confirmed ectopic pregnancy or undiagnosed mass
c. Uncontrolled hypertension (BP >160/100 mm of Hg)
d. Cardiovascular diseases like angina, valvular heart disease, arrhythmia
e. Severe liver, renal and respiratory disorder
f. Coagulopathy or the patient is under anticoagulant therapy
g. Uncontrolled seizure disorder.

Q. What are the common side effects of the drugs used for early termination of pregnancy?

Ans. Nausea, vomiting, pain lower abdomen, bleeding, diarrhea, chills, headache, dizziness and fatigue.

Q. Choice between medical and surgical abortions?

Ans.
a. MVA is used for termination of pregnancy, if GA is < 8 weeks. As it is a surgical procedure, it may be associated with risks of infection, perforation of uterus, incomplete abortion, and uterine synechiae.
b. Medical abortion by mifepristone and misoprostol is favorable (95%), if pregnancy is <7 weeks (49 days), but it may be used for

induction of abortion up to 9 weeks and success rate depends upon multiple factors such as the regimes used, dosage schedule, and route of administration and side effect of the drugs.
  c. MVA is a quick procedure but medical abortion takes longer time for total completion and the blood loss is less in the former compared to the later, if it is uncomplicated.
  d. Surgical abortion is preferred, if patient wants concurrent ligation.
  e. First counseling of the patient about the procedures and final choice depends upon the patient's choice and also counsel the patient if there is failure of medical induction, continuation of pregnancy may be harmful.
  f. Medical abortion, if it is incomplete may end in surgical procedure.

Q. What is drug failure?

Ans. True drug failure (1–3%) means the presence of fetal cardiac activity 2 weeks following mifepristone and misoprostol administration or need of surgical intervention like surgical curettage and surgical evacuation for any reason as per decision of doctor.

Repair of Cervical Tear (Figures 3.44A and B)

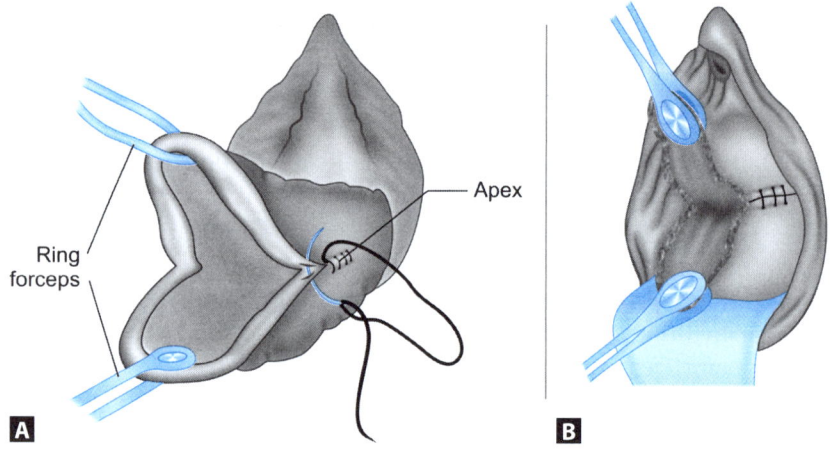

Figures 3.44 A and B: (A) Repair of cervical tear starting from apex; (B) Interrupted sutures applied

> **Note**
> After delivery, if the uterus is hard, well-contracted but profuse bleeding per vagina exists; think of maternal soft tissue injury.

Q. How do you identify the cervical tear?

Ans. a. Catheterize the bladder, if it is full.
  b. Gently grasp the cervix with sponge holding/ring forceps.

Obstetric Operations and Interventions

  c. Apply the forceps on both the sides of the tear and gently pull in various directions to see the entire cervix (Usually the tear is lateral).
  d. Ask the assistant to give fundal pressure.
  e. If the lateral tear is not visible, put the Sims speculum to retract the lateral vaginal wall and cervix is pulled in opposite direction.

Q. How do you repair cervical tear?

Ans. a. The tear is sutured with chromic—0 catgut or polyglycolic suture.
  b. Interrupted sutures are placed at 0.5 cm apart from the apex by taking full thickness of the cervix.
  c. Continuous suture starting from the apex may also be applied.
  d. If the apex is difficult to reach:
      i. Put stay suture below and go upward by traction and suture the upper edge of the tear.
      ii. If it is difficult, grasp the apex with artery forceps/ring forceps and leave the forceps for 4 hours *in situ*. After 4 hours, open the forceps partly but do not remove. After another 4 hours remove the forceps completely.
      iii. If it is extended deep into the vagina (beyond vaginal vault)—laparotomy is needed.

Paracervical Block (Figure 3.45)

Q. What are the indications?

Ans. a. Dilatation and curettage operation.
  b. MVA operation.

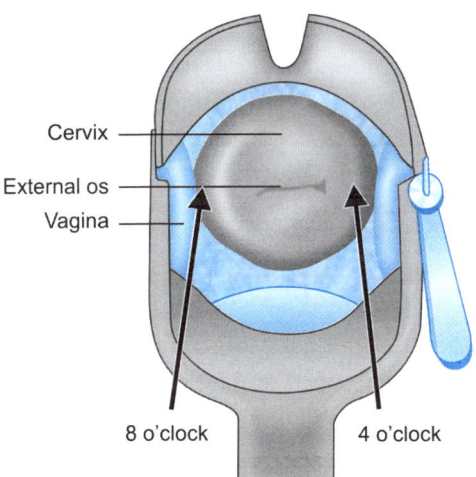

Figure 3.45: Paracervical block

Q. What is the procedure of paracervical block?

Ans. It is a simple effective procedure. Prepare 20 mL of 0.5% lignocaine solution without adrenaline and insert a 3.5 cm, 22 gauge needle to inject the lignocain solution into the mucosae of cervix not deeper than

3 mm at either 4- and 8 o'clock position and wait for 2–4 minutes for the effect of anesthesia.

Q. What are the complications?

Ans. Allergic reaction, hematoma at the site of injection (rare), convulsion and death, if IV injection of lignocain occurs.

Pudendal Block (Figures 3.46A and B)

Q. What are the indications?

Ans. a. Instrumental or breech delivery
b. Episiotomy and repair of perineal tears.

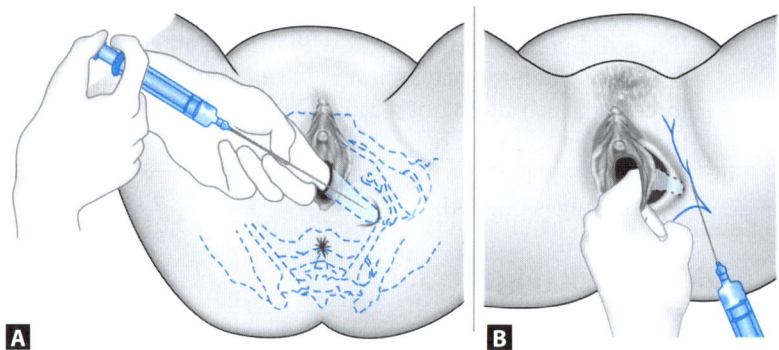

Figures 3.46 A and B: (A) Vaginal approach of pudendal block; (B) Perineal approach of pudendal block

Q. Procedure.

Ans. Prepare 40 mL of 0.5% lignocain solution without adrenaline and inject 30 mL of it by using a 15 cm, 22 gauge needle to block the pudendal nerve as it passes through the lesser sciatic notch. The rest 10 mL is used for perineal injection during repair of tears.

Approach:
1. Perineal approach—through the perineum
2. Vaginal approach—through the vagina, which requires a special needle guide (trumpet) for protection of the provider's finger:

Vaginal Approach (Figure 3.46A)
a. Use the left index finger to identify the left ischial spine through the vaginal wall.
b. Through a guide, by using the right hand, a needle is inserted in the vagina and directed laterally and posteriorly to the left ischial spine. Keep the finger tip near the end of the needle guide to avoid needle stick injury.
c. Place the needle just below the tip of the ischial spine.
d. The needle is penetrated through the vaginal mucosa and advanced into the sacrospinous ligament, where resistance is felt.

Obstetric Operations and Interventions

e. If aspiration is negative for blood, 3–5 mL of 0.5% lidocaine is injected and the needle is advanced for further 0.5–1 cm. If aspiration is again negative, 5–7 mL of solution is injected
f. The needle is withdrawn into the guide and reposition the guide, so that it is just above the ischial spine
g. Vaginal mucosa is penetrated and an aspiration of blood is again done, and if no blood is aspirated, inject 5 mL of lignocain solution.
h. A total of 10–15 mL is injected on each side. Approximately 10 minutes are required for anesthesia to occur
i. The same procedure is repeated on the other side
j. Infiltrate the perineal skin.

Perineal approach (Figure 3.46B):
First of all inject the perineal skin by xylocain solution on either side at a point between anus and ischial tuberosity. The index and middle fingers in the vagina guides the needle through the perineal tissue and identifies the ischial spine. Inject 10 mL of lignocain solution deep to the under margin of ischial spine. A further 5 mL is placed medial to the ischial tuberosity where pudendal nerve lies in the Alcock's canal. Then infiltrate the skin of perineum and labium majus beside vagina. The same procedure is repeated on the opposite side. Total amount of 0.5% lignocain injected should not exceed 40 mL.

Q. How do you avoid lignocain toxicity?

Ans.
a. Dilute solution is to be used (0.5%)
b. Addition of adrenalin when more than 40 mL of lignocain is used
c. Use lower effective dose
d. Observe maximum dose
e. Avoid IV injection.

Q. What is the maximum safe dose of lignocain?

Ans.

Drugs	Maximum dose (mg/kg body weight)	Maximum dose for 60 kg adult (mg)
• Lignocain	4	240
• Lignocain + adrenalin: 1:200,000 (5 µg/mL)	7	420

Q. How do you prepare lignocain of 0.5%?

Ans. Lignocain is commercially available as 2% or 1% strength and requires dilution before its use. The dilution should be made to 0.5% for most of the obstetric procedure and it gives maximum benefit with least toxicity.

Combine
 Lignocain 2%, one part
–Normal saline or sterile distilled water, three parts
or
–Lignocain 1% one part
–Normal saline/sterile distilled water, one part.

Q. What is the advantage of adding adrenalin with xylocain solution?

Ans. a. Less blood loss
b. Longer effect of anesthesia (1–2 hours)
c. Less risk of toxicity as the absorption is slower into the circulation.

> **Note**
> Adrenalin is necessary when more than 40 ml of local anesthesia is required for larger surface area to reduce the absorption rate and toxicity.

Q. How do you prepare 0.5% lignocain solution containing 1:200,000 adrenalin?

Ans.

Desired amount of local anesthesia	NS	Lignocain 2%	Adrenalin (1:1000)
20 mL	15 mL	5 mL	0.1 mL
40 mL	30 mL	10 mL	0.2 mL
100 mL	75 mL	25 mL	0.5 mL
200 mL	150 mL	50 mL	1.0 mL

> **Note**
> Normal saline (NS), insulin syringe should be used for accurate measurement of adrenaline.

Dextrose solution should not be used to dilute it for fear of infection.

Prenatal Diagnosis

A. Screening for chromosomal abnormalities (Downs' syndrome) is discussed in USG chapter
B. Screening for neural tube defects (NTDs).

Q. What is the most important marker for screening of neural tube defect?

Ans. Maternal serum alfafeto protein (MSAFP). In the USA, a screen positive cut-off 2.5 MoM (multiples of the median) is commonly used as a screen positive rate of approximately 5%.

> **Note**
> USG is very much necessary before MSAFP screening to verify the GA, multiple gestation, IUFD, and to improve the false positive rate.

Q. What is the time for screening of NTDs?

Ans. It should be optimally performed between 16–18 weeks of gestation but it can be done between 15–20 weeks.

Q. What are the conditions associated with the elevated MSAFP?

Ans. Open NTDs, sacrococcygeal teratoma, multiple gestation, ventral wall defects—Gastroschisis and omphalocele, esophageal and duodenal atresia, renal agenesis, congenital nephrosis, polycystic kidney disease, hydrops or ascites, LBW, cystic hygroma, placental leak, retroplacental hemorrhage and maternal hepatoma.

Obstetric Operations and Interventions

Q. What are the conditions associated with lower MSAFP?

Ans. Chromosomal trisomies, gestational trophoblastic diseases (GTDs), fetal death, increased maternal weight, overestimated gestational age.

> **Note**
> All women with MSAFP positive should have USG to rule out the risks of open neural tube defect and other fetal anomalies.

Q. What other tests are mandatory for MSAFP elevated cases?

Ans. USG to rule out certain risks mentioned above, amniotic fluid—for i. AFP (raised); ii. Acetyl cholinesterase (presence of which is diagnostic of fetal NTDs); iii. Cytogenetic analysis of amniocytes.

Q. What are the indications of invasive prenatal diagnostic testing?

Ans. Abnormal biochemical screening result, fetal anomaly diagnosed by USG, Increased nuchal translucency (> 3 mm), cystic hygroma, previous fetal/child chromosomal anomaly, parents are carrier of monogenic disorders like Tay-Scachs disease, huntington disease, myotonic dystrophy and on parent request for fetal karyotyping.

> **Note**
> Single gene disorder affects both sexes equally.

Q. What are the invasive prenatal diagnostic procedures?

Ans. Chorionic villus sampling, amniocentesis, percutaneous umbilical blood sampling.

1. Chorionic Villus Sampling (CVS)

Q. What are the indications of CVS?

Ans.
a. DNA analysis for diagnosis of single gene disorder without culture [Thalassemia major, hemophilia, Duchenne muscular dystrophy (DMD) (where males are affected, not the female when relevant gene is present on x-chromosome)].
b. Early karyotype (increased maternal age, previous aneuploidy, parental balanced trans location and fragile X-syndrome).
c. Biochemical enzyme study from cells for inherited metabolic disorder [Phenyl ketonuria, mucopolysaccharoidosis, Gaucher's disease, aminoaciduria].

Q. What is the timing of CVS?

Ans. About 8–12 weeks, however, the optimum time to perform the procedure is 11–12 weeks to minimize the teratogenic effect of CVS.

Q. What are the different techniques of CVS?

Ans.
a. *Transcervical:*
Under all aseptic precaution the flexible catheter is slowly introduced into the cervical canal and directed to the placental area under

continued USG guidance on the suprapubic area. The stylet is withdrawn and a 20 mL syringe containing 3 ml of heparinized culture media is attached to the free end of the catheter and suction is applied, to get 10–25 mg of villus material (20 mg sample is ideal for cytogenetic analysis, larger sample 20–40 mg of tissue may be required if direct molecular and biochemical studies are to be performed in addition to cytogenetic studies). Contents of catheter and syringe are flushed into petri dish and examined.

b. *Transabdominal:*
Aseptically, 18 or 20 gauze needle is passed into the long axis of the placenta under continuous USG guidance through the abdominal skin, uterus to the edge of the trophoblast. Thick part of the placenta away from the cord insertion is chosen and care should be taken not to pierce the amniotic sac. After removal of the stylet, villi are aspirated into the 20 mL syringe containing tissue culture media. Unlike transcervical CVS, transabdominal CVS can be performed throughout pregnancy.

> **Note**
> *Posterior placenta in a retroverted gravid uterus is especially amenable to transcervical approach whereas transabdominal approach would be preferable in all other cases involving anterior placenta in the anteflexed uterus and fundal placenta.*

CVS sample in culture media is transferred to genetic laboratory for analysis. The direct culture is done immediately by utilizing trophoblastic tissues (rapidly dividing cells). It is more error prone (mitotic error) and for additional risk of contamination by maternal tissue, the interpretation may be difficult. The second type of culture is a long-term culture by using mesenchymal core and is highly accurate. Maternal tissue around the villi is usually removed under dissecting microscope and DNA is extracted for single gene disorder. A PCR technique is used for detection of mutation on genes. Presence or absence of SRY-gene (specific to Y-chromosome) for detection of DMD.

> **Note**
> *Rh-negative patient should receive 100 µg of anti-D globulin.*

Q. What are the complications?

Ans. 1. Procedure-related complications:
  a. Infection (more common in transcervical route), bleeding and leaking per vagina
  b. Mild uterine cramp
  c. Abortion—2 %(0.5–1%)
  d. Limb defect—0.1%, when sampling is done in 56 and 63 days.

Obstetric Operations and Interventions

> **Note**
> A follow-up of USG should be done four days after CVS to ensure the fetal well-being.

2. *Diagnosis related complications*:
   a. Maternal cell contamination
   b. Chromosomal mosaicism (1–2%).

2. Amniocentesis

Q. What are the indications of amniocentesis?
Ans.
a. Maternal age >35 years
b. Birth of previous child with chromosomal defect, genetic metabolic disease, hemoglobinopathies, fetal malformation, hemophilia.
c. Family history of mental retardation, any other genetic disease and neural tube defect.
d. Congenital infections.
e. Spectrophotometric analysis of amniotic fluid bilirubin in Rh-isoimmunized mother.

Q. What is the exact timing of amniocentesis?
Ans. The ideal timing of amniocentesis is 16–18 weeks as the amniotic fluid volume is sufficient (200–250 mL) and viable amniotic fluid cells are greatest. Some of the centers also offer early amniocentesis at 11–14 weeks of gestation for prenatal diagnosis and in case of detection of any abnormality MTP may be done easily. Sometime, amniocentesis is also done in third trimester to note fetal lung maturity (L/S ratio), uterine infections, and fetal anemia.

Q. What are the disadvantages of early amniocentesis?
Ans. In early amniocentesis lesser amount of fluid is taken, technically difficult, lesser number of amniocytes should be available for diagnostic purpose, increased rate of fluid leak, and chances of pulmonary complications are high. Besides, the incidence of hip dislocation, RDS, neonatal pneumonia is also very high.

Q. Procedure?
Ans. Under USG guidance a 22–23 G spinal needle is introduced aseptically through maternal abdomen into the amniotic sac and 15–20 mL of amniotic fluid is aspirated through the sterile syringe. Needle-tip should be away from fetal face and cord and insertion through the placenta is avoided. The amniotic fluid in a sterile tube (without any additive) is sent to genetic laboratory to determine chromosomal constitution or to diagnose mutation of single gene, biochemical defects or open neural tube defects (alpha-fetoprotein is high).

Q. What are the complications?
Ans. *Maternal*: Uterine infection, bleeding, cramp and spotting

Fetal: Pregnancy loss (0.5%), amniotic fluid leak (1.2%), Preterm premature ruptue of membranes (PPROM) in 3% of cases and preterm delivery is 8%.

3. Percutaneous Umbilical Blood Sampling (PUBS)/ Cordocentesis (Figure 3.47)

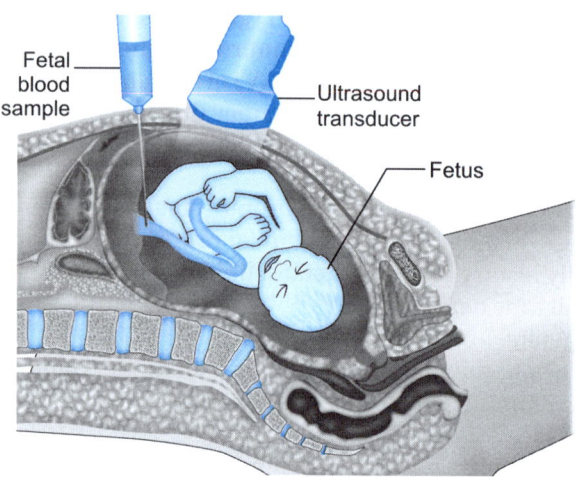

Figure 3.47: Cordocentesis

Q. What are the indications?
Ans. Diagnostic:
   a. Chromosomal analysis
   b. Single gene defect—Thalassemia, hemophilia, DMD, fragile 'X' (most common cause of mental retardation)
   c. Other hematological disorder like thrombocytopenia
   d. Congenital infections—TORCH
   e. Hemoglobin and hematocrit investigations such as Rh- isoimmunization and nonimmune hydrops
   f. Fetal blood gas analysis.

   Therapeutic:
   Intrauterine transfusion, drug therapy and stem cell transplant.

Q. What is the timing of cordocentesis?
Ans. It is done in 17–18 weeks of gestation as the cord vessel diameter is good, and if any gross defect is noted the termination of pregnancy is easier.

Q. How do you proceed for cordocentesis?
Ans. Under USG guidance localization of placenta and placental origin of cord should be determined first as it is comparatively fixed and is the best site for cordocentesis. Under aseptic precaution, the spinal needle (21–22G) is introduced with continuous guidance of USG through mother's abdomen and needle tip is advanced towards puncture site

Obstetric Operations and Interventions

avoiding injury to fetal structure. When the needle tip reaches the cord a sharp tap is made over the wall to achieve penetration into the vessel. Fetal blood sampling is taken from the umbilical artery; however, the umbilical vein is preferred because it is larger and less likely to be associated with fetal bradycardia when punctured. Stylet is withdrawn and 2–4 mL of fetal blood is aspirated. After aspiration needle and stylet is taken out and close monitoring of fetal heart rate is necessary. Prophylactic antibiotics and anti-D globulin should be administered in Rh negative mother. In order to confirm that the sample is of fetal origin the mean corpuscular volume (MCV) of the sample should be assessed. The fetal blood cells (140 fl) are larger than maternal cells (80 fl). The MCV of a sample of fetal blood should be above 100.

> **Note**
>
> Anesthetic agents such as atracurium/vencuronium 0.1 mg/kg can be injected to induce fetal paralysis and stop fetal movements, if required. This, however, is not necessary where placenta is attached on the anterior wall of uterus.

Q. What are the complications?

Ans. *Mother:* Bleeding, chorioamnionitis, emergency LSCS.

Fetus: Transient bleeding from puncture site, cord hematoma, fetal bradycardia, PPROM.

Chapter 4

Maternal Pelvis and Fetal Skull

PELVIS

Q. Describe an articulated pelvis.

Ans. *Articulated pelvis is composed of:*
   a. Iliac bones (2)
   b. Sacrum (5 pieces joined together)
   c. Coccyx (4 pieces).

Q. Which joints are involved in the pelvis?

Ans. a. Two sacroiliac joints
   b. Sacrococcygeal joint
   c. Symphysis pubis.

Q. Describe the pelvic brim.

Ans. From before backwards upper border of symphysis pubis, pubic crest, pubic tubercle, pectineal line, iliopubic eminence, arcuate line, sacroiliac articulation, ala of the sacrum and sacral promontory. The same things are orderly present on the opposite side.

Q. What is true pelvis?

Ans. The part of the pelvis below the pelvic brim (Figure 4.1).

Q. How do you hold the articulated pelvis?

Ans. a. Hold the articulated pelvis with the incisures of the acetabulum pointing directly downward as the normal position of the pelvis in erect woman.
   b. The same result is achieved when the anterior superior spines of ilium and the pubic tubercles are placed in the same vertical plane.
   c. Angle of inclination is 55° with the horizontal line (see later).

Q. What are the different parts of true pelvis?

Ans. Inlet, cavity, outlet.

Q. What is the length of symphysis pubis and sacrum?

Ans. Symphysis pubis—4 cm
   Sacrum-promontory tip to coccyx (straight line depth 10 cm, curved depth 12 cm).

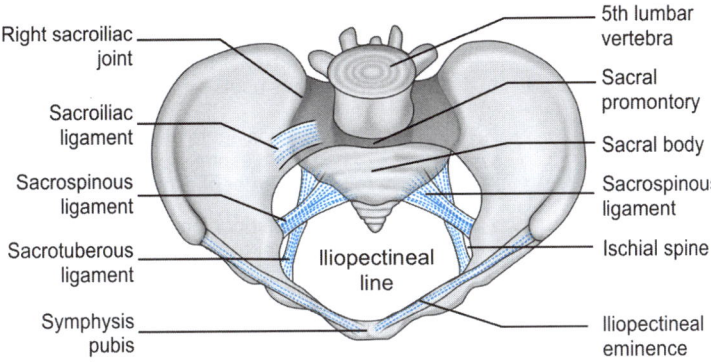

Figure 4.1: Bony pelvis showing important landmarks and ligaments

Q. What is the shape of pelvic inlet?

Ans. Reniform, i.e. transversely oval.

Q. What is inclination of pelvis?

Ans. In erect posture, the plane of pelvic inlet makes an angle of 50° to 60° (usually 55° with the horizontal line) (Figure 4.2).

Q. What is sacral angle?

Ans. It is the angle formed by plane of brim and first two pieces of sacrum (normal >90°). Narrow sacral angle—flat sacrum in funnel pelvis.

Q. What is the importance of pelvic inlet?

Ans. It affects engagement. High inclination or increase in angle of inclination due to sacralization of 5th lumbar vertebra, causes delay of engagement and favors occipitoposterior. Low inclination may occur in lumbarization of first piece of sacral vertebra. This favors early engagement.

Q. What is the diameter of pelvic inlet?

Ans. 1. *Anteroposterior (AP) diameter or the conjugate diameter or true conjugate*: The distance between middle of the inner margin of the upper border of symphysis pubis to the center of sacral promontory. The diameter is 11 cm (Figures 4.2 and 4.3).
2. *Obstetrical conjugate*: The distance between the midpoints of sacral promontory behind to the point 1 cm below the upper margin of posterior surface of symphysis pubis in front. It is the shortest AP diameter, measurement is 10 cm.
3. *Diagonal conjugate*: Distance from middle of the lower border of symphysis pubis to the midpoint of sacral promontory, measurement is 12 cm. It is clinically measured. The obstetrical conjugate = Diagonal conjugate—2 cm, i.e. 12 cm–2 cm = 10 cm (symphysis pubis width = 2 cm) (Figure 4.2).
4. *Transverse diameter*: It is the distance between the two points furthest apart on the pelvic brim over the iliopectineal lines (midpoint between iliopectineal eminence and sacroiliac joint). This crosses

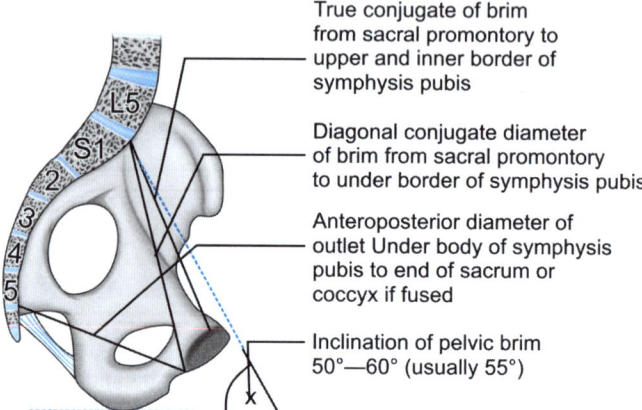

Figure 4.2: Shows vertical plane of pelvic inlet and different anteroposterior diameter of pelvic inlet and outlet

the true conjugate in its middle third usually posterior to the center. It measures 13 cm (Figure 4.3).
5. *Oblique diameter:* It is the distance between one sacroiliac articulation to the opposite iliopectineal eminence. Right and left denotes the sacroiliac joints from which it starts. It measures 12 cm (Figure 4.3).
6. *Sacrocotyloid diameter:* It is the distance from the midpoint of sacral promontory to the iliopectineal eminence on either side. It measure 9.5 cm. It represents the space occupied by the biparietal diameter (BPD) of the head while negotiating the head of fetus in flat pelvis.

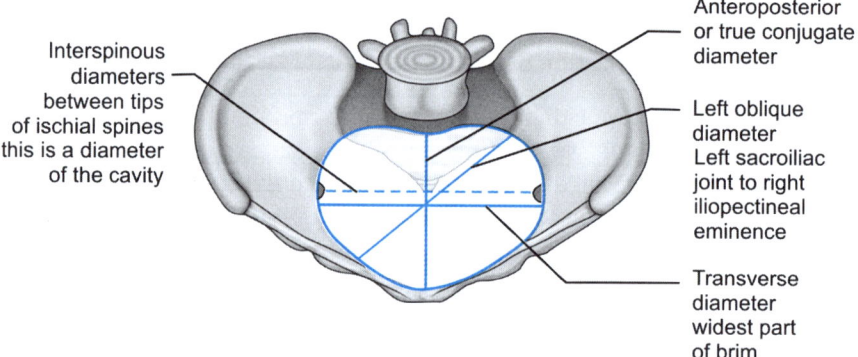

Figure 4.3: Shows different diameters of bony pelvis (true conjugate diameter, left oblique diameter and interspinous diameter)

> **Note**
> *Contracted inlet is diagnosed if AP diameter is less than 10 cm or the transverse diameter is < 12 cm.*

Q. What is the cavity?

Ans. *Boundaries*:
In front—pubic bones

Behind—anterior surface of sacrum
Each side—inner surface of ischial and iliac bones
Above—pelvic brim
Below—plane of least pelvic dimension (PLD).

Q. What is the plane?

Ans. Plane of mid cavity (Plane of greatest pelvic diameter starts from mid pubis to the junction of S2 and S3) (Figure 4.4B).

Q. What are the diameters?

Ans.
a. Anterioposterior diameter from the center of posterior surface of symphysis pubis to the junction of S2 and S3 behind.
b. Measurement is 12 cm.
c. Transverse and oblique diameter cannot be measured accurately because of intervening soft tissues over obturator foramina. Measurement is 12 cm.

Q. What is pelvic outlet?

Ans. Boundaries
- It is a diamond—shaped space
- Anteriorly—pubic arch
- Laterally—ischial tuberosities and sacrotuberous ligament
- Posteriorly—tip of the coccyx if fused or end of the sacrum.

Plane
- Lower border of symphysis pubis through the ischial spines to the tip of 5th piece of sacrum. It is the narrowest plane of pelvis (PLD) (Figure 4.4B).
- Dimension of PLD (plane of least pelvic dimension)
- Transverse diameter—distance between the tip of ischial spines, measurement is 10.5 cm (Figure 4.3)
- Anteroposterior diameter is from the middle of inferior border of symphysis pubis to the end of sacrum, measurement is 11.5 cm
- Posterior sagittal diameter—distance between the same point of the sacrum and the midpoint of bispinous diameter; measurement is 5 cm.

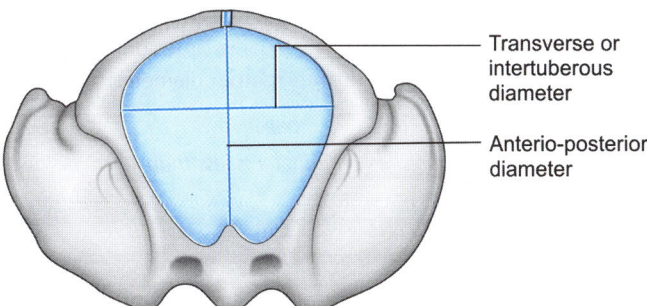

Figure 4.4A: Showing anatomical outlet with different diameters

> **Note**
>
> Mid pelvis is likely to be contracted when the sum of interischial spinous and posterior sagittal diameter of the mid pelvis (normally 10.5 + 5 cm = 15.5 cm) falls to 13.5 cm or below or when interischial diameter is smaller than 8 cm
> Management : Elective cesarean section.

Q. Anatomical outlet of pelvis (Figures 4.4A and B).

Ans. Anteroposterior diameter is middle of inferior border of symphysis pubis up to the tip of the coccyx behind. Measurement is 13 cm with the coccyx pushed back in 2nd stage of labor. In normal position of coccyx, the measurement is 2.5 cm less (i.e. 9.5–11.5 cm) when the tip of the sacrum is considered as the fixed point on the posterior aspect.

Transverse diameter—distance between the inner border of ischial tuberosities, measurement is 11 cm. (It is clinically measured by 4 knuckles of a closed fist, which fits well in between the inner margins of ischial tuberosities). If this diameter is 8 cm or less pelvic outlet is contracted.

Posterior sagittal—part of AP diameter, which lies behind the transverse diameter, measurement is 8.5 cm (It is clinically assessed by measuring the distance between sacrococcygeal joint and margin of anus).

> **Note**
>
> Vaginal delivery depends upon the length of posterior sagittal diameter in obstructed labor in midpelvis.

Q. What is obstetrical outlet?

Ans. It is the segment of the pelvis bounded above by plane of least pelvic dimension (PLD) and below by the anatomical outlet.

> **Note**
>
> Anatomical outlet may be linked by two triangles. The interischial diameter forms the base of both. The sides of anterior triangle are pubic rami, and its apex the inferior posterior surface of the symphysis pubis. The posterior triangle has no bony sides but is limited at its apex by the tip of last sacral vertebra (not the tip of the coccyx) (Figure 4.4B). Outlet contraction without concomitant midpelvic contraction is rare.

Q. What are the diameters of pelvis?

Ans. Pelvic diameters are present in centimeter (Table 4.1).

Table 4.1: Diameter of pelvis

	Anteroposterior (cm)	Oblique (cm)	Transverse (cm)
Inlet	11	12	13
Cavity	12	12	12
Outlet	13	–	11

Q. What is the importance of PLD (Plane of least pelvic dimension)?

Ans. a. Origin of levator ani muscles.

b. Internal rotation of occiput.
c. Forward curvature of pelvic axis.
d. Station '0'.
e. Obstetric curve of carus directed upwards from the level of ischial spine.
f. Pudendal nerve block by the guideline of ischial-spine.
g. Deep transverse arrest may occur at this plane.

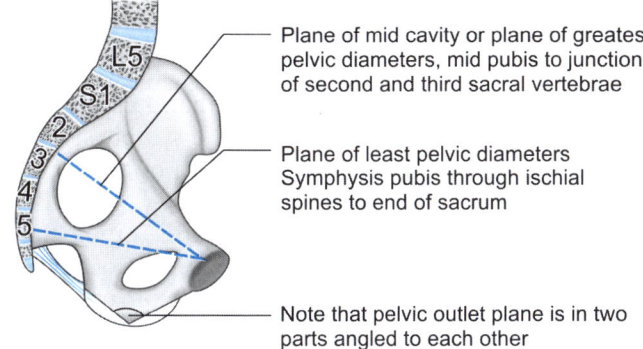

Figure 4.4B: Diagrammatic representation of different planes of pelvic

Q. What are the different types of pelvis?
Ans. Gynecoid (50%), anthropoid (20%), android (25%), platypelloid (5%).

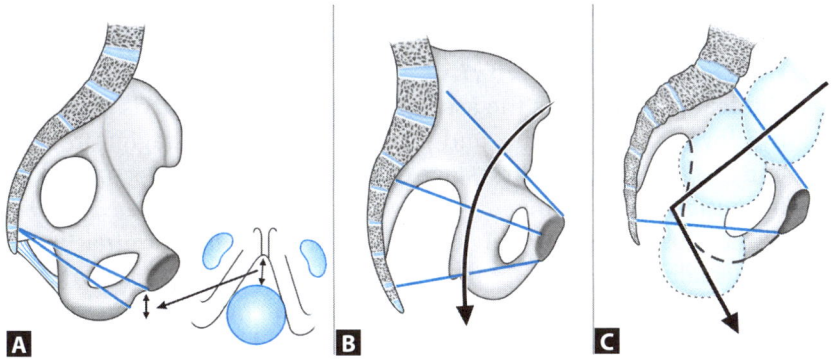

Figures 4.5A to C: Pubic arch: (A) Waste space of Morris; (B) Anatomical pelvic axis; (C) Obstetrical pelvic axis

Q. What is subpubic angle?
Ans. It is formed by approximation of the two descending pubic rami. It measures normally 90° or more.

Q. What is pubic arch?
Ans. Arch is formed by descending pubic rami of both sides and is of obstetric importance than subpubic angle, clinically it is assessed by placing 3 fingers side by side.

Q. What is waste space of Morris?

Ans. The narrow the pubic arch, the fetal head is displaced backwards and less the room available for it. Normally, subpubic arch is rounded and less space is wasted under symphysis pubis when a round disc of 9.4 cm of diameter (diameter of well-flexed head) is placed under the pubic arch, the distance between the lower borders of symphysis pubis and circumference of disc is measured. This measurement is waste space of Morris and should not exceed 1 cm in normal pelvis (Figure 4.5A).

Q. What is the available anteroposterior diameter of outlet? What is its clinical importance?

Ans. When the waste space of Morris is greater than 1 cm the anterior point of AP diameter of outlet extends below the symphysis pubis and the distance between the said point and the tip of the sacrum is called available AP diameter of outlet (Figure 4.5A).
Clinical importance: If the waste space of Morris is more than 1 cm due to narrow subpubic angle, the available anteroposterior diameter of outlet becomes less, fetal head passes by injuring perineum or may get arrested.

Q. What is obstetric pelvic axis?

Ans. Through this axis the fetus negotiates in the pelvis. It is uniformly curved directed downwards and backwards up to the ischial spine and then directed abruptly forwards (Figure 4.5C).

Q. What is anatomical curve of carus?

Ans. Anatomical pelvic axis is formed by joining the mid points of AP diameter of inlet, cavity and outlet. It is uniformly curved with the convexity fitting with the concavity of sacrum (Figure 4.5B).

Q. What is clinical pelvimetry?

Ans. Clinical pelvimetry is the assessment of maternal pelvis aseptically by gloved fingers (index and middle) through the vagina from the end of 37 weeks to the first stage of labor (Bladder and rectum should be empty).

Clinical pelvimetry or pelvic assessment by digital examination
It is usually assessed in terms of inlet (brim), mid pelvis and outlet.

Pelvic brim: By measuring the diagonal conjugate (DC in cm) and palpation of fore pelvis (posterior surface of pubis, iliopectineal line).

Mid pelvis: Shape of the sacrum (curved/straight), the width of the sacro-sciatic notch, side wall of the pelvis, prominence of ischial spine and distance between them.

Pelvic outlet:
a. Estimation of the distance between ischial tuberosities (TDO—usually about 10 cm).
b. Palpation of coccyx to determine its orientation and mobility.
c. Assessment of sub-pubic angle to be >90° and subpubic arch.
d. Narrow or normal posterior sagittal diameter.
e. The convergence or divergence of pelvic side walls.
(See also the long case of primigravida with floating head).

Maternal Pelvis and Fetal Skull

Q. What is normal female pelvis?

Ans. It is gynecoid in type with normal diameter at all levels of pelvis.

Q. What are the shapes of the brim in different types of pelvis and specify their clinical significance?

Ans. a. *Gynecoid:* Round brim, labor is expected to be normal.
b. *Android:* Heart-shaped, occipitoposterior position is common and due to funnel shaped pelvis deep transverse arrest is very common.
c. *Anthropoid:* Oval, persistent occipitoposterior position is common.
d. *Platypelloid:* Transversely oval. There is difficulty in engagement of fetal head.
e. *Small gynecoid pelvis:* All pelvic diameters are proportionately small, so there is delay in every stage of labor.

> **Note**
> *Different types of female pelvis (see Appendix 4).*

Q. What are the different abnormalities of the pelvis?

Ans. a. *Naegele's pelvis*: One ala of the sacrum is absent developmentally.
b. *Robert's pelvis*: Both the ala of the sacrum is absent developmentally.
c. *Rachitic pelvis*: This was common in ricketic patient, inlet is reniform in shape but nowadays it is uncommon due to routine supplementation of vitamin D.
d. *Kyphoscoliosis*: Pelvic deformity is due to the disease like TB and rickets of vertebral column.

FETAL SKULL

Q. What are the bones forming the fetal skull (Figure 4.6)?

Ans. a. Two parietal bones
b. One occipital bone
c. One frontal bone
d. Two temporal bones.

Q. What are the different sutures (Figure 4.7)?

Ans. a. *Sagittal suture*: between the two parietal bones, running antero-posteriorly between two fontanelles.
b. *Lambdoid suture*: runs transversely outward from posterior fontanelle between the parietal bones and occipital bone.
c. *Coronal suture*: extends outwards from anterior fontanelle running between parietal and frontal bones.
d. *Frontal (metopic) suture*: lies between two halves of frontal bones.

Q. What is anterior fontanelle? Why is it important?

Ans. a. It is called bregma (Figure 4.7).
b. Located at the junction of sagittal, coronal and frontal sutures.
c. Diamond-shaped, soft membrane filled area of 3 cm × 2 cm.
d. Ossified at the age of 18 months.

Importance
1. Accommodates brain growth.
2. Facilitates molding.
3. Position denotes the degree of flexion and extension of head.
4. Depressed in dehydration and bulged in raised intracranial tension noted after delivery.

Q. What is posterior fontanelle?

Ans. a. It is also called lambda (Figure 4.7).
   b. Located at the junction of sagittal and lambdoidal sutures.
   c. Its floor is membranous and closes at term.

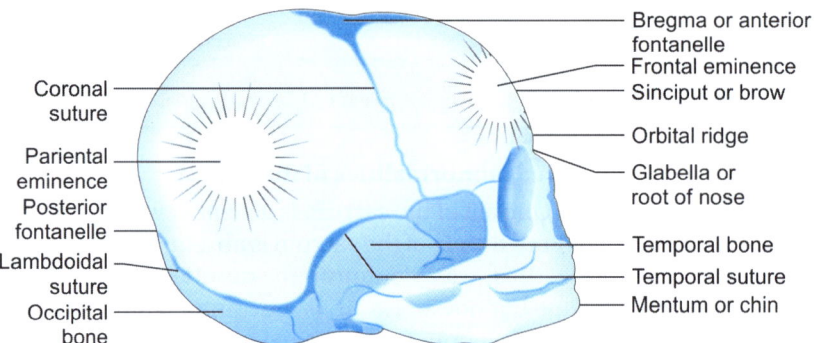

Figure 4.6: Fetal skull showing different landmarks of obstetrical significance

Q. What are the landmarks of fetal skull (Figures 4.6 and 4.7)?

Ans. a. **Occiput**: It is the part of the fetal skull bone lying below the posterior fontanelle (limited to occipital bone).
   b. **Sinciput**: Area bounded by supraorbital ridges and glabella inferiorly and bregma and coronal suture superiorly.
   c. **Vertex**: Diamond shaped area between anterior fontanelle and coronal sutures, posterior fontanelle and lambdoid sutures and the two parietal eminences laterally.
   d. **Glabella**: The elevated area between orbital ridges.
   e. **Nasion**: The root of the nose.
   f. **Parietal eminence**: The bossed area of the parietal bones.
   g. **Vault**: From orbital ridges to the nape of the neck [frontal (2), parietal (2) and occipital (1), temporal bones (2) and wings of sphenoid]. It is compressible.
   h. **Brow**: It is the area bounded on one side by anterior fontanelle and coronal suture and on the other side by root of the nose and supraorbital ridges of both side.
   i. **Face**: It is the area bounded on one side by root of the nose and supraorbital ridges and on the other side by junction of floor of mouth and neck.

Maternal Pelvis and Fetal Skull

Q. Diameters of fetal skull and other important diameters (Figure 4.8).

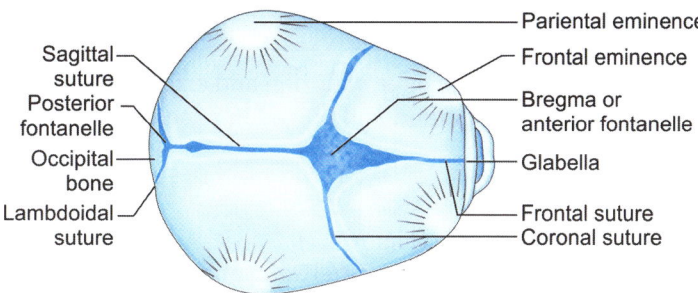

Figure 4.7: Fetal skull showing important sutures, fontanelles

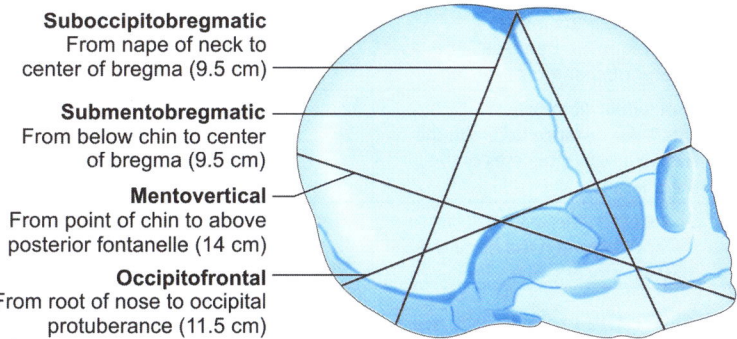

Figure 4.8: Different diameters of fetal skull

Diameter	Measurement	Obstetric significance
a. *Biparietal diameter (BPD)* Distance between the two parietal eminences	9.5 cm	Largest transverse diameter of the skull
b. *Bitemporal* The distance between the two anteroinferior end of coronal suture	8.0 cm	Shortest transverse diameter of the skull
c. *Suboccipitobregmatic* From nape of the neck to the center of the bregma	9.5 cm	Engaging diameter in vertex presentation in completely flexed head
d. *Suboccipitofrontal* From nape of the neck to the anterior end of bregma or center of sinciput	10 cm	Incompletely flexed vertex
e. *Occipitofrontal* From occipital protuberance to the root of the nose	11.5 cm	Extended head
f. *Mentovertical* From mid point of chin to the highest point of sagittal suture	14 cm	Brow—it does not engage, no mechanism of normal labor

Contd...

Contd...

Diameter	Measurement	Obstetric significance
g. Submentovertical Extends from junction of neck and lower jaw to the highest point on the sagittal suture	11.5 cm	Face—incompletely extended
h. Submentobregmatic Extends from junction of neck and lower jaw to the center of bregma	9.5 cm	Face—completely extended
i. Supersubparietal diameter It extends from a point placed below one parietal eminence to a point placed above the other parietal eminence of the opposite side	8.5 cm	For engagement of head in platypelloid pelvis
j. Bitrochanteric diameter This extends between the two greater trochanters of the femur	10.5 cm	It engages in breech presentation
k. Bisacromial diameter This is the distance between the two acromian processes of the scapula.	12.0 cm	
l. Bimastoid diameter Distance between the tip of the mastoid process	7.5 cm	The diameter is incompressible

Q. What are the circumferences of fetal head in specific positions?

Ans. See below.

Circumference	Measurement (cm)
Suboccipitobregmatic × Biparietal (Well-flexed vertex)	28.0
Occipitofrontal × Biparietal (Deflexed vertex, OP position)	33.0
Mentum-vertical × Biparietal (Brow position)	35.5

Q. What is the difference of caput succedaneum and cephalhematoma?

Ans.

Caput succedaneum	Cephalhematoma
Site—localized swelling on the scalp due to stagnation of fluid beneath the girdle of contact	Subperiosteal hematoma
Onset—present at birth	Appears a few hours after birth
Position—may lie on suture	Limited by suture lines to the skull bones
Feel—soft, pits on pressure	Soft but does not pits on pressure
Size—gradually increases during obstructed labor	Biggest at birth but reduces gradually
Disappear—in 24 hours	After 4 to 12 weeks
Occurs—after rupture of membrane	Not related with rupture of membrane

Q. What is the treatment of cephalhematoma and caput succedaneum?

Ans. No treatment is required in both the conditions.

Q. What are the complications of cephalhematoma?

Ans. a. Jaundice of neonates
b. Rarely infected, in case of abscess, it requires surgical drainage.

Q. What is molding?

Ans. Overlapping of two fetal skull bones due to prolonged compression during the passage through the birth canal.

Molding occurs first at the junction of occipitoparietal bones and later at the parietoparietal bones. During normal delivery, an alteration of 4 mm skull diameter commonly occurs and it disappears within a few hours after birth.

Q. What are the degrees of molding?

Ans. a. Zero—if the bones are apart.
b. '+'—if they are overlapping.
c. '++'—if they overlap but can be reduced by digital pressure.
d. '+++'—if they overlap but cannot be reduced by pressure.
Two scores can be added together and scored out of total "6".

Q. What is the importance of molding?

Ans. a. Slight molding is beneficial for normal delivery.
b. Extreme molding causes tearing of tentorium cerebelli leading to intracranial hemorrhage and subdural hemorrhage.
c. Shape of the molding is very much helpful for information about the position of head occupied in the pelvis.

Q. What are the conditions where molding is absent?

Ans. a. Baby delivered by elective CS
b. Breech presentation
c. Precipitate labor
d. Postmaturity—as the sutures are almost closed.

Q. How do you hold a dummy fetus in LOA, ROP, ROA, LOP Breech and transverse lie before pelvic brim?

Ans. Place the legs, arms and fetus in flexed attitude and hold the trunk in left hand with head above the pelvic brim. Right hand will flex the head so that chin comes towards chest.

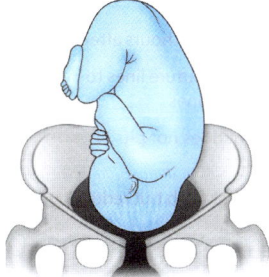 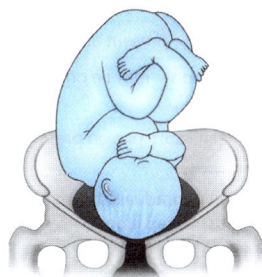

Figure 4.9: Left occiput anterior (LOA)   **Figure 4.10:** Right occiput posterior (ROP)

LOA (Figure 4.9):
Next place the occiput pointing towards left iliopubic eminence on left/anterior quadrant of pelvis.

ROA (Figure 4.13): Occiput is pointed towards the right iliopubic eminence on right anterior quadrant of pelvis.

ROP (Figure 4.10):
Occiput is kept in right posterior quadrant pointing towards the right sacroiliac joint.

LOP (Figure 4.13): Occiput is kept in left posterior quadrant pointing towards left sacroiliac joint.

Q. How do you hold fetal skull on pelvic brim?

Ans.
a. Put the index finger of right hand in foramen magnum of fetal skull and hold the bony pelvis in left hand by placing fingers in greater sciatic notch before and sacrum behind.
b. Flex the finger in the foramen magnum.
c. Direct, vault of the skull towards pelvic brim and place occiput towards left iliopectineal eminence in LOA.

Q. How do you hold dummy in other abnormal presentation?

Ans. Face: Place fetal head in extension in face presentation. The mentum is related to the iliopubic eminence and glabella or fore head to the opposite sacroiliac joint in left mentun anterior (LMA) and right mentum anterior (RMA) positions (see Figure 5.6A for LMA)

Brow: Head lies in between in full flexion and full extension.

Breech: The podalic end will come first in the pelvic brim

LSP: The sacrum of fetus is on left sacroiliac joint of pelvis (Figure 4.11A)

LSA: Sacrum is directed towards the left iliopubic eminence.

RSA: Sacrum directed towards the right iliopubic eminence.

Transverse lie: The position is determined by the direction of the back, which is the denominator. It may be (a) Dorso-anterior (60%)—the flexor surface of fetus fits well in the convexity of maternal spine, (b) Dorso posterior—chances of fetal extension is common with increased risk of arm prolapse (c) Droso-superior (d) Dorso-interior. According to the position of fetal head the fetal position may be right or left (common).

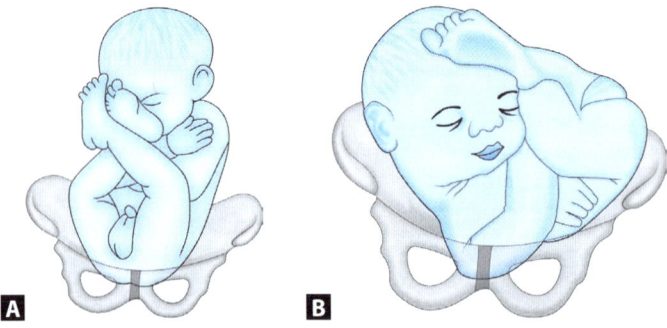

Figures 4.11A and B: Abnormal presentation: (A) Breech (LSP); (B) Transverse lie (Dorso-posterior)

Maternal Pelvis and Fetal Skull

Q. Different presentation of fetal head in relation to pelvis.

Ans. See Figure 4.12.
LOA LOT LOP
ROA ROT ROP.

Q. What is girdle of contact?

Ans. Fetal head circumference of vertex and face passes through true pelvis. This circumference of fetal head is the girdle of contact. Shape and diameter of circumferences of fetal head may vary in different presentations.

Q. What are the changes in fetal head in labor?

Ans. a. Molding
b. Caput succedaneum—It is due to the pressure effect of dilating cervical ring and rigid vaginal outlet. It gives an idea of the position of head in the pelvis and degree of flexion.

Q. What is presentation and presenting part (PP)?

Ans. The part of the fetus that lies over the pelvic inlet is presentation, e.g. cephalic (96.3%), podalic (breech—3.2%), shoulder and others (0.5%). The first fetal part that is accessible at the internal os at the time of bimanual pelvic examination are the PP, e.g. in cephalic presentation, presenting parts may be vertex (96%), brow and face.

Q. What is denominator?

Ans. The arbitrary fixed point of the presenting part (PP).

Presenting parts	*Denominator*
Vertex	Occiput (outside the presenting part)
Face	Mentum
Breech	Sacrum
Shoulder	Scapula (acromian)
Brow	No (according to some frontal eminence).

Q. What is the fetal position?

Ans. It is the relation of the denominator to the different quadrant of pelvis (Figure 4.12).

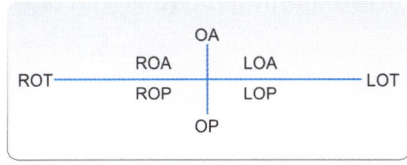

Figure 4.12: Fetal position, the orientation of the presenting vertex within the maternal pelvis (eight positions of vertex)

Q. How do you diagnose presentation and position of fetus?

Ans. *Several diagnostic methods are:*
a. Abdominal palpation (Leopold's maneuvers) (see history taking in obstetrics)
b. Vaginal examination

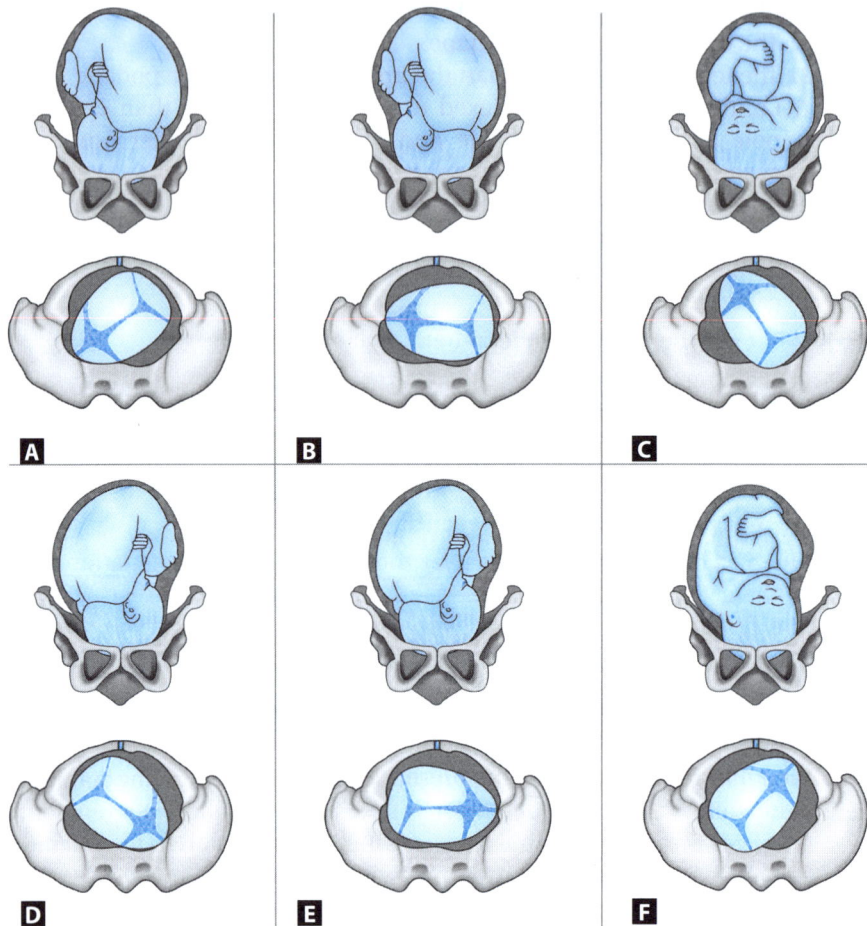

Figure 4.13: Position of fetal head in relation to pelvis: (A) LOA: Left occiput anterior; (B) LOT: Left occiput transverse; (C) LOP: Left occiput posterior; (D) ROA: Right occiput anterior; (E) ROT: Right occiput transverse; (F) ROP: Right occiput posterior

    c. Combined examination
    d. Auscultation of FHS and in certain doubtful cases USG or radiography or CT scan.

Q. What is oblique lie?
Ans. The fetal and maternal axis may cross at 45° angle, called, oblique lie, which is unstable and may become longitudinal (99% labor at term) or transverse during labor.

> **Note**
>
> *Lie of fetus: It is the relation of long axis of fetal spine with that of maternal spine.*
> *a. Longitudinal lie: Long axis of fetal spine lies parallel to the maternal spine (99.5%);*
> *b. Transverse lie: Spine of fetus lies at right angle to maternal spine (0.3%).*

Maternal Pelvis and Fetal Skull

Q. What is the reason for predominance of cephalic presentation?

Ans. 1. The uterus is pyriform in shape.
2. The fetal head is larger than the breech but the entire podalic pole, i.e. the breech and its flexed extremities is bulkier than cephalic pole and is more movable and make use of roomier fundus—accommodation.
3. The cephalic pole is comprised of the fetal head only and occupies the less roomy area.
4. As the fetal head is heavier, it comes down to the bottom of uterine cavity—Gravitation.

Q. Why LOA is common than ROA?

Ans. In LOA, the sagittal suture lies on right oblique diameter and in ROA, the sagittal suture lies on left oblique diameter. The left oblique diameter is encroached by rectum.

Q. Which diameters are of 9.5 cm in fetal head?

Ans. BPD, suboccipitobregmatic, and submentobregmatic.

> **Note**
> Sacro-cotyloid diameter of maternal pelvis is also 9.5 cm.

Q. Which diameter is good for normal delivery—Suboccipitobregmatic, or submentobregmatic and why?

Ans. Of course the suboccipitobregmatic diameter as it is the engaging diameter in cephalic presentation in completely flexed head. In submentobregmatic diameter the presenting part is face which is completely extended and engagement is delayed in face as the long distance between the mentum and biparietal diameter (BPD) is 7 cm where as this measurement from BPD to occiput is only 3 cm which favors early engagement for normal delivery.

> **Note**
> Facts in relation to the engagement of vertex: If the lowest part of the occiput is at or below the level of ischial spines, the head is usually but not always engaged since the distance from the plane of pelvic inlet to the level of ischial spines is approximately 5 cm in most pelvis and the distance from the biparietal plane of the unmolded fetal head to the vertex is about 3–4 cm. Under these circumstances the vertex cannot possibly reach the level of spines unless the BPD has passed the inlet or fetal head is elongated by molding and formation of a caput. So in severe molding and large caput cases the head may not be engaged or BPD may not pass through pelvic inlet.

Chapter 5

Normal Labor and Labor in Malposition and Presentation

Q. Demonstrate the mechanism of normal labor in left occiput anterior (LOA) (by dummy and pelvis).

Ans. First hold the dummy (in flexed attitude) by right hand and pelvis by left hand carefully.

1. *Engagement*: Vertex of fetal head enters the pelvic brim with occiput lying in relation to left iliopectineal eminence, sinciput at right sacroiliac joint and sagittal suture lying on right oblique diameter of pelvis. The engaging transverse diameter is biparietal diameter (BPD) (9.5 cm) and anteroposterior (AP) diameter of fetal head (Suboccipitobregmatic—9.5 cm).

2. *Descent and flexion*: Descent is a continuous process. Move the head down to the pelvic cavity keeping the sagittal suture on the right oblique diameter of pelvis and occiput on left anterior quadrant till vertex reaches up to the level of ischial spine.

3. *Internal rotation*: Move the fetal head with occiput anterior 1/8th of a circle (45°) below the level of ischial spine from left to midline, so that occiput comes below the pubic arch.
   The internal rotation is followed by further descent until occiput passes beyond symphysis pubis in flexed attitude of fetal head. Occiput is now free at the sub-pubic arch.

4. *Extension*: Extension of fetal head by right hand–vault (vertex and forehead), and face is brought free out of pelvic outlet.

5. *Restitution*: Just rotate the delivered head by right hand for 45° to the left.
   (During normal delivery after birth of fetal head in left occiput anterior (LOA), occiput rotates 1/8th of a circle on the left side to undo the twist in the neck caused by internal rotation of head).

6. *External rotation*: Rotate the free head another 45° on the same direction of restitution and face directed to the right side (right thigh as in normal labor). This corrects internal rotation of shoulder at the pelvic brim to bring the bisacromial diameter in relation with the anteroposterior diameter of pelvic outlet. After delivery of head see cord round the neck *in vivo* and slip the cord over the head of it is loose, or cut the cord in between clamps if it is tight.

Normal Labor and Labor in Malposition and Presentation

7. *Delivery of the shoulders*: Bring the anterior shoulder below the symphysis by pressing head towards the perineum so that it hitches under symphysis pubis and then lift the fetal head by holding in between palms and bring out posterior shoulder. During delivery abrupt or powerful force is avoided to avest brachial plexus injury in vivo.
8. Rest of the trunk is delivered by lateral flexion.

> **Note**
> *Practice normal labor in right occiput anterior (ROA) by dummy and pelvis.*

Q. What is synclitism?
Ans. In early labor, vertex engaged at transverse diameter of pelvic brim. Position is like left occiput transverse (LOT) or right occiput transverse (ROT).

Q. What is asynclitism?
Ans. It is a condition when the sagittal suture of fetal head lies nearer to the symphysis pubis or sacral promontory.

Q. What is anterior asynclitism and posterior asynclitism?
Ans. In multigravida, the sagittal suture lies near the sacral promontory (anterior asynclitism, anterior parietal obliquity or Naegele's obliquity). In primigravida due to tight abdomen, the sagittal suture of fetal skull lies near the symphysis pubis and posterior parietal bone lies lower than anterior one (posterior asynclitism or Litzmann's obliquity).

Q. How does descent of head occur in labor?
Ans. Descent of head is brought about by one or more forces after engagement:
1. Pressure of amniotic fluid
2. Direct pressure of fundus on breech with contraction
3. Bear down effort of maternal abdominal muscles
4. Extension and straightening of fetal body.

Q. Why flexion of head occurs in normal labor of occiput presentation?
Ans. Due to uterine contraction the buttocks of fetus are pushed by the fundus and fetal axis pressure is generated. The head can be imagined as a lever (the atlanto-occipital joint acts as a fulcrum) with the short posterior arm from fulcrum to occiput and long anterior arm (from fulcrum to chin). As the fetus is pushed downward the short posterior arm moves down ward, meets with the less resistance and occiput descends more than the forehead, resulting flexion (Figures 5.1A and B).

Q. Why internal rotation occurs in normal labor?
Ans. a. Slopping character of pelvic floor (the levator ani muscles with other soft tissues of pelvic floor) forms a curved gutter directed downwards, forward and inwards towards the midline. When head is flexed, occiput reaches the pelvic floor first (mechanism discussed above) and stretches the levator ani and when contraction goes

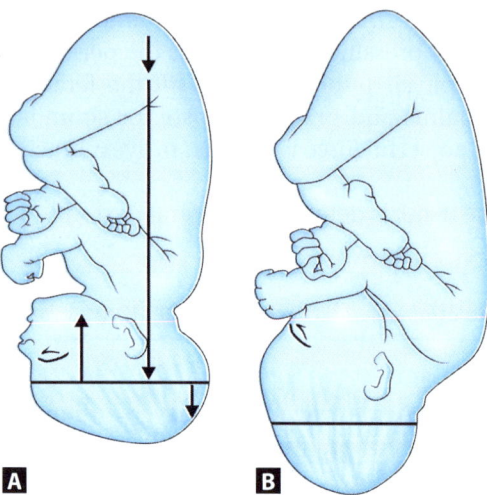

Figures 5.1A and B: (A) Lever action producing flexion of the head reducing occipito frontal to B; (B) Suboccipito bregmatic diameter

off, the elastic recoil of levator ani brings the occiput towards the midline. The process is repeated until the occiput becomes anterior (Hart's rule).
b. *Shape of the pelvis*: The pelvic floor is deficient anteriorly due to wide pubic arch. The part of the head which moves forward is moving in the direction of least resistance.
c. Unequal flexibility of the different parts of fetus.

Q. Active management of third stage of labor (AMTSL).

Ans. Third stage begins after the delivery of baby. The active management of third stage consists of three activities for prevention of postpartum hemorrhage (PPH), anemia and decreased need for blood transfusion. It also decreases the length of third stage of labor.
a. *Uterotonic drug*:
  i. Injection syntocinon, 10 units, IM, just within 1 minute after delivery of the baby by ensuring the fact that there is no other baby inside the uterus. It acts within 2 to 3 minutes to reduce PPH (WHO) (commonly used).
  ii. Misoprostol—3 tab (200 μg) should be given immediately after delivery of the baby by sublingual/oral/PR (Not a good route).
  iii. IV Methergine (0.25 mg) just after delivery of anterior shoulder of baby; it should not be used in hypertensive disorder and organic heart disease (Not used now routinely). It also causes increased incidence of diastolic blood pressure, nausea, vomiting, increased pain and increased use of analgesic from the time of birth to hospital discharge.
b. *Controlled cord traction (CCT) for delivery of placenta*: In AMTSL, wait for 2-3 minutes for strong uterine contraction and then CCT should be done. If placenta does not descend during 30–40 seconds, the attempt must be stopped. Gently hold the cord and reattempt

again until the uterus is well contracted. As the placenta is delivered hold it in between two palms and turn it until the membranes are twisted and then pull to complete the delivery of placenta.

Following delivery of placenta, examine carefully, both maternal and fetal surface to note whether there is missing of any cotyledons and membrane or there is any torn membrane with blood vessels, and also note umbilical cord for two arteries and one vein and its attachment to the placenta. In any abnormalities of the placenta, pathologic evaluation is warranted.

c. *Uterine massage*: Helps in contraction of uterus and prevents PPH.

> **Note**
> Chances of retained placenta is high by IV injection methergin use in AMTSL. According to WHO recent guideline, sustained uterine massage is not required in woman who has already received prophylactic oxytocin, however uterine tone assessment is recommended for early detection of uterine atonicity following all deliveries.

Q. How placenta is separated?

Ans. There are two ways of separation of placenta.
  a. *Central separation (Schultz)*: Central portion of the placenta is detached first from its uterine attachment resulting in opening of a few uterine sinuses and accumulation of blood behind placenta. Increase of uterine contraction causes more detachment of placenta and retroplacental hematoma formation until whole placenta is delivered.
  b. *Marginal separation (Matthews-Duncan)*: Separation of the placenta occurs at the margin. With uterine contraction the placenta gets separated.

> **Note**
> The placenta separated through the deep spongy layer of deciduas basalis. Blood loss and hemostasis after placental delivery is achieved by occlusion of blood vessels by contraction and retraction of uterine musculatures and formation of thrombosis.

Q. What are the signs of separation of placenta?

Ans. a. Uterus becomes hard, globular and ballotable.
  b. Gush of bleeding per vaginal (PV).
  c. Apparent lengthening of cord (extravulval portion).
  d. If the fundus of uterus is gently pushed upwards, the cord will not recede into the vagina (Kustner sign).

> **Note**
> In expectant management we should wait for signs of separation of placenta. The disadvantages of this management are:
> i. Third stage of labor is prolonged
> ii. Chances of PPH is high.

Q. What is Brandt-Andrews method?

Ans. The separated placenta is removed by traction on the cord, while other hand maintains pressure on the uterus above the pubic bone upwards and backwards (abdominal hand is most important). Never apply cord traction (pull) without applying counter traction (push) above the pubic bone with other hand. The abdominal hand prevents uterine inversion.

Q. What is the risk of cord traction?

Ans.
a. Tearing of cord.
b. Uterine inversion.

Q. What is the normal loss of blood following normal delivery?

Ans. 250 mL (average) [range: 100 mL–300 mL].

Q. What is the immediate postpartum care?

Ans.
a. Vagina and perineum are looked for any tear.
b. Monitoring of pulse, BP, P/V bleeding (PPH).
c. Uterus—to ensure well-contracted by placing hand on abdomen.
d. The vulva is swabbed down and sterile pad is placed over it to collect the lochial discharge.

Q. When will you discharge the patient following normal delivery?

Ans. Within 48 hours following uncomplicated delivery for management of PPH, if occurs. The other advantage is less exposure to hospital based cross infection to the mother following delivery and breastfeeding practice should also be well established within this period, and to start zero dose immunization [Inj. BCG, oral polio, and hepatitis B vaccine (HBV)].

FLYING QUESTIONS ON NORMAL LABOR

Q. What is normal labor (Eutocia)?

Ans. It is a process of spontaneous onset by which fetus, placenta and membrane are expelled through birth canal after 37 completed weeks of pregnancy, in cephalic presentation (vertex is the presenting part) within 10 to 12 hours from onset of true labor pain without any instrumental aid except episiotomy, and remains low risk throughout labor and delivery and both mother and baby should be in good condition after birth.
Normal labor—37.0 weeks (259 days) to 42.0 weeks (294 days), primi—10–12 hours, multi—6 hours.

Q. How will you diagnose labor?

Ans. Labor is a clinical diagnosis characterized by:
a. True labor pain (Character discussed in case discussion in normal pregnancy at term), i.e. painful uterine contraction at shorter interval.
b. Palpable uterine contraction that increases in frequency and intensity.
c. Dilatation and effacement of cervix.

Normal Labor and Labor in Malposition and Presentation

d. Show –bloody mucus from cervix before onset of labor.
e. Fetal membrane may rupture during the course of labor, however membrane may rupture before the onset of labor leading to sudden gush of water/or watery discharge per vagina.

Q. What is effacement?

Ans. Progressive shortening and thinning of cervix and is recorded in percent. It is caused by merging cervix with the lower uterine segment due to pull of upper active segment. When cervical canal is 2.5 cm, it is 0% effaced, lower part of cervical canal is tubular (50% effaced), but when it is papery thin, 100% effaced.

Q. What are the stages of labor?

Ans. *First stage*: Onset of labor pain to full dilatation of cervix. Primi—10-12 hours; multi—6 hours.
Second stage: From full dilatation of cervix up to the delivery of fetus. Primi—2 hours, multi—1/2 an hour.
Third stage: After the delivery of the baby ends with the delivery of placenta. Time—15 minutes to 1/2 an hour.
Fourth stage: Monitoring two hours after delivery of placenta to detect mainly PPH and other complications. Respiration rate, pulse, BP, vaginal bleeding and uterine hardness are observed every 15 minutes for 2 hours.

Q. How do you assess the progress of labor?

Ans. See the answer in normal pregnancy case discussion.

Q. What is latent phase of labor?

Ans. If the cervix is 1–4 cm and uterine contractions are weak; less than 2 contractions in 10 minutes, but the patient is in first stage of labor. It is characterized by slow cervical dilatation and is variable duration (on an average ~ 8 hours).

Q. What is active phase of labor?

Ans. If the cervix is greater than 4 cm, but orifice of the uterus (os) may not fully dilated, still the patient is in first stage of labor. It has 3 phases and duration 4–6 hours, dilatation rate is of 1 cm/hour
  a. Acceleration phase—(cervical dilatation 3–4 cm) and dilatation rate is 0.6 cm/hour.
  b. Phase of maximum slope (4–9 cm), maximum dilatation of 5 cm, dilatation rate is 1.2 cm/hr in primigravida and 1.5 cm/hr in multigravida.
  c. Deceleration phase—(9–10 cm), dilatation of 1 cm.

> **Note**
> *These subdivisions are rarely used currently. Cervical dilatation is mainly due to a. hydrostatic action of bag of fore water, b. fetal axis pressure. Cervical canal dilates from 2 cm at the onset of labor to 10 cm (full dilatation). A normal cervix dilates 1cm/hr in primigravida and 1.5 cm/hr in multigravida in active labor (after 4 cm of cervical dilatation).*

Q. How do you know that the patient is in second stage of labor?

Ans. Cervix fully dilated (10 cm), bulging of the perineum, gaping of the vagina and anus and head is visible in between contraction.

Q. What will you do when the patient is not in active stage of labor? (Cervix—1-4 cm, uterine contraction is weak, < 2 in 10 minutes)?

Ans. Monitoring of labor every hour:
- Frequency of contraction (once in how many minute), intensity (how strong) and duration (second) of contraction
- Fetal heart sounds (FHS)
- Presence of any emergency signs (difficulty in breathing, shock, bleeding PV)
  Monitoring every 4 hours
  - Progress of labor
  - Progressive descent of the presenting part
  - FHS will descend from above, downward and medially
  - Cervical dilatation, effacement and station
  - Temperature, pulse and blood pressure (BP) of mother
  - Record the time of rupture of membrane and color of liquor
- If after 8 hours, the contractions are stronger and more frequent and there is no progress of labor or cervical dilatation with or without rupture of membrane then it is a case of non-progress of labor, re-assess the pelvis, if fetal distress occurs go for lower segment cesarean section (LSCS)
- If the membrane is already ruptured on admission, but even after 8 hours there is no increase of frequency/intensity of contraction start for induction of labor if there is no obstetrical contraindication.

Q. How do you manage when the patient is in active stage of labor? (If cervix ≥ 4 cm dilated)?

Ans. Monitoring of labor every 30 minutes:
- Look for frequency, intensity, duration of contraction
- Fetal heart rate (FHR)
- Presence of any emergency sign.

Monitor the following every 4 hours:
- Temperature, pulse and BP, and P/V examination for assessment of cervical dilatation and effacement.
- Start partographic chart (Discussed in the chapter of Partogram).

Q. What is the expected length of different phases of labor?

Ans. See Table 5.1

Management of second stage of labor:

Cervix fully dilated, perineum is thin and bulging, anal gaping, the head of the baby is visible at introitus.

1. Monitor the following every 5 minutes:
    a. Frequency, intensity, duration of uterine contraction
    b. Fetal heart sound (FHS)
    c. Perineal thinning and bulging
    d. Descent of the head during contraction.

Normal Labor and Labor in Malposition and Presentation

Table 5.1: Duration of different phases of labor			
Phases of labor	**Average duration (hours)**	**Maximum slope (cm/hour)**	**Upper limit of normal**
Nulliparous labor			
Latent phase	8.60	–	>20 hours
Active phase	4.90	1.2 or less	–
Second phase	0.95	1.0 or less	none†
Multiparous labor			
Latent phase	5.30	–	>14 hours
Active phase	2.20	1.5 or less	–
Second phase	0.24	2.0 or less	none†

† There is no limit to the length of the second phase as long as progress is being made and there is no fetal distress

2. Bearing down effort is required as cervix is fully dilated.
3. Avoid injury to perineum to hasten delivery.
4. Episiotomy is not mandatory in all cases.

Delivery of head:
- Encourage the woman to push only during contraction
- Ask the mother to breathe steadily in between contraction
- Do not give fundal pressure
- A sterile pad is placed over the anus. The sinciput may be felt behind the anus at the tip of the sacrum
- Press the perineum with pad to maintain flexion
- Press downward on the head to promote flexion and allow occiput to slip under pubis
- Crowning of the head—when maximum transverse diameter of the presenting part stretches the perineum and it does not recede back in between contraction
- When head is free, extension is encouraged by placing the head against symphysis pubis and press the perineum by pad (Modified Ritgen's maneuver) and head is delivered.

After delivery of the head:
- Suck the baby's mouth and eyes should be cleaned by sterile cotton swab soaked with normal saline
- Free the cord around the neck if present. If tight, cut the cord in between clamps and if loose, slip the cord over the head.

Delivery of shoulders (Do not be hasty):
- Wait for 1 minute for spontaneous rotation of shoulder.
- Perineal tear can be prevented by delivering one shoulder at a time.
- Apply gentle downward traction until the anterior shoulder appears under pubic arch.
- Then lift the baby up, to deliver the lower posterior shoulder and the anterior shoulder drops down beneath the symphysis pubis.
- The rest of the baby is delivered by lateral flexion.
- Place the baby on tray.

Cutting of the cord:
1. Clamp and cut the cord at 30–60 seconds after birth. This will supply extra amount of blood (80 mL) to neonate and prevent fetal anemia (50 mg of iron to the infant's store). Newborn is not elevated above

the introitus at vaginal delivery or above the abdominal wall at cesarean section.
2. Put the first clamp around the cord 6–8 cm from fetal abdomen and milking towards the newborn is safe and advantageous if rapid cord clamping is clinically indicated. Neither method of early cord clamping or delayed cord clamping after stoppage of cord pulsation are beneficial and later on umbilical cord is tied at 2 or 3 cm from the baby's abdomen and the second clamp should be placed as close to perineum for identification of apparent lengthening of the cord, which is one of the important signs of separation of placenta.
3. Cut the cord in between the clamps with sterile blade/scissors and tie the cord with the presterile disposable clip towards baby's side. Look for oozing of blood after 2 hours. If oozing is present place a second tie between the baby's skin and first tie.
4. Examination of proximal end of cord will prevent clamping part of omphalocele and umbilical hernia.

> **Note**
>
> Tie the cord 2–3 cm from the base and cut the remaining cord. Leave the stump uncovered and dry. The 2010 American Heart Association Neonatal Resuscitation guideline suggest cord clamp delay.

Q. Enumerate the conditions where early cord clamping is necessary.

Ans. Prevention of Rh incompatibility, diabetic baby, asphyxiated baby, during cesarean section (CS) when baby is delivered by cutting placenta (in anterior placenta previa), tight cord round the neck.

> **Note**
>
> Early clamping reduces the risk of phototherapy by 40%.

After delivery of the baby
- Maintain baby's temperature to prevent hypothermia by skin to skin contact with mother after delivery (Kangaroo method) or by covering the baby with blanket after wiping the baby repeatedly. Bathing is not recommended after birth as it causes hypothermia leading to hypoxia, hypoglycemia, poor growth, metabolic acidosis and pulmonary hypertension.
- Note Apgar score at 1 and 5 minutes
- If baby does not cry, resuscitate the baby
- Breastfeeding within 1/2 an hour of normal delivery (or within 2 hours of LSCS)
- Care of the cord—no ointment or sterile water on the cord and inspect the cord 2 hours after ligation for any evidence of bleeding.
- Care of eyes of newborn by separate sterile swab soaked with saline
  - Congenital defects (cleft lip, palate, anal and esophageal atresia, imperforate anus) are looked for.
- Injection Vitamin K prophylaxis 1mg IM after birth to prevent bleeding disorder if the weight of the baby is >1,000 g, but if the weight of baby is <1,000g use it in a dose of 0.5 mg IM.

- Baby passes meconium within 24 hours and 97% of newborn baby void urine within 48 hours
- At birth, BCG, OPV and hepatitis B immunization should be given to the baby.

Q. How do you treat specific labor abnormalities?

Ans. See Table 5.2.

Table 5.2: Treatment of labor abnormalities

Labor pattern	Preferred treatment
Prolonged latent phase (>20 hours in nulli, >14 hours in multi-ineffective uterine contraction)	Therapeutic rest, hydration, pain relief/Oxytocin and amniotomy or CS for urgent problem
Arrest disorder 1. Arrest of dilatation (>2 hour in active phase) 2. Arrest of descent (fails to get station of 1 cm in 1 hour)	With CPD-CS; without CPD-oxytocin With CPD-CS; without CPD-oxytocin, operative vaginal delivery or CS
Protracted active phase Nulliparous <1.2 cm/hour, multiparous <1.5 cm/hour	Oxytocin infusion is not always successful, CS for CPD
Prolonged second stage Fetal head descent <1 cm/hour or duration >2 hours	Operative vaginal delivery or CS

CS, cesarean section; CPD, cephalo–pelvic disproportion

PROGRAMMED LABOR (FOR POSTGRADUATES)

Q. What is programmed labor?

Ans. Pain relief in labor and to document the events during labor on a partogram and reaching the goal of 'safe motherhood' by optimizing obstetric outcome.

Q. Protocols of programmed labor.

Ans. It depends on three pillars:
  a. *Power*: Ensure optimal uterine contraction with the help of oxytocin, if required.
  b. *Pain relief*: Judicious combination of analgesia/antispasmodic medication and epidural analgesia.
  c. *Partogram*: Documentation of progress of labor and timely intervention.
  Identification of start of active phase of labor.

Q. When will you start for programmed labor?

Ans. a. Cervix should be 4 cm dilated and 50% effaced
  b. The fetal head should be engaged
  c. Presence of show
  d. Three contractions in 10 minutes persisting for 35–60 seconds, if pain is not optimal, pitocin infusion.

Q. What is the protocol of management?

Ans. a. Obstetrical examination
  b. Amniotomy—note the color of liquor

c. Obtain a base line FHR
d. Start IV infusion with Ringer lactate (RL)
e. Optimize the pain with oral prostaglandin (PG) tablet, primiprost (0.5 mg) every 1–2 hour or add oxytocin to ensure optimum uterine contraction
f. Optimization of pain relief
   1. *Immediate or short time pain relief:*
      Injection 6 mg pentazocin + 2.0 mg diazepam (1/5th ampoule of Fortwin + 1/5th ampoule of calmpose) diluted in 10 mL of distilled water and give slow IV as a bolus through the infusion tube.
   2. *For long-term pain relief:*
      Injection tramadol—1.0 mg/kg body weight (BW) IM with 1 ampoule of injection Drotin (40 mg) slow IV.
   3. *For pain relief in advanced labor:*
      After 7–8 cm dilatation of cervix, if patient complains of unbearable pain, injection ketamine, 0.5 mg/kg BW, diluted, and give slow IV. In case further analgesia is required, the ketamine dose can be repeated in half the initial amount (0.25 mg/kg BW) at an interval of 20–30 minutes until delivery.
g. Partographic record (discussed on partographic chapter).
h. Active management of third stage by 125 µgm (microgram) of $PGF_2\alpha$ IM after the birth of the baby. This reduces the third stage to 3–5 minutes and blood loss to 50–75 mL only.
i. After delivery add the remaining 4/5th of diazepam and 4/5th Fortwin injection to the mother.
j. Note Apgar score of baby at 1 and 5 minutes.

Q. What are the advantages of programmed labor?

Ans.
a. Shorten the duration of labor
b. In primigravida, active stage reduces from 8 to 5 hours
c. Pain relief in labor
d. Incidence of obstetrics interference are reduced
e. Neonatal outcome is satisfactory
f. Minimum blood loss.

Q. What is the basic concept of Active Management of Labor (AMOL)?

Ans.
a. Comprehensive prenatal education.
b. Admission when cervical dilatation is 2–3 cm with painful, regular uterine contraction.
c. Only nulliparous patients are included.
d. Amniotomy at the time of admission irrespective of cervical dilatation.
e. Frequent cervical examination by nurses (1–2 hours interval) and to ensure progress of labor.
f. High dose oxytocin protocol.
g. One-on-one nurse care for auscultation of fetal heart and continuous fetal monitoring.
h. Mid-forceps or rotational forceps should not be used.

Normal Labor and Labor in Malposition and Presentation

i. Active involvement of obstetrician.
j. Continuous internal audit.

> **Note**
> Primary goal of AMOL:
> a. To prevent prolonged labor.
> b. To reduce the rate of CS.

Labor in Abnormal Positions

Occiput Posterior Position

Occiput posterior (OP) is a malposition of head and occurs in 13% of cephalic presentation. The presenting part is the vertex and denominator is the occiput (Figure 5.2).

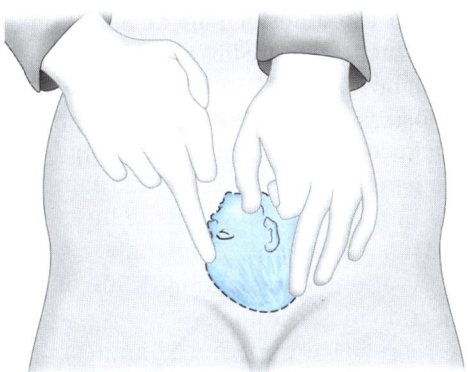

Figure 5.2: Abdominal examination to diagnose sinciput and occiput of fetal head, which are not at the same level. In deflected head it will be at same level

Q. Why ROP is more common than LOP?

Ans. 1. Pelvic colon occupies the left posterior quadrant
2. The uterus is dextrorotated.

Q. What are the causes of occiput posterior?

Ans. 1. *Fault in passage:*
   a. Pendulous abdomen—this is found in multipara.
   b. Anthropoid pelvic brim—favors direct OP.
   c. Android pelvic brim—the transverse diameter of the brim being nearer to the sacrum encourage biparital diameter (BPD) to accommodate posteriorly.
   d. A flat sacrum—with poorly flexed head leads to further deflexion and OP.
   e. Placenta on anterior wall of uterus.
2. *Fault in passenger*—deflexed head, large fetus.
3. *Fault in power*— abnormal uterine inertia.

Q. How do you diagnose OP?

Ans. *Abdominal examination:*
a. Flattening of lower abdomen.
b. Fundal grip—breech is felt.
c. Lateral grip—the fetal back is found on one side and difficult to palpate, the limbs are in front and gives hollowing above the head.
d. Pelvic and Pawlik grip—nonengaged vertex with sinciput and occiput at the same level. (**Que.** How will you examine sinciput and occiput per abdomen? **Ans.** See the Figure 5.2 where sinciput and occiput are not at the same level).
e. Auscultation—FHS is heard on the flank.
f. Vaginal examination—the membrane ruptures early often before labor is well-established. If the membrane is intact it protrudes through the cervix giving finger like fore water and obscure the presenting part. Due to deflexion of head, anterior fontanelle is readily felt in the anterior part of pelvis near the iliopectineal eminence. The sagittal suture lies on right oblique diameter of pelvis in right occiput posterior (ROP) and left oblique diameter of pelvis in left occiput posterior (LOP). Posterior fontanelle is not easily felt till the head is in lower pelvic cavity (Figure 5.3).

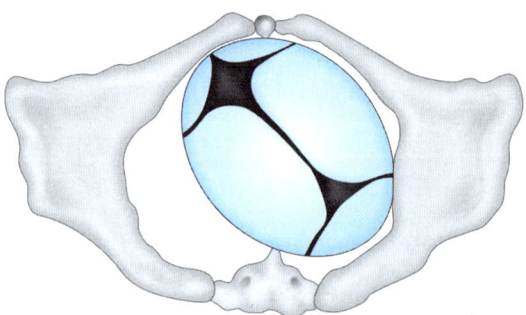

Figure 5.3: Left occiput posterior (LOP)

Q. Mechanism of labor (Figure 5.4).

Ans. *Engagement*: In ROP head engages in the right oblique diameter of pelvis and LOP head engages in the left oblique diameter of pelvis. Engaged diameter of head is occipitofrontal (11.5 cm) or suboccipitofrontal (10 cm). If descent occurs see Figure 5.4 (Favorable side for vaginal delivery) If unfavorable: Deflexion persists which may be:
a. *Mild deflexion*: Anterior rotation of occiput by 1/8th of a circle—deep transverse arrest (DTA).
b. *Moderate deflexion:* Occiput and sinciput touch the pelvic floor at the same time—oblique posterior arrest.
c. *Severe deflexion:* Sinciput touches the pelvic floor first then rotate to 1/8th of a circle under symphysis pubis and occiput is rotated to sacral hollow—occipito-sacral arrest or persistent occiput posterior (POP).

Normal Labor and Labor in Malposition and Presentation

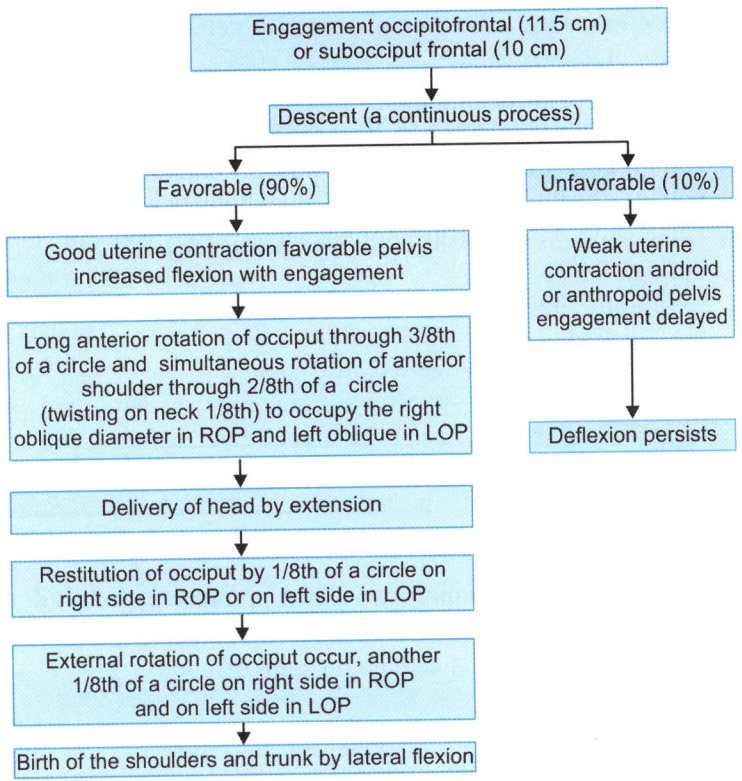

Figure 5.4: Mechanism of labor in occiput posterior position

Q. Is normal delivery possible in POP?

Ans. In some cases of POP, face to pubis delivery occurs with good uterine contraction and adequate pelvis.

Root of the nose stems under the symphysis pubis—vertex and occiput are born by flexion and face is delivered by extension.

Occipitofrontal diameter with BPD lying posteriorly distends perineum and chances of more perineal injury (wide episiotomy is mandatory in this case).

Restitution: The head moves 1/8th of a circle in opposite direction of internal rotation then turn face to look towards the mother's left thigh in ROP and right thigh in LOP.

External rotation: The occiput rotates to the same direction of restitution to 1/8th of a circle placing finally the face looking directly towards left thigh in ROP and right thigh in LOP.

Q. What are the problems of OP during labor?

Ans. a. Occiput posterior leads to dysfunctional labor.
  b. Contraction may be painful accompanied by troublesome backache, uterine contraction is incoordinate and progress is slow.
  c. Good analgesia and epidural block is ideal.

d. Retention of urine is common and catheterization may be required frequently.
e. Mother feels urge to bear down before full dilatation of cervix probably due to pressure on the sacrum and rectum.
f. Premature expulsive force delays progress by causing edema of the cervix and epidural analgesia is again helpful in this condition.

Q. How do you manage a case of occiput posterior position?

Ans. Principle:
1. Early diagnosis
2. Strict vigilance
3. Timely interference.

> **Note**
> OP is not an indication of CS.

Q. When CS is performed?

Ans. In cephalopelvic disproportion (CPD), pregnancy-induced hypertension (PIH), elderly primi mother, post CS pregnancy, big baby, early rupture of the membrane, with no progress of labor.

First Stage
- Patient is in bed
- Anticipate prolonged labor
- Progress of labor is measured by head descent, rotation of back and anterior shoulder towards midline, increased flexion of head, cervical dilation and effacement.
- Late CS is performed in fetal distress, incoordinate uterine contraction, maternal distress and arrest of labor.

Second Stage

In majority of cases anterior rotation is complete and head is delivered or face to pubis delivery in POP with good uterine contraction and adequate pelvis.

Third Stage

Active management of third stage by oxytocics (Injection syntocinon 10 unit IM just within 1 minute after delivery of baby).

Q. What is deep transverse arrest (DTA)?

Ans. When the head is deep in the pelvic cavity and sagittal suture of fetal head is in the transverse diameter or bispinous diameter and there is no progress of labor in 1/2 to 1 hour following full dilatation of cervix in spite of good uterine contraction.

Q. What are the causes of DTA?

Ans. a. Faulty pelvic architecture—prominent ischial spine, flat sacrum and convergent side walls
b. Deflexion of head (Figures 5.5A to C).

Normal Labor and Labor in Malposition and Presentation

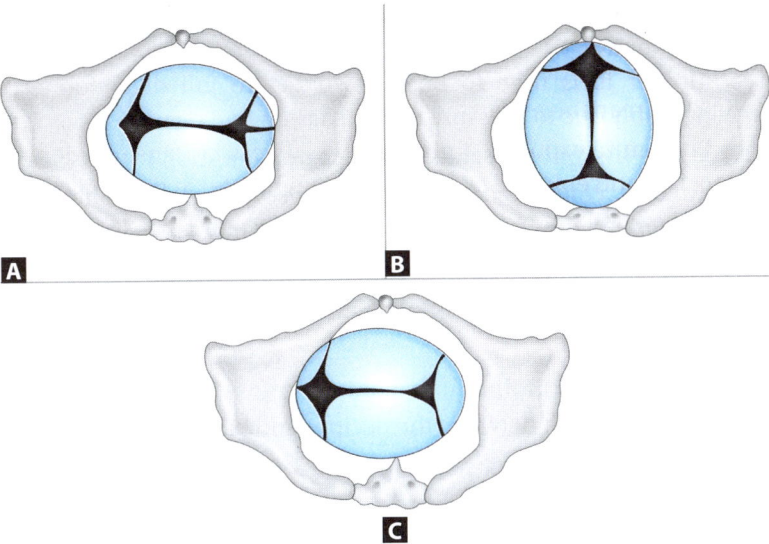

Figures 5.5A to C: Deflexion of head. (A) Right occiput transverse; (B) Persistant occiput posterior; (C) Left occiput transverse

Q. How will you diagnose DTA?

Ans.
    a. Head is engaged
    b. Sagittal suture is in bispinous diameter
    c. Anterior fontanelle is palpable (persistent fetal head deflexion)
    d. Faulty pelvic architecture
    e. Abnormal uterine action.

Q. How do you manage a case of DTA?

Ans.
    a. Fetal and pelvic assessment are mandatory before formulating any line of management.
    b. P/A—size of baby, FHS, engagement of head, amount of liquor.
    c. P/V—station of head, position of sagittal suture and occiput, degree of deflexion of head, molding, caput and assessment of pelvis is to be done.

If vaginal delivery is unsafe:
Fetal distress, fetal head is more than 3/5th palpable per abdomen, big baby, inadequate pelvis—cesarean section.

If vaginal delivery is safe, follow any of the methods below:
1. Application of ventouse is ideal
2. Manual rotation and forceps delivery (see the Chapter 3, Forceps)
3. Forceps rotation and forceps delivery (see the Chapter 3, Forceps)
4. Craniotomy, if baby is dead.

Q. How do you deliver the baby in POP?

Ans. If the head is low down and pelvis is good—forceps delivery, otherwise cesarean section should be performed.

LABOR IN ABNORMAL PRESENTATION: FACE

Q. What is the incidence of face presentation?
Ans. 1 in 300 pregnancies.

Q. What are the common causes of face presentation?
Ans. High parity, contracted pelvis, flat pelvis, fetal abnormality and fetal thyroid enlargement, twisting of the cord several times in the neck.

Q. Can you feel sinciput and occiput in face presentation?
Ans. No, there is hyperextension of fetal head. So, neither occiput nor sinciput is palpable.

Q. On abdominal examination what is the most important finding?
Ans. Groove may be felt between the occiput and back.

Q. How do you differentiate face and breech by PV examination?
Ans. **Face:**
    a. Mouth and malar eminence are not on one line (form a triangle).
    b. Hard alveolar margin is felt.
    c. Sucking effect of mouth may be felt.
    d. Absence of meconium stain on the examining finger.
Breech:
    a. The anus and ischial tuberosity are on the same line.
    b. Soft anal margin.
    c. Anal sphincteric grip is felt.
    d. Meconium stain on the examining finger.

Q. What is the engaging diameter of face?
Ans. Submentobregmatic (9.5 cm) in fully extended head and submentovertical (11.5 cm) in partially extended head.

Q. The submentobregmatic and suboccipitobregmatic are of same dimension 9.5 cm, so why labor is delayed in face presentation?
Ans. a. In normal vertex, suboccipitobregmatic and BPD are in the same plane, but in face presentation, submentobregmatic and BPD are in different planes. The submentobregmatic and bitemporal diameter engages together.
    b. Delay in labor
        1. Weak uterine contraction and poor cervical dilatation due to attitude of extension
        2. Absence of molding of facial bones
        3. *Delayed engagement*: The distance between the biparietal planes to the chin is 7 cm and to occiput is 3 cm.
        4. Late internal rotation.
        5. Arrest may occur at any time.

Q. What is the most common position of face?
Ans. Most common position is left mentum anterior (LMA), as ROP is 5 times more common than LOP. Overall anterior position is more common than posterior position.

Normal Labor and Labor in Malposition and Presentation

Q. Why perineal damage is more common in face delivery?

Ans. Wide BPD (9.5 cm) stretches the perineum and submentovertical diameter (11.5 cm) emerges out of the introitus.

Q. How will you deliver face in mentoanterior position?

Ans. If cervix is fully dilated:
   a. To proceed to normal child birth.
   b. If slow progress and no sign of obstruction, augment labor with oxytocin.
   c. If descent is unsatisfactory, deliver by forceps.
      (So vaginal delivery is possible in chin anterior position).

Q. What will you do in mentoposterior position?

Ans. Chances of vaginal delivery is less (Complete anterior rotation of mentum occurs in only 20% is living)—Lower segment cesarian section (LSCS)
   - Baby is dead— individualize the case—Craniotomy/LSCS.

Q. Why CS is preferred in mentoposterior position?

Ans. In 70–80% of cases there is arrest of labor due to incomplete anterior rotation, nonrotation and short posterior rotation of the mentum. There is no possibility of spontaneous labor in persistent mentoposterior position because the thorax thrust resulting in bregmaticsternal diameter (18 cm or 7 inch) to occupy the pelvic cavity as a result neither flexion nor extension of the fetal head is possible.

Q. Mechanism of face delivery.

Ans. Mentoanterior (Figure 5.6A)
   a. Engagement—right oblique diameter in LMA, left in RMA. Engaging diameter is submentobregmatic (9.5 cm) in fully extended head or submentovertical (11.5 cm) in partially extended head.

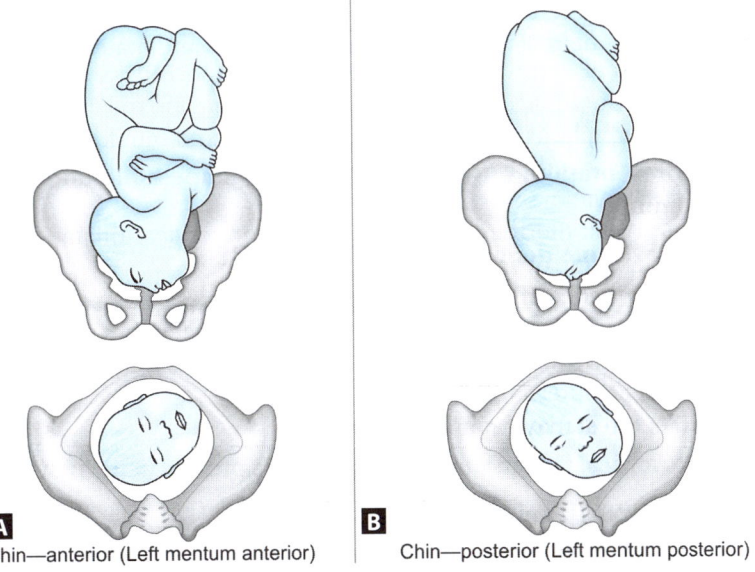

A Chin—anterior (Left mentum anterior) **B** Chin—posterior (Left mentum posterior)

Figures 5.6A and B: (A) Chin anterior; (B) Chin posterior

b. Descent with extension.
c. Internal rotation—mentum rotates through 1/8th of a circle, anteriorly.
d. Further descent occurs till the submentum hinges under the pubic arch.
e. The head is born by flexion (instead of extension as in occiput) delivering the chin, face, brow, vertex and lastly the occiput.
f. Restitution occurs through 1/8th of a circle opposite to the direction of internal rotation.
g. External rotation occur further 1/8th of a circle to the same side of restitution so that face looks towards left thigh in LMA and right thigh in right mentum anterior (RMA) positions.
h. This follows the delivery of anterior shoulder followed by posterior shoulder and rest of the baby is delivered by lateral flexion.

Mentoposterior (Figure 5.6B)
a. Engagement.
b. Descent with extension.
c. Internal rotation—long internal rotation 3/8th of a circle so that submentum comes under the symphysis pubis and delivery occurs as in mentoanterior otherwise there may be mentotransverse or mentosacral arrest.

In mentoposterior presentation, cesarean section is the choice than manual rotation and forceps delivery, if the baby is dead, craniotomy (in experienced hands).

Q. What is the clinical course of labor in face presentation?

Ans. a. Extension of face causes poor ball—valve action in LUS and leads to PROM
b. Cord prolapse
c. Prolonged labor is anntcipitated (causes already discussed)
d. Increased chances of perineal tear as submento-vertical diameter (11.5 cm) stretches the perineum
e. Chances of PPH is high due to atonic uterus and maternal injury.

BROW PRESENTATION

(In brow presentation, engagement is usually impossible and arrest of labor is common)

Q. What is the incidence?

Ans. 0.07%.

Q. What is the etiology?

Ans. Partial deflexion of fetal head, CPD.

Q. What is the diameter of engagement?

Ans. Mentovertical (14 cm), no such diameter is present in the pelvis.

Q. How do you diagnose?

Ans. a. *Clinical*: Diagnosis in late pregnancy is very difficult. It is diagnosed in labor by vaginal examination. Diagnosis is made by frontal suture,

Normal Labor and Labor in Malposition and Presentation

anterior fontanelle, supraorbital ridges, forehead, root of the nose and eyes. The posterior fontanelle, mouth and chin cannot be palpated in the brow presentation.

b. *Ultrasonography (USG)* to exclude major anomalies and macrosomia.

Q. How do you manage brow presentation in labor?

Ans. a. More than 50% of brow presentation converts by flexion to vertex or by extension to face presentation when fetus is small
b. Management of persistent brow presentation:
  i. Vaginal delivery is less than one-third of patient with persistent brow presentation, prefer cesarean section (CS) when fetus is alive
  ii. If labor progress is protracted or arrested—LSCS (80%)
c. Attempt to deliver instrumentally or manipulation of the fetus vaginally to vertex (Thorn's maneuver) or face are dangerous and contraindicated.
d. If fetus is dead—LSCS (lower segment cesarean section)/Craniotomy (in experienced hand).

> **Note**
> Cesarean section should be done in brow presentation.

BREECH PRESENTATION

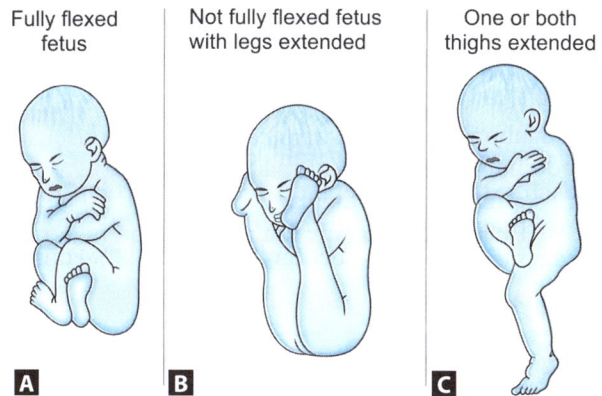

Figures 5.7A to C: Types of breech; (A) Complete or fully flexed breech; (B) Frank breech; (C) Footling or incomplete breech

Q. Define breech.

Ans. When the fetal podalic end presents at the pelvic brim.

Q. Incidence of breech.

Ans. 5% at 34 weeks and 3% at term.

Q. What are the types of breech?

Ans. a. **Complete or flexed breech** (5–12%): Here the lower extremities of the fetus are flexed both at the hip or knee joint, feet are present in pelvis. Common in multigravida (Figure 5.7A).

b. **Incomplete breech:**
   i. *Frank or extended breech (60–70% of all breeches)*: Here the thighs of the fetus are flexed at the trunk, but the legs are extended, common in primigravida (Figure 5.7B).
   ii. *Footling presentation*: Here both the thighs and legs are partially extended with the feet presenting at the brim (Figure 5.7C)
   iii. *Knee presentation (rare)*: Extension at hip joint and flexion of knee joint, knees are presenting part.

Q. How will you diagnose breech?

Ans. Palpation
a. Longitudinal lie
b. Firm lower pole—soft, broad and irregular nonballotable mass
c. Limbs on one side
d. Head at the fundus—hard, smooth, globular and ballotable

Auscultation: FHS is best heard above the umbilicus

PV: No head in pelvis, soft buttocks or feet may be felt; finger may go into the anal canal giving rise to meconium stain of finger where membrane is ruptured.

USG: Differentiation of head and breech, head is readily detected by scan.

CT and MRI: Pelvic architecture and configuration.

Q. Describe the management of breech.

Ans. a. External cephalic version (ECV) in antenatal period or early labor which its discussed in the chapter of version (under obstetrics intervention and operation Chapter 3)
b. Vaginal breech delivery.
   1. Spontaneous (10%)
   2. Assisted—conducted by trained doctor
   3. Breech extraction in fetal distress, cord prolapse and accidental hemorrhage and to deliver second twin
c. Lower segment cesarean section (LSCS) (20–50%) during pregnancy and labor.

> **Note**
>
> *Complicated breech (breech with contracted pelvis, APH, preterm labor, multiple pregnancy, pre-eclampsia, PROM) are indications of elective cesarean section. Other indications of elective CS are discussed later.*

Q. How do you conduct assisted breech delivery in 2nd stage of labor?

Ans. Labor should proceed normally in extended breech
- The mother should be in lithotomy/dorsal position when buttocks are seen at introitus
- The bladder should be empty
  – IV infusion should to be started
- The anesthetist and pediatrician should be present in the labor room
  – Continue FHR monitoring by CTG

- An episiotomy is made when posterior buttock distends the perineum and cervix is fully dilated
- The breech, legs and buttocks should be allowed to deliver spontaneously and pull the cord to exclude short cord and is kept in the sacral bay, but if the breech is arrested at the outlet single groin traction is usually effective (The index finger is to be hooked in the fold of anterior groin and gentle traction should be given towards the trunk than towards the femur for fear of fracture and the traction should be simultaneous with the contraction of uterus and fundal pressure which is very important). In case of difficulty, traction is given on both the groins simultaneously with fundal pressure.

1. Delivery of the Legs

If the legs are flexed they will fall out, but if they are extended they should be lifted out; once access can be gained to the popliteal fossa. If the arrest of buttock is in the mid pelvis then either CS or Pinard's maneuver, if mid pelvis is not contracted. Patient is put under general anesthesia (GA) and maintain full surgical asepsis during the procedure. The hand, the palmar surface of which corresponds to the ventral aspect of the fetus is introduced and first disimpact the buttock so that the anterior one can be pushed up to the level of symphysis pubis (Figures 5.8A to C) for delivery of legs. When delivery of one leg is completed the delivery of the second follows quickly.

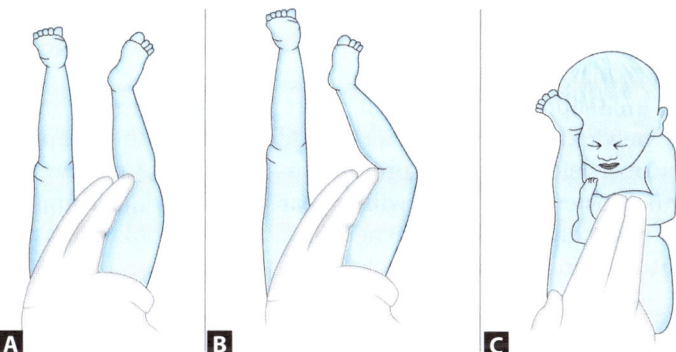

Figures 5.8A to C: Delivery of the legs: (A) Press by middle and index fingers in the popliteal fossa for flexion of the knee and displace it to the side of the trunk (abduction), while other hand presses down the fetal head per abdomen; (B) Fingers are worked along leg towards ankle to encourage further flexion; (C) The ankle is grasped and the foot is swept over the other leg by a movement of adduction—Pinard's maneuver

2. Delivery of the Arm

Generally arms are felt on the chest. When arms are flexed, the vertebral border of the scapula remain parallel to the vertebral column and when arms are extended there is winging of the scapula (parallelism is lost). Allow the arm to disengage one by one, only assist this delivery, if necessary. The delivery proceeds spontaneously as the anterior shoulder blade or scapula appears at the outlet.

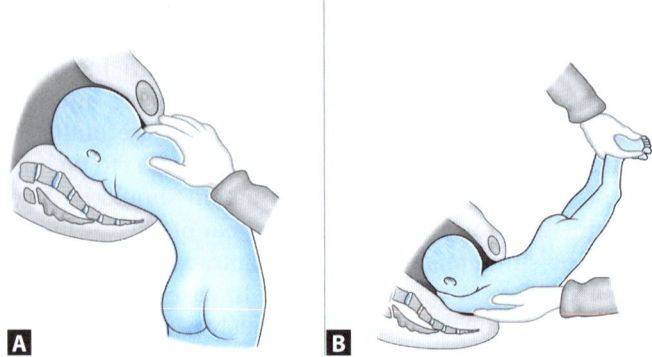

Figures 5.9A and B: Delivery of the arms. (A) Delivery of anterior arm; (B) Delivery of posterior arm

a. The arm is delivered by placing of the appropriate hand (right if the right shoulder) over the clavicle and then round the point of shoulder and then elbow and carrying the forearm free (Figure 5.9A).
b. The ankle is then grasped and lift the buttock towards the mother's abdomen to deliver the posterior arm (Figure 5.9B).
c. If arm does not spontaneously delivered, place one or two fingers in the elbow of the baby's arm and bend the arm, bring the hand down over the baby's face and deliver it.

Lovset's Maneuver (No Anesthesia is Required)

Principle

Due to the inclination of pelvic brim, short anterior wall and long posterior wall of the pelvic cavity, the anterior shoulder is above the symphysis pubis and posterior is below the sacral promontory and if these are now reversed in position, the posterior shoulder will appear just below the symphysis pubis and can be easily delivered. The maneuver should start only when the inferior angle of the anterior scapula is visible under pubic arch.

Procedure

Step 1: Hold the baby by hips (femoropelvic grip keeping the thumbs parallel to the fetal vertebral column) and fingers should rest on anterior superior iliac crest and keep the baby elevated and turn the baby half a circle (180°) keeping the back anterior by applying downward traction at the same time, so that the arm that was posterior now become anterior and can be delivered under the pubic arch and which is then hooked out (Figures 5.10A and B).

Step 2: The trunk is then rotated in a reverse direction keeping the back anterior by applying downward traction to deliver the anterior shoulder under the pubic arch (Figure 5.11).

Q. If the arms are stretched above the head or folded around the neck, how do you deliver the arms?

Ans. a. By Lovset's maneuver (discussed above).
b. *Classical method*: Under GA, the hand is introduced up to the elbow to bring down the arm across the face. While doing the same for

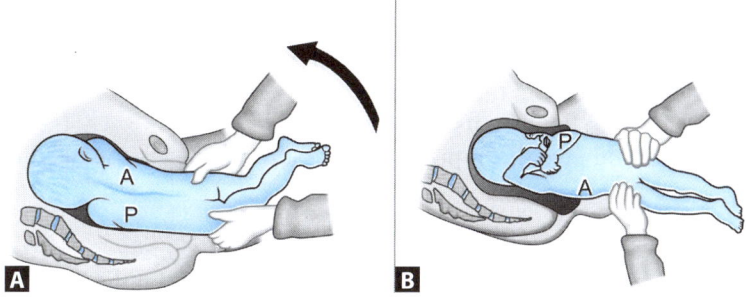

Figures 5.10A and B: Lovset's maneuver process—step 1. (A) Holding the baby by hips; (B) Turning the baby half a circle (180°)
A = Anterior shoulder and P = Posterior shoulder

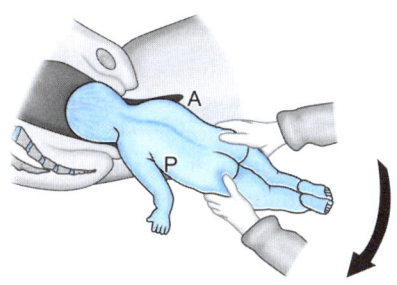

Figure 5.11: Lovset's maneuver process—step 2
A = Anterior shoulder, P = Posterior shoulder process

other arm, sometimes there occurs dorsal or nuchal displacement of arm. In such case a long rotation of the trunk is made in the direction that brings head away from arm.

In nuchal arm:

Procedure: Rotate the fetus through half a circle counter-clockwise so that friction exerted by birth canal will draw the elbow towards the face. If rotation is not possible push the baby upward in an attempt to release it. In desperate cases the nuchal arm is delivered by hooking a finger over it and force the arm over shoulder which may cause fracture of bones.

Q. What will you do if the baby's body cannot be turned?

Ans. If the baby's body cannot be turned to deliver the arm that is anterior first, deliver the shoulder that is posterior
  a. Hold the baby by the ankle.
  b. Move the baby's chest towards the woman's inner leg, the posterior shoulder is delivered.
  c. Deliver the arm and hand.
  d. Pull the back down by ankles, the shoulder that is anterior should now deliver.
  e. Deliver the arm and hand.

3. Delivery of the Head

- Do not be in a hurry, about 5 minutes can be safely allowed between the delivery of the cord and the head
- Allow the baby to hang on its own weight
- Assistant should give the suprapubic pressure to engage the head in the pelvis.

Burns-Marshall Method (Figure 5.12)

When the nape of the neck is visible below the pubic arch lift the baby slowly by its ankle on the mother's abdomen keeping the back of the baby up. The assistant should continue the suprapubic pressure. This allows the head to be delivered in a controlled manner in a state of flexion, with first face, then forehead, then vertex sweeping over the perineum.

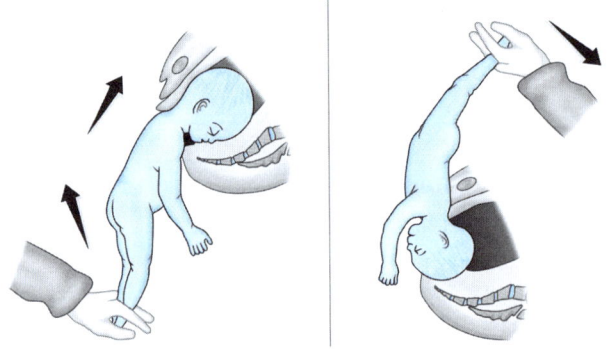

Figure 5.12: Delivery of head by Burns-Marshall method

Delivery of Head by Forceps (Figure 5.13)

Head is delivered by forceps: The assistant is to lift the baby's trunk as much to facilitate introduction of blades from below to occupy the occipito-mental diameter and traction (initially traction of force is downwards, then forwards and finally upwards) is given along the curve of birth canal. Piper's forceps or any forceps having the usual length of the shank can be used. Outlet forceps is never used for this purpose.

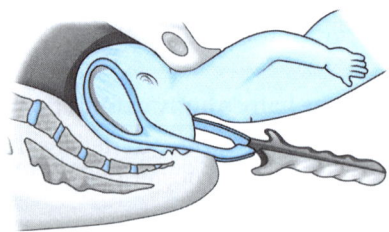

Figure 5.13: Delivery of head by forceps

Advantages

a. Pull is directly on head and not through neck.
b. Flexion is better maintained.

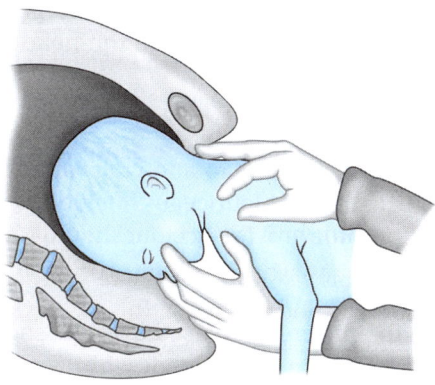

Figure 5.14: Jaw flexion and shoulder traction

c. Mucus can be sucked out from the mouth more effectively.

Ordinary forceps with usual length and shank is effective for this delivery, but Piper forceps is specially designed for this delivery.

*Jaw Flexion and Shoulder Traction
(Mauriceau-Smellie-Veit Technique) (Figure 5.14)*

This method is employed under general anesthesia:
- Lay the baby's face down with the length of the baby over your left hand and forearm.
- The middle finger of left hand is placed in the mouth and the index and ring fingers catch the cheek bones (modification of the original method—The middle and the index fingers of left hand are placed on the malar bones of either side).
- Traction by these fingers promotes flexion of head.
- The index finger and thumb of other hand grasp the left shoulder, the middle finger press the occiput and other two fingers (ring and little fingers) are placed on the child's right shoulder. Traction is given by downwards and backward direction till the nape of the neck is visible under the pubic arch. The assistant should give suprapubic pressure to maintain flexion, then the fetus is carried upward and forward towards mother's abdomen releasing the face, brow and lastly the trunk is depressed to deliver the vertex and occiput.

> **Note**
> In all cases head should be delivered slowly to decrease the risk of damage of brain.

Difficulty with the after Coming Head

Wigand–Martin Maneuver

The body of baby is placed on the stretched arm and the middle finger of that arm is placed in the mouth of the baby to maintain flexion of the head while the index and ring fingers of the same hand are placed on the malar bones to exert traction. A continuous suprapubic pressure is exerted by other hand on the occipital region to force the head down to pelvis and delivery of head.

Occiput Posterior

a. **Rotation method**: In such a case rotation may often be done by grasping the head and trunk as for the Mauriceau-Smellie-Veit technique and they are then pushed up a little and the occiput should rotate forward and the head and trunk must be rotated together to avoid injury to the spine of the baby.
b. **Prague method**: The fingers are placed over the shoulders from behind and outward and upward traction is made while the other hand grasps the legs and the body is swung over the mother's abdomen. Thus, the occiput is born over perineum. There is a risk of stretching of neck and fracture of spine by this method.
c. **Modified Prague maneuver**: If after delivery of the baby occiput remains in posterior direction and attempt to rotate occiput anteriorly is unsuccessful, the delivery of head in persistent occiput posterior (POP) position is done by modified Prague method.

Method

If the chin is down, the ordinary method of passing fingers on the malar eminence of the face of the baby from front and grasping the shoulders with two fingers of other hand from behind should be employed (Mauriceau-Smellie-Veit technique) and the child is pulled backward and when the forehead is fixed against the posterior surface of symphysis pubis the trunk is pulled upwards towards the mother's abdomen and this method is supplemented by suprapubic pressure and episiotomy. This flexes the head and result in delivery of the occiput over the perineum.

> **Note**
> *In dead fetus craniotomy is the alternative.*

An insufficiently dilated cervix:
Delivery of entrapped head (in incomplete dilatation of cervix), baby is alive
a. Gentle downward traction on the shoulder with fundal pressure simultaneously given by the assistant may deliver the baby.
b. In premature or small baby the fingers are passed through the constricted cervix and to reach the chin or face of the baby and the fingers are used as improvised shoe-horn along with the pressure from above and traction from below to deliver the live baby.
c. If this fails general anesthesia (halothane) is used to obtain complete relaxation of the lower segment and pelvic floor. Gentle downward traction on the shoulder may affect the after coming head delivery.
d. If delivery is still unsuccessful Duhrssen's incision must be made in posterior cervix at 6 o'clock to loosen the entrapped head. Sometime additional incisions are necessary at 2 o'clock and 10 o'clock.

Normal Labor and Labor in Malposition and Presentation

e. In dead baby: Allow the baby to hang with weight for full dilatation of cervix and do craniotomy if needed.

> **Note**
> 1. Duhrssen's incision releases the head but its extension in upward direction causes severe hemorrhage, so rarely used in modern obstetrics
> 2. In all cases head should be delivered slowly to decrease the risk of damage of brain in living breech.

Q. What is breech extraction?

Ans. Operative delivery of breech under general anesthesia without any assistance of mother during delay of second stage of labor and in presence of maternal and fetal distress.

Steps

1. One hand is introduced into the uterus and the anterior feet is grasped by the heel (Figure 5.15A) (pulling the posterior limb tends to turn the baby into the sacroposterior position).
2. Downward traction is made on the leg and outside hand, press the head upward (Figure 5.15B).
3. Gentle traction is made on delivered leg until the breech is delivered (Figure 5.15C).
4. Proceed the delivery allowing by Lovset's maneuver for hand delivery followed by delivery of head.
5. Give a prophylactic antibiotic for intrauterine manipulation.

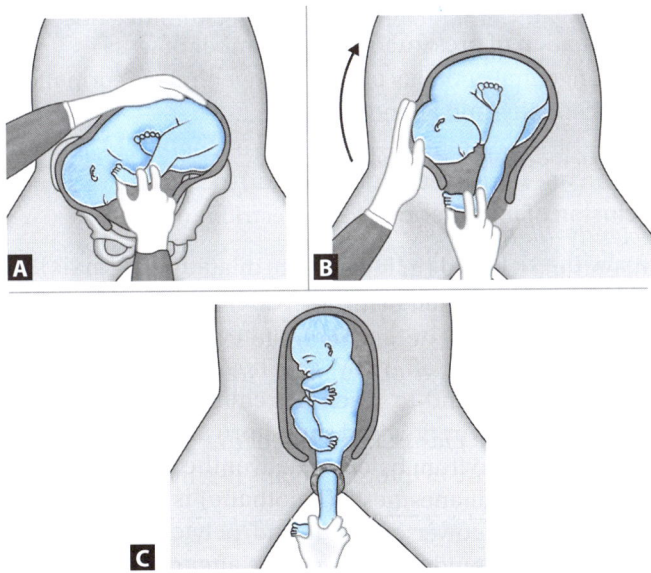

Figures 5.15A to C: Breech extraction: (A) Step 1; (B) Step 2; (C) Step 3 (see the text)

Q. What are the complications of breech extraction?

Ans. a. Uterine rupture
b. Injury of the fetus
c. Infection.

Q. What are the indications of breech extraction?

Ans. a. Delivery of second twin (commonest indication)
b. Prolapse of cord
c. Fetal distress
d. Excessive per vaginal bleeding or abruption placentae
e. Following internal version in cases of oblique and transverse lie.

Q. What are the indications of LSCS in breech?

Ans. a. Large fetus (> 4 kg)
b. Contracted or borderline pelvis
c. Footling breech
d. Preterm breech or severe FGR
e. Bad obstetric history (BOH)
f. No delivery after 8 hours in premature rupture of membranes (PROM)
g. Hypertension, associated PIH, diabetes
h. Elderly primigravida
i. Placenta previa
j. Previous cesarean delivery
k. Cesarean section on demand.

Q. What are the indications of vaginal delivery in breech presentation?

Ans. See X-ray breech.

Q. Role of USG in breech.

Ans. a. Confirmation of presentation and number of fetus
b. Any congenital anomaly of fetus (congenital malformation 8–10%)—hydrocephalus and anencephaly
c. Biometric measurement—BPD, femur length (FL), fetal weight (FW)
d. Flexion or extension of fetal head and location of placenta
e. Exclusion of intrauterine growth restriction (IUGR).

Q. What are the risks to the fetus?

Ans.
- *Head:* Intracranial hemorrhage
- *Neck*: Dislocation of neck, damage to sternomastoid muscles
- *Shoulder:* Dislocation of shoulder, fracture of clavicle, fracture of humerus
- *Injury of brachial plexus*: Erb's-Duchenne paralysis
- *Abdomen*: Rupture of internal organs like liver, spleen and kidney
- *Hip*: Dislocation
- *Femur*: Fracture.

Asphyxia of the baby due to:
a. Cord compression.
b. Retraction of the placental site when the head is still inside.

Normal Labor and Labor in Malposition and Presentation

c. Cord prolapse.
d. Premature attempt of respiration.
e. Delayed delivery of head.

> **Note**
> Fetal hazards can be prevented by:
> i. Adoption of ECV where possible
> ii. Liberal use of LSCS
> iii. Vaginal delivery by skilled obstetrician.

Q. Mechanism of labor.

Ans. The denominator is sacrum and leading part is anterior buttock lie—longitudinal, presentation—breech, position—left serum anterior (LSA).

Mechanism of Delivery of Breech in Left Sacral Anterior (Figures 5.16A and B)

Engagement: Engagement with labor occurs along left oblique diameter of pelvic brim. The sacrum lies on left iliopectineal eminence, the engaging diameter is bitrochanteric (10 cm).

a. Descent is a continuous process until it reaches the pelvic floor.
b. *Internal rotation*: The anterior buttock is rotated forward by 1/8th of a circle towards the symphysis pubis.
c. Further descent occurs and anterior buttock hinges under symphysis pubis.
d. *Lateral flexion*: Lateral flexion of the baby round the pubis allows the anterior buttock to step forward under the symphysis pubis and posterior buttock to slip over the perineum. The breech is delivered.
e. *Restitution*: The anterior buttock rotates back towards its original oblique position.

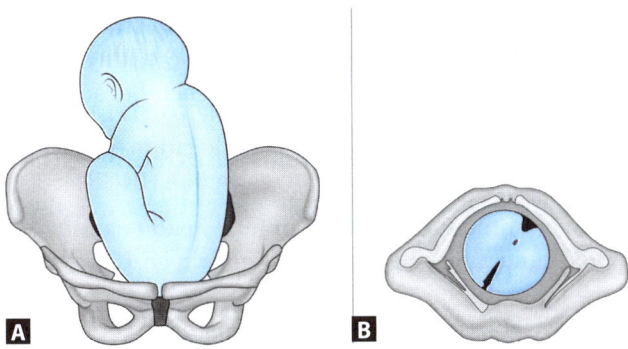

Figures 5.16A and B: Breech in left sacral anterior position (LSA) followed by legs (anterior buttock delivers first followed by delivery of posterior buttock)

Mechanism of Delivery of the Shoulders

- The shoulders now engage in the same pelvic diameter as hip, the left oblique diameter (bisacromian diameter—12 cm)
- Descent continues and the anterior shoulder touches the pelvic floor and rotates forward through 1/8th of a circle along right side of pelvis,

this causes the anterior shoulder to come under the symphysis pubis and other into the hollow of the sacrum
- The posterior shoulder delivers first followed by anterior shoulder
- Restitution: The anterior shoulder moves back to its original oblique position
- External rotation: The anterior shoulder rotates further 45° or 1/8th of a circle laterally so that the baby lies dorsoanterior.

Mechanism of Delivery of Head

As the shoulder is born, the head in the pelvic brim is either transverse or opposite oblique diameter (right oblique diameter) as that occupied by buttocks of the brim (left oblique diameter). The engaging diameter is BPD and suboccipitobregmatic or suboccipitofrontal (10 cm).
- Descent of the head with further flexion.
- Internal rotation of the occiput occurs by 1/8th or 2/8th of a circle at the level of pelvic floor and occiput hinges under the symphysis pubis.
- The head is born by flexion by bearing down efforts of mother, the chin, face and brow are born first and lastly occiput.

Q. In which breech presentation, chances of cord prolapse is high?

Ans. In footling presentation fetal mortality and chances of cord prolapse is high (12%) in comparison to frank breech. In complete breech risk of cord prolapse is 6%.

Q. Why breech is pathological in comparison to cephalic presentation?

Ans. a. The mother has greater risk for perineal tear, fetal and neonatal mortality is 10% when compared to cephalic presentation.
b. In cephalic presentation flexion occurs at the level of cervical spine, thereby reducing the diameter, whereas flexion occurs at lumbar spine in breech which does not help in decreasing diameter.
c. Flexion of trunk is difficult in frank breech because of splinting of head by the legs.
d. There is increased risk of cord prolapse as the breech can not fill the birth canal completely.
e. Insufficient time for moulding of fetal head resulting perineal tear, serious intracranial injury like hemorrhage (ICH) to the fetus in breech presentation.
f. Prolonged labor in breech when compared to cephalic.
g. Increased operative interference in breech, so operative morbidity is high.
h. Injury of the liver or kidney due to incorrect holding of the trunk, but fracture of humerus, and Erbs or Klumpke's palsy are high in breech than vertex presentation.

Q. What are the complications of persistent breech presentation?

Ans. a. Prolapse of cord
b. Congenital anomalies of baby

Normal Labor and Labor in Malposition and Presentation

c. Difficult delivery
d. Increased maternal and perinatal morbidity.

> **Note**
> Persistent breech is common in placenta previa and in uterine anomaly and tumor.

CORD PROLAPSE

Q. What is prolapse of umbilical cord?

Ans. The umbilical cord is in the birth canal below the presenting part or outside the vagina following the rupture of membrane.

> **Note**
> Occult cord prolapse—when the cord descends through the cervix alongside the presenting part; overt cord prolapse—when the cord is infront of the presenting part.

Q. How do you prevent cord prolapse? How do you diagnose it?

Ans.
a. USG to exclude malpresentation and cord position
b. Fetal heart rate monitoring to exclude FHR abnormalities
c. ARM is avoided in non-engaged head
d. ARM is avoided if there is worm like feeling through the intact membrane below the presenting part, with PROM and early rupture of membrane, PV examination is to be done to exclude cord prolapse.

> **Note**
> Cord prolapse is common in transverse lie, prematurity, breech with footling presentation, twin, hydramnios, in free floating head after low rupture of membrane.

Q. How do you manage the case of cord prolapse?

Ans. General management: Give oxygen 5 to 6 L per minute by mask or nasal catheter.

Specific management:

If cord is pulsating and fetus is alive:
Go for rapid per vaginal examination to note the stage of labor (if in first stage of labor, go for urgent cesarean delivery as early as possible for best fetal outcome, confirm fetal heart sound on OT table before starting LSCS).
Temporary measures to decrease the pressure on the cord before LSCS:
- Push the presenting part above the pelvis per vagina to decrease pressure on the cord
- Place the other hand on the suprapubic region to keep the presenting part out of the pelvis
- Once the presenting part is out of the pelvis remove the vaginal hand and keep the abdominal hand until CS

- Sims lateral position or with a pillow under the hip in the trendelenburg position and fill the bladder with normal saline (500 mL)[Vago's Method] is the other alternative procedure
- Salbutamol 0.5 mg IV slowly over 2 minutes to reduce the contraction of uterus.

If second stage of labor:
- Expedite the delivery by forceps with episiotomy in cephalic presentation if the criteria for forceps delivery is fulfilled, otherwise LSCS
- In breech presentation, breech extraction and forceps to the after coming head should be considered, otherwise LSCS
- Resuscitate the baby after delivery.

If baby is dead (no cord pulsation felt):
- No active intervention is necessary in many cases
- Spontaneous vaginal delivery is allowed.

> **Note**
> Process of delivery, which is safe to the mother, should be adopted.

COMPOUND PRESENTATION

Q. What is compound presentation?

Ans. Compound presentation is the presentation when the fetal extremity presents or prolapses by the side of the presenting part like cephalic or breech during pregnancy and labor. Most common incidence is the head with hand.

Others are:
a. Head with foot
b. Head with hand and foot together
c. Breech with hand prolapse.

Q. What are the causes of compound presentation?

Ans.
a. Preterm fetus (commonest) with PROM
b. Contracted pelvis
c. Twin
d. Dead fetus
e. Hydramnios and fetal malformation
f. Abnormal presentation
g. No apparent cause.

> **Note**
> Diagnosis should be suspected with any arrest of labor in the active phase or failure to engage during active labor.

Q. How do you manage head with hand presentation?

Ans. Diagnosis: Antenatally it is very much difficult to diagnose, but when the patient is in labor hand can be felt by the side of the head through membrane or after rupture of membrane hand is prolapsed by the side of the head felt on per vaginal examination

Treatment:

Management depends upon gestational age, pelvic size, high-risk factors and type of compound presentation.
1. No high risk factors and no cord prolapse
   a. Expectant treatment
   In second stage of labor:
      i. Head descends and hand recedes—vaginal delivery
      ii. If hand does not recede, manual pushing of the hand up and head is delivered spontaneously or use of forceps/or ventouse may be needed
2. With high-risk factors or cord prolapse
   a. LSCS, if baby is living
   b. Destructive operation or LSCS if baby is dead
3. Persistent compound presentation with term sized baby LSCS.

Q. What are the fetal and maternal risks?

Ans. Fetal: Cord prolapse and birth trauma
Maternal: Soft tissue damage and obstetric lacerations.

Q. What are the indications of cesarean section in compound presentation?

Ans.
1. Persistent compound presentation with term size baby
2. Contracted pelvis
3. Failure to progress of labor
4. Associated cord prolapse
5. Maternal high-risk factors
6. Fetal compromise.

Transverse lie

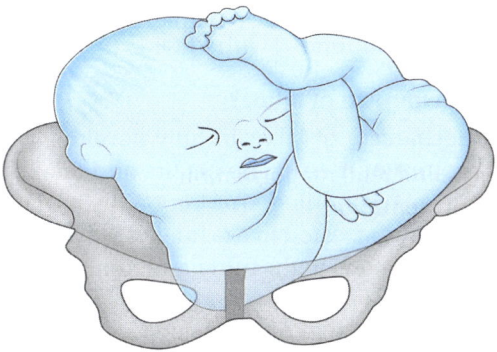

Figure 5.17: Transverse lie (Dorsoposterior)

Q. What is transverse lie (Figure 5.17)?

Ans. Long axis of the fetus is approximately perpendicular to that of mother.

Q. What is the incidence?
Ans. 1 in 322 singleton deliveries (0.3%).

Q. What are the causes of transverse lie?
Ans.
a. Abdominal wall relaxation due to high parity
b. Preterm fetus
c. Placenta previa
d. Uterine anomaly (arcuate septate or subseptate)
e. Hydramnios
f. Contracted pelvis.

Q. How do you diagnose transverse lie?
Ans. Clinically:
Per abdomen
Inspection: The abdomen is unusually wide transversely and uterine fundus extends only slightly above the umbilicus.
Palpation:
  i. Fundal height is less
  ii. *Fundal grip*: No fetal pole is detected in fundus
  iii. *Lateral grip*: Ballotement of head is found in one iliac fossa and the breech in the other. When the back is anterior a hard resistance plane extends across the front of abdominal, while when it is posterior irregular nodulations are felt through the anterior abdominal wall
  iv. *Pelvic grip*: Empty.
Auscultation: FHS is audible much below the umbilicus in dorso-anterior position, where as it is located at a higher level and often indistinct in dorsoposterior position.
Per vagina: In early stage of labor, if the side of thorax can be reached, it may be recognized by 'gridiron' feel of the ribs. With further dilatation the scapula and clavicle are further distinguished on opposite side of the thorax. The position of the axilla indicates the side of the mother towards which the shoulder is directed.
X-ray: See X-ray of transverse lie (Chapter 9)
USG, CT, MRI.

Q. What is the mechanism of labor?
Ans. There is no mechanism of labor in fully developed newborn. If labor progresses, rupture of membrane occurs and fetal shoulder is forced into pelvis and corresponding arm frequently prolapses. In advanced labor the shoulder is arrested in the inlet of pelvis with the head in one iliac fossa and the breech in the other and ultimately in neglected cases the uterus ruptures.

If the baby is small (<800 g) or macerated fetus and the pelvis is large, the fetus is compressed with the head forced against its abdomen and is expelled doubled up with chest and abdomen apposed. The head and feet are delivered last—*Conduplicato corpore.*

Other favorable terminations are (very rare) a. spontaneous rectification to vertex, b. spontaneous version to breech, c. spontaneous evolution—the trunk and breech are delivered followed by delivery of head.

Unfavorable termination in mature fetus is very common.

Q. How do you manage transverse lie?

Ans. See X-ray of transverse lie (Chapter 9).

Neglected Shoulder Presentation

Shoulder is impacted into the pelvis and prolapse of arm and cord occurs following rupture of membrane. A thick muscular band, pathological retraction ring develops just above the thin lower uterine segment. The force generated during a uterine contraction is directed centripetally at and above the level of pathological retraction ring. This stretches the lower uterine segment below and rupture of uterus may occur.

Treatment

a. Cesarean delivery with IV fluid and antibiotics
b. In severe infection or rupture of uterus, cesarean hysterectomy should be done.

> **Note**
> *Transverse lie of a large fetus especially if the membrane is ruptured and the shoulder is impacted in the birth canal usually needs classical cesarean section.*

Chapter 6

Assessment of Fetal Well-being

1. Daily fetal movement count (DFMC).
2. Fetal heart rate (FHR) monitoring.
3. Antepartum fetal surveillance.
4. Fetal distress in labor.
5. Different CTG tracings.

DAILY FETAL MOVEMENT COUNT

a. *Cardiff count to ten chart*: Start count of fetal movement from 9 am to 9 pm and if tenth fetal movement is not felt within 12 hours then go for non-stress test (NST).
b. Count fetal movement 1 hour after breakfast, 1 hour after lunch and 1 hour after dinner and multiply the count by 4 to get the total count in 12 hours. Normal fetal movement is 10 in 12 hours (Table 6.1).

Table 6.1: DFMC-chart

Time	Date	
	14.8.2011	15.8.2011
9–10 am after breakfast	3 movement	1 movement
1–2 pm after lunch	2 movement	-
9–10 pm after dinner	2 movement	1 movement
Movement in 3 hours	7	2
Movement in 12 hours	28	8
Remarks	Good	Bad

FETAL HEART RATE MONITORING

Accurate recording of uterine activity and fetal heart rate (FHR) pattern are an essential part of fetal monitoring.

Electronic Fetal Monitoring (EFM)
a. External cardiotocography (CTG)
b. Internal CTG—not discussed here.

Assessment of Fetal Well-being

Advantage of electronic fetal monitroing over clinical monitoring
- Can detect hypoxia/fetal distress early
- Improves perinatal mortality
- Decreases intrapartum fetal death
- Medicolegal documentation

Disadvantages
- High cost of the instrument
- LSCS rate is high for false interpretation.

External Cardiotocography

Plays a certain role in antepartum testing—NST, CST and also intrapartum evaluation of fetal distress.

Uterine contraction are measured by a displacement transducer (Tocodynamometer) placed on maternal abdomen, close to right cornu of uterus and another transducer for fetal monitoring is placed at the site of located fetal heart sound (FHS) on mother's abdomen. It displays the frequency of uterine contraction and FHR pattern and its relation to uterine contraction. The strip moves at a rate of 1 cm/minute though it is possible to move 2–3 cm/minute. *The following parameters are studied:*
1. Baseline FHR.
2. Beat-to-beat variability.
3. Long-term variability (LTV) of baseline FHR.
4. Acceleration of FHR with fetal movement.
5. *Uterine contraction*: Frequency, amplitude and duration.
6. Change of baseline FHR with uterine contraction.
7. Deceleration—Early, late, variable and prolonged in intrapartum monitoring.

Normal Fetal Heart Rate Pattern

The graph (Figure 6.1) shows FHR pattern monitored during delivery.

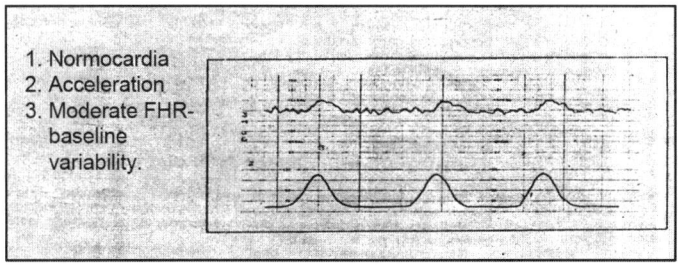

Figure 6.1: Normal fetal heart rate pattern during delivery

FETAL DISTRESS AND MONITOR

Causes of Fetal Distress

Maternal Factors

Maternal hypoxia (heart disease, asthma), hypotension (bleeding, supine hypotensive syndrome), vascular spasm, (eclamptic seizure, vascular diseases).

Uterine Factors

Excessive uterine contraction, rupture of uterus, uterine anomaly.

Placental and Umbilical Cord Factors

Placental dysfunction—diabetes, post-term pregnancy, pregnancy-induced hypotension (PIH), premature separation of placenta, placenta previa, prolapse of the cord, cord round the neck, true knots, velamentous insertion of cord.

Fetal Factors

- Prematurity, fetal anemia, congenital heart disease.
- Intrauterine growth restriction (IUGR).

Mechanism of Fetal Heart Rate Variation

Heart of the fetus is developed by the second week of gestation and heart beat begins between the 4th and 5th week of gestation and at 6th week it is observed by ultrasonography (USG) (abdominal).

1. Occlusion of arterial blood flow, due to compression of umbilical cord causes rise of blood pressure (BP) in the fetus, exciting the baroreceptors in the carotid artery, fetal aortic arch causing tension of vagus nerve and rapid reduction of FHR.
2. Under low partial pressures of oxygen (pO_2) the sympathetic nerve system is excited by chemo receptors in carotid bodies, which sometimes increases the FHR (tachycardia); in some cases it directly excites the vagus nerve, reduces FHR causing bradycardia and again hypoxia in heart muscles causes bradycardia.
3. Chemoreceptors also react to pH value and carbon dioxide (CO_2) concentration and under fetal distress various changes in FHR occur, as a result of different complicated mechanisms.

CLASSIFICATION, CAUSES AND MECHANISM OF FETAL HEART RATE PATTERN

Acceleration (Figure 6.2)

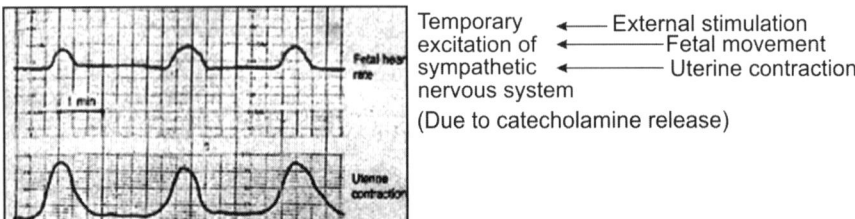

Figure 6.2: Acceleration of FHR

Deceleration (Figure 6.3)

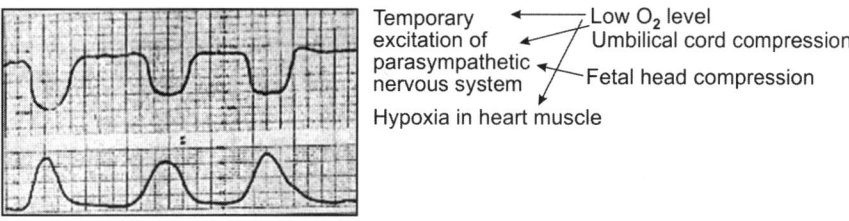

Figure 6.3: Deceleration of FHR

Tachycardia (≥160 bpm) (Figure 6.4)

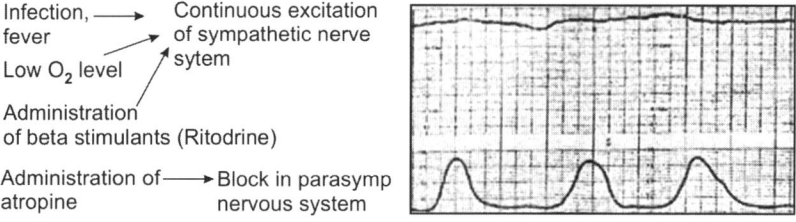

Figure 6.4: Tachycardia

Bradycardia (≤110 bpm) (Figure 6.5)

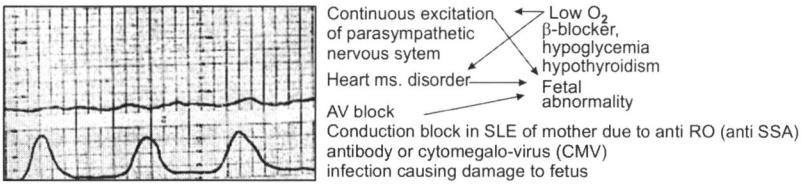

Figure 6.5: Bradycardia

Increased Fetal Baseline Variability (Figure 6.6)

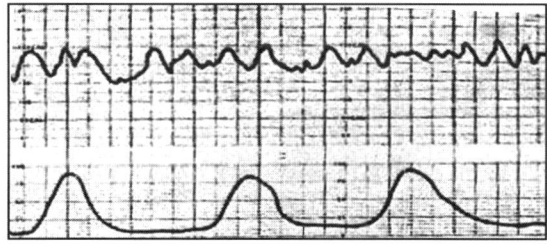

Figure 6.6: Increased fetal baseline variability

Mechanism: *Excitation of autonomic nervous system*

1. Acute low oxygen (O_2) level.
2. Umbilical cord compression.
3. External stimulation.

Premature ventricular contraction: Low O_2 level and fetal abnormality.

Loss of FHR Base-line Variability (Figure 6.7)

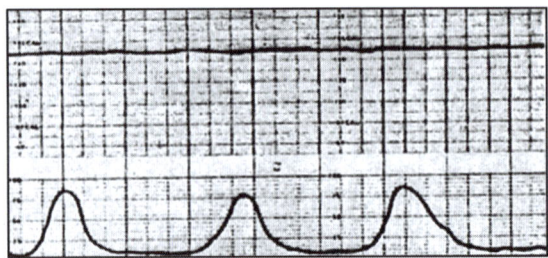

Figure 6.7: Loss of FHR baseline variability

Mechanism: *Inhibition of autonomic nervous system*
1. Sleeping phase of fetus.
2. Drugs-analgesics, anesthetics, barbiturates, and magnesium sulfate.
3. Anencephaly and premature baby.
4. Acidosis.
5. Severe low O_2 level.

Inhibition of heart muscles: Drugs, acidosis, severe low O_2 level.

Sinusoidal Pattern (Amplitude of 5–15 bpm and a frequency of 2–5 cycle/minute) (Figure 6.8)

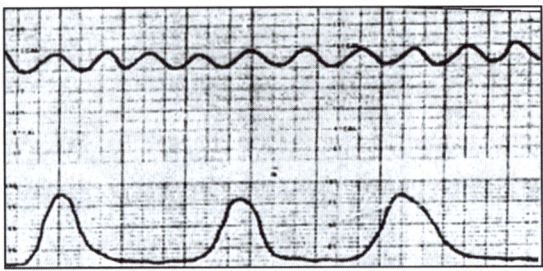

Figure 6.8: Sinusoidal pattern

Mechanism: *Disturbance of autonomic nervous system*
1. Fetal anemia.
2. Low O_2 level.
3. Acidosis.

Table 6.2: The FHR baseline (Basal FHR)		
Sl. No.	**Baseline variation**	**FHR**
1.	160 bpm or more	Tachycardia
	180 bpm or more	Severe tachycardia
	160–180 bpm	Mild tachycardia
2.	110–160 bpm	Normocardia
3.	110 bpm or less	Bradycardia
	100–110 bpm	Mild bradycardia
	100 bpm or less	Severe bradycardia

Fetal Heart Rate Pattern During Delivery
1. Baseline FHR (Table 6.2)
2. Temporary FHR variation
3. Fetal heart rate baseline variability.

Fetal Heart Rate Decelerations

Hon (1975) described a classification of deceleration, which has been internationally accepted.

Early Deceleration

Occurs almost the same time with uterine contraction (Figure 6.9). The peak of the uterine contraction coincides with the lower point of deceleration pattern and the return of baseline, when the contraction ends (mirror image). This pattern were said previously physiological due to compression of head, but it may occur also due to temporary disruption of the blood flow through the umbilical cord, as well as head compression. Care must be taken if there is severe decrease in the FHR and if it continues. Early decelerations seldom go below 100 bpm.

Late Deceleration

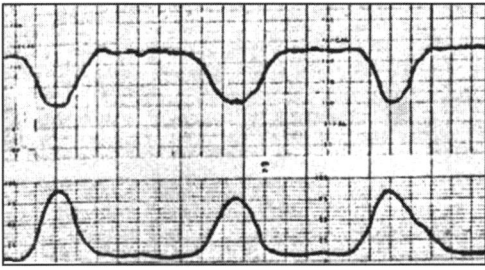

Figure 6.9: Early deceleration

Late deceleration begins after uterine contraction (Figure 6.10). The lowest FHR occurs after the uterine contraction has peaked and recovery of the deceleration pattern is after the uterine contraction is ended. A lag time exists between the uterine contraction and beginning of the FHR deceleration. This is often seen if the fetus is in low oxygen condition and placental insufficiency. During uterine contraction, the placental perfusion is decreased and decline fetal pO_2. When fetal pO_2 level is 15–18 mm of Hg, it triggers chemoreceptors and baroreceptor reflex. Initially centralization of blood volume (favouring perfusion to brain, heart, and adrenals) occurs by vasoconstriction in the vascular beds of limbs and gut. The resultant increase in peripheral resistance provokes reflex deceleration of FHR. Repetitive hypoxemia and centralization of blood volume, as evidenced by late deceleration may force hypoperfused tissue to convert for aerobic to anaerobic metabolism (early accumulation of pyruvate, lactate) which diffuse and cause metabolic acidosis, asphyxia and death of fetus.

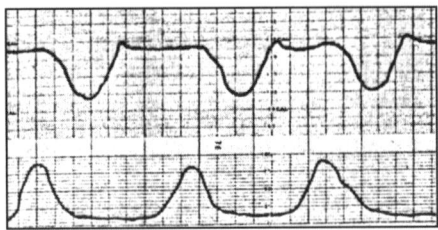

Figure 6.10: Late deceleration

Variable Deceleration

Its onset to uterine contraction is variable (Figure 6.11). Its shape is variable and duration is variable. The FHR drops below 100 bpm, occasionally to only 60–70 bpm. This is seen in cord compression. Characteristics of variable decelerations (V-shaped deceleration) include rapid descent and recovery, good baseline variability, and accelerations at the onset and at the end of contractions (i.e. shoulders). Umbilical vein is first occluded resulting in decreased venous return, relative hypovolemia, can reflexly increase FHR (shoulder) just before the onset of deceleration. Then occlusion of UmA, increase in peripheral resistance, elevation of fetal BP and baroreceptors mediated slowing of fetal heart rate pattern can lead to an attempt to return BP normal.

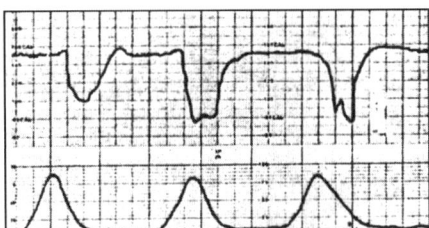

Figure 6.11: Variable deceleration

Severe variable deceleration: The deceleration pattern lasts for > 60 seconds and depth of deceleration is 70 bpm.
Mild variable deceleration: The deceleration pattern lasts for <30 seconds and the depth of deceleration is less than 70 bpm.
Moderate: Duration 30–60 seconds depth is < 70 bpm.
As cord compression is relieved, at times resulting in transient tachycardia or 'overshoot' at the end of deceleration due to reverse sequence of events. Shoulders are not part of variable decelerations.

Non-periodic Acceleration

This pattern sometimes classified as variable deceleration, has no direct relationship to the uterine contraction and is due to compression of umbilical cord (Figure 6.12).

Acceleration

Fetal heart rate temporarily increases by 10–15 beats per minute and lasts for 15 seconds or longer. There is a direct relationship to the uterine contraction

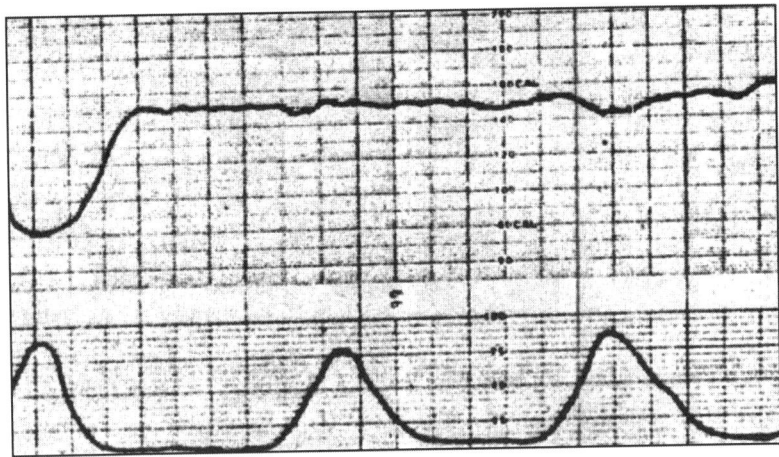

Figure 6.12: Non-periodic acceleration

and movement of fetus. This is due to increase catecholamine release and decreased vagal stimulation. The frequency is decreased by narcotics, magnesium sulfate ($MgSO_4$), atropine, prematurity and fetal distress. There is decreased rate of acceleration with the use of betamethasone to pregnant mother for fetal lung maturity (Figure 6.13).

Fetal Heart Rate Variability

Basal fetal heart rate pattern: The normal FHR is 110–160 bpm. The rate is defined as the average between the peaks and depression. Tracing of FHR of term normal fetus shows small, rapid, rhythmic fluctuations, with amplitude of 5–15 bpm. These fluctuations are superimposed on the basal FHR and are often referred to as beat-to-beat variability. Normal variability (5–15 bpm) represents intact nervous pathway through the cerebral cortex midbrain, vagus nerve and cardial conduction system variability is influenced by GA, fetal sleep, maternal medications, fetal acidosis and fetal tachycardia.

Short-term Variability

Short-term variability (STV) is a beat-to-beat variation of FHR from one beat to another. It can be measured accurately only with a fetal electrocardiography (ECG). It cannot be measured visually. Usually computer analysis is done; the normal range is between 5 and 15 bpm. Parasympathetic tone primarily affects the short-term beat to beat variability (Figure 6.14).

Long-term Variability (Figure 6.15)

Long-term variability (LTV) is associated visually from FHR tracing. Sympathetic stimulation is the strongest determinant of LTV and acceleration of heart rate. The oscillatory changes, which occur during the course of one minute are called LTV. When FHR varies 2–6 cycles per minute on the FHR tracing, it is called normal. When width of variation decreases to 5 bpm or less, it has clinical importance of fetal distress during delivery.

FHR variability is considered normal or average, when short-term or long-term variability is present and the difference between peak and toughs of LTV is 5–25/minute. Increased variability >25 bpm is uncommon and it may reflect increased catecholamine release in early fetal hypoxia. So, careful evaluation of the tracing is very important. Decreased variability <5 bpm is due to fetal central nervous system (CNS) activity for fetal sleep or due to administration of analgesics, $MgSO_4$, calmpose, atropine to mother. Betamethasone transiently decreases the FHR variability which returns to pretreatment status by the 4th–7th day. The movement of fetus after injection of corticosteroid may also be less transiently for 3–4 days for conservation of energy.

A good beat-to-beat variability normally indicates good fetal reserve and decrease or absence of beat-to-beat variability indicates fetal distress.

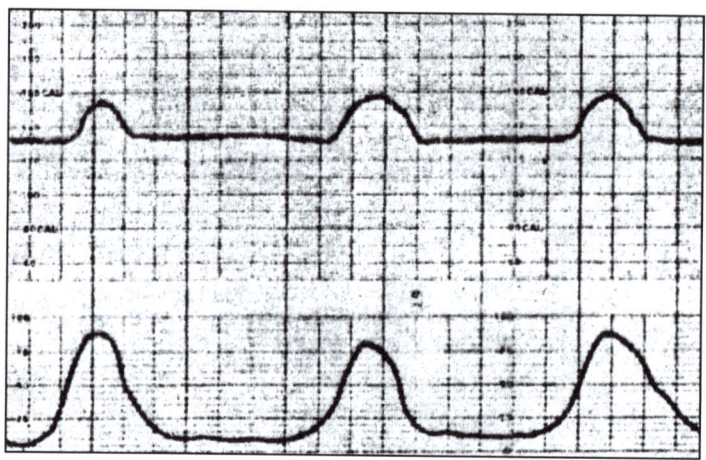

Figure 6.13: Acceleration

Classification of LTV (Hammacher) (Figure 6.15)

The term applied for fetal heart rate variation (FHRV)
   a. Silent pattern   <5 bpm
   b. Decreased variability   5–10 bpm
   c. Normal variability   10–25 bpm
   d. Saltatory   >25 bpm

> **Note**
> In an ideal normal CTG tracing: Short-term and long-term variability must be present.

Sinusoidal Pattern

A special type of LTV undulating wave form alternating with a flat or smooth baseline FHR. It is extremely significant finding and implies severe fetal jeopardy and impending fetal death in hemolytic anemia and hypoxia of fetus (*see* Figure 6.8).

Assessment of Fetal Well-being

FHR pattern during pregnancy (Antepartum)—a. DFMC, b. NST, c. CST, d. BPP, e. Doppler velocimetry.

Non-stress test (screening test)

Acceleration of FHR associated with fetal movement is the usual indication in a normal healthy condition. NST is recommended by 32–34 weeks of GA.

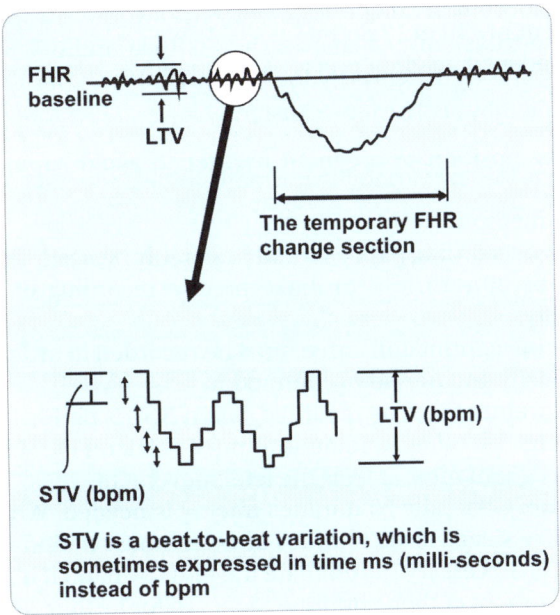

Figure 6.14: Short-term variability (STV) and LTV on FHR baseline

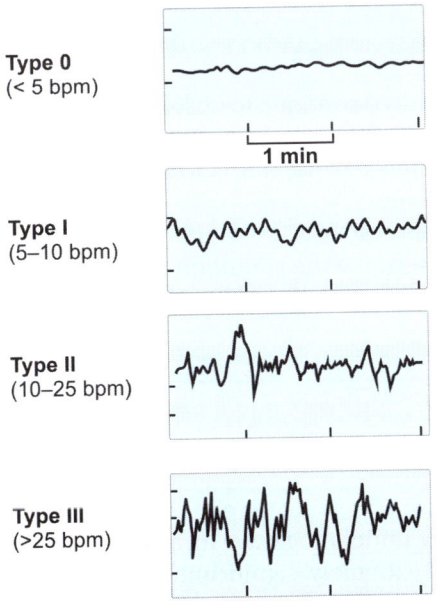

Figure 6.15: Long-term variability

Conditions where NST is preferable:
1. High risk cases: Pregnancy-induced hypertension, diabetes with pregnancy, post-term pregnancy where the fetal condition may be jeopardized during pregnancy.
   Other conditions—IUGR, SLE, APLAS, hemoglobinopathies, BOH (Bad obstetrical history—High-risk factors of previous pregnancy may likely to affect present pregnancy).
2. Fetal kick count <10 in 12 hours
3. Unexplained fetal death in previous pregnancy.

Methods

1. Semi-sitting position of pregnant mother to avoid supine hypotensive syndrome.
2. Recording method
   a. Large size recording paper should preferably be used. The paper speed should be 30 mm/min to make precise recording of FHR baseline variability.
   b. The uterine contraction curve must be recorded in order to determine the intensity and period of contraction.
   c. Fetal movement is to be recorded, when NST is performed—the usual way to check fetal movement is to put a mark on the recording paper, when pregnant mother feels the fetal movement.

Recording time: Generally 20 minutes tracing is needed. When the fetus is quiet or in active sleep, 40–60 minutes or even longer period is necessary to record. It may be necessary to stimulate the fetus by hand if it does not move for 40 minutes or longer then continue to record for further 20 minutes.
Diagnostic criteria: See Table 6.3
Visual acoustic stimulation (VAS) of 80 Hz and 82 db is sometimes helpful for FHR acceleration.

Management

- If NST is reactive then continue to observe the proceeding carefully.
- If NST is non-reactive, repeat the NST 2 times/day. If persists, go for back-up biophysical profile score, if it is less, lower segment cesarian section (LSCS) is to be done.
- Contraction stress test (CST) should be used occasionally, when it is impossible to determine the condition of fetus by NST and to determine, whether it is possible to deliver through the vagina by labor induction or LSCS.

> **Note**
> NST is a test for condition of fetus but CST is a test for uteroplacental function.

Table 6.3: Diagnostic criteria of NST

NST diagnosis	Diagnostic criteria	Management
Reactive	2 or more acceleration of 15 bpm persisting for 15 second in 20 minutes. tracing	Observe proceeding

ANTEPARTUM FETAL SURVEILLANCE (FLOWCHART 6.1)

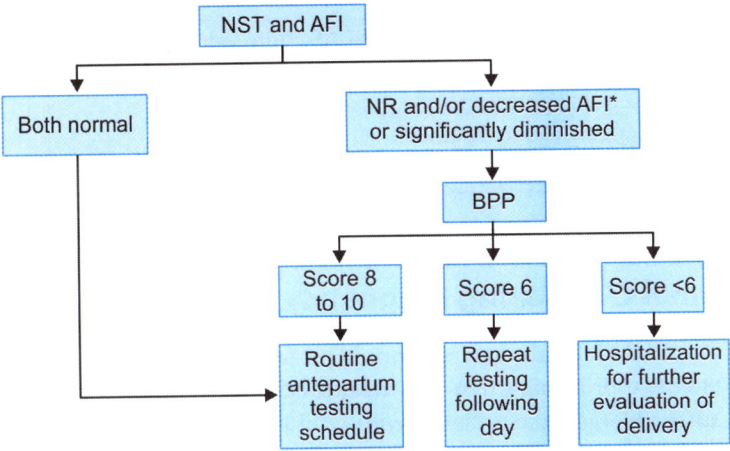

Flowchart 6.1: Antipartum fetal surveillance by NST, AFI and BPP

Abbreviations: NST—Non-stress test; NR—Normal; AFI—Amniotic fluid index; BPP—Biophysical profile; * If fetus is matured and AFI is reduced, delivery should be considered before further testing is undertaken. BPP and AFI—See the chapter of USG.

Example of Actual CTG

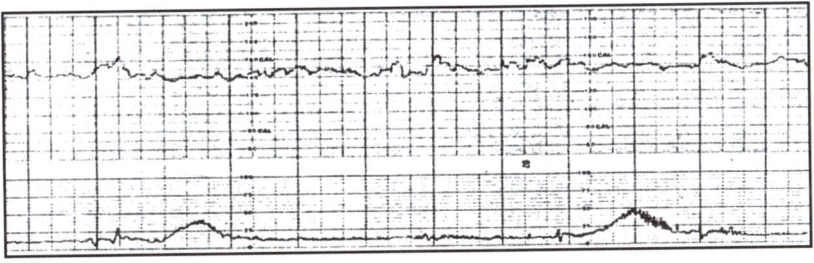

Figure 6.16: Normal CTG during labor

Normal CTG During Labor

Age: 25 years, Primi mother, GA of 40 weeks, normal CTG in first stage of delivery.

Fetal heart rate baseline: 140–150 bpm, variability of FHR baseline 10 bpm, acceleration observed with no deceleration. Delivery finished 8 hours later. Neonate 3,008 g, Apgar score 9 (Figure 6.16).

Normal CTG during Pregnancy (Reactive NST) (Figure 6.17)

Primi mother, age 26 years, GA-38 weeks, UC external, NST was conducted as mother is a case of diabetes mellitus (DM) with intrauterine growth restriction (IUGR). There is acceleration associated with fetal movement (FM) and no deceleration. FHR baseline 150 bpm. Variability is adequate.

Uterine contractions occur spontaneously at 39 weeks of GA and delivery was normal, neonatal wt 2.3 kg, Apgar score 9.
- Mark for fetal movement

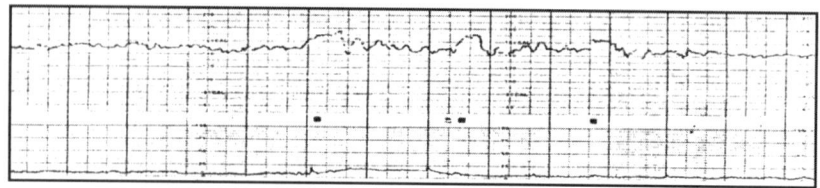

Figure 6.17: Normal CTG during pregnancy

Abnormal CTG During Pregnancy

Non-reactive NST

Age—28 years, primipara, GA—34 weeks, NST was conducted in DM with IUGR, no acceleration associated with fetal movement. Variability on FHR-baseline is also small, after one day, a late deceleration pattern was noted and CS was performed (Figure 6.18).
- Mark the fetal movement.

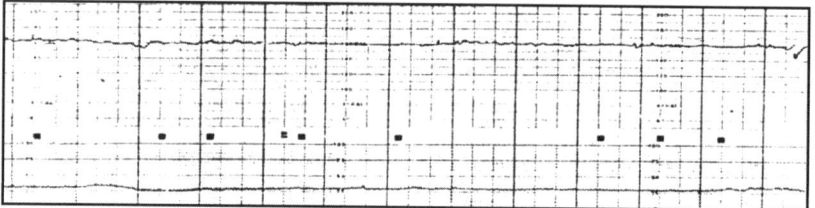

Figure 6.18: Non-reactive NST

Treatment of Fetal Distress in Labor: Ideally baby should be delivered whithin 30 minutes

Steps are to be taken before any definitive measures:
1. Change of position of mother—Left lateral position.
2. Oxygenation of mother—100% of oxygen, 5 to 6 liter/minute.
3. Supervision of uterine contraction—Omit syntocinon drip and administer uterine relaxant, if necessary.
4. Start IV line with RL/NS as dextrose solution causes lactic acidosis in anaerobic condition.
5. Scalp blood pH measurement if the facility is available.
6. Lower segment cesarean section or forceps delivery is needed according to the condition.

Practical Implications of Scalp Blood pH (Flowchart 6.2)

Contraindication of fetal blood sample (FBS):
a. Prematurity (< 34 weeks)
b. Maternal infections (HIV, Hepatitis virus)
c. Fetal bleeding disorder (e.g. hemophilia).

Assessment of Fetal Well-being

Flowchart 6.2: Intrapartum-fetal monitoring and management of fetal distress

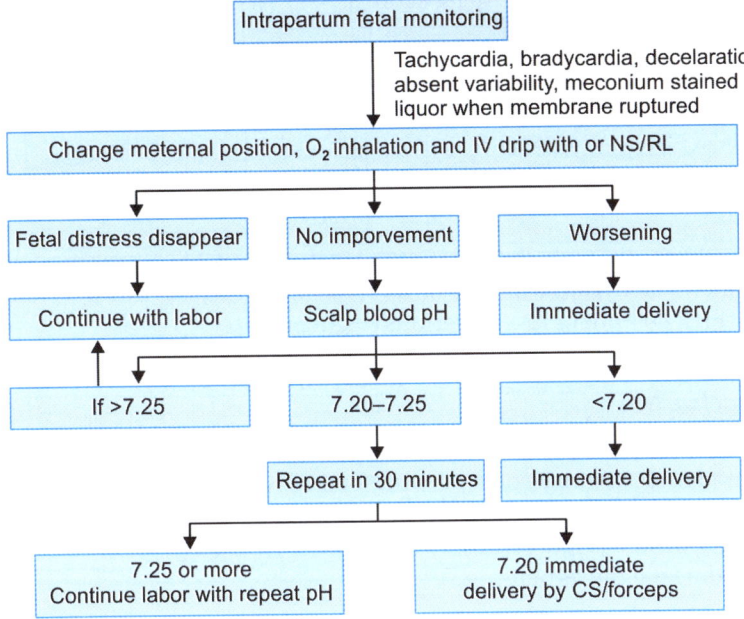

> **Note**
> 1. Scalp blood PH measurement–not used frequently recently for cumbersome procedure, technical inaccuracy, uncomfortable to the patient and repated sample is required.
> 2. Other methods of (intrapartum evaluation):
>   a. Percutaneous umbilical blood flow sampling
>   b. Fetal scalp stimulation by vibroacoustic stimulation and digital scalp stimulation are less invasive and when there is acceleration following stimulation, academia is unlikely and labor can continue
>   c. Fetal pulse oxymetry: Determines fetal oxygen saturation
>   Procedure: The sensor is placed against fetal cheek transcervically when membrane is ruptured.
>   Interpretetion:
>   • Normal: 40–70%
>   • Cut off value: <30% corresponds to pH 7.2
>   • >30% saturation even in presence of non-reassuring
>   • FHR tracing indicates normal fetal oxygenation.
>   d. Lactate level in fetal blood sampling: Normal fetal scalp lactate is <2.8 mmol/L; 2.9 mmol/L-3.08 mmol/L is suspicious and >3.08 mmol/L is abnormal. It is not routinely used in practice.

EXAMPLES OF SOME ABNORMAL FETAL HEART RATE BASELINE

Tracings in CTG

Severe tachycardia (Tachycardia with FHR baseline of 195 bpm) and bradycardia was noted 1 hour later and LSCS was performed (Figure 6.19).

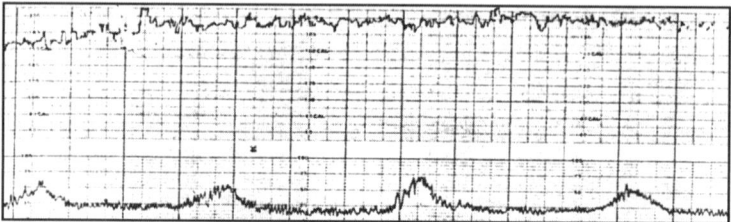

Figure 6.19: Severe tachycardia

Severe tachycardia with deceleration—Treatment of LSCS was performed immediately, tachycardia is not in favor of fetal distress, but deceleration pattern (FHR 80 bpm or less) is serious (Figure 6.20).

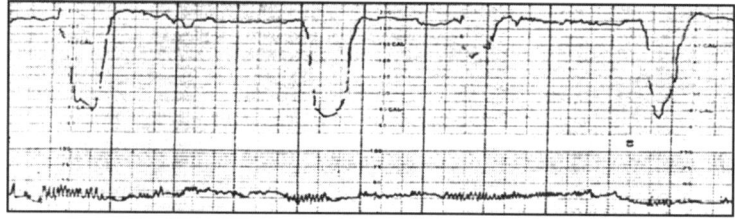

Figure 6.20: Severe tachycardia with deceleration

Mild bradycardia with a FHR baseline of 110 bpm, no deceleration was noted. The pregnant mother was hospitalized, NST was performed. After spontaneous uterine contraction began at a GA of 42 weeks, fetal distress becomes obvious and CS was performed (Figure 6.21).

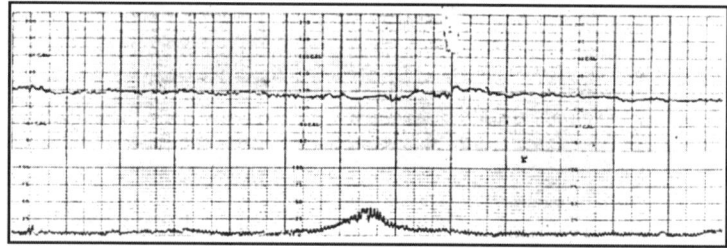

Figure 6.21: Mild bradycardia

During first phase FHR baseline was 150 to 160/minute due to O_2 inhalation and change of posture, bradycardia disappeared temporarily and then occurred again—LSCS was done 1 hour later (Figure 6.22).

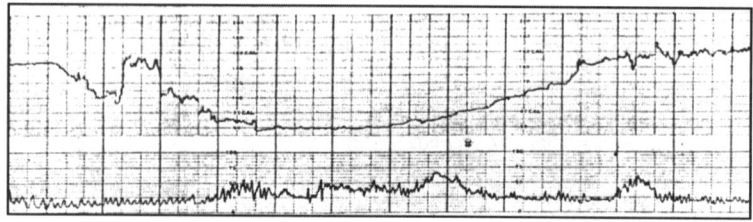

Figure 6.22: Severe bradycardia

Assessment of Fetal Well-being

Fetal heart rate baseline variability > 30 bpm and related to umbilical cord factor (Figure 6.23) when variable deceleration was severe, forceps delivery was performed.

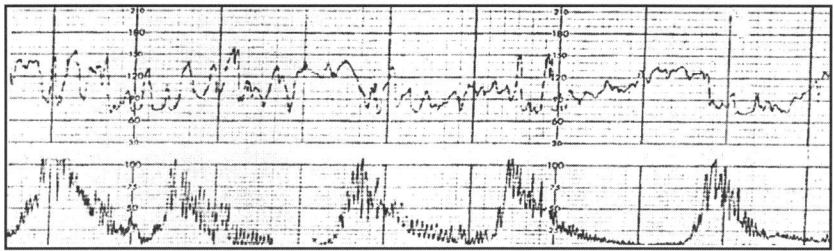

Figure 6.23: Increased fetal baseline variability

FETAL HEART RATE DECELERATION

In Labor: CTG Tracings

a. Early deceleration (Figure 6.24)
b. Late deceleration (Figure 6.25)
c. Variable deceleration (Figure 6.26)

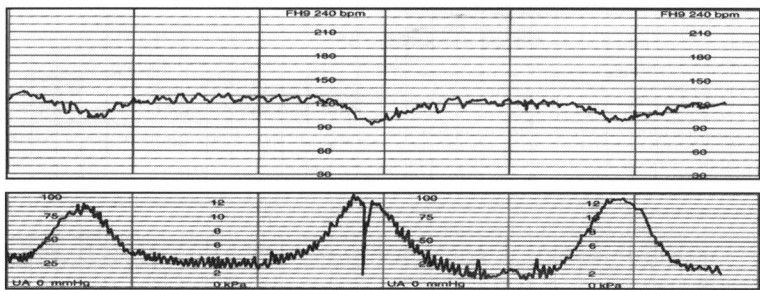

Figure 6.24: Early deceleration

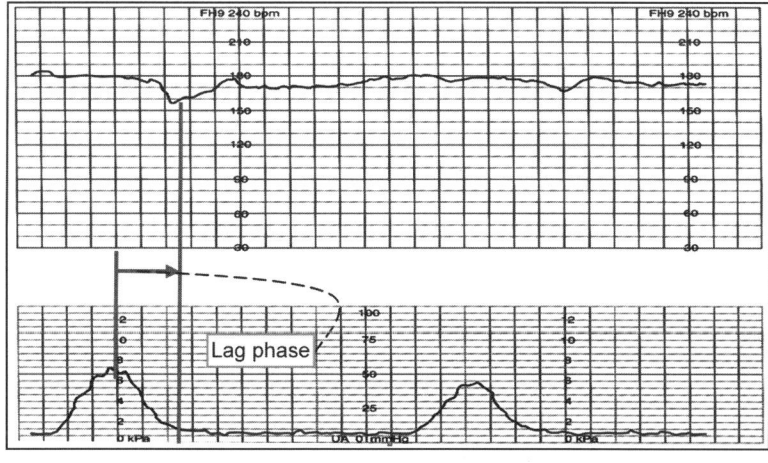

Figure 6.25: Late deceleration

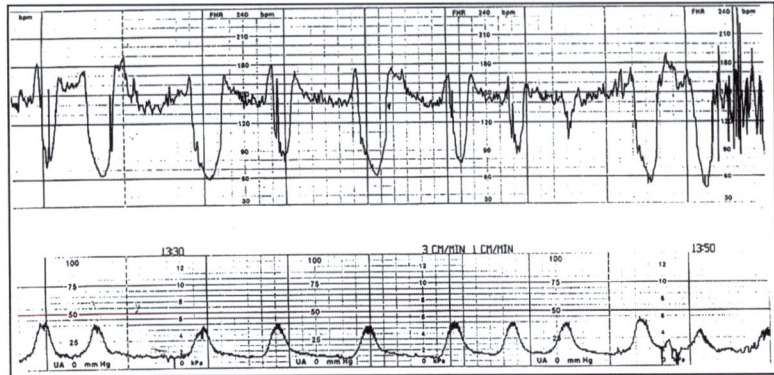

Figure 6.26: Variable deceleration

The last deviation pattern is FHR 50 bpm with duration of 4 minutes, so diagnosis is fetal distress. Rapid delivery by forceps as cervix is fully dilated (Figure 6.26).

Abnormality in Uterine Action (Figure 6.27)

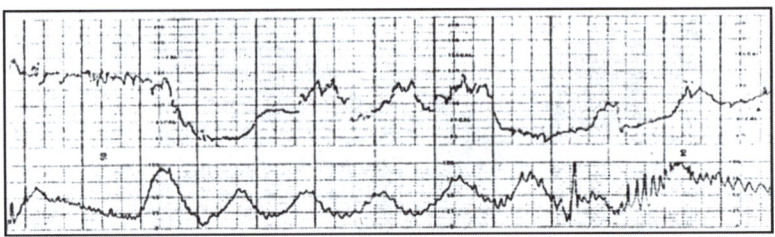

Figure 6.27: Hyperactive uterine contraction

- Age—28, primimother, GA—40 weeks of labor was done by oxytocin infusion.
- A severe deceleration pattern due to hyperactive uterine contraction, however the deceleration pattern disappeared when the infusion was discontinued. A severe variable pattern reappeared later and LSCS was performed.
- *Neonate*: 3,000 g, Apgar score 9.

FOR POSTGRADUATES

Categorization of Fetal Heart Rate Traces

RCOG and NICE guideline 2001—Universal Classifications of CTG into normal, suspicious and pathological categories (Tables 6.4 and 6.5).

Table 6.4: Categorization of Fetal heart rate traces	
Category	Definitions
Normal	A CTG where all four features fall into the reassuring category
Suspicious	A CTG with one feature classified as non-reassuring and the remaining features classified as reassuring
Pathological	A CTG with two or more features classified as non-reassuring or one or more classified as abnormal

Assessment of Fetal Well-being

Table 6.5: Classification of fetal heart rate features

Features	Baseline (bpm)	Variability (bpm)	Deceleration	Acceleration
Reassuring	110–160	>5	None	Present
Non-reassuring	100–109 161–180	<5 for 40–90 minutes	Early deceleration Variable deceleration Single prolonged decelebration up to 3 minutes	The absence of accelerations with an otherwise normal trace
Abnormal	<100 >180 sinusoidal ≥10 minutes	<5 for 90 minutes	Atypical variable decelerations, late decelarations, single prolonged deceleration for > 3 minutes	Cardiograph are of uncertain significance

FETAL ECG WAVE FORM ANALYSIS (ST ANALYZER—STAN) (FIGURE 6.28)

ST analyzer or STAN helps to identify fetal hypoxia by detecting the ST segment of the fetal electrocardiograph (ECG), which reflects myocardial hypoxemia. In response to hypoxia, there is a catecholamine surge from fetal adrenal glands, leading to peripheral vasoconstriction and redistribution of blood to the central organs, tachycardia and glycogenolysis in the myocardium. The influx of glucose with potassium into the cells causes change (increase in) the T-wave. Fetal hypoxia causes progressive rise in T-wave height and develops elevated S-T segment of the fetal ECG (Figure 6.29). The change is reflected by the increase in T/QRS ratio which reflects hypoxia and appears before neurological damage of fetus. If the hypoxic insult is short lasting, it is termed **episodic** T/QRS rise and if hypoxia is long lasting (over 10 minutes), it is termed **baseline** T/QRS rise.

Used in conjunction with fetal electronic monitoring (EFM), this technique may help us to detect fetus that shows reaction to hypoxia. Unlike the scalp pH, STAN provides information about the oxygen status in myocardium which may also reflect cerebral oxygenation. CTG with STAN helps in monitoring of fetal hypoxemia and reduces operative delivery than CTG alone. With excessive fetal movement there may also be adrenaline surge which may result **episodic** T/QRS and rise in ST events. In this case CTG would show normal tracing with acceleration and so, the ST events should be ignored.

> **Note**
> - Tests of peripheral acidosis like fetal scalp blood sampling, scalp lactate or oxygenation (pulse oximetry) do not adequately reflect the central oxygenation of the fetus.
> - STAN is a test of central oxygenation when it is used in combination with CTG.

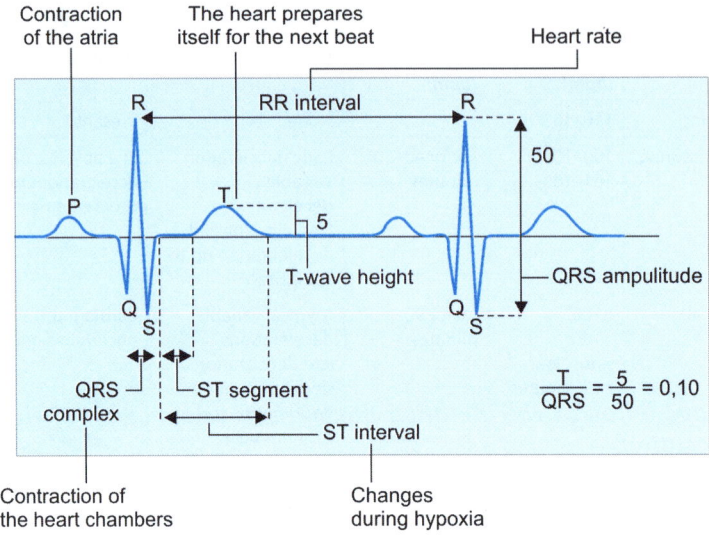

Figure 6.28: Fetal ECG complex

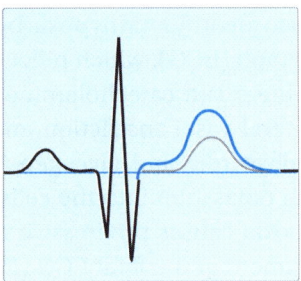

Figure 6.29: Increased T-wave amplitude (blue) in adrenaline surge and hypoxic/anaerobic metabolism

Conclusion

a. The goal of antepartum fetal surveillance is prevention of fetal death due to asphyxia and avoidance of unnecessary intervention.
b. Fetal surveillance is often warranted in high risk pregnancies, most common being IUGR, PIH, DM, multiple pregnancy and post datism.
c. *Antepartum fetal testing are*:
   1. Daily fetal movement count (DFMC)
   2. Non-stress test (NST)
   3. Contraction stress test (CST)
   4. Biophysical profile (BPP)
   5. Maternal uterine artery Doppler ⎫ See USG, Chapter 8
   6. Fetal umbilical artery Doppler ⎭
d. In labor CTG tracing, scalp blood pH measurement, fetal pulse oximetry, fetal scalp lactate and ST analysis of fetal ECG are important.
e. Admission CTG—Short CTG recording for 20 minutes at admission to identify unrecognized '*at risk*' fetuses and to categorize into low and high risk groups. If the admission test is normal and if the patient is not under oxytocin induction or epidural analgesia, the risk of fetal hypoxia in next three hours is very low. Current evidence does not support routine admission test for low risk woman as there is no benefit.

Chapter 7

Partograph

(We have followed the modified partograph adopted by World Health Organisation)

Q. What is partograph?

Ans. A graphical recording of progress of labor and salient features of mother and fetus.

Q. What is the modification of World Health Organization (WHO) partograph?

Ans. World health organization modified and made the partograph easier. The latent phase of labor has been removed and the plotting on the partograph begins from active phase of labor when cervix is 4 cm dilated.

> **Note**
> For more simplification the graphical record of descent of head is omitted in partographic chart.

Q. What are the indications of partogram?

Ans. a. All primimothers
b. High-risk pregnancies
c. Occipito posterior position
d. Borderline contracted pelvis.

Q. What are the instructions for plotting the partograph?

Ans. a. **Patient's information:** Name, gravida, parity, hospital number, date and time of admission, time of ruptured membrane.
b. **Fetal condition:** Fetal heart rate (FHR) should be counted every 30 minutes for full 1 minute and count should be done immediately after uterine contraction. When FHR is greater than 160 bpm or <110 bpm, it results in fetal distress. Each of the small box of vertical column of a partograph represents ½ hour interval.
c. **Amniotic fluid:** Record of color of amniotic fluid at every vaginal examination:
- Intact membrane (marked 'I')
- Clear liquor ('C')
- Meconium stained ('M')

- No liquor ('A')
- Blood stained liquor ('B').
  d. **Mouldings:** Sutures apposed (+), sutures overlapped and reducible (++), sutures overlapped and not reducible (+++).
  e. **Cervical dilatation:** Assessed at every vaginal examination, and marked with an 'X'. Begin plotting on the partograph at 4 cm.

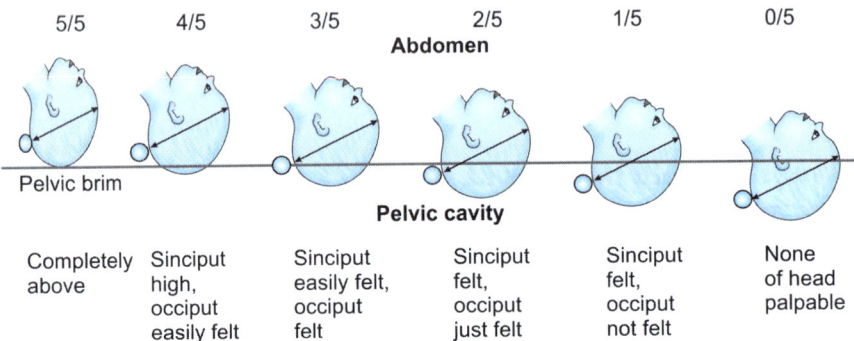

Figure 7.1: Descent assessed by abdominal palpation

> **Note**
> The recording of the descent of head is omitted in the more simplified partograph.

  f. **Alert line:** A line started from 4 cm dilatation to the point of expected full dilatation at the rate of 1 cm/hour.
  g. **Action line:** A line parallel to the 4 hours to the right of alert line.
  h. **Descent of the head:** Relation of the head in relation to pelvic brim and symphysis pubis (Rule of 5th by Crickton) (Figure 7.1).
  i. **Hours:** Refers to the time passed, since onset of active phase of labor (observed or extrapolated).
  j. **Time:** Record actual time.
  k. **Contractions:** Chart every 1/2 hour, palpate the number of uterine contractions in 10 minutes and their duration in seconds.

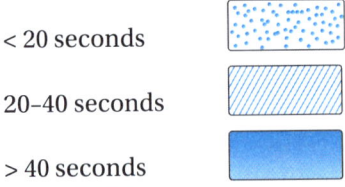

> **Note**
> To note the onset, duration, disappearance and intensity of uterine contraction, the palm is placed on the uterus and the degree of firmness during contraction gives the idea of intensity.

  l. **Oxytocin:** Record the amount of oxytocin per volume intravenous (IV) fluid in drops/minute every 30 minutes when used.
  m. **Drugs given:** Record any additional drug.

Partograph

n. **Pulse:** Record every 30 minutes and mark it with dot (•).
o. **Blood Pressure:** Record every 4 hours and mark by arrows (↕).
p. **Temperature:** Record every 2 hours.
q. **Protein acetone and volume:** Record every hour when urine passed.

Summary of monitoring of observations recorded in partogram

Pulse	30 minutes
BP	4 hourly
FHR	30 minutes
Uterine contractions	every 30 minutes
Temperature	every 2 hours
Urine	every hour if possible.

> **Note**
>
> *Do not use partograph in the following conditions:*
> *a. Gross CPD*
> *b. Severe Preeclampsia/eclampsia*
> *c. Antepartum hemmorrhage (APH)*
> *d. Severe anemia (Hb <7 g %)*
> *e. Multiple pregnancy*
> *f. Malpresentation*
> *g. Preterm labor*
> *h. Fetal distress*
> *i. Intrauterine fetal death (IUFD)*
> *j. Previous cesarean section.*

Interpretation of Figure 7.2

Primigravida was admitted in the latent phase of about 5 am.
- Fetal head 4/5th palpable
- Cervix—dilated 2 cm
- Three contractions in 10 minutes each lasting for 20 seconds.

Normal maternal and fetal conditions.

> **Note**
>
> *Because the woman is admitted in latent phase, this information is not plotted on the partograph. Cervical dilatation is plotted on alert line. If the patient is seen for the first time at 5 cm dilatation, the first marking should be 1 hour after 0 hour. This applies to 6 cm, 7 cm and so on when it is marked at 2-hour, 3-hour and so on after 0- hour.*

At 9:00 am
- Fetal head 3/5th palpable.
- Cervix dilated 5 cm.
- Four contractions in 10 minutes each lasting for 35 seconds.

> **Note**
>
> *The woman was in active phase of labor and the information is plotted on the partograph, cervical dilatation is plotted on alert line.*

At 11:30 am
- Fetal head 2/5th palpable.
- Four contractions in 10 minutes, each lasting for 45 seconds.

At 1:00 pm
- Fetal head is 0/5th palpable.
- Cervical dilatation is progressed at the rate of > 1 cm/hour and cervix is fully dilated.
- Five contractions in 10 minutes lasting for 45 seconds.

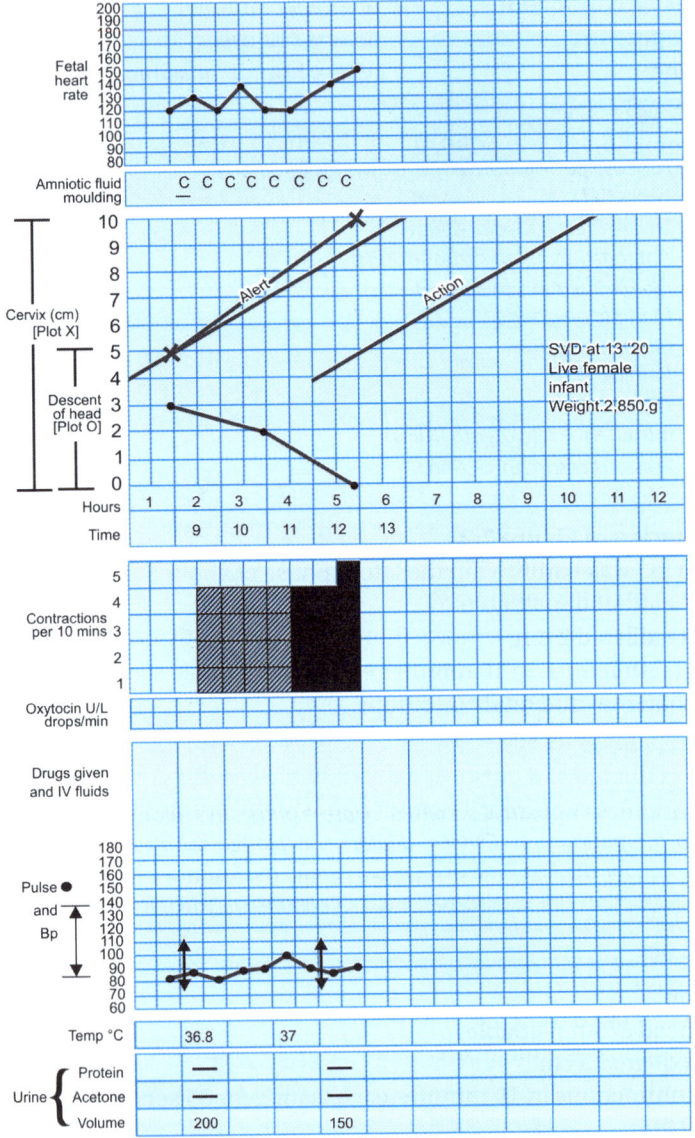

Figure 7.2: Sample partograph of normal labor

Name Mrs. X—Gravida 2, Para 1 + 0
Hospital No.—45539, BMC

Partograph

Date of admission—01.08.2008
Time of admission—5:00 am

Representation of Partograph

Time	Pulse rate (PR)	Blood pressure (BP)	Temp	Per abdomen (P/A)	Fetal heart rate (FHR)/ others
9 AM	90	–	–	4 contraction in 10 minute each lasting for 35 second	120/minute
11–30 AM	100	–	–	4 contractions in 10 minutes each lasting for 45 seconds	120/minute
1 PM	90	–	–	5 contraction in 10 min lasting for 45 second	150/minute

1:20 p.m.– vaginal delivery
(In examination please point out all the compartments of the graph)

Illustrations of unsatisfaction progress of labor by sample of partographic analysis (*Courtesy:* EMOC training modules)

Interpretation of Figure 7.3

> **Note**
>
> *The partograph was not adequately filled out and this example demonstrate inappropriate management of prolonged labor. The diagnosis of prolonged labor was evident at 2 pm and labor should have been augmented with oxytocin by that time.*

The woman was admitted in active labor at 10:00 am
- Fetal head palpable 5/5
- Cervix dilated 4 cm
- Inadequate uterine contraction (2 in 10 minutes, each lasting for <20 seconds).

At 2:00 pm
- Head palpability still 5/5
- Cervix dilated to 4 cm and to the right of alert line
- Membranes ruptured(R) spontaneously and amniotic fluid is clear (see 'C' in Figure 7.3)
- Inadequate uterine contraction (1 in 10 minutes, each lasting for <20 seconds).

At 6:00 pm
- Head is still 5/5 palpable
- Cervix dilated 6 cm
- Contraction is still inadequate (2 in 10 minutes, each lasting for <20 seconds).

At 9:00 pm
- FHR 80/minute
- Amniotic fluid stained with meconium (see 'M' in Figure 7.3)
- No further progress in labor.

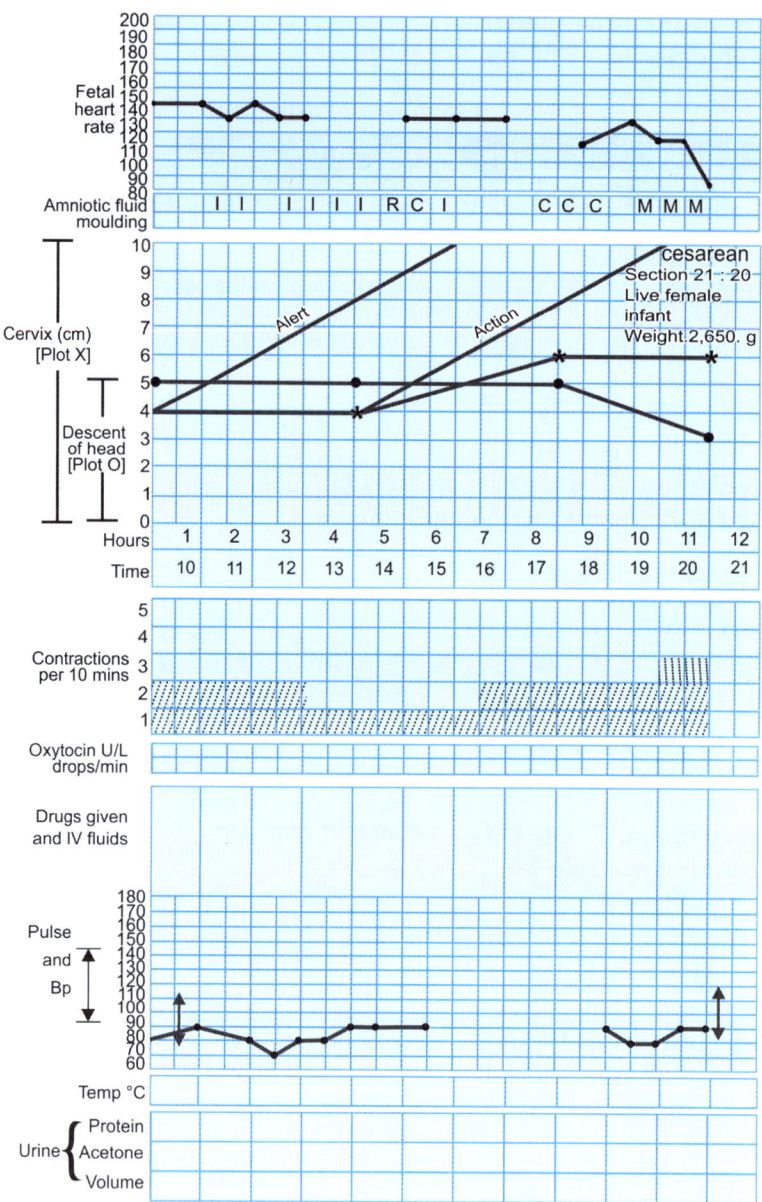

Figure 7.3: Partograph showing prolonged active phase of labor

Name Mrs M—Gravida 1 Para 0 + 0
Hospital No—65329, BMC
Date of admission—02.03.2009
Time of admission—10:00 am
Ruptured membrane—13:30 hours

At 9:20 pm
- Cesarean section was performed due to fetal distress.
For representation of partograph see the table

Partograph

Time	Pulse rate (PR)	Blood Pressure (BP)	Temp	Per abdomen (P/A)	Fetal heart rate (FHR)/ others
2:00 pm	80	110/70	–	1 contraction in 10 min lasting for < 20 second	140/minute
6:00 pm	90	110/70	–	2 mild contractions in 10 min lasting for < 20 second	130/minute
9:00 pm	90	–	37°C	3 contractions in 10 minute lasting for < 20 sec	<90 minute

Liquor-meconium stained
At 9:20 pm lower segment cesarian section (LSCS) for fetal distress

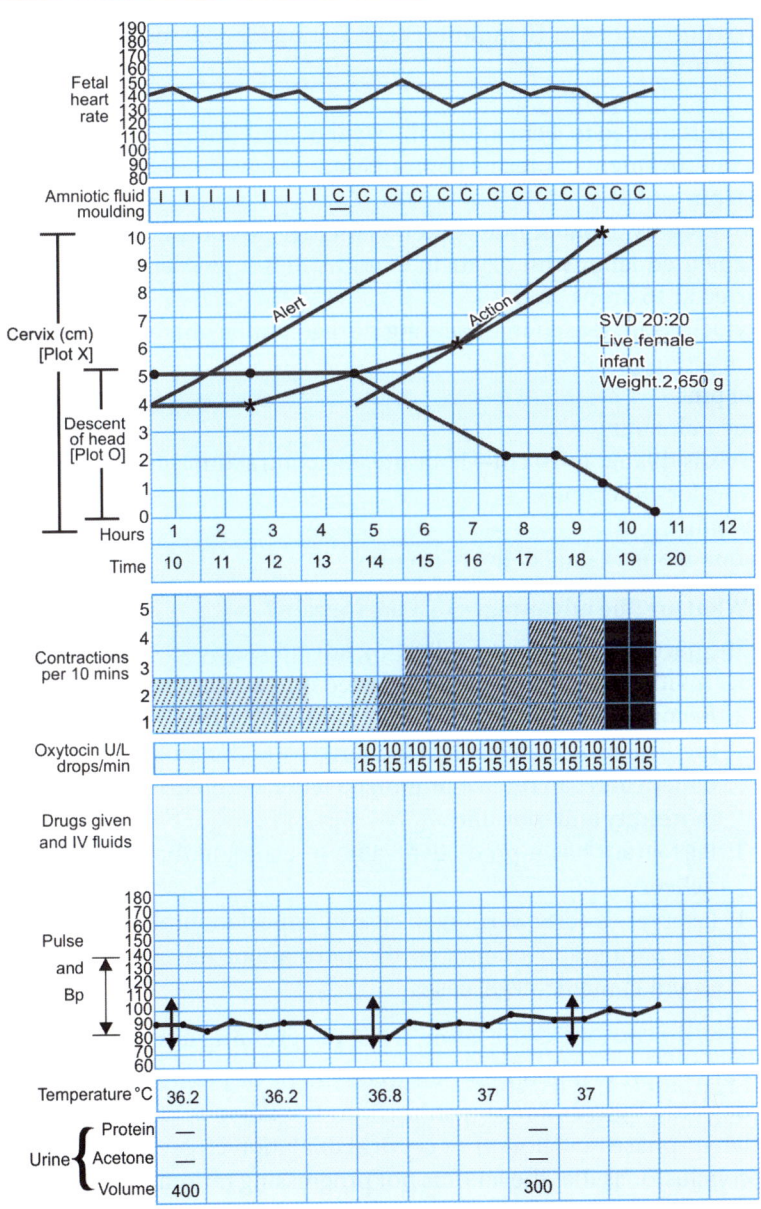

Figure 7.4: Partogram showing inadequate uterine contraction corrected with oxytocin

Name	— Mrs N Gravida 1, Para 0 + 0
Hospital No.	— 394392, BMC
Date of admission	— 02.05.2008
Time of admission	— 10:00 am
Ruptured membrane	— 13:30 hours.

Interpretation of Figure 7.4

The woman is admitted at 10:00 am
- Fetal head palpability 5/5
- Cervix is dilated to 4 cm
- Two contractions in 10 minutes, each lasting for < 20 seconds.

At 12:00 pm
- Fetal head palpability 5/5
- Cervix is dilated to 4 cm and to the right of alert line
- No improvement of uterine contraction.

At 2:00 pm
- Poor progress of labor due to inefficient uterine contraction
- Augmented labor with oxytocin 10 units in Ringer's lactate (RL). IV fluid started at 15 drops/minute
- Oxytocin is increased in escalating dosage until a good pattern of uterine contraction was established.

At 7:00 pm
- Head palpability 1/5
- Cervix is dilated to 10 cm—Four uterine contractions in 10 minutes, each lasting for 45 seconds.

At 8:20 pm
- Spontaneous vaginal delivery occurs.

Q. What are the advantages of a partogram?

Ans. The partogram offers the following advantages:
1. Total information may be recorded on a single sheet.
2. Records are straight forward and objective, both nursing and medical staffs can see it at a glance—the prognosis of labor of each patient and can reduce prolonged labor, cesarean delivery, perinatal morbidity and mortality.
3. Partogram has a predictive value to estimate the expected time of delivery.
4. It serves as early warning in case of important problem.
5. The partograph maintains the permanent record of labor and is useful in medicolegal cases.

Q. How do you assess the labor, if not progressing normally?

Ans. Partograph is a good tool for assessment of progress of labor. When despite of good uterine contraction, the labor is in latent phase (the latent-phase is >8 hours) or cervical dilatation crosses the alert line, the conclusion is that the labor is not progressing normally.

So abnormal progress of labor is divided into 3Ps':

a. **P**ower-related: Poor uterine contraction

b. **P**assage-related: Contracted pelvis and CPD
c. **P**assenger-related: Big baby, hydrocephalus

> **Note**
>
> *Paperless partogram: It is the partogram without paper and action should be taken 4 hours after alert estimated time of delivery (ETD) when cervix dilates 1 cm/hour in active phase of labor. For example if the dilatation of cervix is 4 cm at 7 am, ETD will be at 1 pm (full dilatation =10 cm), while action time will be at 5 pm.*

Q. What is prolonged labor?

Ans. It is an active labor with regular uterine contractions, without adequate cervical dilation or descent of the presenting part but lasts for more than 12 hours without delivery.

What are Causes of Prolonged Labor
a. In-coordinate uterine contractions, uterine inertia
b. Cephalopelvic disproportion (CPD) or fetopelvic disproportion. (CPD cannot be judged before 37 weeks as the head is not reached the birth size), pelvic tumor.
c. Malpresentation, malposition, big baby, congenital anomaly of fetus.

Q. How do you treat prolonged labor?

Ans. Selective and judicious low artificial rupture of membrane (ARM) with or without syntocinon or operative delivery by LSCS. Active management of PPH in third stage of labor.

Q. What is obstructed labor?

Ans. Secondary arrest of cervical dilatation and descent of the presenting part in spite of good uterine contractions, or the fetus cannot descend downwards due to mechanical obstruction at inlet, cavity or outlet of the pelvis.

Q. What are causes of obstructed labor

Ans. a. CPD (commonest), contracted pelvis, big baby
b. Malpresentation (brow, mentoposterior)
c. Pelvic tumor.

Q. How do you diagnose and manage a case of obstructed labor?

Ans. *History:* Age (teen age), parity (multipara or not), previous stillbirth, duration of labor and progress of labor, time of rupture of membrane, color of liquor.

General examination: Physical exhaustion, dehydration causing tachycardia, fever or features of shock (due to sepsis or ruptured uterus).

Abdominal examination: Fetal head is above pelvic brim, or below, size of fetus, strong uterine contractions followed by absent uterine contractions—due to exhaustion (primi) and rupture of uterus (multi), bandl's ring (depression across the abdomen at about the level of umbilicus and above it, the uterus is retracted and below it, the lower segment is distended), fetal distress.

Vaginal examination: Edema of vulva, vagina—dry and hot, severely molded head, large caput, malpresentation, incomplete or complete dilatation of cervix, edematous lip of the cervix, ballooning of lower uterial segment, cervix is poorly applied to the presenting part, high up head or malpresentation.

Management:
Cervix—dilated (= 4 cm) after 8 hours of regular contraction and the woman is still not delivered for >12 hours. If the mother is exhausted, start the following:

a. i. Rehydration with RL or normal saline and catheterize bladder
   ii. IV antibiotics,
   iii. No wait and watch policy by oxytocin,
   iv. Cesarean section, if the baby is living and head high up,
   v. Incompletely dilated cervix, head high up, lower segment cesarean section (LSCS) is to be done even if the baby is dead.
   vi. Head low down—baby dead—craniotomy is the method of choice when cervix is fully effaced and os is fully dilated.
b. After instrumental delivery, look for rupture of uterus and continuous catheter drainage is mandatory for 10 days to avoid vesicovaginal fistula (VVF).
c. Active management of PPH.

Q. What are the effects of such labor on mother and fetus?

Ans. *Mother*: Exhaustion, dehydration, acidosis, genital sepsis, rupture of uterus, PPH and shock.

Fetus: Asphyxia, acidosis, intracranial hemorrhage (ICH), infection.

Chapter 8

Ultrasonography in Obstetrics

INTRODUCTION

[if any ultrasonography (USG) plate is given in examination, start the demonstration of the plate in the following way:
a. Color of the plate: Black and white or colored
b. Route: Transabdominal/vaginal
c. 2- DUS or 3-DUS (three-dimensional ultrasound)
d. Features of the USG figure
e. Finally diagnosis

If the plate of Figure 8.1A is displayed: Say it is a transabdominal black and white 2-D USG plate showing, bladder, uterus and ring within the uterus. Final diagnosis: Early intrauterine gestational sac in 2D scan].

Early Diagnosis of Pregnancy

Gestational Sac

First visualized from 33 to 35th day of last menstrual period (LMP) (5th week). It appears as a spherical ring, which is non-echogenic with prominent ring of echoes. It is 6–8 cm in diameter at 15th week of gestation (Figures 8.1A and B).

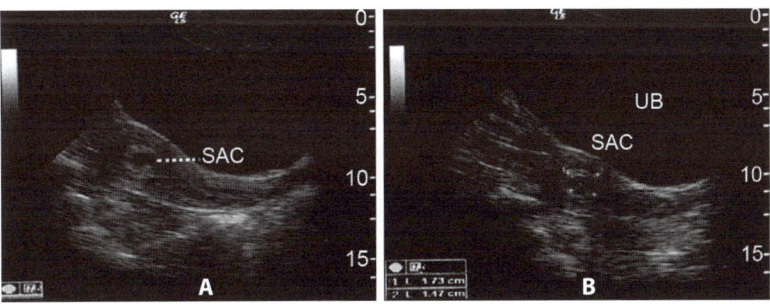

Figures 8.1A and B: USG of gestational sac

By endovaginal sonography (EVS), the gestational sac (GS) within the decidua is visualized by approximately 4.5 weeks menstrual age, when the mean sac diameter (MSD) is 2.5 mm.

Determination of gestational sac: By this, normal growth can be seen:
At 5 weeks—8 mm, then increase by 1 to 2 mm per day
At 6 weeks—14 mm
At 7 weeks—25 mm
At 8 weeks—34 mm

Morphologically, identification of double decidual sac sign (DDSS) is the best method for differentiating true sacs with pseudo sac due to concentric echogenic ring of decidua capsularis and parietalis by a hypoechogenic space.

Yolk Sac

In GS, a small round or oval and a uniformly thick echogenic wall appears, i.e. yolk. The yolk sac has echogenic periphery with a fluid-filled center. It often appears before appearance of amnion or embryo. It is a confirmatory sign of true gestational sac and appears at 5 weeks detected by TVS.

The yolk sac is involved in transfer of nutrients to the embryo, hematopoiesis and in formation of primitive gut. Using EVS, the yolk sac should always be visualized, when the mean sac diameter (MSD) is at least 8 mm. The yolk sac grows at a rate of 0.1 mm per mm of growth of MSD before 15 mm MSD, after which it grows at a rate of 0.03 mm per mm growth of MSD.

Yolk sac should never exceed 5.6 mm in diameter. Yolk sac is an indicator of poor outcome if it is:
a. Too small
b. Too large >6 mm
c. Thick walled
d. Irregular and solid.

Fetal Pole

Firstly visualized at 5th week. It appears as bright echogenic streak. Between 6–7 weeks of normal gestation, fetal pole was imaged in 50% of subjects and between 7–8 weeks, in 82.6% of subjects. By 8th completed week, fetal pole was imaged in all subjects (Figure 8.2).

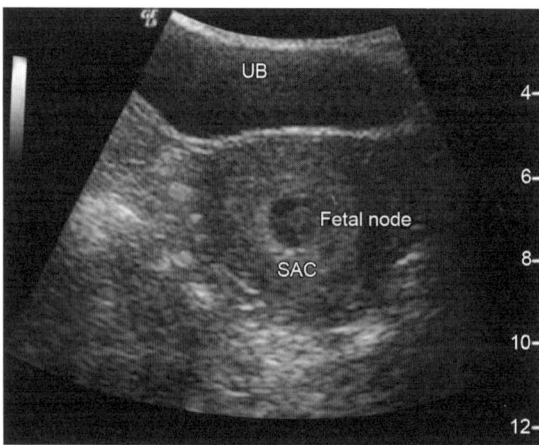

Figure 8.2: USG showing fetal pole

Fetal Heart (Figure 8.3)

Fetal heart can be picked up from 6th weeks in (42 days of amenorrhea). Between 7th and 8th week, heart motion was detected in 97% of cases perabdominal ultrasonography (USG). The heart motion could be translated to M-mode for better perception. Appearance of fetal pole without cardiac activity is a sign of abnormal pregnancy.

By endovaginal scanning (EVS) at 5th week, embryonic heart rate is 123 bpm and by 9th week, it is 171 bpm.

Measurement of Crown Rump Length (CRL) (Figure 8.4)

Once the embryo is visible, the measurement of CRL supercedes GS measurement.

This is the maximum longitudinal length between the fetal poles. This method is used up to 14 weeks. The reproducibility is 1.2 mm in 95% of the population and accuracy is ± 4 days of the estimated date of delivery.

It can be measured as 10 mm at 7 weeks, 83 mm at 14 weeks.

For a rough calculation: Fetal age in weeks = CRL in cm + 6.5, accuracy: ±5–7 days.

> **Note**
> CRL (between 6–14 weeks) is very useful for calculation of gestational age measurement in later part of pregnancy.

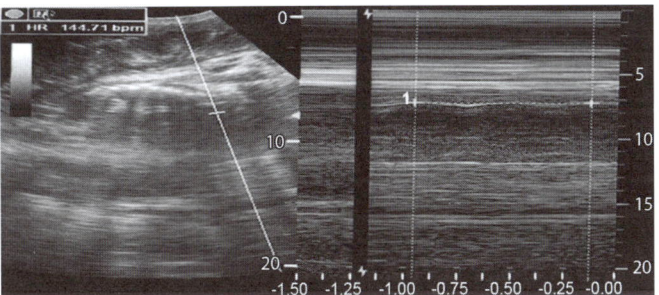

Figure 8.3: USG showing fetal heart rate

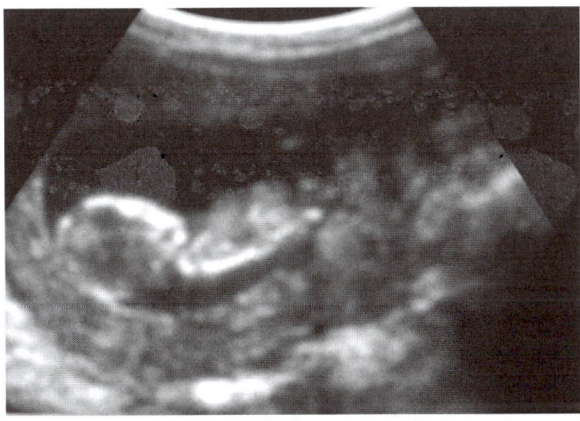

Figure 8.4: USG showing CRL

FIRST TRIMESTER PREGNANCY PROBLEMS

Blighted Ovum or An-embryonic Sac

Presence of an embryonic GS is the most frequent cause of spontaneous abortion.

Features

a. Presence of GS of diameter ≥20 mm or more on TAS in which no fetal pole is visible or gestational sac (>25 mm) with no embryo.
b. If sac is <20 mm on first examination, then failure of GS occurs to increase at least 75% over a period of 1 week.
c. If gestational sac is accurately known, then failure to locate fetal pole occurs by 8 weeks from LMP.
d. With accurate menstrual date, the GS is small for date.
e. Appearance of sac, which is quite irregular in shape and thin walled.
f. Presence of fluid, fluid level in GS and the separation of sac from the uterine wall (subchorionic hematoma).

Abortions

Threatened Abortion

Ultrasonography has prognostic value in this case. USG demonstrates healthy GS (regular sac with bright echogenic rim), a measurable CRL with definite fetal heart motion, a normal fetus sac ratio and a normal placental implantation—the prognosis for achieving a term pregnancy is very good. In this, cervix is closed and there may be blood in vagina.

Inevitable Abortion

If the cervix is open, then size of uterus corresponds to the period of gestational age. Gestational sac lies in the lower pole.

Incomplete Abortion

If some product is visualized in the uterine cavity and no fetal cardiac activity and no definite GS is seen.

Complete Abortion

If uterine cavity is empty.

Missed Abortion

If the pole is seen, but fetal cardiac motion is not visualized. USG is able to identify an embryo without a heart beat from 6 weeks onwards. The traditional definition of missed abortion is fetal death before 20 weeks without expulsion of the fetus for at least 8 weeks afterwards, is at present inappropriate (Figure 8.5).

Twin Pregnancy (Figures 8.6A and B)

Sonographic diagnosis of twin pregnancy was made earliest at 6th week by visualizing two fetal sacs and the quadruplets was diagnosed earliest at 9th week. Two fetal heads can be detected at 14th week. USG Doppler heart motion can identify two fetal heart sounds at 14 weeks.

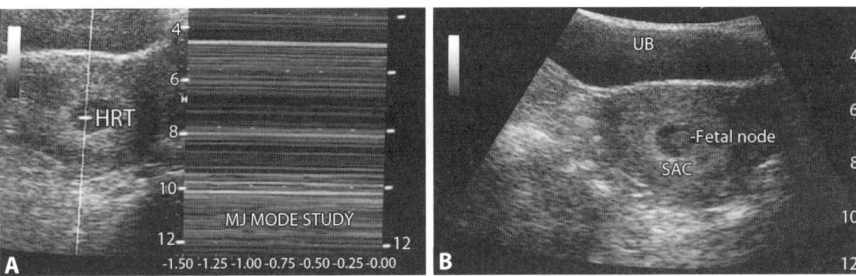

Figure 8.5: Missed abortion with no FHR

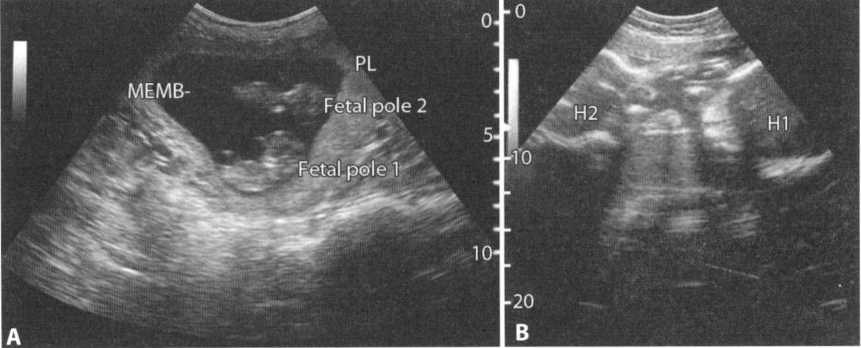

Figures 8.6A and B: Twin pregnancy pole (A) Fetal pole 1 and fetal pole 2 (B) Fetal head (H1), fetal head (H2)

Vanishing Twin

When one sac undergoes embryonic resorption.

Incidence: 13–78% (mean 21%) before 14 weeks of GA

The finding of USG examination of pyramidal area of placental tissue at the peak of insertion of separating membrane between twins the so called 'Lambda sign-twin peak' suggests dichorionic-diamniotic twin pregnancies. *Labeling of multiples*: The sac closest to cervix is labeled 'A', one, then labels B, C, D in anticlockwise direction from the left (Figure 8.7).

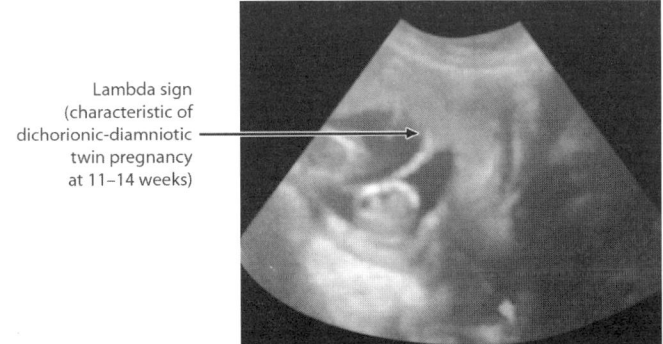

Figure 8.7: Twin peak sign
(A triangular portion of placenta is insinuated between amniochorion layers)

> **Note**
> T-sign in USG helps in diagnosis of monochromic diamniotic gestation. 'T' is formed by the point at which amnion meets the placenta, so contains no placental tissue.

Ectopic Pregnancy

If the GS is visualized inside the uterus then one may be assured that the case is not of ectopic gestation. False negative sign, i.e. intrauterine pseudogestational sac may be visible within the uterus in ectopic pregnancy (Figure 8.8).

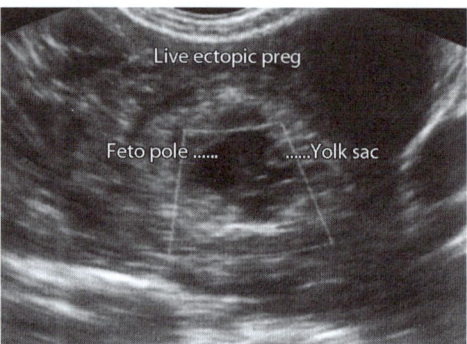

Figure 8.8: EVS—shows a live ectopic pregnancy *(For color version, see Plate 2)*

Causes of Pseudo Sac

i. Presence of blood clot in the uterine cavity
ii. The decidual lining may appear as a well-defined spherical and apparently fluid-filled structure
iii. May result from thick proliferative endometrium. So,
    a. Empty uterus sign or fluid in endometrial cavity surrounded by a single decidual layer instead of double decidual sac
    b. Free pelvic fluid (blood)
    c. Direct positive signs, including adnexal mass, cystic or semicystic with lots of internal echoes, adnexal pregnancy and living embryo.

If uterus is empty, presence of human chorionic gonadotropin (hCG) hormone in urine with adnexal mass or fluid in pouch of Douglas (POD)—proves ectopic gestation.

Color flow Doppler (CFD): Adnexal peritrophoblastic flow is defined as high velocity, low resistance flow separated from the ovary. Vascularity of tubal ring may aid in diagnosis of unruptured tubal ectopic pregnancy.

The true gestation sac must be differentiated from pseudo sac which is often seen in ectopic pregnancy (see below).

Features	True sac	Pseudo sac
Situation	Eccentric in uterine cavity	Central in endocavity
Margins	Double decidual ring	No hyperechoic ring
With uterine peristalsis	No change in shape	Changes in shape
On Doppler	Peripheral vascular ring	No peripheral vascularity

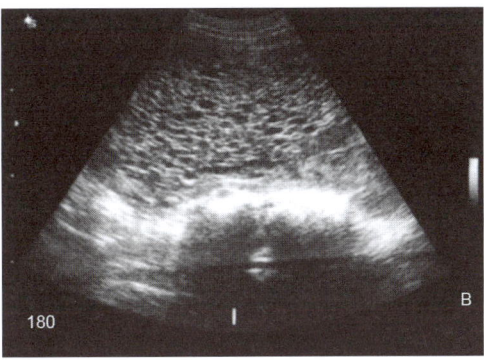

Figure 8.9: USG shows snow storm appearance

Trophoblastic Disease

Hydatidiform mole gives appearance of a clearly translucent echogenicity within the uterine cavity. It must be emphasized that the classical sign 'snow storm' appearance is not always visualized in all cases of molar pregnancy (Figure 8.9). The diagnostic accuracy has been estimated to be over 98%. Invasive trophoblastic disease can also be detected and secondaries in liver and brain can be picked up early. The lutein cysts can be visualized as multicystic adnexal mass in 40–50% of cases (Differential diagnosis of snowstorm appearance: (i) Missed abortion, (ii) Degenerated fibroma of uterus).

FOR POSTGRADUATES

PREGNANCY OF UNKNOWN LOCATION (PUL)

It can be diagnosed in 8–31% of cases when pregnancy test is positive, but it is not visualized on USG. If location of pregnancy can not be determined by USG, hormonal markers and their interpretation is essential. In majority of cases, a single measurement of hCG will not be diagnostic. The discriminatory zone and serial β-hCG measurement is important.

a. Increased serial hCG >66% over baseline value at 48 hours apart in first 48 days of gestation, there is probability of the intrauterine pregnancy (IUP). Scan is repeated after 2 weeks.
b. If increased serial hCG is <66% at 48 hours apart or there is plateauing hCG, possibility of ectopic pregnancy (EP) is high. So close monitoring with serial hCG and TVS until diagnosis is made or hCG falls below 15 IU/L.
c. In majority of cases when serum β-hCG level is above discriminatory zone (≥1500 IU/L), probable ectopic pregnancy can be diagnosed by vaginal USG or laparoscopy, but the problem arises at lower serum hCG level or in smaller number of cases when an USG diagnosis can not be made.

> **Note**
> *Discriminatory zone may vary among institutions but if the discriminatory level is >1500 IU/L an intrauterine pregnancy is noted in 92% of cases compared to 28.6% of cases when levels were below 1500 IU/L.*

d. If hCG level is <500 IU/L, pleatuing, negative TVS and laparoscopy, there may be more chances of persisting PUL which needs methotrexate 50 mg/m² for treatment and serum hCG level subsequently resolved.

> **Note**
>
> *Concept of discriminatory zone (DZ): it is the minimum serum beta- hCG level above which the gestational sac should always be detected in a normal intrauterine pregnancy. With transabdominal sonography the DZ was at higher side (6,000–6,500 IU/L), while with the development of high frequency endovaginal sonography the DZ is decreased to 1,000–2,000 IU/L. Depending on the sensitivity of ultrasonic equipment and experience of ultrasonographer, the β-hCG representing the discriminatory zone may be lower.*

Fetal Anomalies

Diagnosis of gross anomalies, such as cystic hygroma and large cranial cyst, can be made in first trimester. Many severe anomalies may have a normal sonographic appearance in the first trimester. The most dramatic example is anencephaly, which may only become evident after ossification of the calvarium that occurs at 12th week of menstrual age.

Anencephaly is the absence of cranial vault (acrania) and much of the brain showing frog facies as the orbits become protruding structures. There was no forehead or calvarium (Figure 8.10).

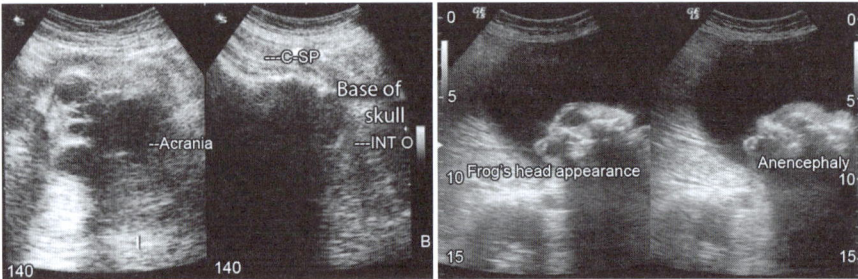

Figure 8.10: USG shows frog faces (diagnosis: anencephaly) (Acrania: It is a totally non-ossified skull vault bones, diagnosed after 11 weeks)

The cerebral hemisphere and mid brain are usually completely absent, leaving remnants of the forebrain and generally well formed medulla. In the first trimester the only sonographic feature is acrania and CRL may be reduced. In the second and third trimester, the diagnosis is evident and typical frog facies is noted. It is very much important to exclude amniotic band as an etiology of anencephaly and recurrence risk is high in periconceptual folic acid deficiency.

Ovarian and Uterine Tumors

Associated ovarian and uterine tumors can also be diagnosed.

USG IN SECOND AND THIRD TRIMESTER

During pregnancy it is desirable to perform USG at least once at around 18–20 weeks of gestation for targeted fetal congenital anomalies scan.

Determination of Gestational Age

1. Biparietal diameter (BPD)
2. Head circumference (HC)
3. Femur length (FL)
4. Abdominal circumference (AC)

When two or more parameters are used to determine gestational age, significant improvement is observed to single parameter.

Biparietal Diameter (Figure 8.11)

Biparietal diameter (BPD) can be measured after 12 weeks onwards. The planes in which BPD is measured are:
a. Transaxial plane
b. At the level of thalamic nuclei
c. At the level of cavum septum pellucidum
d. Slit-like third ventricle in the midline
e. The parietal bone should be equidistant from midline
f. Measure widest diameter from outer skull table of anterior parietal bone to inner skull table of posterior parietal bone
g. The plane of BPD should be at right angle of the midline.

Growth rate
- 3–4 mm/week between 13–20 weeks
- 3 mm/week between 21–28 weeks
- 2–3 mm/week between 29–32 weeks
- 2 mm/week after 32 weeks.

Use of BPD: Estimate GA, fetal growth rate (FGR), fetal weight (FW), structural abnormality of the head, e.g. anencephaly, hydrocephaly, acrania, encephalocele, etc.

Errors of BPD measurement:
a. Can occur due to incorrect plane
b. Deeply engaged head, breech, transverse lie and deflexed head

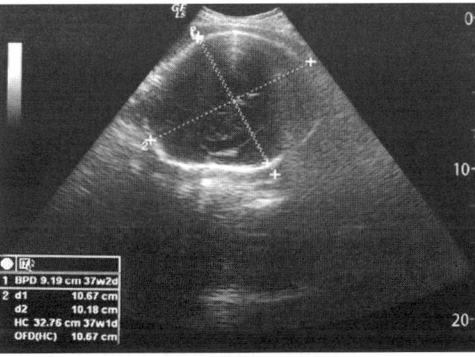

Figure 8.11: USG—BPD and HC

c. Observer's error
d. Transducer pressure may compress the fetal skull diameter.

Accuracy of BPD measurement: Before 28 weeks, variation in GA was 28 weeks ± 10 days. After 28 weeks, variation was 28 ± 21 days (3 weeks). The rate of growth of BPD begins to fall-off slightly <2 mm/week in the last trimester of pregnancy. Hence, accuracy of prediction of GA from BPD falls with increasing gestational age.

Cephalic index remains constant throughout pregnancy and they can be used to check the accuracy of BPD measurement.

$$\text{Cephalic index (CI)} = \frac{\text{BPD}}{\text{OFD}} \times 100$$

Occipitofrontal diameter (OFD) is measured from the midpoint of frontal bone to the midpoint of occipital bone similar to BPD plane.
Normal CI = 75–85%
Dolichocephaly CI = < 75%
Brachycephaly CI = > 85%

Corrected BPD (cBPD): BPD and OFD are used to adjust for variations in head space (c BPD) = sqare root of BPD × OFD +1.26.

Head Circumference (Figure 8.11)

Head circumference (HC) is also measured in the same plane of BPD, outer skull table is used to measure the AC, the accuracy is ± 2 to 3 weeks. It is ideal to be measured in case of dolicocephalic and brachycephalic head. If HC is <2 SD for that period of gestational age, possibility of microcephaly should be kept in mind. In later part of pregnancy, HC is better indicator than the BPD, because it is more shape dependent measurement than the BPD and not affected by molding.

Measurement of HC = (BPD + OFD) × 1.62

HC too large: Hydrocephalus, hydraencephalus, intracranial hemorrhage, short limb dystrophies, tumor.
HC too small: Anencephaly, cerebral infarction, synostosis, microcephaly vera.

Abdominal Circumference

Abdominal circumference (AC) (Figure 8.12B) is measured in transaxial plane. The plane should be circular, showing lumber spine and taken at the level of bifurcation of main portal vein in right and left branches. It is a poor prediction of GA. Sensitivity is same as BPD, but better prediction of GA from 36 to 42 weeks.

AC = 1.57 × (AP diameter + transverse diameter)

If AC <5th percentile for the period of gestation, it suggests FGR, whereas >95th percentile to the period of gestation, signifies macrosomia. The absence of stomach bubble is diagnostic of esophageal atresia and presence of double bubble shadow signifies duodenal atresia.

AC too large: GI tract obstruction, obstructive uropathy, ascites, hepatosplenomegaly, congenital nephrosis, abdominal tumor.

AC too small: Diaphragmatic hernia, omphalocele, gastroschisis, renal agenesis.

Femur Length

Femur length (FL) (Figure 8.12A) is measured from greater trochanter to lateral condyle of femur. Exclude the head and neck of femur. Do not include distal femoral epiphysis. Growth rate after 28 weeks would be little less than 2 mm/week. After 28 weeks, FL is a better parameter than BPD.

GA given is ± 2 weeks.

Ultrasonography Derived FW

By use of BPD and AC, the fetal weight (FW) is calculated and in 90.5% of cases the accuracy is within ±300 g.

Appearance of Epiphyseal Bone Centers

In 95% of all cases
- Distal femoral epiphysis (DFE): >33 weeks of GA
- Distal femoral epiphysis (DFE) >5 mm: >35 weeks of GA
- Proximal tibial epiphysis (PTE): >35 weeks GA
- Proximal humeral epiphysis (PHE): >38 weeks GA

Different ratios: The following ratios must be measured:
1. BPD/OFD (cephalic index)
2. HC/AC: HC/AC >1 before 36 weeks of GA
   HC/AC = 1 at 36 weeks
   HC/AC < 1 after 36 weeks
   Deviation from normal is suspicion of hydrocephalus, microcephaly or asymmetrical intrauterine growth restriction (IUGR).
3. *FL/AC (Ponderal index)*: Normally, it is 20–24% and on an average 22%. If it is >24%, then intrauterine growth restriction (IUGR) is suspected.

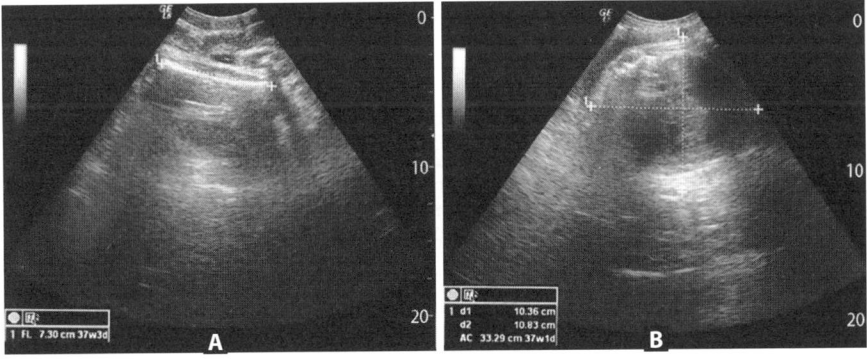

Figures 8.12A and B: (A) Femur length; (B) Abdominal circumference

Placenta

At 12th week, placenta is visualized as low level echo all around. Basal plate, chorionic plate and placental substance can be identified.

Grannum's Classification

Grade 0: Fine echogenic pattern with well-defined homogeneous chorionic plate, basal layer is devoid of echogenic density.

Grade I: Many subtle undulation in the previous smooth, straight chorionic plate and a few scattered echogenic areas in the placental substance. Basal layer is devoid of any echogenic density.

Grade II: Chorionic plate develops more marked indentation. The placental substance becomes partially divided by 'comma like separations' that originates from the areas of previous indentation of the chorionic plate. The echogenic densities within placental substance become dense and the basal plate develops inner echoes within it either broken or as a straight line. It is the hallmark of Grade II placenta.

Grade III: The septation arising from the chorionic plate extends through the placental substance to the basal layer. They also become highly echogenic as a result of calcium deposition. In addition, echo spared (fall out areas) may develop normally in the placenta during third trimester.

There is also acoustic shadow in the placental substance. Fibrinoid deposits appear as cystic areas in the placental substance.

Grade 0—before 30 weeks
Grade I—at 31.1 weeks (40% of the placenta have grade I at term)
Grade II—at 36.36 weeks (45% of the placenta have grade II at term)
Grade III—at 38.04 weeks (15% of the placenta have grade III at term).

At 42 weeks, placenta with uncomplicated pregnancy 55% have grade II, 45% have grade III.

Placental Thickness

Diminished with advancing gestational age
Grade I—3.8 cm; Grade II—3.6 cm; Grade III—3.4 cm

If >4cm—Diabetic mother, Rhesus (Rh) isoimmunization, nonimmune hydrops fetalis, fetus with congenital anomalies, syphilis.

> **Note**
> Placentomegaly—'HAD IT'
> H—Hydrops; A—Abruption; D—Diabetes mellitus; I—Infection; T—Triploidy

Thin placenta—3 cm in IUGR, renal agenesis, oligohydramnios, pre-eclampsia with placental infarcts, chromosomal anomalies.

Lung maturity—It is done at 37 weeks completed.

Grade I—65% have matured L/S ratio.

Grade II—87.5% have matured L/S ratio.

Grade III—100% have matured L/S ratio.

Placental Grading of Medical and Obstetrical Complications

Grade III placenta before 35 weeks is suggestive of IUGR with or without pregnancy-induced hypertension (PIH).

Grade 0 after 32 weeks may be because of diabetes and Rh-isoimmunization.

Placenta Previa

Placenta previa patient must have full bladder to visualize relationship of placenta with internal os. Around 16–20 weeks roughly, 25% of the placenta lies near internal os, but diagnosis should not be made by this time. Repeat scan should be done at 28 weeks in the absence of bleeding or earlier, if bleeding occurs because in later months of pregnancy with the formation of lower segment, the placenta migrates away from the internal os.

Diagnostic accuracy in 3rd trimester is 90% but there is an average false positive result in 10% of cases. In the last few weeks of pregnancy, sonar placentography is difficult in posterior placenta and in patients with oligohydramnios. If transabdominal scan is unclear transvaginal scan should be done.

Abruptio Placentae

The sonogram may demonstrate either a retroplacental hematoma as a sonolucent area behind placenta or there may be a hematoma dissected beneath the chorionic membrane and recognized as a sonolucent area between the membrane and uterine wall.

In revealed type, USG is helpful to differentiate the condition from placenta previa by localizing placenta.

Abnormalities of the cord (Single umbilical artery) the best way to confirm cord vessels number is the identification of umbilical arteries on either side of fetal bladder.

Hydramnios and Oligohydramnios

By measuring amniotic fluid index (AFI), measure largest pocket in 'cm' in each of the four quadrant of uterus or abdomen. Summation of amniotic fluid pocket in four quadrants gives AFI in cm form that period of gestation (Table 8.1).

Liquor pocket measurement: Deepest vertical pocket of the fluid, which is free of cord and any feat parts, measured in cm (Figure 8.13).

Table 8.1: Measurement of liquor pocket and AFI

Amniotic fluid index (AFI)		Liquor pocket
<5 cm	Oligohydramnios	<2 cm
5–8 cm	Borderline low oligohydramnios	
8–18 cm	Normal	2–8 cm
18–24 cm	Borderline high	
>24 cm	Polyhydramnios	> 8 cm

Diagnosis of Intrauterine Fetal Death

Measurement of BPD twice with an interval of 4 days to find reduction of about 5 mm or lack of fetal motions (fetal cardiac activity, fetal movements, FBM) is +ve diagnosis of intrauterine fetal death (IUFD).

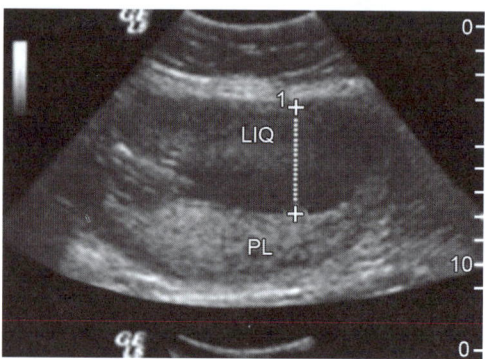

Figure 8.13: Liquor pocket and placenta

Integrity of Previous Cesarean Section Scar

In case of LSCS, look for previous CS scar. A scar <2.5 mm thick is a weak scar. It is a thick linear echogenic shadow traversing whole myometrium at the level of internal os

Biophysical profile score (BPS)—Testing should not later than 32–34 weeks of gestational age until delivery. It is a specialized type of ultrasound examination that was originally described by Manning and Colleagues. Do not perform BPP within 48–96 hours of administration of corticosteroid because it decreases BPP. Biophysical profile is given in Table 8.2.

Modified biophysical profile (MBPP) = NST + amniotic fluid volume (AFI) by USG, which is an indicator of long-term function of the placenta and takes only 10 minutes to perform.

Interpretation of MBPP:

a. MBPP is normal when NST is reactive and AFI is more than 5 cm. It is repeated once in a week or earlier, if clinically indicated.
b. MBPP is abnormal, if NST is nonreactive and AFI is ≤5 cm.
   When this test is abnormal, a CST, or full BPP can be performed as a back-up test.
   The use of weekly CST, biweekly NST, biweekly BPP should result in perinatal mortality rate of 0.4–3 per 1000 livebirths within 1 week of normal test.
   Figure 8.14 shows USG of normal craniovertebral junction and cerebellum.

Congenital Defects of Fetus

Central Nervous System

Anencephaly, hydrocephalus, microcephaly, holoprosencephaly (incomplete development of forebrain or prosencephalon), Dandy-Walker malformation (cerebellar vermis is absent the cerebellar hemisphere is separated, and there is a dilated 4th ventricle occupying the posterior fossa), encephalocele [herniation of meninges and CSF (meningocele) and if the brain tissue is present—encephalomyelocele], spina bifida.

> **Note**
> NST—Short-term marker of fetal status, AFI—Marker of long-term placental function.

Table 8.2: Biophysical profile

Criteria	Score 2	Score 0
NST	Reactive	NR
AFI	>5 cm	< 5 cm
FBM (Fetal breathing movement)	At least 1 episode of FBM of 30s in 30 minutes	Absent or no episode FBM of <30 s in 30 minutes
Gross body movement	3 discrete body movement or 1 limb movement in 30 minutes	Absent or < 3 fetal movement
Fetal tone	At least one episode of active extension and flexion of fetal limbs or trunk. Opening and closing of hand is considered as normal tone	Either slow extension or with return to partial flexion or movement of limb in full extension or absent fetal movement
Interpretation	Score— Maximum = 10; Minimum = 0	
8–10	Without oligohydramnios = normal	
6	Suspicious and test repeated within 24 hours	
<6	Increased perinatal mortality and morbidity	
Score	*Recommended Management*	
8–10	Repeat in one week (DM, Post-dated pregnancy—repeat twice weekly—no intervention)	
4–6	If fetal pulmonary maturity is assured, delivery is favored; otherwise repeat within 24 hours. If persistent score of 4–6 or if pulmonary maturity is certain, delivery; otherwise treat with steroids and delivery must be undertaken within 48 hours	
0–2	Evaluate for immediate delivery; in case of certain pulmonary, immaturity steroid is given and deliver in 48 hours	

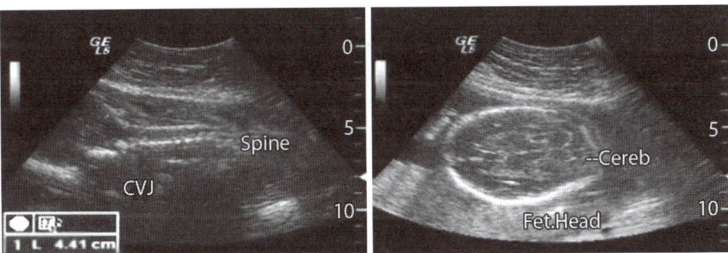

Figure 8.14: USG showing craniovertebral junction and cerebellum

Hydrocephalus

Hydrocephalus—Ventriculomegaly of lateral cerebral ventricles with or without dilatation of 3rd or 4th ventricles. Mild or borderline ventriculomegaly is usually defined as transverse atrial width of lateral cerebral ventricles of 10–15 mm (normal 7–10 mm).

> **Note**
> Chroid plexus normally touches both the walls of the lateral ventricle, but when it fails to touch both the wall, think of ventriculomegaly. In that case measure the distance between the medial border of lateral ventricle to medial border of chroid plexus, it has to measure less than 3 mm in normal ventricle.

Down Syndrome/Screening for Fetal Aneuploidy

Down syndrome: An increased size of nuchal translucency (NT= 0.37 cm at 12 weeks) due to cardiac failure in skeletal deformity, abnormality in extracellular matrix, delayed development of lymphatic system.

Nuchal Translucency (NT)- Normal value (1.2 to 2.4 mm at CRL 45 mm to 1.9–2.7 mm at CRL of 84 mm)

It is a fluid-filled space which appears behind the fetal neck and it is increased in Down syndrome and also increases with gestation. In case of first trimester screening, if the fetal NT is ≥3.5 mm (normal: 1–2 mm). Patient should be offered a targeted USG and fetal echocardiogram. In addition to nuchal translucency other USG parameters of Down syndrome are:
   i. Absence of fetal nasal bones
   ii. Increased resistance to blood flow in the ductus venosus (DV)
   iii. Presence of tricuspid regurgitation.

At 11–14 weeks—NT (high), Free (f) β-hCG (high—2.0 × normal), PAPP-A (low—0.4 × normal)[Combined screen].

Triple screen test: MSAFP (f) β-hCG and unconjugated estriol (uE3) At 14–20 weeks—Quad test—AFP (low, 0.75 × normal), uE3 (low, 0.72 × normal), β-hCG (high, 2.0 × normal), Inhibin -A (high, 2.0 × normal) Table 8.3.

Table 8.3: Biochemical marker profile in second trimester Aneuploidy

Marker	T21	T18	T13	Turner
AFP	Low	Unchanged	Increase	Decrease
hCG	High	Very low	Normal	Very high
uE3	Low	Low	Normal	Decrease
Inhibin-A	High	Unchanged	Normal	Very high

Skull—Brachycephaly and strawberry shape.
Fetus with spina bifida may have cranial signs like small BPD, frontal bone scalloping called 'Lemon sign', elongation and downward displacement of cerebellum (Banana sign).
Face—Cleft, ear, eyes, nose, tongue, micrognathia
Neck—Nuchal translucency, cystic hygroma

Gastrointestinal Tract

Omphalocele, duodenal atresia (double bubble shadow), diaphragmatic hernia, fetal ascites.

Cardiovascular System

Congenital heart disease.

Excretory

Renal dysplasia, hydronephrosis, hydroureter, posterior urethral valve obstruction, renal agenesis, multicystic dysplastic kidneys.

Figure 8.15 shows normal fetal stomach, spine, umbilical cord and kidneys.

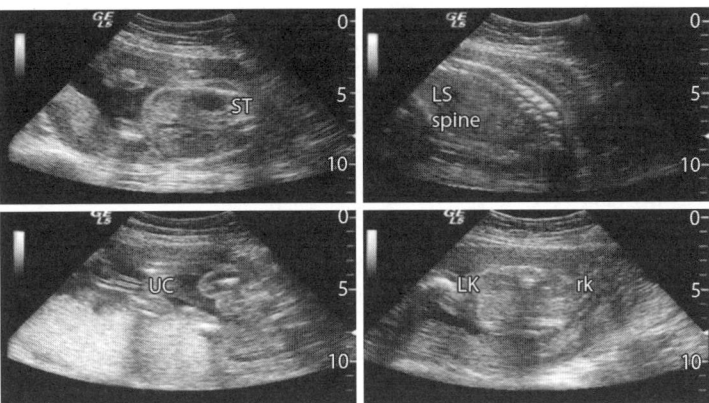

Figure 8.15: USG showing fetal stomach, spine, umbilical cord (UC) and kidneys

Skeletal dysplasia (See all 4 limbs with fingers and toes): Achondroplasia, dyschondroplasia, bone disease—osteogenesis imperfecta, hand and foot anomalies.

USG in Invasive Procedure

- Amniocentesis—at 15-16 weeks of GA (20-30 mL fluid)
- Chorionic villus sampling (CVS)—9-12 weeks
- Cordocentesis—after 17 weeks of GA to remove the blood from the cord.

For Therapeutic Purpose

a. Intrauterine blood transfusion in severe Rh-isoimmunization
b. Shunt operation in hydrocephalus—ventriculoamniotic
c. Fetal suprapubic catheterization to relieve hydronephrosis due to urethral obstruction
d. Selective killing of abnormal fetus by injecting hypertonic saline or KCl solution through umbilical artery or heart in multiple pregnancies (triplet/quadruplet). The dose of KCl is 0.2–0.5 mL solution into the heart. In monochorionic (MC) twin KCl is contraindicated and cord occlusion technique is used for selective fetal reduction to prevent cotwin demise.

Diagnosis of Cervical Incompetence

1. *Cervical length:* Average cervical length of non-pregnant cervix = 2.5 cm when compared to 3.7 cm for pregnant cervix. The pregnant cervix is rarely >6 cm in length. Shortening of the cervix in the absence of any other changes does not alter the prognosis of pregnancy as this is a physiological phenomenon of the mid trimester.
2. *Width of internal os:* This should be <0.5 cm. A measurement of 1.5 cm or more during first trimester and greater than 2 cm during 2nd trimester is diagnostic and woman at risk of cervical incompetence found to have a cervical canal diameter >6 mm is observed in patients who require circlage, aborted or had a preterm birth.

3. *Bulging of the membrane:* USG can detect bulging of membrane into the endocervical canal prior to pregnancy loss.

Cervical Insufficiency

- If cervical length is ≥30 mm, the risk of preterm delivery is low and no intervention is necessary
- Identification of short cervix (<25 mm) in the second trimester in women with prior preterm birth should alert the examiner to the possibility of cervical insufficiency and increased risk of recurrent spontaneous preterm birth
- These women benefit from ultrasound induced circlage operation prior to 24 weeks of gestational age.
  Initiate TV ultrasound cervical length (CL) at 14 weeks
    - If CL is ≥30 mm repeat every 2 weeks upto 23 weeks
    - If CL is 25–29 mm repeat every 1 week until 23 weeks
    - If CL is < 25 mm prior to 24 weeks, offer circlage operation.

ULTRASONOGRAPHY DOPPLER

Doppler signals may be obtained by three types of waves:
1. Continuous wave: Here Doppler employs probes with two crystals, one for receiving and one for transmitting signals.
2. Pulsed wave: It uses only one crystal, which operates as both a transmitter and a receiver. It is more expensive and less mobile than continuous wave. They are essential in studies of uterine blood flow.
3. Color flow mapping: Modifies direction and intensity of blood flow within a vessel and which are indicated by different colors.
   - Blue indicating flow away from transducer
   - Red orange—flow towards transducer
   - Mosaic pattern—red orange or blue green represents flow in several directions indicating turbulence.

Qualitative Analysis (Figure 8.16)

1. It is not dependent on angle of insonation.
2. Flow velocity waveform of different vessels can also be differentiated.
   S/D ratio
   RI (Resistance index) = $S-D/S$
   PI (Pulsatility index) = $S-D/A$

> **Note**
> Umbilical artery Doppler indices should be measured after 23 weeks of gestation.

S = Peak systolic velocity due to cardiac contraction
D = End-diastolic velocity, which depends on vessel wall compliance, peak flow, heart rate and vascular impedance
A = Average velocity over the cardiac cycle.
PI and RI are useful when diastolic flow is absent.

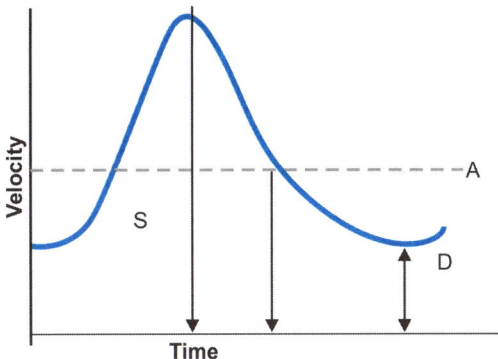

Figure 8.16: Doppler velocity waveform of artery UmA, MCA

Q. Why do you choose MCA for measuring blood flow velocity?

Ans. MCA supplies 80% of blood flow in fetal brain and undoubtedly very sensitive to hypoxemia. To measure the velocity of blood flow accurately, it is essential to achieve an angle of zero degree between USG beam and direction of blood flow and this can be achieved easily in MCA. Hence, real velocity is measured. The compensatory mechanism of increased MCA-PSV in fetal anemia is due to a combination of decreased blood viscosity, leading to increased venous return and cardiac preload and the peripheral vasodilatation that result from fall in blood O_2 content. MCA-PSV is very much useful nowadays for:
  a. Prediction of fetal anemia.
  b. Improved management for the isoimmunized fetus in Rh negative mother by reducing the number of invasive tests (amniocentesis, fetal blood sampling) and its complications.
  c. It is also used for follow-up of fetus after intrauterine transfusion to assess the need of subsequent transfusion.

QUESTIONS ON DOPPLER IN FETAL HYPOXIA

Q. What is hypoxemia?
Ans. Decrease in oxygen content of fetal blood.

Q. What is hypoxia?
Ans. Decrease in oxygenation at cellular level.

Q. What is asphyxia?
Ans. Hypoxia with metabolic acidosis.
In anoxia—umbilical artery (UmA) Doppler flow shows increased S/D ratio or PI (greater than 1.5) and absent or reversed end-diastolic flow.
Interpretation (Figures 8.17A and B):
a. RI of MCA/UmA = 0.75/0.47 = 1.59, i.e. >1(normal), but if the ratio is < 1— hypoxic fetus; PI of MCA/ PI of UmA=1.29/0.61=2.1 (normal as the value is greater than 1.08)

b. S/D ratio of UmA = 94.07/49.94 = 1.88, i.e. < 3 (normal), but if the ratio is > 3—compromised fetus.

In IUGR, the color flow doppler is used to detect compromised fetus. Due to fetoplacental insufficiency detected by decreased diastolic flow or reversal of end-diastolic flow in UmA doppler, the hypoxic fetus spares its brain, heart and adrenals, which will result in drop in resistance in many areas. Here MCA end-diastolic flow rises resulting in a waveform that resembles normal uterine artery. The increase in end-diastolic flow is a fetal adaptive mechanism to preserve the brain. In decompensated state of fetus, if acidosis progresses this adaptive mechanism fails and end-diastolic flow is decreased before death of fetus. In late onset, IUGR- MCA changes precedes UmA, but before 30 weeks UmA abnormality precedes MCA changes.

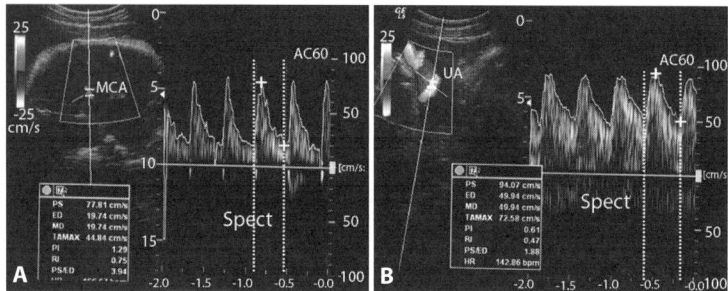

Figures 8.17A and B: (A) Blood flow in MCA (MCA-PI = 1.29, RI = 0.75); (B) Blood flow in umbilical artery (UmA-PI = 0.61, RI = 0.47) *(For color version, see Plate 3)*

Estimation of fetal venous circulation at ductus venosus (DV) level provides more detailed information on the fetus heart and information on the fetal acid-base balance status. Appropriate evaluation of blood flow through the DV can provide an opportunity to deliver the IUGR baby prior to the onset of acidosis, which is most correlative to mortality and long-term morbidity (See USG Doppler in IUGR Case discussion).

Uterine Artery Doppler

a. Normal uterine artery waveform—Good systolic peak, good diastolic flow, and no early diastolic notch (Figure 8.18A).
b. Abnormal uterine artery waveform—Steep sharp systolic peak, poor diastolic flow, early diastolic notch (Figure 8.18B).

The uterine blood flow increases 10- to 12-fold due to invasion of trophoblasts in the spiral arteries within the myometrium and decidua and 50% increase in maternal volume, so diastolic notch in uterine waveform decreases after 20 weeks. If normal trophoblastic invasion and modification of spiral arteries are interrupted, the placental perfusion is decreased due to narrow diameter of the branches of uterine artery resulting increased impedance to flow within the uterine arteries and a notch is produced in the diastolic component.

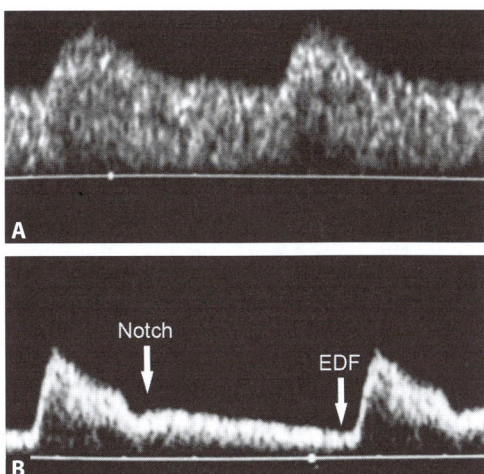

Figures 8.18A and B: Uterine waveform at 24 weeks of GA, uterine artery doppler showing end-diastolic flow (EDF). (A) Normal uterine artery waveform; (B) Abnormal uterine artery waveform, notch in early diastole

Doppler interrogation is performed between 21 to 24 weeks in the prediction of preeclampsia and or IUGR (Figure 8.18), where diastolic notch persists.

> **Note**
> *Doppler velocimetry is not a useful screening test for the detection of fetal compromise and is not recommended as a screening test in the general obstetric population. It is an adjunct method of fetal assessment in association with other method of fetal monitoring in high-risk cases of pregnancy.*

FOR POSTGRADUATES

ROLE OF DOPPLER IN PREGNANCY

Q. What are the uses of color flow Doppler?

Ans.
1. To find out vascular resistance in placental circulation and prediction of pre-eclampsia.
2. To find out the effects of high resistance in fetal circulation.
3. For decision making in high-risk pregnancy like IUGR, fetal anemia, twin-twin transfusion (TTT) syndrome.
4. For detection of unruptured ectopic (living)—ring of fire around the sac.

Q. Which vessels are used for detection of fetal hypoxia?

Ans. Common vessels involve are:
Arteries: Uterine artery, umbilical, middle cerebral, thoracic artery
Veins: Ductus venosus, umbilical vein, inferior vena cava.

Q. What is the principle of Doppler?

Ans. Doppler shift is the change of frequency and wavelength of a sound wave when reflected from a moving object. This principle is used to study the pattern of blood flow in vessels.

Flowchart 8.1: Principle of Doppler

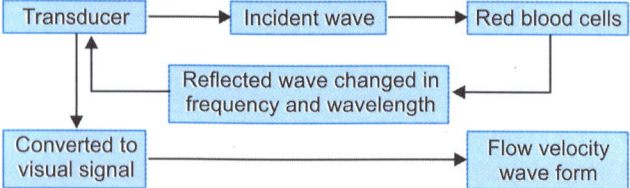

Arterial Doppler

- *Uterine artery*: Determine utero-placental condition (Discussed above).
- *Umbilical artery (UmA)*: Determine feto-placental blood flow
- The vessel is visible by ultrasound at 6–7 weeks of gestational age and does not show any diastolic flow till 10 weeks of gestation. The volume of UmA increases with advancing gestation, so the vascular resistance gradually decreases and the number of tertiary stem villi and arterial channels are also increased in the feto-placental compartment, thereby decreasing the impedance in the UmA. This decrease in vascular resistance allows a continuous forward blood flow in UmA through out the cardiac cycle. It shows a high diastolic flow and a low PI. (Normal UmA study- S/D <3, RI= S-D/S= 0.5–0.7) (Figures 8.19A to C).

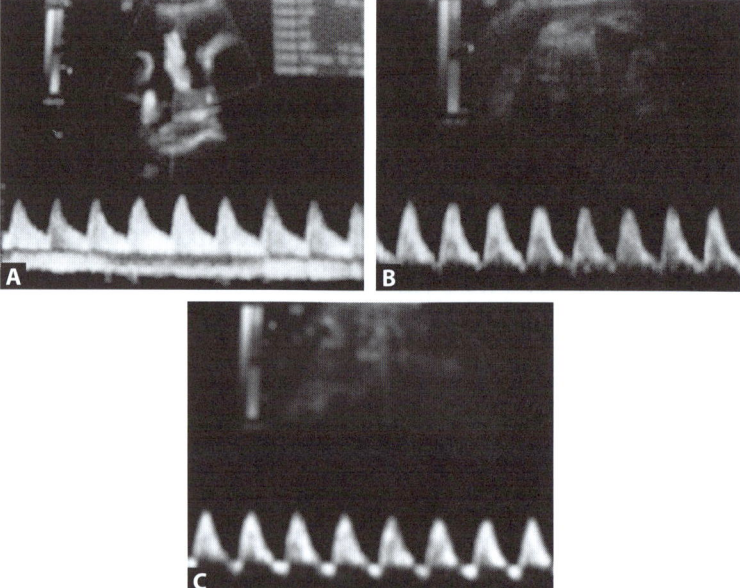

Figures 8.19A to C: (A) Normal umbilical artery Doppler, (B) Absent end-diastolic flow in UmA, (C) Reversed end-diastolic flow in UmA *(For color version, see Plate 3)*

In placental pathology, there is impedance to the blood flow in the UmA, which is more pronounced in diastolic phase. Hence abnormal waveform in the UmA is an early sign of fetal impairment.

The most important diagnostic UmA Doppler waveform is the state of end-diastolic velocity: Absent, end-diastolic velocity (AEDV) [S/D

>3, RI >0.7 and PI –increased, impending hypoxia] or reversed end-diastolic velocity (REDV) [Ominous sign of fetal hypoxia]. In high-risk pregnancies (PIH, IUGR), if GA is greater than 34 weeks in presence of AEDV and REDV, prompt delivery is needed and absent end-diastolic frequency (AEDF) precedes late deceleration (CTG) in fetal hypoxemia by 12 days (range 0–49 days).

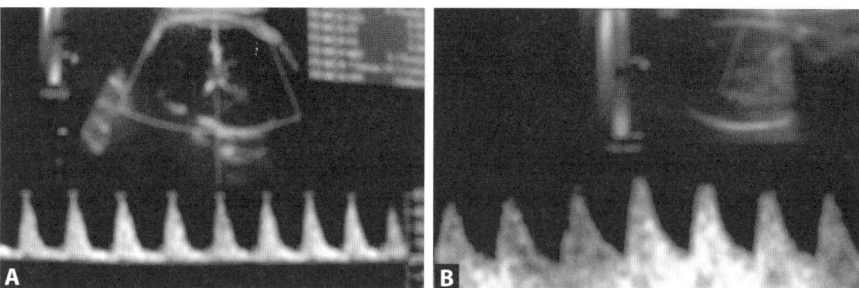

Figures 8.20 A and B: Middle cerebral artery. (A) Normal middle cerebral artery wave form, (B) Redistribution of MCA in a case of severe IUGR (brain-sparing effect) *(For color version, see Plate 3)*

Middle cerebral artery: Determine fetal condition (Figures 8.20A and B) It is very much important in fetal Doppler assessment for its easy accessibility and high sensitivity for detections of IUGR and related complications. In healthy fetus, MCA has a high resistance flow and has a high PI index and S/D ratio is always higher than UmA (S/D) [Normal study of MCA: RI>0.7; PI>1.3].

In hypoxic fetus, there is increased blood supply in the brain, myocardium and adrenal glands and reduction in blood flow in kidneys, GIT and lower extremities. The centralization of circulation causes low impedance in MCA and shows increased blood flow in diastole due to vasodilatation. So, there is decrease in PI (<1.3) and decrease in RI (<0.7). Due to severe oxygen deficiency, there is sudden rise of middle cerebral artery PI, RI and vascular dilatation may be suppressed by cerebral edema. American College of Obstetrics and Gynecology (2012) recommends that MCA has neither been evaluated in randomized trial nor adopted as standard practice in the management of growth restriction. The utility of MCA Doppler to aid the timing of delivery is uncertain.

Cerebroplacental Doppler ratio (CPR)

It is the ratio of pulsatility indices (PI) of MCA and that of the UmA. It suggests both placental status (umbilical artery) and fetal response (MCA). It is a good predictor of fetal oxygenation status at birth and outcome of babies in high-risk pregnancies.

PI of MCA/ PI of UmA must be >1.08 during pregnancy, below which it is abnormal.

Venous Doppler

Umbilical vein

It is pulsatile in early pregnancy due to physiologic decrease in ventricular compliance but resolves in 8–13 weeks. From 15 weeks, it is

nonpulsatile, monophasic flow pattern in normal fetuses. Monophasic pulsatility (systolic peak) is found in fetuses with severe hypoxia.

Ductus venosus: Determine fetoplacental condition and more detailed information of fetal heart (Figures 8.21A and B).

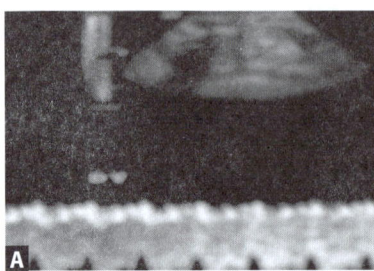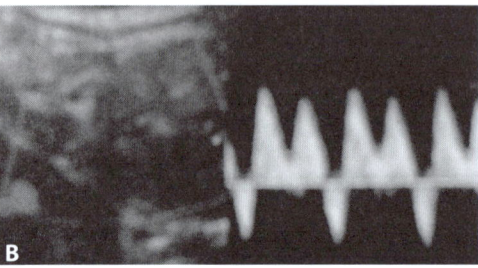

Figures 8.21 A and B: (A) Normal ductus venosus with Doppler waveform, (B) DV waveform with reversed a-wave *(For color version, see Plate 4)*

DV has triphasic waveform representing flow during systole (S wave), diastole (D wave) and atrial systole (a- wave) [see long case of IUGR (Chapter 10)]. DV has the highest forward velocity allowing most oxygenated blood to by pass liver and directly enter the heart, where it is directed through the foramen ovale towards the cerebral circulation.

In response to severe hypoxia, dilatation of DV occurs and allows a larger proportion of umbilical venous flow to pass into the right atrium through the foramen ovale and into cerebral circulation in order to maintain highly oxygenated blood to the brain.

Abnormal indices are: (i) abnormal PI, (ii) abnormal S/A ratio, iii. abnormal peak velocity indices (PVI). Abnormal or reversal blood flow during atrial contraction (a-wave) signifies failure of fetal circulatory compensation to supply proper oxygenated blood to vital organs. So abnormal DV waveform (reversal of a-wave) indicates early delivery otherwise intrauterine fetal demise may occur.

> **Note**
>
> *ACOG (2013) recently concluded that that Doppler assessment of vessels other than UmA has not been shown to improve perinatal outcome and that its role in clinical practice remains uncertain.*

Q. What is the side effect of Doppler?

Ans. It is generally not done in first trimester of pregnancy for thermogenic effect.

> **Note**
>
> *Ultrasound effect: No significant effect on fetus*
> - *Temperature elevation (heating by US absorption)*
> - *Positive and negative (rarefactional) pressure*
> - *Cavitation, heating, pressure, free radical were developed*
> - *Streaming*
> - *Red cell stasis by standing wave.*

Chapter 9

X-ray in Obstetrics

The X-ray has harmful effect on the developed fetus and also maternal ovaries. It is not widely used nowadays due to the advent of ultrasonography (USG), but it should be kept minimum with good antenatal care, if required. Exposure to less than 5 rads has not been associated with an increase in fetal anomalies or pregnancy loss.

> **Note**
> *Though X-ray is not a useful gadget of investigations in modern obstetrics, the readers must read all the questions and answers of different X-rays set in this Chapter for answering questions of long cases, specimens and flying orals that are asked frequently in practical examination.*

BREECH PRESENTATION

Q. Describe the X-ray.

Ans. This is the straight X-ray of lower abdomen and pelvis of a pregnant woman showing fetus in breech presentation (Figure 9.1).

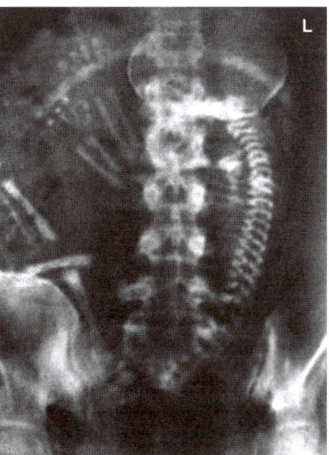

Figure 9.1: X-ray showing breech presentation

Q. Describe the presentation.

Ans. It is a breech with extended legs—frank breech.

Q. What is the incidence of breech presentation?

Ans. 3–4% after 34 weeks.

Q. What are the causes of breech presentation?

Ans.
a. Prematurity—most common
b. Polyhydramnios and oligohydramnios
c. Uterine malformation
d. Multiple pregnancy
e. Fetal anomaly—hydrocephalus
f. Placenta previa
g. Contracted pelvis.

Q. Which variety is common in primigravida?

Ans. Frank breech due to high uterine muscle tone.

Q. What is uncomplicated breech?

Ans. Where breech presentation is the only abnormality.

Q. What is complicated breech?

Ans. Breech with pregnancy-induced hypertension (PIH), placenta previa, contracted pelvis.

Q. What is habitual breech?

Ans. If a woman has consecutive three breeches.

Q. What are the causes of habitual breech?

Ans. Congenital malformations of uterus such as septate, sub-septate or bicornuate uterus cause habitual abortiobreech.

Q. When X-ray should be done in breech presentation and why?

Ans. At 37–38 weeks for confirmation of:
a. Diagnosis of breech
b. Type of breech
c. Contracted pelvis
d. Congenital mal formation of fetus—hydrocephalus
e. Hyperextended neck of fetus
f. Size of fetus
g. Multiple pregnancy.

Q. What are the indications of cesarean section (CS) in breech presentation?

Ans.
a. Large fetus (> 3.5 kg)
b. Contracted/borderline pelvis/fetopelvic disproportion
c. Footling presentation
d. Preterm breech (as the head is comparatively large) and breech with any complications and high risk factors such as PIH, diabetes, elderly primigravida, placenta previa, post CS pregnancy, history of infertility

X-ray in Obstetrics

   e. Not delivered within 8 hours after premature rupture of membrane (PROM)
   f. Skiagram shows extension of fetal head greater than 90°, vaginal delivery causes 90% incidence of fetal spinal cord transection, so CS (Cesarean section)
   g. Bad obstetrical history (BOH).

Q. What are the indications for safe vaginal delivery?

Ans. a. Doctor must be trained in breech delivery
   b. Weight of fetus less than 1.5 kg or less than 3.5 kg
   c. No gross fetopelvic disproportion
   d. It should be frank or complete breech (no footling presentation) with flexed head
   e. There should be no associated high-risk factors in the present pregnancy.
   f. Intrauterine fetal death (IUFD).

Q. Why LBW <1.5 kg is delivered by LSCS?

Ans. This is because of problems of birth asphyxia, trauma and head trapping due to incompletely dilated cervix causing poor perinatal outcome.

Q. How do you manage hyperextension of fetal head in breech presentation?

Ans. It can be diagnosed by X-ray (classically called star-gazing fetus) and by measurement of craniospinal angle in USG. There is a risk of lower cervical spinal cord injury of the fetus due to excessive stretching of the spinal cord at the time of vaginal delivery. There may be chances of tear of dura and epidural hemorrhage. So hyperextension of fetal head is best managed by elective cesarean section.

Q. How will you distinguish foot and hand vaginally?

Ans. *Foot:* If the fingers are run from ankle to toes, the heel is still apparent; toes are normally equal in length.
Hand: If the fingers are run from wrist to palm, the feeling of heel is absent, fingers are equal and thumb is separate.

Q. What is Zatuchni-Andros scoring for breech delivery?

Ans. See Table 9.1.

Table 9.1: Zatuchni-Andros scores			
Sign	**0 point**	**1 point**	**2 point**
Parity	Primigravida	Multipara	
GA	39 week or more	38 weeks	37 weeks or less
Estimated fetal weight	3,630 g	3,629–3,176 g	< 3.175 g
Previous breech	None	One	2 or more
Dilatation (cm)	≤2	3	≥4
Station	Above and at –3	–2	Below and at –1

If the score is 3 or less, delivery by LSCS

Q. What are the principles of vaginal breech delivery?

Ans. Remember the following points while conducting a breech delivery:
- Adequate pelvis
- Extended breech and estimated fetal weight (EFW) 1500–3500 g
- Well-flexed head on USG or X-ray
- Uncomplicated breech
- Perform all the maneuvers gently without the use of undue force
- Do not pull the baby from below, rather push the baby from above
- Discourage the mother from bearing down prematurely till the cervix is fully dilated
- Passage of meconium does not indicate fetal distress
- Regular monitor the progress of labor and the fetal condition, as in normal labor and delivery
- Presence of pediatrician and anesthetist are very important in labor room
- [For other related questions, see the section on 'breech delivery' (Chapter 5)].

HYDROCEPHALUS

Q. Describe the X-ray.

Ans. This is a X-ray of pelvis and lower abdomen showing a fetus with a very large head, base of the cranial vault are thin, the suture lines are widened and fontanelles are larger. The fetus is in breech presentation (Figure 9.2A).

Q. Can it be present in cephalic presentation?

Ans. Though hydrocephalus is common in breech presentation, it may occur in cephalic presentation too (Figure 9.2B).

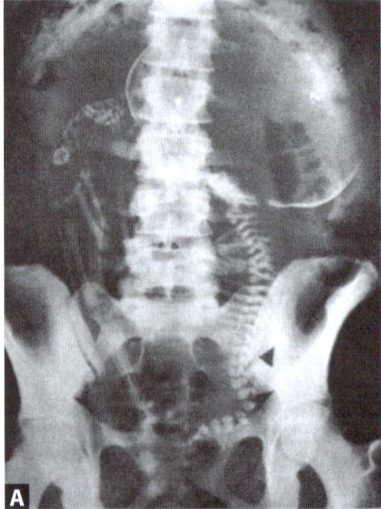 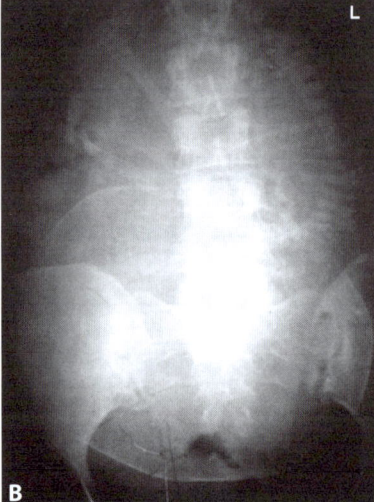

Figures 9.2A and B: X-ray showing: (A) Hydrocephalus in breech presentation; (B) Hydrocephalus in cephalic presentation

X-ray in Obstetrics

Q. What is hydrocephalus?

Ans. Hydrocephalus is the distension of brain and skull due to the increase of pressure by CSF in ventricles.

Q. What is the incidence of hydrocephalus?

Ans. 1 in 2,000 deliveries.

Q. What is the pathophysiology of hydrocephalus?

Ans. Cerebrospinal fluid (CSF) is produced in choroid plexus in lateral ventricle, which is poured to 3rd or 4th ventricles through the median and lateral foramina of the 4th ventricle into the subarachnoid space. If the flow of CSF is obstructed, the pressure in the ventricle increases and fetal head enlarge—obstructive hydrocephalus.

Q. What is the cause of hydrocephalus?

Ans. Multiple genetic factors, i.e. polygenic or environmental by TORCH infection. 'TORCH' stands for:
- **T**oxoplasmosis
- **O**ther infections such as hepatitis B, Syphilis
- **R**ubella
- **C**ytomegalovirus
- **H**erpes simplex virus.

Q. What other congenital defect may be associated with it?

Ans. It may be associated with spina bifida.

Q. How will you diagnose it clinically?

Ans. a. Height of the fundus may be greater than period of amenorrhea.
b. Hydramnios may be associated with it.
c. The fetal head felt at the fundus or at lower pole of uterus and appears very big and tense.

Q. How will you confirm the diagnosis?

Ans. By USG (see USG, Chapter 8) or X-ray.

Q. How do you manage the case?

Ans. *Breech Presentation*

The baby is allowed to deliver spontaneously/or by assisted vaginal delivery and the arrested head can be decompressed by perforating the suboccipital region using a perforator or a sharp-pointed scissors under the guidance of two fingers covering anterior vaginal wall and explore the uterus after the procedure.

Other Methods

Perform laminectomy in the cervical region to open the spinal canal. Drew Smythe catheter is introduced through the opened spinal canal to the ventricle to drain the fluid. If spina bifida is present, introduce the Drew Smythe catheter through the opening to the ventricle to drain the fluid (CSF).

In Cephalic Presentation

The pregnancy, is induced by intracervical PGE_2 gel and when cervix is 3–4 cm dilated decompress the head by introducing a lumbar puncture needle through the vagina into the lowest part of the vault of the skull. This facilitates collapse of the head and subsequently engagement and delivery. If the patient is not in labor or cervical orifice (os) is closed, then decompress the head through the abdominal route by lumbar puncture (LP) needle between symphysis pubis and umbilicus. Bladder must be emptied before hand.

Q. What is the role of intrauterine surgery?

Ans. Various type of shunt operation is done nowadays when the fetus is *in utero*, only when there is no chromosomal or structural deformity of fetus. A shunt is placed between CSF and liquor amnii, thus preventing destruction of brain tissue from CSF pressure.

> **Note**
>
> *Always consider vaginal delivery in breech and cephalic presentations with gross hydrocephalic baby by craniocentesis. If labor is allowed without craniocentesis rupture of uterus may occur. LSCS is preferable in borderline case of hydrocephalus after counseling for advancement of pediatric surgery like shunt operation.*

TRANSVERSE LIE

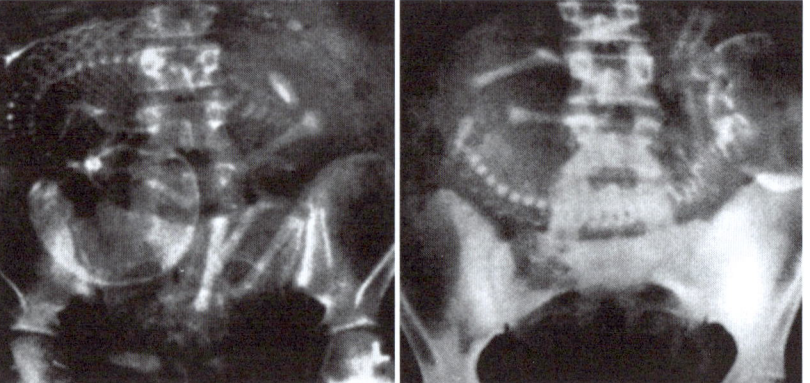

Figure 9.3: X-ray showing transverse lie

Q. Describe the X-ray.

Ans. This is a X-ray of lower abdomen and pelvis of a pregnant woman showing a fetus in transverse lie (Figure 9.3).

Q. What is transverse lie?

Ans. Long axis of fetus lies transversely to long axis of uterus.

Q. What is the presenting part of transverse lie?

Ans. Most common presentation is shoulder.

Q. How will you identify shoulder by per vaginal examination in labor?

Ans. The shoulder is identified by humerus, scapula, acromion process, axilla, coracoid process, clavicle and ribs. All these cannot be felt at a time.

X-ray in Obstetrics

> **Note**
> *Prolapse of an arm is common in shoulder presentation in labor.*

Q. What are the causes of shoulder presentation?

Ans. *Maternal:* Multiparity—laxity of uterus and abdominal wall, placenta previa, contracted pelvis, arcuate or sub-septate uterus, pelvic tumor.
Fetal: Prematurity, intrauterine growth restriction (IUGR), Twins, Polyhydramnios.

Q. What are the problems of transverse lie?

Ans. a. Premature rupture of membranes (PROM)
b. Cord prolapse/hand prolapse
c. Infection
d. Obstructed labor
e. Operative interference
f. Ruptured uterus
g. Intrauterine fetal death (IUD).

> **Note**
> *There is no mechanism of labor in transverse lie with average-sized fetus and pelvis. If left uncared for, it leads to obstructed labor causing rupture of uterus with clinical evidence of dehydration, pallor, acidosis, shock and sepsis and is called 'Neglected shoulder presentation'. Rupture is very common in multiparous women.*

Q. What is complicated shoulder presentation?

Ans. Shoulder presentation along with antepartum hemorrhage (APH), contracted pelvis, PIH.

Q. How will you manage the case?

Ans. a. Complicated cases—lower segment cesarean section (LSCS)
b. LSCS should also be done in:
   1. Mature baby before the onset of labor
   2. Mature and live baby in labor
   3. If signs and symptoms of impending rupture are present.
c. If membrane is ruptured, liquor is drained, the uterus compresses the fetus, then any manipulation is dangerous—LSCS is the choice even the baby is dead.
d. External cephallic version (ECV) may be tried in early labor.
e. *Destructive operation (Decapitation/Evisceration)*: If the baby is dead and surgeon is confident enough for doing such operations, otherwise cesarean section.
f. Internal version—never.

> **Note**
> *Cesarean section is the treatment of choice in transverse lie. See also the destructive operations.*

Q. What happens in neglected cases?

Ans. Rupture of uterus leading to maternal and fetal death.

Fetal Maturity

Q. Describe the X-ray.

Ans. This is a straight X-ray of lower abdomen and pelvis in pregnant woman carrying a fetus in cephalic presentation (Figure 9.4).

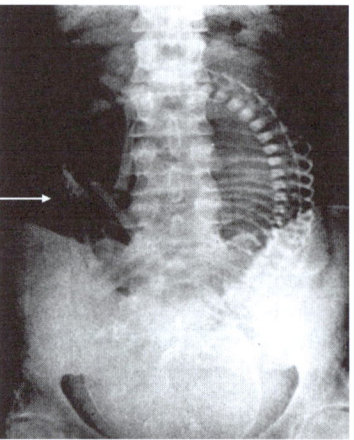

Figure 9.4: X-ray showing fetus in cephalic presentation

Q. Why the X-ray was taken?

Ans. This is taken to diagnose the maturity of fetus considering presentation and size of fetus.

> **Note**
> It can also be diagnosed by fetal biometry by USG.

Q. What are the signs of maturity in X-ray?

Ans. At 36th week—the lower femoral epiphysis can be seen, but upper tibial epiphysis is absent. At 38th week—the lower femoral epiphysis are clearly seen and upper tibial epiphysis (arrow) can be seen. So, the fetus is probably of 38 weeks maturity.

Q. Can any other ossification centre be used to diagnose fetal maturity?

Ans. The ossification centre of cuboid bone appears at 40th week, but it is difficult to detect.

Q. How can you diagnose postmaturity by X-ray?

Ans. If the tibial center is larger than femoral center, the fetus is postmature.

Q. How can you assess fetal maturity in other way?

Ans. a. Clinical examination—SFH measurement, abdominal girth: Fetal weight by Johnson's formula, feeling of the skull bones by P/A examination.

b. *Ultrasonography*: Serial biparietal diameter (BPD), femur length (FL), abdominal circumference.
c. *Amniotic fluid*:
   1. *Mature fetal skin*: Presence of orange cells—these cells are shredded from the mature fetal skin. They are stained orange with Nile blue sulfate.
   2. *Maturity of fetal kidney*: Creatinine level > 2 mg/dL indicates fetal maturity.
   3. *Maturity of fetal lung*: *Lecithin*: Sphingomyelin (L:S) ratio 2:1 or more indicates fetal lung maturity. *Shake test*: Amniotic fluid is shaked well with ethanol in a test tube, frothy bubbles appear in the test tube, L: S is 2 : 1 or more.
   4. Presence of phosphatidyl glycerol also indicates fetal lung maturity.

> **Notes**
> 1. Fluorescent polarization: The automated assay measures the surfactant-to albumin-ratio by uncentrifuzed amniotic fluid and gives result in 30 minutes. A ratio of ≥50 with commercially available TDX-FLM test predicts lung maturity in 100% of cases. Recently, TDX FLM II is used to test the pulmonary maturity, with a threshold ratio of 55 mg/g.
> 2. Radiological maturity in all cases is only accurate within ± 2 weeks. This is not much better than clinical assessment or USG parameters.

ANENCEPHALY

Q. Describe the X-ray.

Ans. This is an X-ray of lower abdomen and pelvis of a pregnant mother showing a fetus without the vault of the skull (Figure 9.5).

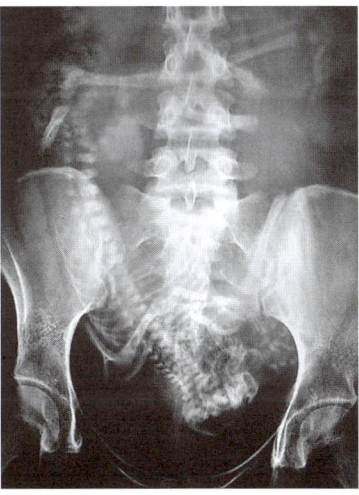

Figure 9.5: X-ray showing anencephaly

Q. What is anencephaly?

Ans. The vault of the fetal skull is absent but the facial portion is normal. Brain is not well-developed and pituitary gland is either absent or hypoplastic.

Q. What is the incidence of anencephaly?

Ans. 1 in 1,000 births.

Q. In which sex, is it common?

Ans. Usually the sex of the baby is female (70%).

Q. Why is it common in female?

Ans. The brain is not developed, pituitary cannot secrete adrenocorticotropic hormone (ACTH) hormone, so the adrenal cortex cannot be developed properly (the androgenic steroid from adrenal cortex is responsible for development of male external genitalia in normal male fetus). So in anencephalic baby due to the deficiency of androgenic steroid, the phenotypical sex is female.

Q. What are the causes of anencephaly?

Ans. The exact cause is unknown. It is polygenic in origin. Genetic and environmental factors are important, viral infections are also responsible. Folic acid deficiency is a contributory factor.

Q. How will you diagnose a case of anencephaly?

Ans. *Clinically:*
  a. Cephalic pole cannot be palpated properly
  b. Hydramnios is present
  c. Face presentation.

  Investigations:
  a. USG at 12–18th week (diagnosed by mass of brain tissue—'Shower cap')
  b. X-ray
  c. Maternal serum AFP at 15–20th week (AFP ≥2.5 MoM).

Q. Why hydramnios is common in anencephaly?

Ans. a. *Exposed choroid plexus*: This causes large volume of CSF to be added in liquor
  b. Defective deglutition
  c. *Absent posterior pituitary*: Due to deficiency of antidiuretic hormone (ADH), a large volume of fetal urine is produced, which increases the liquor volume.

Q. What are the complications of anencephaly?

Ans. a. Hydramnios (70%).
  b. Malpresentation—breech or face.
  c. Premature labor when associated with hydramnios.
  d. Shoulder dystocia.
  e. Obstructed labor when head and shoulder engage together.

Q. How do you manage the case?

Ans. Termination of pregnancy, if diagnosed early in 2nd trimester. Induction of labor is done by artificial rupture of membrane (ARM) with or without syntocinon, if diagnosed later. The uterus is most often refractory to syntocinon because of low level of estriol. If the cervix is unfavorable PGs may be used to ripen the cervix.

Q. What are the dangers of labor?

Ans. a. *Shoulder dystocia*: The small cephalic pole passes through the undilated cervix resulting shoulder dystocia.
b. Soft tissue injury due to bony spicules of the cephalic pole.
c. *Accidental hemorrhage*: By separation of placenta due to low ARM in polyhydramnios.

Q. Why prolonged pregnancy is anticipated?

Ans. Absence of fetal pituitary with oxytocin hormone (which initiates labor) may cause prolonged pregnancy.

Q. How will you manage shoulder dystocia?

Ans. By cleidotomy.

Q. Which presentation is common in anencephaly?

Ans. Face presentation.

MULTIPLE PREGNANCY

Q. Describe the X-rays.

Ans. This is a straight X-ray of abdomen and pelvis of a pregnant woman showing two fetuses, both of them are in cephalic presentation (Figure 9.6A) and the other shows first breech and second cephalic (Figure 9.6B).

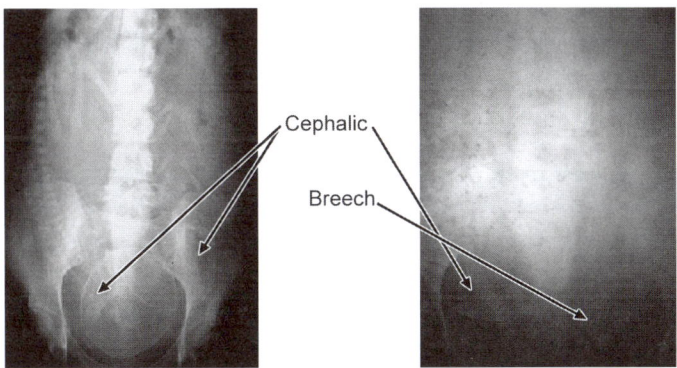

Figures 9.6A and B: (A) X-ray shows two fetuses with head presentation; (B) X-ray shows two fetuses; first breech, second cephalic

Q. Has X-ray any advantage over USG to diagnose twin pregnancy in later months of pregnancy?

Ans. It has following advantages:
a. Better for idea of position and presentation

b. In later months, USG may miss the diagnosis of multiple pregnancy unless the sonologists are conscious about the possibility
c. Two fetuses may not be present in the same frame of USG
d. Conjoined twin is better diagnosed by X-ray.

> **Note**
> See the other questions as mentioned in case discussion of twin pregnancy.

Q. What is the route of delivery in twin pregnancy when:
a. Twin A and Twin B both is vertex (Figure 9.7A)?
b. Twin A vertex and twin B breech (Figure 9.7B)?
c. Twin a non-vertex (breech) and twin B (cephalic) (Figure 9.6B)?
d. If both babies are transverse (Figure 9.7C) or first baby is transverse?

Ans. a. When both the presentation of twins is vertex, always vaginal delivery is preferred considered if there is no obstetrical contraindications. After delivery of first baby presentation of second baby is confirmed as change of presentation may occur in 10–20% of cases. VLBW baby <1500 g and even twin B is substantially larger, but if presentation is cephalic, safe and successful vaginal delivery is possible.
b. Vaginal delivery of twin A(first baby), followed by vaginal delivery of twin B(second baby) either by assisted breech delivery or breech extraction according to the condition. External cephalic version may also be performed after delivery of first baby.
c. Vaginal delivery in twin A (first baby) if breech is problematic as there may be chance of interlocking between vertex of second baby to the after coming head of first breech. Not only that, breech in the first twin may extend the head during vaginal delivery which may cause cervical spine injury. Twin A (first baby), if breech better option is cesarean section.
d. If first baby is transverse or both are transverse, always do LSCS.

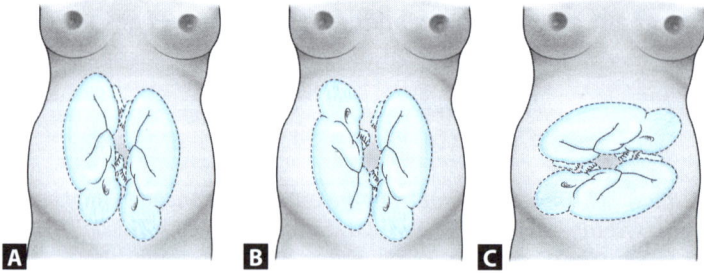

Figures 9.7 A to C: Fetuses. (A) Both vertex; (B) Vertex-breech; (C) Transverse-transverse

Q. What are the causes of death in monochromic twins in 2nd or 3rd trimester?

Ans. a. Cord accident
b. Twin-to-twin transfusion syndrome (TTTS)

c. IUGR (selective)
d. Placental abruption and twin reversal arterial perfusion
e. Congenital anomaly of babies.

Q. Congenital anomaly of one twin—what options can be chosen?

Ans. Counseling with possible risks:
   a. Pregnancy may be allowed to continue in minor defects or non-lethal to other twin
   b. Pregnancy may be terminated, if the patient wishes
   c. Selective termination of the anomalous fetus may be done in major defect or affect the unaffected twin.

> **Note**
> In monochorionic twin selective reduction may result in death of the other one and cord occlusive technique is the method of choice. In dichorionic twin (DC), feticide is done by KCl solution injection in the fetal heart.

Q. What are the adverse effects on living fetus or mother, if one baby is dead in late trimester (>20 weeks)?

Ans. Fetus
   a. Death of one twin is associated with 20–25% increased risk of death in remaining twin
   b. Preterm delivery is common in both mono- and dizygotic twin
   c. Neurological damage (periventricular encephalomalacia)
   d. Monozygotic gestation with monochorionic membrane—embolization of toxic product through vascular anastomosis and these pregnancies require special and frequent evaluation. Fetus may have ischemic end organ injury frequently neurologic (cerebella necrosis, hydrocephalus, encephalomalacia, microcephaly).

Mother
   a. Coagulation defects in the blood secondary to the degenerated product from the circulation of dead fetus
   b. Maternal coagulopathy though uncommon carries serious adverse effect.

> **Note**
> It is a well-known fact that twins are conceived more often than born, but after the first trimester, the incidence of twin varies between 0.5% and 6%.

Q. What will be the fate of single intrauterine demise in twin pregnancy in very early trimester?

Ans. Early pregnancy loss < 20 weeks (vanishing twin syndrome) and fetus papyraceus usually continue without any serious complications of mother and surviving fetus, but close observation is necessary.

Q. How will you manage, if one baby of twin dies in later months of pregnancy?

Ans. Counselling with possible risks and supports are important

Dichorionic: No intervention upto term, unless there is maternal/fetal indication of delivery.
  a. Frequent assessment of surviving fetus by USG, BPP, Doppler flow study (MCA-PSV) and FHR-monitoring, fetal blood sampling for detection of acid-base status if facilities are available.
  b. Evaluation of structural anomalies and growth determination is mandatory of surviving twin by serial USG.
  c. Serial assessment of coagulation profile of mother. DIC is to be corrected by blood and plasma transfusion, as required but is not a necessary indication of delivery. Coagulopathy is uncommon as the baby is delivered within a few weeks.
  d. Delivery is indicated for standard obstetric reason, but only in stable maternal hemodynamic condition. Steroids may be given for early pulmonary maturity. Some prefer delivery at 34 weeks.
  e. Pediatric support is necessary after delivery.

Monochorionic: A single fetal demise in monochorionic twin is urgently delivered whether fetal maturity is present or not and hypoxic/ischemic end organ injury of co-twin occurs immediately after death of sibling.

> **Note**
> USG/MRI during pregnancy and 3–4 weeks after IUD is helpful to detect cavitations and fetal brain atrophy in living fetus of monochorionic twin.

Q. Why the incidences of triplet are high now-a-days?

Ans. Incidence of triplet is high nowadays due to following reasons:
  a. Increase in the treatment of infertility by ovulating agents.
  b. Assisted reproductive technology (ART).

Q. How will you reduce the incidence of triplet?

Ans. Incidence of triplet can be reduced by:
  a. Controlled induction of ovulation
  b. Limit the number of embryo transferred in assisted reproduction technique
  c. Embryo reduction to lower the pregnancy complications.

Q. What are the methods of multifetal pregnancy reduction (MFPR)? When do you perform it? Which route is preferred and why?

Ans. The routes of multifetal reduction are:
  a. USG-guided transvaginal—sac perforated and aspirated
  b. Transabdominal—sac perforated percutaneously, Time: 10-13 weeks of GA. Transabdominal route is preferred as chances of infection are less.

> **Note**
> MFPR is usually delayed till 13 weeks when nuchal translucency (NT) can identify fetus with the lower risk of aneuploidy to be left intact. The first step is to assess chorionicity, CRL and exclusion of anomalies are mandatory before MFPR.

Q. What are the complications?

Ans. Chances of abortion are 12% and PMR is 8%.

> **Note**
> a. Important outcome is evident in multifetal pregnancies when selectively reduced for quadruplets (high fetal order), but for triplet pregnancy, the procedure does not necessarily improve the pregnancy outcome.
> b. Multifetal pregnancies resulting from selective reduction born earlier than nonreduced pregnancies.
> c. Selective fetal reduction is contraindicated in twin pregnancies.
> d. For selective fetal reduction intracardiac injection of 1–2 mEq of potassium chloride is given to the fetal heart under USG guidance.
> e. Ethnic and moral problem.

Q. Which type of twin pregnancy is associated with hydramnios?

Ans. Monozygotic twin.

Q. Is the incidence of congenital defect high in multiple pregnancy?

Ans. Increased incidence of congenital defect (2-3 times higher) than in single tone pregnancy and congenital defects are more common in MZ (monozygotic) than DZ (dizygotic) twin.

Q. What are the congenital defects of baby in twin pregnancy?

Ans.
a. Conjoined twin
b. Neural tube defect
c. Hydrocephalus
d. Congenital heart disease
e. Chromosomal abnormality
f. Single umbilical artery
g. Acardius fetus (heart does not develop):
   It is of 4 types due to TRAP sequence:
   i. *Acardius amorphous*: It is a shapeless mass
   ii. *Acardius acormus*: Head develops but lower portion of body does not develop (rarest type)
   iii. *Acardius anceps*: Head and face partially develops
   iv. *Acardius acephalus*: No cephalic structures
h. Parasitic twin.

Q. Why congenital malformation occurs in twin pregnancies?

Ans.
a. Defects resulting from twinning itself—conjoined twin, acardiac twin
b. Defects resulting from vascular interchanges—microcephaly, cerebellar necrosis, multicystic encephalomalacia.
c. Defects as a result of crowding—club foot, congenital hip dislocation.

CONJOINED TWINS (SEE THE SPINE)

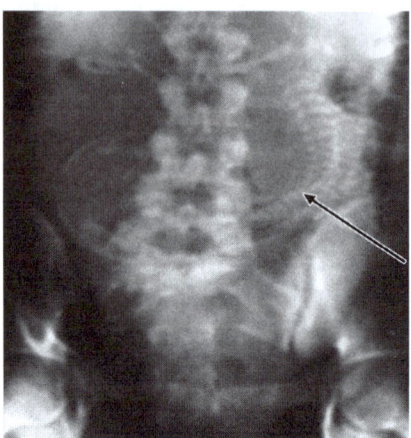

Figure 9.8: X-ray of conjoined twins (see the arrow for spines)

Q. How do you diagnose conjoined twins by X-ray (Figure 9.8)?

Ans. a. The relative positions of head and the spines remains unchanged in different skiagrams taken at different times
b. Spine of the two fetuses are either very close or joined together.

> **Note**
> 3D-USG can diagnose the condition early in pregnancy.

Q. What is the cause of conjoined twins?

Ans. Imperfect separation of monozygotic twins after 13 days of fertilization.

Q. What are the different types of conjoined twin?

Ans. a. Thoracopagus: Fusion at chest(40%)[see Figure 9.7]
b. Omphalopagus: Fusion at anterior abdominal wall (33%)
c. Pyopagus: Fusion at buttocks (18%)
d. Ischiopagus: Fusion at ischium (6%)
e. Craniopagus: Fusion at head (2%).

Q. How will you manage conjoined twins?

Ans. Vaginal delivery is possible when it is grossly preterm but nevertheless majority advocates LSCS as obstructed labor is common. After delivery pediatric surgeon will take decision regarding separate operations.

Q. What is the method of delivery in triplets and quadruplets?

Ans. Premature labor is very much common. Vaginal delivery is possible in triplet pregnancy though CS is the method of choice. Delivery by CS is invariably the method of choice in quadruplet pregnancy as prematurity, IUGR, and malpresentation are common.

INTRAUTERINE FETAL DEATH (IUFD)

Q. Describe the X-ray.

Ans. Straight X-ray of abdomen and pelvis showing radiological evidence of IUFD.

Q. What are the radiological findings of IUFD?

Ans.
 a. Overlapping of the skull bones—Spalding's sign (Figure 9.9)
 b. Hyperflexion (Bell's sign) or hyperextension of vertebral column (due to softening of the ligaments)
 c. Crowding of the ribs
 d. Presence of gas shadow in the heart or great vessels (12 hours of fetal demise)
 e. Edema of the soft tissue giving a halo around the cranium (Devel's halo sign).

Q. Why Spalding's sign appears?

Ans. Due to softening and liquefaction of brain materials.

Q. When does Spalding's sign appear?

Ans. Usually 1 week after IUFD.

> **Note**
> USG can diagnose IUFD very early than X-ray by identifying absence of FHR.

Q. Why does the gas shadow appear?

Ans. After fetal demise a mixture of CO_2, O_2, N_2 liberates during maceration, 45% of gas shadow appears after 12 hours—Robert's sign (it is not common).

Q. What is Bell's sign?

Ans. The fetus is in an attitude of hyperflexion due to loss of muscle tone, resorption of amniotic fluid, reduction of uterine size and crowding of ribs.

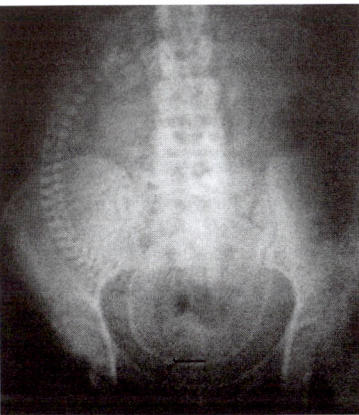

Figure 9.9: X-ray showing overlapping of skull bones (Diagnosis of IUFD)

Q. What is the difference between Spalding's sign and molding?

Ans. See Table 9.2.

Table 9.2: Difference between spalding's sign and molding	
Spalding's sign	**Molding**
a. Occurs in dead fetus	a. Living fetus
b. Occurs before the onset of labor	b. During labor
c. Irregular overlapping of skull bones	c. Regular pattern overlapping between parietal bones or parietal and frontal bones

Q. What is IUFD?

Ans. Antepartum fetal death after 20 weeks of gestation.

> **Note**
> *Some consider age of viability is 22 weeks of gestation.*

Q. What are the common causes of IUFD?

Ans. Maternal:
a. Diseases associated with pregnancy—PIH, APH, eclampsia
b. Maternal diseases—HSRM (Heart disease, severe anemia, renal disease, malabsorption syndrome), uncontrolled diabetes, high fever, malaria, jaundice, SLE, APLAS, drugs—quinidine,

Fetal—prematurity, postmaturity, Rh-isoimmunization, IUGR, intra-uterine infections (TORCH), congenital anomalies.

Placental cause—chronic placental insufficiency and oligohydramnios, placental anomaly and cord accident.

Idiopathic.

Q. What are the causes of recurrent fetal death?

Ans. Women with diabetes (uncontrolled), Antiphospholipid antibody syndrome (APLAS), carrier of single gene mutation are at increased risk of recurrent fetal death. *Other causes:* Essential hypertension (not controlled by drugs), chronic nephritis and SLE.

Q. How will you diagnose IUFD?

Ans. *History of*: Loss of fetal movement, brownish discharge per vagina may or may not be present.
On examination: Fundal height is less, liquor may become small in volume, no active fetal movement
FHS: Absent.
Per vaginal: Overlapping of the cranial bones, head feels soft, dirty brown discharge
Confirmation by USG: Loss of fetal heart movement
X-ray: Spalding sign.

Q. Which investigations are done in case of IUFD?

Ans. a. **Routine: Blood**—Hemoglobin percent, Group and Rh, total leukocyte count (TLC), differential leukocyte count (DLC), blood glucose (Fasting and PP), VDRL, HbSAg, HIV-1 and 2,
b. Routine urine, microscopy and C/S

c. For hypofibrinogenemia—see the investigations later
d. Postmortem examination of fetus and placenta

> **Note**
>
> Other laboratory evaluation:
> a. 3 mL of fetal blood from umbilical cord or heart.
> b. If blood can not be obtained, then at least one of the following:
>   i. Placental block (1 × 1 cm) below the cord insertion
>   ii. Umbilical cord 1.5 cm long
>   iii. Fetal tissue from costo-chondral junction or patella without skin tissue is washed with normal saline and sent in ringer lactate (not in formaline solution) for cytogenetic analysis.

Q. How do you detect hypofibrinogenemia?

Ans. a. Weekly estimation of serum fibrinogen.
 b. Bleeding time (BT), clotting time (CT), platelet and clot observation test (bedside method).

Q. How do you perform clot observation test?

Ans. a. 2 mL of venous blood is taken in a dry test tube and keep it in closed fist to make it warm and after 4 minutes tip the tube slowly to see, if clot is forming and again every 1 minute until the blood close.
 b. This test provides a rough idea of fibrinogen level.
 c. If clotting time is < 6 minute, then fibrinogen level is more than 150 mg%.
 d. If clot fails to form after 7 minutes and the clot is poor or soft—fibrinogen level is probably 100–150 mg%.
 e. If no clot forms within 30 min, the fibrinogen level is less than 100 mg%.

Q. How do you manage a case of IUFD?

Ans. a. Early medical induction as IUFD is diagnosed by USG very early.
 b. Previously protocol was wait for 2 weeks for spontaneous delivery following IUFD after counseling the attendants of the patient. Coagulation profile should be carefully noted during conservative management of 2 weeks when the time of IUFD is not certain.
 c. *If labor fails*: Medical induction only (no surgical induction/ARM for fear of infection) by:
   i. IV oxytocin in escalating dosages
   ii. Cerviprime gel to dilate the cervix
   iii. Tab misoprostol orally or per vaginally [(The RCOG green-top guideline: If GA >27 weeks, 25 µg of misoprostol initially followed by 25–50 µg per vagina at an interval of 4 hours (4 such), if GA is < 26 weeks 100 µg P/V every 6 hours)]
 d. LSCS is rarely indicated.
 e. Management of PPH, if it occurs.

> **Note**
>
> In postcesarean IUFD, first counsel about the increased risk of uterine rupture irrespective of the methods used for inducing labor: if GA > 26 weeks, PGs should be avoided for fear of uterine rupture, but a low dose oxytocin or a standard Foley's catheter may be used for cervical ripening, but if GA < 26 weeks, misoprostol may be used (50 µg, 6 hourly, maximum 5 doses per course).

Q. What are the complications of IUFD?

Ans. a. Psychological upset of mother and family
b. Coagulation disorder (due to hypofibrinogenemia)—generally occurs after 4 weeks
c. Infection leads to gas gangrene. Renal failure and hepatic failure in severe cases may occur.

Q. What are the possibilities, if after repeated induction; baby fails to come out per vagina?

Ans. Consider secondary abdominal pregnancy or ruptured uterus.

Q. What is stillbirth and stillbirth rate?

Ans. It is defined as (WHO) the death of fetus after 22 completed weeks of gestation having fetal weight >500 g or crown heel-length 25 cm or more.

Stillbirth—antepartum deaths (macerated/fresh) + intrapartum death (fresh)

Stillbirth rate is calculated as late fetal death (>20 weeks) in a year divided by livebirths plus stillbirths multiplied by 1000.

For international comparison

$$\text{Stillbirth rate} = \frac{\text{Fetal deaths weighing over 1000 g at birth during the year} \times 1000}{\text{Total livebirths + stillbirths weighing over 1000 g at birth during the year}}$$

Q. What are the causes of intrapartum stillbirth?

Ans. Antepartum death—as stated above
Intrapartum—acute fetal distress, traumatic vaginal delivery, intracranial hemorrhage, birth asphyxia, congenital malformation, umbilical cord accidents.

Q. Which tests are recommended for evaluation of recurrent stillbirth?

Ans. Lupus anticoagulant screen, anticardiolipin antibody (ACA), factor V-leiden mutation, prothrombin G20210A mutation, protein-C, protein-S and antithrombin III deficiency, if facilities are available and USG.

Q. How much is the level of fibrinogen in blood?

Ans. a. Fibrinogen level in non-pregnant women is 200–400 mg%
b. Fibrinogen level in pregnant mother is 400–600 mg%
c. Change is 50% during pregnancy
d. Critical value is considered to be 100 mg% (plasma).

> **Note**
>
> *High fibrinogen level during pregnancy is very much helpful as fibrinogen is activated to form fibrin mesh which covers the old placental site following placental separation after vaginal delivery. This results in 10% reduction in the concentration of clottable fibrinogen following a normal vaginal delivery.*

Chapter 10

Obstetric Cases

HISTORY TAKING

Write the history on pregnant mother's own words, but examination findings in weeks.
a. Name
b. Age
c. Address
d. *Gravida(G)*: Total number of pregnancies—present and past, irrespective of period of gestation.
e. *Parity(P)*: Number of previous childbirth after the age of viability, e.g. $G_{gravida} \ P_{viable\ births\ +\ abortion}$
   - First pregnancy gravida 1 (G_1) para (P) $_{0+0}$
   - 2 children, no abortion, woman is pregnant, $G_3 P_{2+0}$
   - 2 children, one abortion at 4 months, female is pregnant again, $G_4 P_{2+1}$
   - 2 children are living, one died soon after birth, one ectopic pregnancy at 3 months, female is pregnant again, $G_5 P_{3+1}$, LI-2.
   - A woman who delivers twin in first pregnancy is still gravida-1, para-1.

   Other nomenclature:
   Example: $G_4 P_{3-0-0-3}$ (Gravida –4 pregnancies)
   Parity: mnemonic (FPAL)   'F-P-A-L'
   Full term   3
   Preterm   0
   Abortion   0
   Living   3
f. Religion
g. Duration of marriage
h. Date of admission
i. Date of examination.

CHIEF COMPLAINTS IN CHRONOLOGICAL ORDER

1. Pregnancy of 9 months (do not say 36 weeks)
2. Bleeding per vagina for 3 days

3. Frequency of urination for 2 days
4. Pain lower abdomen for one day.

History of Present Pregnancy

Elaborate the Chief Complaints

- History of early present pregnancy-nausea, excessive vomiting, bleeding per vagina (PV)
- History of mid pregnancy—any history of urinary infection, operation for cervical incompetence, date of quickening
- History of late pregnancy—swelling of feet, bleeding PV (pain less or associated with pain), dribbling of liquor, pain abdomen and description of pain in details
- Number of antenatal check-up
- Immunization of injection T toxoid
- Bleeding whether associated with pain or painless, color of the bleeding to differentiate placenta previa, accidental hemorrhage, show frequency of urination-associated with lower abdominal pain, fever, vomiting
- If pain in abdomen, elaborate the pain by the acronym COLDERR; C—Character of pain (sharp, dull, crampy); O—Onset (sudden or gradual, cyclic or constant); L—Location (localized or diffused); D—Duration (for how much time the pain is present); E—Exacerbations (which activities or movement make the pain worse); R—Relief (which activities or movement or medications make the pain better); R— Radiation (any radiation of pain in back, groin, flank) Pain also is to be differentiated from true or false labor pain.

Past History

a. Past obstetrical history (Table 10.1)

Table 10.1: Past history of obstetrics

Year	ANC	Pregnancy	Labor	Puerperium
1980	Booked	Uncomplicated	ND at 40 weeks	*Mother*: Uncomplicated, *Baby*: Sex, BW, congenital defect, Apgar score, alive/dead, if dead then cause of death, stillborn-fresh or/macerated, if alive-breast feed/artificial feed, status of immunization
1984	Unbooked	Severe pregnancy-induced hypertension (PIH)	Low forceps at 39 weeks	Non-union of episiotomy wound, Baby: living and take other points

Abbreviations: ND = Normal delivery; BW = Birth weight of baby

b. *Past medical history:*
   Tuberculosis (TB), rickets, rheumatic fever, heart disease, hypertension, diabetes, epilepsy, asthma allergy to any drug, history of blood transfusion, corticosteroid therapy, injection anti-D globulin in Rhesus (Rh)-isoimmunized mother.

c. *Past surgical history:*
   General surgery for example appendicitis
   Gynecological surgery for example discharge (D/C); disseminated intravascular coagulation (DIC); pelvic floor repair (PFR); repair of vesicovaginal fistula (VVF) and current procedural terminology (PT).

Family History

Diabetes mellitus (DM), hypertension, TB, blood dyscrasia, multiple pregnancy.

> **Note**
> *Obstetric family history as a predictor of obstetric complications like pre- or post-term birth, pre-eclampsia, or operative delivery, gene-environment interactions can provide prenatal care.*

Menstrual History

1. Age at menarche
2. Cycle—days
3. Duration—days
4. Flow-average/scanty/heavy
5. Pain lower abdomen—yes/no
6. 1st day of last menstrual period (LMP)
7. Expected date of delivery (EDD).

Calculation of EDD—Naegele's Rule:
a. By adding 9 calendar month + 7 days in normal cycle (28 days) with first day of LMP
b. Come back 3 calendar months from the month of LMP and then add 7 days with the 1st day of LMP, e.g. calculate the EDD when the 1st day of LMP is on 2nd July, 2008 EDD, 9th April, 2009.

> **Note**
> *Ovulatory or fertilization age is typically 2 weeks shorter.*

Personal History

Sleep, bowel, bladder habit, addiction of tobacco, alcohol, etc. use of any contraception, how long trying for baby, education of mother and husband as well, family-joint/nuclear, number of child, diet vegetarian/nonvegetarian—adequate or poor, family income or socioeconomic status.

> **Note**
> *It is a recognized fact that some obstetric syndromes (preterm birth, PROM, pre-eclampsia, abnormal labor, IUGR) are more likely to recur in an woman over successive pregnancies.*

Examination

- Consciousness and alertness
- Built—obese, average, thin
- Nutrition—Good/average/poor
- Height—meters   BMI = kg/m² (Prepregnant weight or weight in early trimester)
- Weight—kg
- Gait—limping or normal

Pallor: Site of examination—lower palpebral conjunctiva, dorsum and tip of the tongue, nailbed, palm and palmar creases, sole and skin (multiple sites are to be examined). Koilonychias—the nailbed becomes spoon shaped instead of convexity.

Jaundice: Site of examination—upper bulbar conjunctiva, under surface of the tongue, hard and soft palate, palm, sole and skin (multiple sites are to be examined) in a good day light.

> **Note**
>
> Jaundice: Yellowish discoloration of mucous membrane and skin when the serum bilirubin level is >2 mg %, (normal bilirubin: 0.8–1 mg%; latent jaundice: serum bilirubin level is 1–1.9 mg%; clinical jaundice: Serum bilirubin level is >2 mg%).

Edema: Both legs are examined. The site for edema to be examined is over the medial maleolus and anterior surface of lower third of tibia. The area is to be pressed for 15–30 second and feel depression in pitting edema on the leg. Varicosities also are to be noted in the legs (*Causes of edema—*
a. Physiological: Disappear at rest,
b. Pathological: Pregnancy-induced hypertension (PIH), anemia, hypoproteinemia, congestive cardiac failure (CCF), nephritic syndrome).

Others: Neck gland, neck veins, condition of the thyroid-physiological enlargement occurs in 50% of cases, cyanosis. Pulse/respiration/temperature and blood pressure (do not forget to take weight and measure blood pressure (BP) in examination).

Measuring the Blood Pressure

Instruments: Mercury sphygmomanometer (MS)—gold standard; Callibrated aneroid device—can be used; Automated BP machine is not good.

a. By Palpatory Method

For systolic BP measurement
1. Ask the patient to lie comfortably or in sitting position.
2. Woman should be tilted to left side when she lies down.
3. Place the sphygmomanometer on a flat surface at the level of woman's heart.
4. Ensure that the pointer on dial is at zero.
5. Fix the appropriate inflatable cuff (breadth is of 1.5 times the circumference of the arm) on the upper part of either arm after removing the clothing. The lower border of the cuff should be at 2.5 cm from the cubital fossa.

6. Feel the brachial artery over the cubital fossa or radial pulse by left hand.
7. Inflate the cuff by pressing the rubber bulb till you do not feel the pulse—increase the pressure by 10 mm Hg above the level at which the pressure disappeared.
8. Deflate gradually till you feel the pulse to reappear again—the level at which pulse reappear is systolic.

b. By Palpatory Method

Both systolic and diastolic pressure can be measured by stethoscope.
1. Deflate the cuff by loosening the screw of rubber bulb and now raise the pressure again to 30 mm Hg above the level at which the radial pulse will no longer be palpable.
2. Place the stethoscope on cubital fossa; lower the BP by 2 mm Hg at a time till you start hearing repetitive thumping sound. The reading at which sound start firstly (Korotkoff-1), is systolic blood pressure (SBP).
3. Continue lowering the BP until the sound first gets muffled and finally disappeared. The reading at which the sound finally disappears (Korotkoff-V) is diastolic blood pressure (DBP).
4. Note the SBP/DBP in mm Hg.
5. In some cases, the sound disappears at '0'; in that case appearance of muffling sound (Korotkoff-IV) should be designated as DBP.

> **Notes**
> - If DBP is persistently less than 40 mm of Hg use muffling or fourth sound and make a note
> - BP is consistently high in one arm, refer to the arm which records higher BP.

Systemic examination: Heart, lung, liver, spleen.

Cardiac examination: The heart should be examined systematically. Heart should be auscultated at the apex and its base. Heart sounds, murmurs, and clicks should be characterized.

Pulmonary examination: Lung field is also examined systematically thoroughly. Wheezes, rales, ronchi and bronchial breath sounds should be recorded.

Obstetrical Examination

Female attendant is necessary for male students.

Breast

See the nipple (cracked/depressed), skin condition of areola, the purpose is to correct abnormality. Breast examination for establishment of breastfeeding in puerperium is not mandatory according to National Institute for Health and Care Excellence (NICE) guideline.

Abdomen—expose the part to be examined properly with prior consent of woman

Inspection:
- Description of swelling—anteroposterior or transversely oval
- Undue enlargement of uterus
- Presence of any scar tissue

- Condition of umbilicus—flat or everted
- Linea nigra and presence of striae
- Presence of ring worm.

Palpation: Avoid palpation during Braxton-Hicks contraction or contraction during labor.
- Superficial palpation—temperature of the skin of abdomen or any hyperesthetic zone
- Deep palpation.

Fundal height:
1. Ask the pregnant mother to evacuate the bladder and dextrorotation is to be corrected by tilting the uterus towards the midline of abdomen.
2. Ask the pregnant mother to lie on her back with flexed hip and knee with slight tilt on left side by pillow underneath the back to avoid supine hypotensive syndrome.
3. The examiner should stand on the right side of abdomen.
4. The examiner's hand must be warm and should be placed on the abdomen till the uterus is relaxed. Do not poke the uterus by fingertip.
5. Now place the ulnar border of left palm on the woman's abdomen parallel to the symphysis pubis—start from xiphisternum (lower end of sternum) and proceed downwards gradually towards symphysis pubis, lifting your hand each step down till you finally feel resistance, which is uterine fundus. Correct dextrorotation of uterus with back of other hand, if present.

> **Note**
> Height of the fundus can also be determined by the method of percussion starting from xiphisternum. The percussion note becomes resonant (due to hollow intra-abdominal organs) until it reaches uterine fundus downwards. The dull note appears at uterine fundus.

6. Mark the level of the fundus by skin marking pencil. By using a measuring tape, measure in centimeter from the upper borer of symphysis pubis to the markings at the top of the fundus keeping the legs of the pregnant mother straight and not flexed (Figure 10.1A).

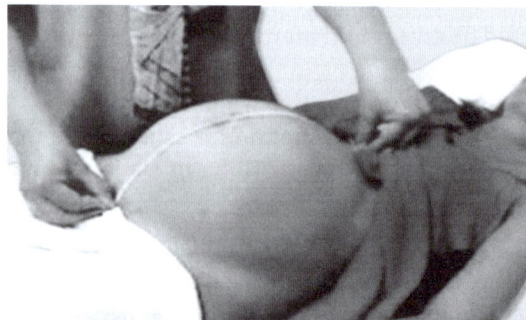

Figure 10.1A: Symphysis fundal height measurement
(For color version, see Plate 4)

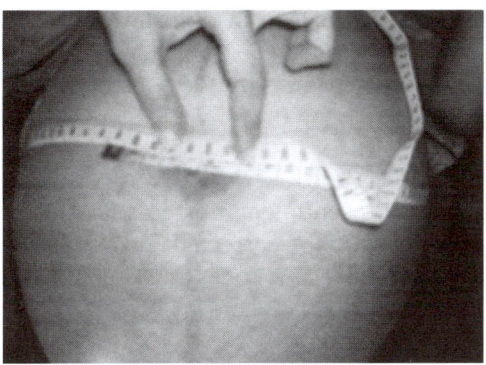

Figure 10.1B: Measurement of abdominal girth at the level of umbilicus *(For color version, see Plate 4)*

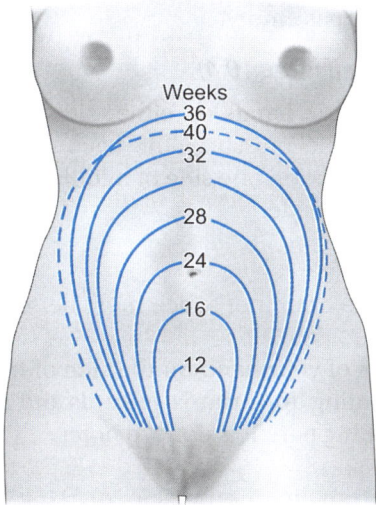

Figure 10.2: Normal fundal height

After 24 weeks of gestation, fundal height (in cm) corresponds to the gestational age (GA) in weeks (within 1–2 cm deviation). *Pre-requisites*: Bladder should be empty and uterus should be on midline (Figure 10.2)

- At 12th week—just palpable above symphysis pubis
- At 16th week—lower 1/3rd of the distance between symphysis pubis and umbilicus
- At 20th week—lower 2/3rd of the distance between symphysis pubis and umbilicus
- At 24th week—at the level of umbilicus
- At 28th week—lower 1/3rd of the distance between umbilicus and xiphisternum
- At 32nd week—2/3rd of the distance between umbilicus and xiphisternum

- At 36th week—at the level of xiphisternum
- At 40th week—below the level of 36 weeks, but the flanks are full. The height of uterus becomes less as the presentation entire into the pelvis.

Pelvic Grips (4 in number)

To determine the lie and presenting part of fetus. Ask the patient to evacuate the bladder, dextrorotation is to be corrected and ask the woman to lie on her back with partial flexion of hips and knees and keep the legs slightly apart.

Fundal Grip (Figure 10.3)

Face of the doctor should be towards the mother's face. Palpate the uterine fundus by laying both hands on the side of the fundus to determines, which pole of the fetus is in the fundus.
- Breech—soft, broad, irregular non-ballotable mass
- Head smooth, hard, globular, ballotable mass
- Transverse lie—the grip is empty.

Lateral or Umbilical Grip (Figure 10.4)

Place the palms of both the hands on either side of uterus at the level of umbilicus and apply gentle pressure. The back of the fetus—feels like a continuous hard, flat surface on one side of midline and the limbs are felt as irregular knob like on other side.

First Pelvic Grip (Figure 10.5)

To perform this grip, the examiner's face must be towards the foot end of mother.

Keep both the palms of your hand on the side of the uterus with fingers held close together pointing downwards, inwards and medially, and palpate to recognize the presenting part. It is done to note:

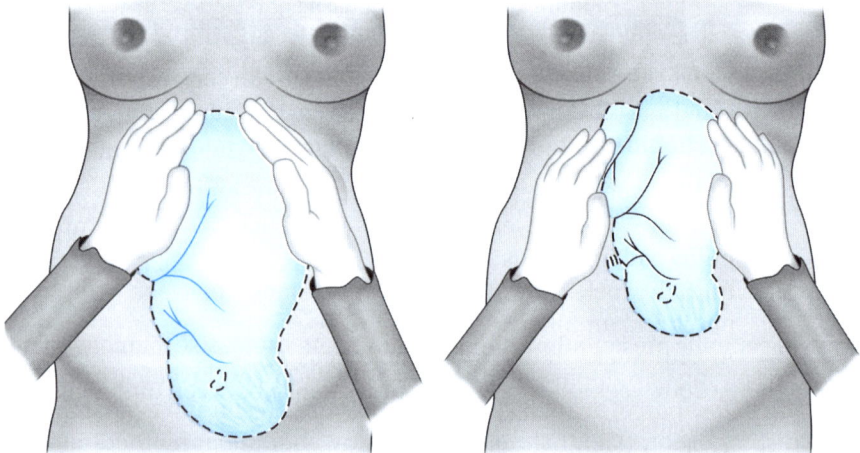

Figure 10.3: Fundal grip **Figure 10.4:** Lateral grip

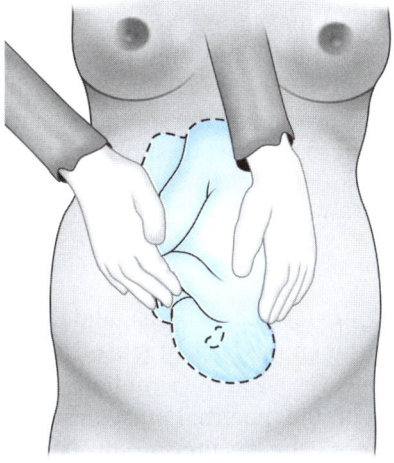
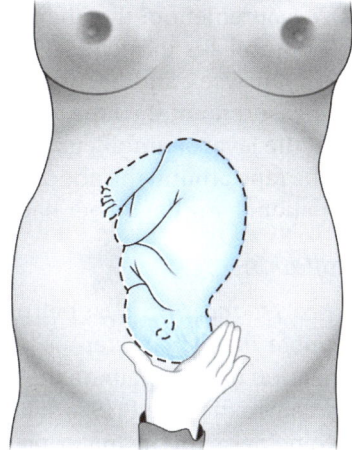

Figure 10.5: First pelvic grip   **Figure 10.6:** Second pelvic grip

a. Presentation—if cephalic (feels like a hard, rounded mass, which is ballotable).
b. If presentation is cephalic then note the attitude of head—flexed, deflexed or extended (the occiput lies lower than sinciput in well-flexed head).
c. Whether the presenting part is engaged or not

> **Note**
> *If the pregnant mother cannot relax her muscles, ask her to flex the leg slightly more and more palpate in between deep breaths*

Second Pelvic (Pawlick's) Grip (Figure 10.6)

Spread your hand widely over the symphysis pubis with the ulnar border of the right hand touching the symphysis pubis. Try to approximate the thumb and fingers putting gently and deep pressure over the lower part of uterus, the presenting part can be felt in between fingers and thumb. Determine, whether it is breech or head. In transverse lie, the grip is empty. Mobility of the presenting part is also determined by gripping the presenting part and try to move it to see whether it is engaged or not.

> **Note**
> *In Leopold's maneuvers the order of grips are: 1. Fundal grip; 2. Lateral grip; 3. Pawlick grip/superficial pelvic grip (first pelvic grip); 4. Second pelvic grip/deep pelvic grip.*

Q. What is engagement?

Ans. In cephalic presentation when the maximum transverse diameter of the presenting part, biparietal diameter (BPD) crosses the pelvic brim and 2/5 or less part of the head is felt per abdomen. Testing for cephalopelvic disproportion (CPD) should be done by abdominal method after 37 weeks of gestation, if head is not engaged in case of primi mother (for details see the long case of primigravida with floating head).

Q. How do you measure abdominal girth?

Ans. Measurement of the abdominal girth by a measuring tape at the level of umbilicus in inch. At 30th week it is 30 inch and then increase by 1 inch/week and become 40 inch at 40th week. For abdominal girth, measurement the tape was repositioned to encircle the woman's waist at the level of umbilicus without applying excessive pressure to tighten the tape around the abdomen. The measurement is performed with the patient lying flat on her back with legs extended (Figure 10.1B).

Auscultation

Fetal heart sound (FHS): Use bell of stethoscope or fetoscope to auscultate FHS. Remember the FHS in utero is best heard through the back of fetus. During auscultation of FHS, palpate the maternal pulse as a routine simultaneously and note whether the FHS is synchronous with the maternal pulse or not. If FHS coincides with the maternal pulse, it is not FHS. It is uterine soufflé. If it is asynchronous with the maternal pulse, then it is FHS. Count the fetal heart sound and maternal pulse separately for 1 minute.

For normal cephalic presentation, the FHS is best heard midway between the line joining the umbilicus and anterior superior iliac spine on the side where the back is, in occiput posterior position the FHS is audible further laterally. In breech, the FHS is best heard above the umbilicus; in transverse lie—dorsoanterior position, the fetal heart sound is best audible around the umbilicus.

Vaginal examination is not allowed in undergraduate examination. Initially, the index and middle fingers of the one gloved hand should be introduced into the patient's vagina and vaginal examination in late pregnancy provides certain valuable informations such as presentation, presenting part, station of the presenting part in relation to ischial spine; estimate pelvic capacity and identifies pelvic architecture, softness, effacement and dilatation of cervix, position of cervical opening to the fetal head, the presence or absence of membrane and the color of amniotic fluid (See Vaginal Examination in Obstetrics later on).

Investigations

- Blood for hemoglobin percentage (Hb%), blood group and Rh, Venereal Disease Research Laboratory (VDRL) or Rapid Plasma Reagin (RPR) test, Oral glucose challenge test (OGCT) for detection of GDM [75 g glucose irrespective of fed state of mother, single blood sample is to be taken after 2 hours], hepatitis B surface antigen (HbSAg), human immunodeficiency virus (HIV)-1 and 2, in prevention of parent to child transmission of HIV.
- Urine for routine examination (R/E) and culture and sensitivity (C/S) [if pus cell is high > 5 high-power field (HPF) including colony count]
- Stool for ova, cysts and parasite (OCP) examination
- Ultrasonography (USG)—at 16–18 weeks to exclude congenital defect of fetus
- What is your case?
- Say the summary and then diagnosis.

- What is your diagnosis?
- Say the diagnosis only and not summary.

Vaginal Examination in Obstetrics

Procedure

a. Ask the pregnant mother to evacuate the bladder, do not catheterize as a routine.
b. Position of mother-dorsal with legs drawn up with knees and thighs are semiflexed.
c. The doctor should wear sterile gloves on both hands.
d. Vulva is inspected for any swelling sore, discharge and edema.
e. Separate the labia with left index finger and thumb and wash introitus with cotton swab-soaked with savlon from above downwards by single use and not from below upwards to avoid anal contamination.
f. Now introduce gloved index and middle finger of right hand inside the vagina gently, the thumb remains abducted and ring and little fingers are flexed.
g. The left hand is placed over the lower abdomen.

During Pregnancy

a. To confirm the diagnosis of early pregnancy
b. To exclude the pelvic pathology like fibroid uterus, ovarian tumor
c. For assessment of pelvis after 37 weeks
d. In antepartum hemorrhage (APH), examination is to be done in OT where everything is ready for lower segment cesarean section (LSCS).

During Labor

a. To diagnose the onset of labor
b. To note the progress of labor (PV examination at 4 hour interval)
c. In abnormal labor
   i. With rupture of membrane to exclude cord prolapse
   ii. Arrested labor with maternal and fetal distress
d. Before any operation—forceps or ventouse.
   During puerperium: Done 6 weeks later in normal puerperium.

Some Important Points regarding Vaginal Examination in Labor

a. The first vaginal examination in a woman with symptoms suggestive of labor will be done when she has uterine contraction lasting for 20 seconds and occur at least once every 4 minutes.
b. Active labor is defined as the stage of labor when cervix is fully effaced and at least 4 cm dilated.
c. Vaginal examination should be repeated every 4 hours, if the woman is in active labor at the initial assessment and after 6 hours, if patient is not in active labor.
d. Vaginal examination may be done earlier, if there are significant FHR abnormalities.

Some Important Points Regarding USG in Pregnancy

- At least one ultrasound for congenital anomalies should be done in 18–20 weeks of pregnancy (Basic essential care)
- Ultrasound evaluation once in each trimester (additional care)
- Because of low lying placenta detected at 20 weeks another transabdominal scan at 36 weeks and if transabdominal scan is unclear a transvaginal scan should be offered
- Pregnant women should be offered an early USG scan to determine GA assessment, multiple pregnancy, anembryonic sac, early screening of Down's syndrome and reduce the need for induction of labor after 41 weeks.

NORMAL PREGNANCY AT TERM

(Case discussion)

Summary and Diagnosis

Mrs XX, G1 P0 + 0, aged 25 years with no antenatal check-up admitted with the c/o pain in lower abdomen and on examination only mild pallor was noted and her BP is normal (120/80 mm of Hg) at the time of examination. Obstetrically, the pregnancy is at 40 weeks of gestation, longitudinal lie, cephalic presentation with engaged head. FHS is 150/min regular, liquor volume is good with normal uterine tone. P/V examination is not done for undergraduates, but for postgraduates note down the findings.

Provisional diagnosis: Primigravida with engaged head at term.

Discussion of the Case

Q. What is the importance of age?

Ans. In which age pregnancy occurs is very much important. If pregnancy occurs in teen age group or after 30 years (elderly primi mother) it carries some risk during pregnancy, so these two groups are included in high-risk cases of pregnancy.

Q. What is elderly primigravida and its complications?

Ans. If pregnancy occurs >30 years. Complications are miscarriage, Down's syndrome, hypertensive disorder, IUGR, preterm labor, VTE and pulmonary embolism, GDM.

Q. What is grand multipara? What are the complications?

Ans. It relates to a pregnant mother who has got previous 4 or more viable births. Complications—anemia, unstable lie, abruptio placentae, uterine rupture, PIH, multiple pregnancy, CPD, PPH, subinvolution.

> **Note**
>
> *Some important definitions: Nulligravida—A nulligravida is a woman who is not now and never has been pregnant; nulliparous—A nullipara is a woman who has never completed a pregnancy beyond an abortion; Primipara—A primipara is a woman who has been delivered once of a fetus or fetuses who reached the stage of viability.*

Obstetric Cases

Q. What are the causes of pain abdomen during pregnancy?

Ans. *Obstetrical causes:*
- *Early*: Abortion, ectopic pregnancy, hydatidiform mole, and acute hydramnios
- *Late*: True labor pain, acute fulminant toxemia, abruptio placentae, impending rupture of uterus.

Non-obstetrical causes:
- Medical—pyelitis, cystitis
- Surgical—acute appendicitis, acute pancreatitis, duodenal perforation, intestinal obstruction and volvulus
- Gynecological—retention of urine, red degeneration of fibroid.

Q. How do you diagnose pallor? Define anemia?

Ans. See the different sites for pallor as in history taking. Pallor and anemia are not same. Pallor is the clinical diagnosis whereas anemia is diagnosed practically by laboratory or of Hb%. (To convert grams of Hb into percentage multiply grams by 7; e.g. 9 g = 9 × 7 = 63%). Anemia means qualitative and quantitative diminution of Hb and RBCs in peripheral blood in relation to age and sex of the patient (see case discussion of anemia in pregnancy).

Q. What are the methods of Hb estimation?

Ans. Sahli's method, cyanmethemoglobin method, Haemaccel method, WHO approved color scale.

Q. How will you detect edema?

Ans. a. By pressure of thumb on the dorsum of the foot, medial malleolus, lower end of tibia 1 inch above the ankle joint and pressure should be given on both legs at the same time persisting for 30 seconds. Depression of skin surface—pitting edema.
b. Occult edema is detected by taking weight gain.

Q. What is normal weight gain during pregnancy?

Ans. Total weight gain in pregnancy is 10–11 kg (1 kg = 2.204 lbs).
1–2 kg in—first trimester
0.2 kg/week—in second trimester
0.5 kg/week in third trimester
or 0, -1, +1, 4, 4, 5, 5, 3, 3 lbs in each month.

> **Note**
> According to NICE guideline, serial weight measurement in pregnancy is not mandatory until indicated.

Q. What is abnormal weight gain?

Ans. Rapid weight gain of more than 5 lbs in a month or more than 1 lb/week in later months of pregnancy is significant. Excess weight gain causes PIH, preterm delivery, LBW and macrosomia in some women.

Q. How do you calculate the rate of weight gain?

Ans. Weight gain = $\dfrac{wt_t - wt_{t-1}}{GA_1 - GA_2}$

where, wt = Weight, GA= Gestational age in weeks, 't' is the time of most recent measurement, 't−1' time of previous measurement, e.g. if body weight is 135 lbs at 20 weeks of GA, and 139 lbs at week 25, then

Weight gain (lbs/week) = $\dfrac{139 \text{ lbs} - 135 \text{ lbs}}{25 \text{ week} - 20 \text{ week}} = 4/5 = 0.8$ lbs/week

It is applicable in 2nd and 3rd trimester as in 1st trimester the rate of weight gain is low.

> **Note**
> Poor weight gain is associated with LBW and more complications in pregnancy.

Q. How do you calculate maternal blood volume in pregnancy?

Ans.

$$\text{Nonpregnant blood volume (mL)} = \dfrac{\text{Height (inches)} \times 50 + \text{Weight (pounds)} \times 25}{2}$$

Pregnancy Blood Volume

- Average increase is 30–60% of calculated nonpregnant volume
- Increases across the gestational and plateau at approximately 34 weeks
- Average increase is 40–80% in multiple pregnancy
- Average increase is less in pre-eclampsia
- Blood volume decreases in acute hemorrhage (APH, PPH).

Q. What is body mass index (BMI)?

Ans. BMI = wt/ht^2 = kg/m^2 or lbs/in^2 (weight is pre-pregnancy weight or weight in very early trimester).

Q. Pre-pregnancy BMI and ideal weight gain during pregnancy?

Ans. According to Food and Nutrition Board of the Institute of Medicine (IOM)

BMI Kg/m²	Weight for height status	Recommended weight gain
< 19.8	Underweight	28–40 lbs
19.8 – 26	Normal weight	25–35 lbs
26–29	Over weight	15–25 lbs
> 29	Obese	15 lbs

Q. How do you measure the BP?

Ans. Discussed in history taking.

Q. When do you say a pregnant mother is hypertensive?

Ans. When the BP is >140/90 mm of Hg.

Obstetric Cases

Q. How do you ascertain the duration of pregnancy?

Ans.
a. Date from first day of last menstrual period
b. Uterine size is to be determined in very early part of antenatal check-up (within 12 weeks of pregnancy)
c. Date of quickening-first perception of fetal movement in multi gravida is 16 weeks and in primigravida is 18 weeks
d. Height of the fundus and symphysio-fundal (S-F) measurement in cm (1 cm/week after 24 weeks).

e. McDonald formula = $\dfrac{\text{S-F measurement in cm}}{3.5}$ = Duration of pregnancy in lunar months.

For example, If S-F length is 30 cm, then 30/3.5 = 8 and ½ lunar months = 34 weeks

f. Clinical examination of size of fetus, volume of liquor, and uterine tone per abdomen.
g. Measurement of abdominal girth.
h. USG—Fetal BPD, FL and other parameters discussed in USG in obstetrics.

Q. How do you determine the fetal age?

Ans.
a. Determine the fundal height
b. Symphysio-fundal (S-F) height measurement
c. Clinical estimation of fetal size and hardening of skull bones by pelvic grip
d. Determine the fetal weight by:
  1. **Johnson's formula**
     Fetal weight (in g) = [Fundal height (fh) (in cm) – n] × 155
     n = 12, if vertex is above ischial spine; n = 11, if vertex is below ischial spine.
     where fh: fundal height measured from the upper border of pubic symphysis
     If patient's weight is > 91 kg (200 lbs), 1 cm is subtracted from the fundal height as in the following example, fh = 30 cm station = – 2. Therefore (30–12) × 155 = 2790 g, the calculation is accurate within 375 g in 75% of newborn.
  2. **Dare's formula**—Fetal weight (g) = SFH × AG, where (SFH: symphysio-fundal height, AG: Abdominal girth). All are measured in 'cm'.
  3. **USG parameter**— more accurate, estimated fetal weight (EFW) is usually within 10% of actual fetal weight but fallacy is higher in preterm and SFD babies.
     For formula, see the long case of IUGR.

Q. How do you calculate EDD in a patient with 21 days cycle or 34 days cycle?

Ans. In 21 days cycle, Naegele's formula 'minus 7 days'
In 34 days cycle, Naegele's formula 'plus 6 days'

So, EDD = LMP + nine calendar months + 7 days (± additional days, if any).

> **Note**
> Incidence of delivery on expected date (ED) is 4%; ED ± 1 week is 50%.

Q. Is it possible that the pregnancy at 38 weeks and the height of fundus is 34 weeks?

Ans. It is possible. Possible causes are wrong date, IUFD, IUGR, transverse lie, leakage of liquor.

Q. Is it possible that pregnancy at 34 weeks and the height of fundus is 38 weeks?

Ans. Yes, possible. Causes are wrong date of LMP, hydatidiform mole, multiple pregnancies, hydramnios, concealed accidental hemorrhage, big baby, pelvic tumor.

Q. How do you determine the fetal presentation and position?

Ans. By abdominal grips (clinically), USG.

Q. Show me the different abdominal grips?

Ans. See the diagrams in obstetrical history taking.

Q. Which abdominal grip is more informative?

Ans. First pelvic grip (but in Leopold's maneuver 2nd pelvic grip). Informations are presentation, attitude (flexed or deflexed) and engagement of head.

Q. What are the evidences of engagement of head?

Ans.
a. Engagement means the descent of BPD through the pelvic brim.
b. Head is not mobile, both poles sinciput and occiput can not be felt per abdomen, however sincipital pole can be felt with difficulty when the head is engaged.
c. Examining hand in the first pelvic grip remains parallel.
d. 2/5th or less will be felt abdominally.
e. Vaginal examination can palpate the leading part of head at the level of ischial spine.

Q. What is the evidence of nonengagement?

Ans.
a. Both poles of head are palpable per abdomen or 3/5th head palpable above maternal symphysis.
b. Head can be moved from side to side.
c. Examining hand can be converged below the presenting part.
d. Vaginal examination shows the leading part of the presenting part is above ischial spine.

Q. What do you mean by term, preterm and post-term birth?

Ans. Preterm—birth before 37 completed weeks; Term—37–42 weeks (normal pregnancy is 40 weeks/280 days); Post-term—42 weeks or more.

Q. How do you know the attitude of head?

Ans.
a. Occiput lying below the sinciput—fully flexed vertex presentation
b. Ociput and sinciput lying at the same level-deflexed head (Brow)
c. Sinciput lying below the occiput—completely deflexed head (face).

> **Note**
> Attitude—In cephalic presentation, it refers to degree of flexion of the fetal head (Figures 10.7A to C).

Q. How do you advise the patient to come for antenatal visit?

Ans. *In normal pregnancy*
- < 12 weeks—once
- 12–28 weeks—every 4 weeks
- > 28–36 weeks—every fortnight
- 36 weeks or more—every week.

Q. What is a booked case?

Ans. Women who has attended antenatal check-up at least on 4 occasions in pregnancy (by WHO). (Minimum 4 visits):
a. First visit within 12 weeks or as soon as the pregnancy is known
b. Second visit between 14–26 weeks
c. Third visit between 28–34 weeks
d. Fourth visit: Between 36 weeks to term.

Q. What are the benefits of prenatal care/booked case?

Ans.
a. Detection and management of high risk cases during pregnancy
b. Regular supervision of pregnant mother
c. Education of the mother regarding diet and nutrition, intake of tetanus toxoid, and avoidance of smoking, alcohol or other illicit drugs

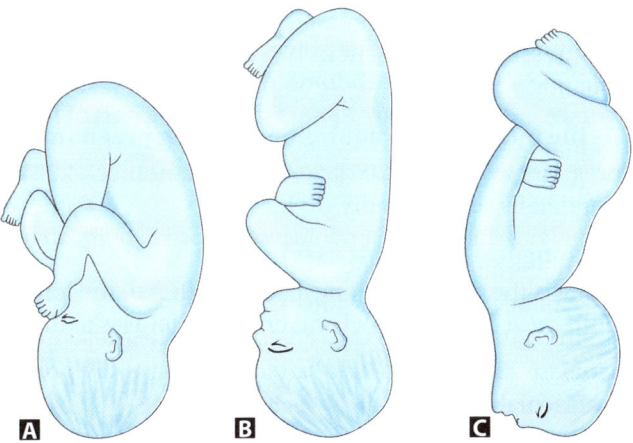

Figures 10.7A to C: Attitude of fetal head. (A) Fully flexed vertex; (B) Deflexed head; (C) Completely deflexed or extended head

d. To impart physiological and psychological support for labor and breastfeeding
e. Can reduce maternal and perinatal morbidity and mortality.

Q. What are the limitations of prenatal care?

Ans. Inspite of good prenatal care, it cannot prevent PROM, cord prolapse, unexplained IUFD, APH (due to placenta previa) and PPH.

Q. A patient came to the antenatal clinic on 15th September and her LMP is on 10th March. How do you calculate the duration of pregnancy?

Ans.
March 31–10	22 days
April	30 days
May	31 days
June	30 days
July	31 days
August	31 days
September	15 days

190 days/7 = 27 weeks 1 day

Q. What are the sounds that can be heard in pregnant abdomen?

Ans. Fetal heart sound, uterine soufflé, funic souffle, and intestinal sound. Fetal heart sound is the surest sign of pregnancy.

Q. What is uterine soufflé?

Ans. It is a soft-blowing murmur produced by the passage of blood through the enlarged uterine vessel and is synchronous with maternal pulse.

Q. Besides pregnancy can it be present in other condition?

Ans. Yes, it may be present in fibroid uterus.

Q. What is funic soufflé?

Ans. It is a soft-blowing murmur synchronous with FHS. It is due to rush of blood through the compressed umbilical arteries caused by knots twists or pressure. It is present in 15% cases of labor and diagnostic sign of pregnancy.

Q. What is the total calorie requirement during pregnancy?

Ans. Non-pregnant women—2200 kcal, Pregnant mother—2200 + 300 = 2500 kcal (For details see Appendix –01).

Q. Is the lie longitudinal in this case?

Ans. Yes. The lie is the relation of long axis of mother to the long axis of fetus. Here both the axis are parallel and breech of fetus is at the upper end of uterus.

Q. What is the presentation and presenting part?

Ans. The part of the fetus which occupies the lower pole of the uterus is called the presentation of fetus. The part of the presentation which overlies the internal os and is felt by the examining finger through the cervical opening is called the presenting part. So, cephalic is the presentation but vertex (most common) is the presenting part, similarly brow and face is the presenting part of head presentation.

Q. Which vaccines are contraindicated in pregnancy? Which are indicated?

Ans. All live vaccines are contraindicated—BOYS MMR (B—BCG, O—oral polio, oral typhoid, Y—yellow fever, S—smallpox, MMR—mumps, measles and rubella). Indicated vaccines are: (a) Injection Toxoid—1st dose—At first contact with woman of child bearing age or as early as possible in pregnancy (at 1st ANC visit), second dose is atleast 4 weeks later after first dose. (b) Antirabies vaccine, if necessary (c) Hepatitis-B vaccine, if necessary.

Q. Why the patient is admitted in this case?

Ans. The patient is admitted as she is at term pregnancy with c/o lower abdominal pain and I will have to differentiate whether it is true labor pain or false labor pain. If pain persists re-examine after 6 hours, if there is cervical effacement and dilatation–diagnose labor. If no cervical change–diagnose false or pre-labor. If pain subside—observe for 24 hours.

Q. What is Braxton-Hicks Contraction?

Ans. In early pregnancy, the uterus undergoes irregular contraction that are painless. In second trimester, these contractions may be palpable by bimanual examination. It is nonrhythmic, intensity varies between 5-25 mm of Hg. In the last week of pregnancy, these occur at 10–25 minutes and attain some degree of rhythmicity. In 75% of cases, women with 12 or more of these contractions per hour were diagnosed with active labor within 24 hours. It is absent in secondary abdominal pregnancy.

Q. How will you differentiate true or false labor pain?

Ans. *Contraction of true labor pain:*
    a. Occur at regular interval
    b. Interval gradually shorten
    c. Intensity gradually increases
    d. Discomfort in back and abdomen
    e. Progressive dilatation and effacement of cervix
    f. Show.

Contraction of false labor pain:
    a. Occurs at irregular interval
    b. Intervals remain long
    c. Intensity remain unchanged
    d. Discomfort chiefly in lower abdomen
    e. Cervix does not dilate
    f. No show
    g. Usually relieved by sedation or enema.

Q. If the patient is in true labor pain, what will you do?
Ans. I will asses the uterine contraction, progress of labor, maternal and fetal condition, if all are good, I will go for normal delivery, if there is no cephalopelvic disproportion (CPD).

Q. If the patient is in false labor what will be the line of management?
Ans. As the mother is at term pregnancy, I will wait for 41 weeks and then assess Bishop score and pelvis. If the Bishop score is poor, induce by intracervical PGE_2 gel or by oxytocin. DFMC, recording of BP, external fetal monitoring is mandatory, when the pregnant mother remains in the hospital.

Q. How do you diagnose labor?
Ans. a. Painful and intermittent uterine contraction with increasing frequency and intensity.
b. Show—blood-stained mucus per vagina from cervical os before onset of labor and digital examination.
c. Dilation and effacement of cervix.
d. Does not depend upon leaking of fetal membrane or bulging of bag of fore water in intact membrane.

Q. What is show?
Ans. Profuse cervical secretion with mild oozing of blood from cervical os due to rupture of capillary vessels from decidual surface caused by separation of membrane due to stretching of lower uterine segment (LUS).

Q. How do you confirm onset of labor?
Ans. a. Regular painful uterine contraction of >20 seconds duration and atleast once in every 10 minutes.
b. Progressive cervical dilatation and effacement
c. Cervical dilatation ≥4 cm.

Q. How do you note progress of labor? or How do you assess the progress of labor ?
Ans. (Start from abdominal finding)
P/A
a. Increasing strength, frequency, and duration of uterine contraction
b. Head palpability per abdomen in relation to symphysis pubis, i.e. descent of the head (by rule of fifth, e.g. 5/5; 4/5; 3/5; 2/5; 1/5; 0/5)
c. Lowering of the fetal heart sound
P/V—Dilatation of cervix and taken up, level of presenting part (station) [Dilatation of the cervical os is measured in cm; 1 finger = 1.25 cm and effacement (shortening of cervical length) in%].
Vaginal examination protocol in assessment of progress of labor:
a. Every 4 hours in active phase (cervix >4 cm dilated)
b. Every 2 hours when cervix is >7 cm dilated
c. Every 2 hours when labor is augmented by oxytocin
d. Every 1 hour when cervix is >1 cm dilated
e. In dysfunctional labor every 2 hour

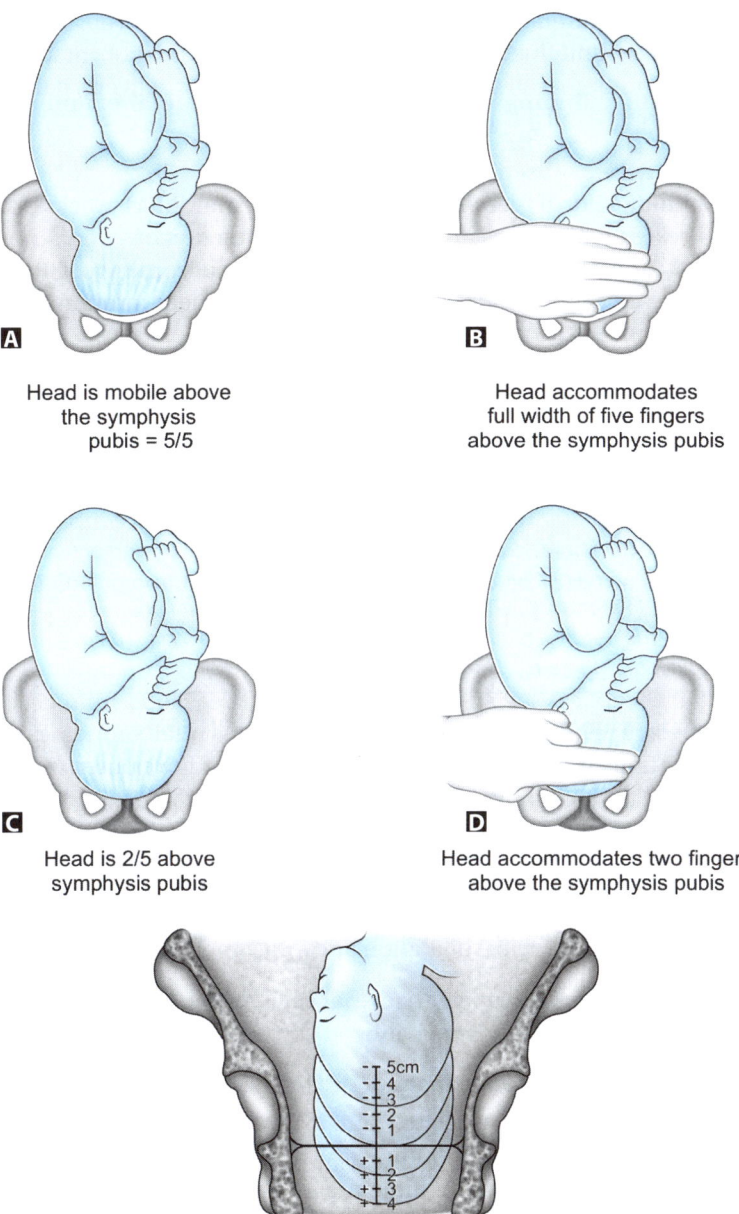

Figures 10.8 A to E: (A to D) Measurement of head palpability in fifth by abdominal palpation; (E) Station of head in cm by P/V examination

Per abdomen (Figures 10.8A to E)
    a. *Head palpability measurement*: It is measured in terms of 'fifths' of the fetal head palpable above the maternal pubic symphysis, only in OA position.

b. The measurement relies on term fetal diameter (basovertical) of 9–10 cm and finger's width of 2 cm.

Q. What other findings are noted during per vaginal examination in labor?

Ans.
a. Presence or absence of bag of fore-water
b. Liquor color, if membrane is ruptured or after ARM
c. Presentation and molding in cephalic presentation
d. Position of the presenting part—determined by palpating the suture lines and fontanel in relation to pelvis (in head presentation) and pressure of the presenting part on the cervix.
e. Caput formation and molding according to presentation and position.

> **Note**
>
> *Level of presenting part—Assessed in relation to ischial spine (on vaginal examination 'zero' is the level of ischial spine) that is in the mid pelvis and estimation in 'cm' is done above or below 'zero'. The leading part of presentation is 'Zero' (0) means just engaged. If above the ischial spines, the distance are started in minus figure (−1 cm, −2 cm, −3 cm, −4 cm and floating); if below the spine, the distance are in plus figure (+1 cm, +2 cm, +3 cm, +4 cm, and on the perineum) (Figure 10.8E).*

Q. What is premature rupture of membrane (PROM) and PPROM?

Ans. PROM is the rupture of fetal membrane before the onset of labor. In most cases, it occurs near term, but when membrane ruptures before 37 completed weeks of gestational age, it is known as preterm PROM (PPROM). High-risk factors:
1. Polyhydramnios
2. Previous history of PPROM
3. Bicornuate uterus
4. Infection—chladymia or bacterial vaginosis
5. Bleeding P/V in late pregnancy.

Q. What are the different causes of PROM?

Ans. Different factors are associated with PROM:
a. Infection causing amnionitis, cervicitis
b. Polyhydramnios and multiple pregnancy
c. Cervical conization or circlage
d. Fetal anomalies
e. Low socioecnomic status
f. Maternal trauma
g. Smoking.

Q. How do you diagnose it?

Ans. By history, physical examination and selective laboratory tests:
History
a. Reporting of gush of fluid with continued leakage
b. Pain abdomen, bleeding per vagina, recent intercourse, fever

Physical examination and laboratory test:
a. P/S—Examination is done in aseptic precaution, gush of fluid on coughing and cord prolapse should be excluded and high vaginal swab should be taken for C/S
b. A sterile pad placed over vulva—soaked with amniotic fluid
c. If facilities are available
   - *Nitrazine test*: Touch of nitrazine paper in amniotic fluid becomes yellow to blue as amniotic fluid is alkaline (pH = 7.0–7.5), whereas vaginal fluid is acidic (pH 4.5–5.5). It is associated with high false-positive rates related to cervicitis, vaginitis (bacterial vaginosis), and contamination with blood, urine, semen, or antiseptic agents.
   - *Fern test*: Amniotic fluid when dried crystallized and leaves a fern-leaf pattern. Spread some fluid pooled in the vagina on a glass slide and let it dry. Examine under microscope for ferning (crystalline pattern is due to the presence of sodium chloride and protein in amniotic fluid).
   - Examination for lanugo hair and fetal epithelial cells stained with Nile blue.
   - AmniSure: It is a rapid test for the presence of placental alpha microglobulin-1(PAMG-1) protein found in high levels in amniotic fluid and extremely low level in cervical and vaginal fluid in absence of ruptured membrane.

Procedure: A sample of cervicovaginal fluid is collected using a sterile swab (no speculum) and eluted into a vial containing solvent for 1 minute. The test strip is then placed in a solvent, allowing the sample in the vial to move through the membrane by capillary action. The pad region of the test strip has 2 zones, 1 containing anti- PAMG-1 antibodies (test zone) and the other containing anti-IgG (positive control zone). If PAMG-1 is present in the sample, it will interact with the capture antibody forming antigen-conjugate complexes that can be seen as a visible line. In the absence of antigen, no visible line will form.

The positive test confirms the presence of of ruptured membrane.

> **Note**
> P/V examination should never be done unless indicated as it may cause intrauterine infection and preterm labor due to prostaglandin release.

Q. How will you manage the PROM?

Ans. Admit the pregnant women with PROM in hospital.
Evaluate diagnosis, fetal maturity, liquor amount, cervical status, and infection. On admission, P/V examination should be done only.
   i. In labor pain
   ii. Abnormal lie
   iii. Meconium-stained liquor

        iv. Fetal distress
        v. Cord prolapse
        vi. Before induction of labor
    – Steroid—Betamethasone 12 mg IM every 24 hours (two doses) (Repeatation of the dose after 48 hours is ineffective)
    – Antibiotic—Erythromycin is preferable for 10 days as amoxicillin and clavulanic acid may cause neonatal necrotizing enterocolitis for abnormal microbial colonization in gastrointestinal tract. It should be avoided in women at risk for preterm delivery.
    – FHR monitoring twice daily clinically or by CTG in term baby
    – Four hourly temperature chart
    – Repeated P/V examination should not be done
    – USG scan for fetal maturity and liquor volume
    – Examination of phosphatidyl glycerol from liquor for detection of lung maturity.

    If GA is <34 weeks conservative management by the protocol as mentioned above but when signs of chrioamnionitis (characterized by fever, tender uterus, foul-smelling vaginal discharge) appear, terminate the pregnancy irrespective of gestational age of fetus.

    GA 34–37 weeks: If membrane is ruptured for >10 hours, give prophylactic antibiotic (Injection ampicillin—1 g × 6 hourly, IV metrogyl infusion (400 mg) × 8 hourly, Injection gentamicin (80 mg) IM × 12 hourly), then assess cervix. If there is beginning of labor, delivery is to be done vaginally under antibiotic coverage and if no signs of infection is noted following delivery, discontinue antibiotic. If cervix is unfavorable, liquor volume is low and failed induction is noted or fetal distress appears—LSCS after giving first dose of antibiotic.

Q. What is the role of tocolytic therapy in preterm PROM?
Ans. Limited data are available. It is not unreasonable to administer a short course of tocolysis after preterm PROM to allow initiation of antibiotics, corticosteroid administration and maternal transport, although this is controversial, but long-term tocolytic therapy is not beneficial.

Q. Do you use corticosteroid in presence of infection?
Ans. No.

Q. Effect of PROM on mother.
Ans. a. Infection—Intrauterine or puerperal sepsis
   b. Placental abruption
   c. Preterm delivery.

Q. Effect of PROM on fetus?
Ans. a. Preterm baby and their complications (RDS, intracerebral hemorrhage (ICH) which can be prevented by antenatal steroids)
   b. Neonatal pneumonitis or sepsis
   c. Pulmonary hypoplasia and fetal compression syndrome
   d. Prolapse or compression of umbilical cord
   e. Cerebral palsy.

Magnesium sulfate may be used to reduce the risk of cerebral palsy. As an antioxidant, it reduces the proinflammatory cytokines and increases cerebral flow and prevents large fluctuations in blood pressure. It can be given immediately before delivery.

> **Note**
>
> *Amnioinfusion has no definite role in PROM. If labor does not start within 12–24 hours after prelabor rupture of membrane in term pregnancy, induction of labor should be started by syntocinon drip where cervix is favorable, otherwise PGs (oral-misoprostol/PGE2 intracervical gel for unfavorable cervix) or cesarean section according to the condition.*
> - *If PROM occurs before 25 weeks, induction vs expectancy should depend upon GA of mother's desire. Use of steroids is controversial as no beneficial effect is achieved in this gestational age, rather invites infection. Antibiotic use for 7 days may prolong pregnancy but use of tocolytics are controversial.*
> - *If PROM occurs at 33 weeks, liquor is very scanty, fetal weight ≥1800 mg on USG, give steroid if no chorioamnionitis and deliver by LSCS.*

CASE DISCUSSION ON RH-NEGATIVE MOTHER

Summary: Mrs DF aged 22 years, G2 P0 + 1 at 40 weeks of gestation admitted in the hospital in the last night with the complain of lower abdominal pain for last 2 days.

Her LMP was on dd/mm/yy and EDD is on dd/mm/yy. The previous pregnancy was ended by spontaneous abortion at 10 weeks of pregnancy followed by evacuation and check curettage. Her blood group and Rh is B negative and husband's blood group is B positive which were noted from previous obstetrical record. She received 100 mcg of anti-D globulin IM within 24 hours following evacuation. In the present pregnancy indirect coomb test (ICT) was done on two occasions at 28 and 36 weeks of pregnancy during antenatal check-up and the test is found negative and is associated with mild pallor, BP-normal (120/80 mm of Hg). On obstetrical examination, GA is 40 weeks, lie longitudinal, presentation of fetus is head with no CPD, FHS positive, regular, with adequate amount of liquor.

Per vaginal examination (not allowed in undergraduates) cervical os-2 cm; cervix-fully taken up, membrane +, PP-cephalic, LOA, pelvis adequate.

Provisional diagnosis: Unimmunized Rh-negative pregnancy at term.

Case discussion:
Natural history of Rh-Isoimmunized mother:
- The first baby is generally not affected unless she is already been isoimmunized by previous Rh-positive transfusion of blood and blood products, but according to grandmother's theory (see later in the case discussion) the first fetus may be affected in utero.
- The second baby is born anemic requiring treatment of anemia
- A severely anemic baby may require exchange transfusion
- History of hydrops fetalis, intrauterine fetal death (IUFD).

Q. What is the incidence of Rh -ve mother in India?
Ans. 5 to 10% (South India—5%, North India—10%).

Q. If husband is homozygous Rh +ve (DD) and wife is Rh -ve (dd) what will be the possibility of Rh typing of baby?
Ans. All babies are Rh-positive (Dd).

Q. If father is heterozygous Rh +ve (Dd) and mother is Rh -ve (dd), what will be the possibility of fetal Rh typing?
Ans. 50% chances of Rh-positive (Dd) and 50% chances of Rh-negative baby (dd).

Q. What is isoimmunization?
Ans. Isoimmunization is the production of antibody in an individual in response to the antigen derived from another individual of same species provided the first one lacks antigen.

Q. Why incidence of Rh-incompatibility is low practically?
Ans. Rh-incompatibility occurs in 10% of cases practically, cause is not definitely known, but possible explanations are:
  a. Inborn inability to respond to the Rh-antigen stimulus
  b. Associated ABO group incompatibility (Presence of anti-A and anti-B antibodies in O negative mother destroys fetal Rh antigen and non-immunogenic)
  c. Variation in strength of Rh-antigen stimulus
  d. Volume of blood entering in maternal circulation (0.1 mL is the critical sensitizing volume).
  e. Insufficient transplacental passage of fetal antigen and maternal antibody.

> **Note**
> The risk of immunization is 3% with 0.1 mL of fetal RBCs; 25% with 0.25–1 mL of fetal RBCs and increases to 65% with >5 mL of RBCs.

Q. Why generally the first baby is escaped from isoimmunization?
Ans. The initiation of antibody formation starts in the first Rh-incompatible pregnancy. Although small number of fetal red blood cells (RBCs) go into maternal circulation during pregnancy, the important immunizing dose is usually received by the mother at the time of delivery when placenta is compressed or separated. For this reason, Rh-sensitization is uncommon in first pregnancy.

Q. What are the different types of antibody formation?
Ans. 1. Saline agglutinin [Immunoglobulin M (IgM)]: Generally, appears 7 days after stimulation and agglutinate Rh+ cells suspended in saline. It is a large molecule and does not cross the placenta.
  2. Albumin antibody [Immunoglobulin G (IgG)]: It is a small molecule appears 21 days after stimulation and cross the placenta attacks Rh-positive red cells of baby. It agglutinates Rh-positive red cells in plasma, serum and albumin.

Obstetric Cases

> **Note**
> The antibody has no effect on Rh –ve fetus.

Q. What is Kleihauer Betke (K-B) test?

Ans. The presence of fetal cells in maternal circulation can be demonstrated by this test. Fetal Hb is more resistant than adult Hb in acid elution. When a blood film is stained following elution, the dark red fetal cells will stand out against adult 'GHOST' cells (colorless). The fetal RBCs counted in 50 low power field (LPF). So, 80 fetal RBCs in 50 LPF = 4 mL of fetal blood and requires 100 mcg of anti-D globulin. A dose of 300 µg can neutralize FMH of 30 mL and 15 mL of fetal RBCs FMH. If the volume of fetomaternal hemorrhage (FMH) is >30 mL of fetal whole blood an additional 10 µg of anti Rh-D immunoglobulin should be administered in each additional mL of fetal blood by IM route over 24 hours.

Q. What are the complications of Rh isoimmunization?

Ans. On mother:
a. Pre-eclampsia
b. Hydramnios
c. Large placenta—due to proliferation of villi by anoxia

On fetus: In most severe cases (when deficit of hemoglobin exceeds below 6 mg/dL) hydrops fetalis develops due to extensive infiltration of the liver by erythropoietic tissue leading to portal hypertension by parenchymal compression of the portal vessels and hypoprotinemia caused by impaired protein synthesis.

Hydrops fetalis: Severity of anemia causes cardiac failure with widespread edema, ascites and pleural effusion diagnosed by USG.

However, timely detection and treatment may prevent fetal death in 90% of cases.

In less severe degree:
- Icterus gravis neonatorum
- Congenital anemia of newborn-characterized by:
  a. Hemolytic anemia (Hb < 10 g/dL).
  b. Liver enlarged—by proliferation of erythroblastic tissues.
  c. Spleen enlarged by destroying RBCs and producing new cells.

Q. What is kernicterus?

Ans. When bilirubin level is raised by ≥20 mg/100 mL (>340 micro mole/liter, fetal bilirubin crosses the blood-brain barrier and causes necrosis of neurons especially in basal ganglia. The baby is lethargic, refuses to suck, convulsion, rolling eyes and head retraction may be seen.

Q. How do you prevent isoimmunization?

Ans. 1. *By active immunization*: Rh +ve fetal RBCs will produce antibody in maternal circulation. The aim is to hide the D-antigen, so that maternal immune system cannot recognize them as 'foreign' and antibodies will not be formed. This is done by giving the mother anti-D, which attaches itself to D antigen of fetal RBCs making them unrecognizable by immune system and therefore incapable of stimulating antibody formation.

Dose: 300 μg (3 × 500 = 1500 IU) following delivery; 50–100 μg before 12 weeks of GA and 300 μg thereafter in nonimmunized Rh-negative mother.

2. *To prevent fetomaternal hemorrhage (FMH)*:
   a. During cesarean section (CS) minimal spill of blood in the peritoneal cavity and routine manual removal of placenta is prohibited.
   b. Prophylactic ergometrine administration should be withheld.
   c. Prior sonography to localize placenta before amniocentesis.
   d. Avoid external cephalic version (ECV) under general anesthesia.
   e. Manual removal of placenta should be done gently if necessary.

Q. Can you prescribe anti-D globulin during pregnancy?

Ans. It can be used in a non-sensitized mother during pregnancy routinely. 100 μg anti-D globulin at 28 weeks and again at 34 weeks of GA or a single dose of 300 μg at 28-weeks and again within 72 hours following delivery (300 μg) though the baby is weakly Rh +ve. Some however reserve this for invasive procedure such as amniocentesis, ECV, or in other episodes of placental separation such as threatened miscarriage, APH. The dose being estimated according to the GA and volume of blood, but 300 mcg of anti-D globulin is sufficient (this covers sensitization by 15 mL of fetal RBCs or 30 mL of fetal whole blood) but 10 mcg additional anti-D should be given for every additional 0.5 mL fetal RBCs in maternal circulation.

> **Note**
> a. FMH in first trimester of pregnancy is 5%, 16% in second trimester, 29% in 3rd trimester and 50% after delivery.
> b. A woman with weak D (also known as Du-positive) need not receive anti-D.
> c. 50–100 μg anti-D injection should be given after all sensitizing events in first trimester (miscarriage, TOP, ectopic pregnancy).

Q. How do you calculate the dose of anti-D globulin? or Tests of fetomaternal hemorrhage?

Ans. a. By Kleihauer-Betke test
b. Flow cytometry and rosetting technique are alternative technique for quantifying the size of fetomaternal hemorrhage (FMH). Determination of volume of FMH and dose of Anti-D globulin:

The amount of fetomaternal hemorrhage can be calculated from the results of Kleihauer Betke acid elution test using the formula:

$$\text{Fetal blood volume (volume of FMH)} = \frac{\text{Maternal blood volume} \times \text{maternal hematocrit} \times \text{\% of fetal cells in KB}}{\text{Newborn hematocrit}}$$

Number of vials of Anti-D required = Volume of FMH/30

Alternative method is discussed in the question of 'what is K-B test' previously 80 fetal RBCs in 50 LPF = 4 mL of fetal blood and requires 100 mcg (25 µg/mL FMH) of Anti-D globulin.

c. *Free fetal DNA testing in maternal serum*: PCR which picks up fetal DNA from one cell in maternal serum by non-invasive way. It can detect fetal genotype.

> **Note**
> If 300 mcg anti-D globulin is given without a test for quantitative fetomaternal hemorrhage, a few women each year in India will receive less protection than they should when FMH exceeds 30 mL of whole blood (1% of pregnancy).

Q. How do you manage the pregnant mother without antibodies?

Ans.
a. At the first visit of Rh-negative mother, do the blood group and Rh-typing of husband.
b. Screening tests for detection of immune antibodies (indirect Coombs' test).
c. Repeat antibody check-up at 28 and 36 weeks of GA.
d. Administer anti-D globulin routinely during pregnancy
e. *Delivery*: Tendency to over run the EDD is avoided.
   Spontaneous labor is awaited, and if necessary, artificial rupture of membrane (ARM) along with syntocinon for induction or injection syntocinon for augmentation of labor is the method of choice. Active management of 3rd stage of labor is not recommended as uterotonic drugs such as oxytocin, methyl-lergometrine and prostaglandins increase the chance of fetomaternal hemorrhage (FMH).
f. After delivery-mother's blood is tested for antibody check-up and count of Kleihauer. Baby-cord blood is examined for ABO, Rh; Hb%; Coombs' test and bilirubin.
g. Give anti-D globulin to mother, if blood is negative for antibodies and baby is Rh-positive with direct Coomb's test negative within 72 hours after delivery.

Q. How do you manage Rh-negative mother with anti-D antibody?

Ans.
a. First visit—antibody is identified by indirect Coomb's test (ICT) and measured by direct quantization of antibody level (Safe level <4IU/mL).
b. Antibody test repeated monthly or until management decided upon by other investigation, e.g. amniocentesis.
c. Genotype of husband—if father is heterozygous Rh-positive, the possibility of unaffected child exists.
d. Quantitative estimation of albumin antibody—1/16 as a critical one.
e. Amniocentesis.

For amniocentesis:

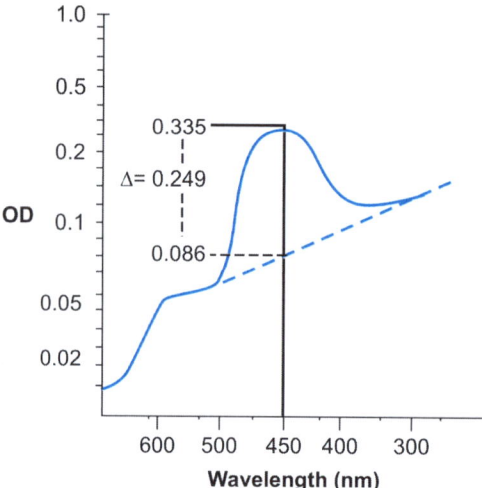

Figure 10.9: Graph of spectrophotometric analysis of amniotic fluid taken from Rh-sensitized pregnancy. The solid line is the plot of the optical density (OD) of the bilirubin-containing fluid across the wavelength on the X-axis. The interrupted line represents the curve expected from amniotic fluid without increased bilirubin. The difference of OD of solid line and interrupted line at 450 nm is δ OD 450 value

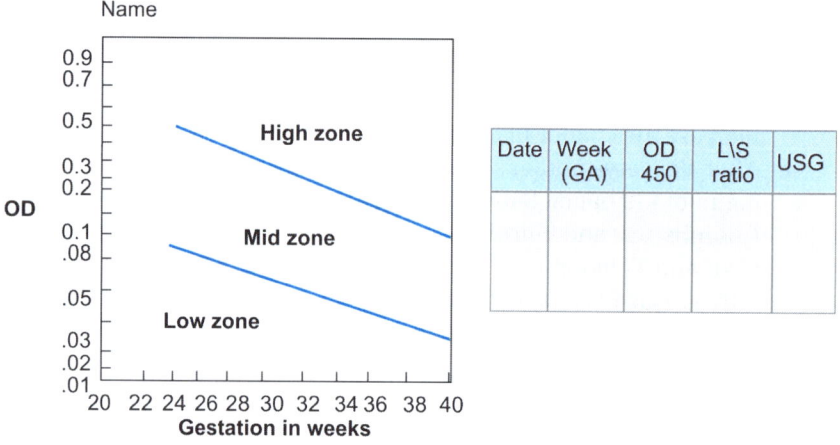

Figure 10.10: Liley graph with linear extrapolation of boundaries to 24 weeks of gestation

Selection Time:
1. No history of previously affected baby—it is to be done at 28 to 30 weeks and second test to be repeated after 3 to 4 weeks
2. Positive history of previously affected baby—it should be done 10 weeks prior to the stillbirth, however, it is useless to perform before 20 weeks.

The bilirubin level in liquor measured by spectrophotometry is a useful prognostic indicator as it reflects the excretions of bilirubin by the baby and the degree of hemolysis. The optical density (OD) of liquor containing bilirubin pigment is observed at 250–750 mµ wavelength. The OD difference at 450 mµ wavelength give the prediction of severity of hemolysis. In the presence of bilirubin, there is a deviation bulge peaking at 450 mµ wavelength (Figure 10.9). The bigger the deviation bulge, the more is the affection of baby. For any given period of gestation the height of spectrophotometric deviation bulge at 450 mµ wavelength falls in one of the three zones when plotted in Liley's chart (Figure 10.10).

If falls in Zone-I (low zone), the baby is unlikely affected and pregnancy continued to term.

If falls in Zone-II (mid zone)—fetus have mild to moderate risk the baby may require premature termination at less than 34 weeks but unreliable for prognosis.

Mid zone is divided into:
a. Lower zone II where expected Hb lies between 11.0–13.9 g/dL
b. Higher zone II when Hb ranges from 8–10.9 g/dL.

Amniocentesis and USG should be repeated within 2–3 weeks. If the value is increased, cordocentesis should be done. If fetal hematocrit is <30%, IUT should be done to increase fetal hematocrit to 45%.

If falls in Zone-III (high zone), if baby is severely affected (Hb<8 g/dL), death is imminent (with in 7–10 days), if pregnancy is greater than 34 weeks termination, or if less than 34 weeks intrauterine transfusion. If intrauterine transfusion is given the aim is to continue treatment to achieve a maturity of 36 weeks before delivery and to increase fetal hamatocrit to about 40%.

> **Note**
>
> *Modified Liley's graph: Liley's graph is applicable only for gestational age of 27 weeks or more. Queenan et al. developed modified Liley's chart (Queenan chart) which can be used for earlier gesatation at 14 weeks. If severe fetal anemia or abnormal amniotic fluid is detected, perform fetal blood sampling and intravascular transfusion in utero is the best method to treat anemia.*

f. *Middle cerebral artery peak systolic velocity (MCA—PSV)*: discussed later

g. *USG*: To detect fetal ascites, edema, indicating severely affected fetus at a very early age in the pregnancy (e.g. less than 20 weeks indicates cordocentesis).

h. *Cordocentesis*: Blood may be obtained from the fetus in patients with history of severely affected rhesus disease and in those in whom USG has demonstrated ascites. A hematological level is at once available and treatment by direct intravascular transfusion can be given, if indicated by the result. If hematocrit < 30% intrauterine transfusion to increase the hematocrit level to 40–45% when conservative management is recommended in GA less than 34 weeks to increase the GA for a couple of weeks. O-Rh-negative blood is needed to increase the hematocrit and the need to be repeated until the fetus is mature to deliver.

i. *Plasmapheresis*: The technique relies on removal of as much antibody as possible from the maternal circulation; the procedure is carried out three to four times in a week removing 1–3 liters of plasma on each occasion. Plasmapheresis can reduce the serum antibody level by up to 75%. At present this strategy has little scope as intrauterine transfusion can be commenced at 18 weeks of gestation, the earliest stage that fetal hemolysis from alloimmunization occurs.

j. *Delivery of fetus*:
- Mildly affected fetus continued to term provided fetal well-being is good.
- Labor induction at 36–37 weeks of GA
- Unfavorable cervix prostaglandine E_2 (PGE_2) gel intracervically
- Continuous intrapartum monitoring and operative delivery when indicated
- *Severely affected baby*: Delivery at 32–34 weeks, pulmonary maturity is demonstrated by amniocentesis L: S greater than 2 or phosphatidylglycerol indicates lung maturity, if lower use of corticosteroid is necessary
- No prophylactic ergometrine
- Quick clamping of the cord for prevention of maternal anti-D transfer to baby
- Manual removal of placenta (MRP), if necessary is to be done gently
- Cord sample is examined for Coomb's test; blood group and Rh, Hb% and serum bilirubin.

> **Note**
> Oxytotic drugs increase the chance of FMH, but better to use for prevention of PPH. FMH can be tackeled by additional prophylaxis of anti-D globulin than standard dose.

Q. What will be the line of management in mild fetal anemia?

Ans. Mild degree of fetal anemia (Hb level not below 12 g%) may not require any treatment and mild degree jaundice responds well to phototherapy as light increases oxidation of bilirubin and excretes through urine. More severely affected baby requires exchange transfusion.

Q. What is exchange transfusion?

Ans. Withdrawal of blood through umbilical vein and its replacement with healthy compatible blood after delivery of baby. It thus correct anemia, reduces high level of circulating bilirubin which would cause kernicterus and washes out free circulating antibodies.

Q. What are the indications of exchange transfusion?

Ans.
- Cord Hb level less than 12 g%
- Serum bilirubin level more than 8 mg%
- Cord bilirubin level 5 mg/dL or more
- Increase in new born bilirubin at the rate of > 1 mg/dL/hour even after phototherapy
- Previously affected baby (kernictarus or severe erythroblastosis)
- Term infants with bilirubin level ≥20 mg/dL

Q. What are the advantages of exchange transfusion?
Ans. Correction of anemia, reduction of high level of circulating bilirubin and washing out of free-circulating antibody.

Q. What are the criteria of ideal donor for exchange transfusion?
Ans. Blood group is O negative; and Hb concentration is 12 g% or more without any communicable diseases. If O negative blood is not available, then Rh-negative blood of either baby's group or mother's group may be given.

Q. How fetal anemia is predicted when fetus is in utero? How do you treat the condition?
Ans. Fetal anemia is predicted by noninvasive method of peak systolic velocity in middle cerebral artery (MCA) by USG doppler and by using a cut-off value of 1.5 times the median, all fetuses with moderate-to-severe anemia were correctly identified with a sensitivity of 100%. Fetal anemia *in utero* is treated by intrauterine transfusion upto 35 weeks.

Q. What is the goal of intrauterine transfusion (IUT)? What are the types of intrauterine fetal transfusion?
Ans. IUT correct fetal anemia in an effort to improve fetal oxygenation and to reduce extramedullary hematopoietic demand which in turn should result in fall in portal venous pressure and improve hepatic function.

Types:
  i. Intrauterine intraperitoneal transfusion (IPT)
  ii. Intrauterine intravascular transfusion (IVT)
  iii. Combined

Q. Intrauterine intraperitoneal transfusion (IPT)?
Ans. Indication: It is done in selected cases (if GA <35 weeks) to continue pregnancy for a couple of weeks.
Contraindication: Hydrops fetalis because injected red cells are not absorbed from peritoneal cavity.
Type and amount of blood transfused: Blood group, O' Rh-negative.
Calculation of amount: The quantity is calculated as number of weeks of gestation over 20 multiplied by 10. For example, at 34 weeks the amount of blood transfused is 14 × 10 = 140 mL.

Packed RBCs are absorbed by lymphatic of the peritoneum and reduces fetal anemia.

Advantage: Technically easy, effective in absence of hydrops, indicated where IVT is difficult and large volume can be administered.
Disadvantage: Fetal hematocrit determination is not possible, slow RBC absorption—correction is delayed, unsuccessful in hydrops, intra-abdominal organ damage with possible occlusion of intra-abdominal portion of umbilical vein leading to IUFD.

Q. When cordocentesis or IVT is indicated?
Ans. If serial USG reveals hydrops and in severe fetal anemia (hematocrit <30%) cordocentesis or IVT should be arranged immediately. The goal is to reach a fetal hematocrit of 40–55%

The following formula can be used to calculate the volume of blood to be transfused

$$= \frac{\text{Fetoplacental volume} \times (\text{Hematocrit final} - \text{Hematocrit initial})}{\text{Hematocrit in transfused blood (usually 80\%)}}$$

Fetoplacental volume = fetal weight (g) × 0.14 e

If initial hematocrit is 20%, estimated fetal weight is 1000 g, then volume of blood transfusion will be 140 × (50−20)/80 = 52.5 mL. Usually 40–60 mL of blood is given in one sitting.

> **Note**
> After transfusion fetal hematocrit may be reduced to 1% (0.33 g of Hb) due to disease process, fetal anemia should be monitored by MCA-PSV for subsequent transfusion at 2–3 weeks interval, if required. When Hct is >30%, it is repeated every 1–2 weeks till 35 weeks.

Advantage: Fetal hematocrit determination is possible, complete and rapid correction of anemia, only method of treatment in hydrops fetalis.
Disadvantage: Difficult procedure, fetomaternal hemorrhage, sudden cardiac overload, cord hematoma, fetal loss.

> **Note**
> After the fetal transfusion, fetal ascites is relieved first followed by placentomegaly.

Q. What is the noninvasive method of prediction of fetal anemia in Rh-isoimmunized mother?

Ans. By Middle cerebral artery-peak systolic velocity (MCA-PSV) method in cm/sec (see ultrasound Doppler) in relation to GA (weeks) are plotted in one or several zones with established guidelines.

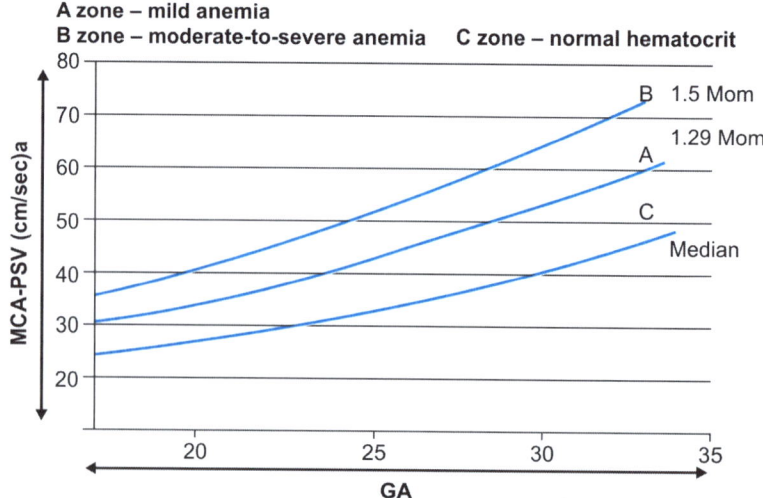

Figure 10.11: Graph showing relation of middle cerebral artery peak systolic velocity (MCA-PSV) and GA

Peak systolic velocity of MCA is used to predict moderate-to-severe fetal anemia from maternal red cell isoimmunization for the following reasons:
a. MCA responds rapidly to hypoxemia
b. As hematocrit rises, PSV in MCA decreases
c. PSV measurement of the MCA were compared to the severity of anemia and using a cut-off value of 1.5 times the median all fetuses with moderate and severe anemia were correctly identified with a sensitivity of 100% in the prediction of moderate-to-severe anemia and a false positive value is only 12% (see the Figure 10.11).

MCA-PSV is measured on weekly basis and plotted on the graph developed by Mary et al. until a level of 1.50 MoM is reached; a point at which fetal blood sampling with possible transfusion are indicated.

MCA-PSV measurement has no discriminative power after 35 weeks of gestation and after 2/or more fetal transfusions. After intrauterine transfusion (IUT), the characteristics of fetal blood are altered due to the infusion of adult red cells which are smaller and less rigid and these display an increased tendency for RBCs aggregation. Therefore, it becomes pertinent to use MCA-PSV after IUT. When the fetal maturity is reached (usually ≥ 35 weeks), fetus is delivered and baby is sent to NICU.

Rh-negative mother: Antenatal management by MCA-PSV method (start from 18–20 weeks up to 35 weeks) (Figure 10.12)

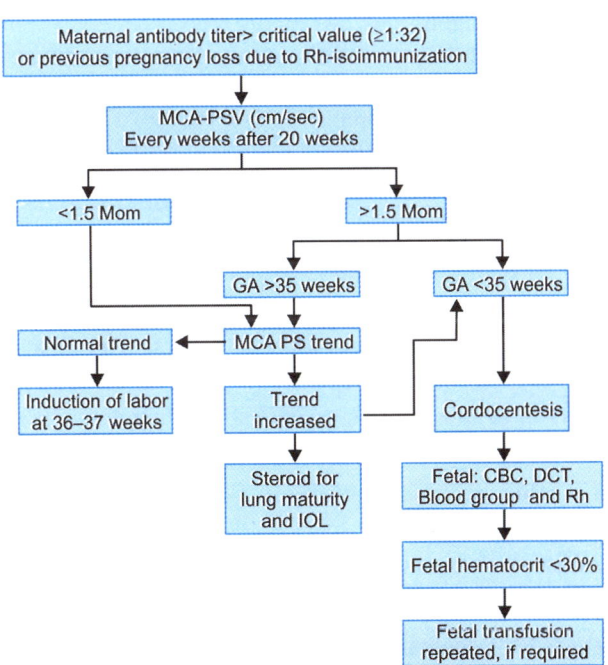

Figure 10.12: MCA—PSV method

Abbreviations: GA = Gestational age; Mom = Multiple of median; IOL = Induction of labor, DCT= Direct Coomb test, MoM-measurement of PSV/expected PSV

> **Note**
> After 35 weeks of gestational age, there is a high false positive rate of fetal anemia, a normal velocity should be followed with a repeated measurement. If the elevated level is noted, Δ_OD_{450} of liquor should be measured to determine whether delivery is indicated or not.

Q. What are the indications of fetal blood sampling (FBS)/transfusion?

Ans.
a. Severe fetal anemia detected by USG
b. Increased ICT titer >4 fold of previous titer
c. MCA-PSV ≥1.5 MoM
d. Previous IUD due to Rh-disease
e. Neonates received exchange transfusion in previous pregnancy.

Q. What are the different types of anti-D Ig preparations?

Ans. Monoclonal anti-D and Polyclonal anti-D immunoglobulins may produce a weak positive –1:1 to 1:4—indirect coombs titer in the mother. This is harmless and should not be considered with development of alloimmunization.

Monoclonal anti-D:
1. Limitless quantity as it can be prepared in laboratory
2. Capable of clearing of RBCs from circulation and apparently helps in suppressing immunization
3. It cannot cover all epitopes
4. Human monoclonal antibodies BRAD-3 and BRAD-5 can prevent weak Rh D-antigen.

Polyclonal anti-D:
1. The accepted safer anti-D prophylaxis throughout the world
2. Made from human plasma
3. Cover all epitopes.

> **Note**
> If there is any doubt regarding D-antigen status immunoglobulin should be given.

Q. If Rh-negative mother comes after 72 hours, after delivery with Rh-positive baby what do you do?

Ans. Use anti-D Ig to the mother, even if she comes late. A standard dose within 9–10 days following delivery may give reasonable protection.

Q. If such mother accepts ligation after delivery should you prescribe anti-D globulin?

Ans. Yes, because this woman remarries and may want further pregnancy.

Q. When do you not prescribe anti-D globulin in Rh-negative mother?

Ans.
a. If baby is Rh-negative
b. If mother's Indirect Coomb Test (ICT) is positive or fetus has positive Direct Coomb Test (DCT), then do not give anti-D globulin as the mother is already sensitized.

> **Note**
> a. Occasionally, a female previously typed as Rh-ve is unexpectedly found to be weak D+ve during pregnancy or after delivery. In this condition, the doctor should suspect that the patient's 'new weak D+ve status actually is due to large number of Rh +ve fetal cells in the maternal circulation. If by K-B test fetomaternal hemorrhage is found the mother should be treated with anti-D immunoglobulin.
> b. Anti -D Ig does not protect against the development of other antibodies which can cause hemolytic disease of newborn.
> c. Antibody due to passive anti-D immunoglobulin administration may cross the placenta and results in weakly positive direct Coomb test (DCT) in cord and neonatal blood and despite this, passive immunization does not cause significant fetal or neonatal hemolysis.
> d. Women who are weekly positive for D-antigen (DU) are not considered for risk of hemolysis and do not require anti-D immunoglobulin.

Q. What is grandmother effect?

Ans. In all pregnancies, small amount of maternal blood goes into fetal circulation which can be demonstrated by presence of maternal Rh D-positive DNA molecule in peripheral blood of Rh–negative newborn by PCR test. So isoimmunization may occur in Rh D-negative female fetus due to exposure of Rh D-positive red cells. When such individual reaches adulthood, she may produce anti-D antibodies before or early in her first pregnancy. So, the fetus in first pregnancy may be affected by maternal antibodies that are already present in maternal circulation provoked by grandmother's erythrocyte.

> **Note**
> See also non-immune hydrops and fetal anemia in Chapter 11 (flying questions).

PRIMIGRAVIDA WITH FLOATING HEAD

Summary

Pregnant mother, aged 23 years, G1 P 0 + 0, GA - 38 weeks, admitted with the, complain of (c/o) pain in lower abdomen for one day. On examination (O/E), pallor-mild, BP 130/80 mm Hg, on first pelvic grip the presenting part is head, which is floating, FHS plus regular and liquor is adequate in amount and no cephalopelvic disproportion was noted. P/V: os-closed, cervix is tubular, PP (presenting part) is head and high up, pelvis adequate.

Provisional diagnosis: Primigravida with floating head at term.

Q. What are the common causes of floating head at term?

Ans. a. Contracted pelvis or cephalopelvic disproportion
b. Occipitoposterior position (most common)
c. Malpresentation
d. Big baby
e. Central placenta previa
f. Hydrocephalus

g. Hydramnios
h. Non-formation of lower segment of uterus or tumor in the lower segment
i. Distended bladder and rectum.

In this present case, only CPD is considered.

Q. What is contracted pelvis?

Ans. *Anatomical definition:* When the essential diameters of different planes are shortened by 0.5 cm of the corresponding value.

Obstetrical definition: Shape and size of pelvis are sufficiently abnormal to cause difficulty in vaginal delivery.

Q. What is disproportion?

Ans. It is the state in which the baby is disproportionately big for the pelvis and is due to:
a. Contracted pelvis
b. Large baby, normal pelvis
c. Combination of both factors.

Q. How do you diagnose CPD?

Ans. The diagnosis is made from history, clinical examination and further investigations.

1. *History*: The important points are history of rickets, injury to pelvis and spine or lower limb, poliomyelitis, TB hip or spine.
2. *General examination*:
   a. Height below 5 ft
   b. Short, stocky, obese, hirsute woman
   c. Limping gait.
3. *Obstetrical examination*:
   i. Abdominal:
      a. Pendulous abdomen
      b. The head of the fetus is not engaged (non-engaged head within 2 weeks of term pregnancy. Deeply engaged head rules out the contracted pelvis).
      c. Malpresentation.
   ii. *USG:* To diagnose hydrocephalus, hydramnios, placenta previa, brow presentation, bony or soft tissue tumor.
   iii. *Clinical pelvimetry:* In cephalic presentation, it should be done beyond 37 weeks, but best time for clinical pelvimetry is first stage of labor due to softening of soft tissue of pelvis.

A. Clinical Assessment

Q. How will you assess pelvis?

Ans. Steps:
a. Bladder and rectum should be empty.
b. The examination should be done in dorsal position of pregnant mother.
c. Aseptic precaution with dressing and draping.

Obstetric Cases

d. The gloved left thumb and index finger will separate the vulvae to expose introitus (in right-handed person), and it should be cleaned with savlon swab by one stroke from above downwards and gloved index and middle finger of other hand will be introduced gently inside the vagina and patient is inspired to relax during examination. The internal fingers should be removed after completion of examination.
   1. *Sacrum*: The internal fingers will palpate the sacrum from below upwards to note its length, breadth curvature and also to note sacrococcygeal joint and any prominence on S2-S3 junction. Ala of the sacrum will also be palpated (Figure 10.13A).
   2. *Lateral wall*: Sacrosciatic notch (Figure 10.13B) when it is sufficiently wide admits two fingers, ischial spine—spines are usually smooth (everted and difficult to palpate), side walls of the pelvis (whether it is convergent, parallel or divergent), interischial diameter—Normally, both the spines cannot be touched at the same time, but if they are prominent this will diminish the space available in mid pelvis, iliopectineal line—beaking is suggestive of narrow fore pelvis (android) (Figures 10.13B to D).
   3. *Posterior surface of symphysis pubis*: Normally, smooth rounded curve, but beaking, is suggestive of abnormality.
   4. *Subpubic arch*: Normally, the pubic arch is rounded, which accommodate palmar aspect of two fingers, configuration of arch is more important than pubic angle.

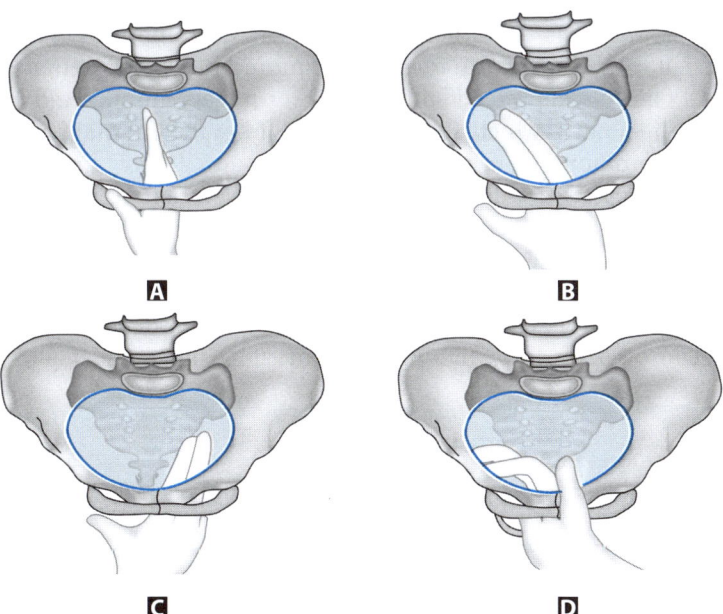

Figures 10.13A to D: (A) Sacrum; (B) Sacrosciatic notch; (C) Ischial spines; (D) The side walls

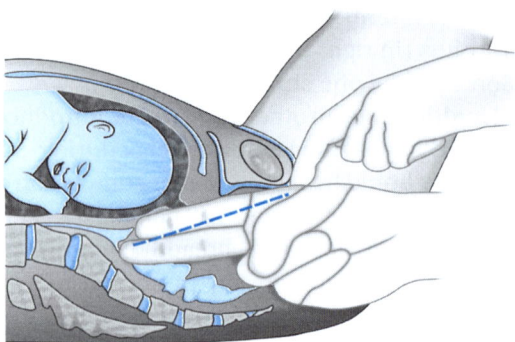

Figure 10.14: Measurement of diagonal conjugate

5. *Diagonal conjugate (DC)*: Normally, the sacral promontory cannot be reached, this indicates that the diameter of pelvic inlet is adequate. At the end of pelvic examination before removing the middle and index fingers, the middle finger impinges on the promontory. The forefinger of other hand marks to the point, where the hand is in contact with the lower border of symphysis pubis. After withdrawing both hands, measure the distance between the point and tip of middle finger with ruler or metallic scale. This is the DC and by subtracting 1.5–2 cm depending upon the height and inclination of symphysis pubis from the measurement of diagonal conjugate, the AP diameter of pelvic inlet (obstetrical conjugate) is obtained (Figure 10.14).

Q. How do you confirm the sacral promontory?

Ans. In normal pelvis, it is difficult to palpate sacral promontory or at best can be felt with difficulty. To reach sacral promontory, the forehand (elbow and wrist) is depressed sufficiently and fingers are directed upwards and the point at which the bone recedes from the internal fingers is the sacral promontory.

Pubic angle: The inferior pubic rami are well-defined in female, but angle roughly corresponds to the fully abducted thumb and index finger. In narrow angle, it corresponds to the abducted middle and index finger (Figure 10.15).

Transverse diameter of outlet (TDO): Four knuckles of clenched fist accommodates, in the medial border of ischial tuberosity (Figure 10.16).

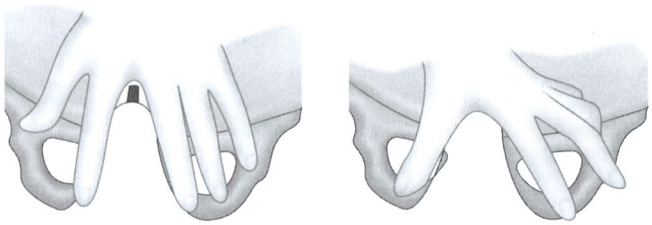

Figure 10.15: The pubic angle

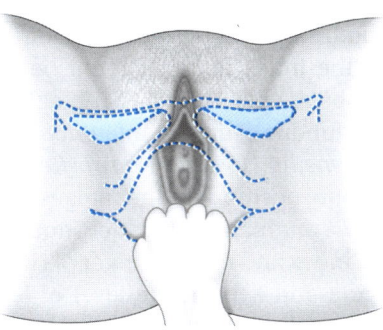

Figure 10.16: Transverse diameter of outlet

B. Radiopelvimetry: In Erect Lateral View

Q. How will you asses the CPD?
Ans. i. Clinical
  ii. X-ray pelvis—anteroposterior and lateral view in erect position
  iii. Cephalometry by:
   1. Clinical
   2. X-ray
   3. CT—More accurate than X-ray and involves less radiation exposure
   4. USG is widely used at present to measure BPD and HC.
   5. MRI to assess pelvic capacity, fetal size, fetal head volume, maternal soft tissues and prediction of vaginal delivery. It has no radiation risk and safe but is more time consuming and costly.

> **Note**
> *Fetal head is the best pelvimeter at term.*

CPD:
Clinical: Assessment per abdomen (a and b)
a. *Abdominal method (It is difficult to perform in high floating head, thick abdominal wall and irritable uterus):* The patient is placed in dorsal position, the thighs are flexed and separated and a pillow is placed under the shoulders. The index and middle fingers are placed over the upper border of symphysis pubis and the fetal head (fetal brow and suboccipital region) is grasped by left hand and pushed in the direction of pelvic inlet (downwards and backwards).
Inference:
No disproportion: The head enters into the pelvic cavity smoothly without touching the fingers on the symphysis pubis.
Borderline: Head can be pushed down a little and slight overlapping of parietal bones evidenced by touch on the under surface of fingers.
Gross disproportion: Head cannot be pushed down and instead the parietal bones over hangs the symphysis pubis displacing the fingers.

b. *Donald's method of detection of CPD per abdomen*: Third, fourth and fifth fingers of both hands are placed at the side to grip the head (occiput and sinciput). The index fingers should be placed over symphysis pubis and thumbs are placed over parietal bones. The assistant will give pressure on fundus of uterus. Inference: as in (a) above

c. *Abdominopelvic method (Muller-Munro-Kerr method):* The patient is placed in lithotomy position under analgesia. The pre-requisites are all same as in PV examination (bladder should be empty and rectum unloaded). The index and middle finger of right hand are introduced inside the vagina and kept at the level of ischial spine, while the thumb of the same hand is placed over the symphysis pubis. The head is then grasped by left hand and is pushed into the pelvic cavity. The extent of the descent of the head is measured by internal fingers, while the thumb estimates the degree of overlapping on the symphysis pubis.

Observation:
1. The head is pushed into the pelvis and touches the internal fingers—no disproportion.
2. The head can be pushed down a little, but not up to the level of ischial spine and there is slight overlapping of parietal bones—borderline disproportion.
3. The head cannot be pushed down instead the parietal bone overhangs the symphysis pubis by displacing the thumb—major degree disproportion.

Drawbacks: (a) In unfavorable cervix it is very difficult to push the head, so it should be done in active labor, (b) It can detect only the disproportion at the pelvic inlet, not at mid cavity and outlet level, (c) It can detect only the shortening of AP diameter than transverse diameter of inlet.

Q. What are the criteria of normal pelvis?

Ans.
a. The sacral promontory cannot be reached
b. The sacrum is well-curved
c. The sacrosciatic notch admits two fingers
d. The side walls are nearly parallel
e. The ischial spines are not prominent and can not be felt at the same time
f. The transverse diameter of outlet admits four knuckles.

> **Note**
> Contracted pelvic inlet; if AP diameter is <10 cm or DC is <11.5 cm; Contracted mid pelvis; if the interischial diameter is <10 cm, the ischial spines are prominent, the pelvic side walls are convergent and sacrosciatic notch is narrow, Contracted pelvic outlet; intertuberous diameter is 8 cm or less, it is usually associated with contraction of midpelvis.

Q. How do you manage a case of CPD?

Ans. By elective cesarean section in gross CPD or by trial of labor in borderline CPD.

Obstetric Cases

Q. When do you choose elective LSCS?

Ans.
1. Major degree of CPD
2. Borderline disproportion with any of the following high-risk factors:
   a. Midpelvic or outlet contraction
   b. PIH
   c. Elderly primigravida
   d. Large baby with post-dated pregnancy.

Q. What is trial of labor? How do you conduct trial of labor?

Ans. Conduction of spontaneous labor in cephalic presentation [Vertex (Vx) is the presenting part] in a case of borderline CPD, with continuous maternal and fetal monitoring to have safe vaginal delivery in an institution, where facilities for cesarean section exists.

Conduction of trial of labor: Selection of patient in borderline disproportion and wait for spontaneous onset of labor, but induction of labor may be performed in selected cases.

First stage:
a. Pregnant mother is kept in bed
b. Evacuation of bladder when necessary
c. Oral water is avoided and maintain IV fluid
   (- When will you go for PV examination in trial of labor?)
d. PV examination
   1. At the onset of labor for assessment of pelvis
   2. To exclude cord presentation
   3. With rupture of membrane to exclude cord prolapse
   4. For assessment of progress of labor 4 hourly in the active phase
   5. Before forceps or ventouse delivery.
   - Augmentation of labor should be done, if the patient is in active phase of labor (i.e. cervix 4 cm dilated) by amniotomy with or without oxytocin infusion according to clinical judgment
e. Careful monitoring of maternal vital signs, fetal well-being, progress of labor (POL) and partogram is mandatory
f. Duration of trial depends on:
   1. Maternal vital signs—P/BP/T/dehydration.
   2. Fetal condition—Fetal heart rate (FHR)/caput/meconium stained liquor/late deceleration, loss of fetal beat to beat variability for a prolonged time, scalp blood pH.
   3. Uterine contraction—duration and frequency are noted clinically in 10 minutes and by cardiotocography (CTG). In normal uterine contraction—labor is allowed to continue.
   4. Progress of labor (POL)—Descent of the presenting part (abdominally and vaginally) and progressive effacement of cervix (examined vaginally).
      - Delayed progress of labor is suggestive of obstruction.
        Good prognostic sign for successful vaginal delivery
        Good uterine contraction, early engagement of head, vertex—anterior position, effaced cervix closely applied to the vertex, no pelvic contraction.

Bad prognostic signs: Weak uterine contraction, slow descent of the head, PROM, uneffaced and partially dilated cervix whIch hangs loosely, occipito posterior position

Second stage:
1. The patient may be delivered normally (30%)
2. Outlet forceps or ventouse delivery (30%)
3. LSCS (40%)

Trial forceps: It is attempted in case of borderline pelvis by an experienced surgeon, where the BPD passes below the midpelvis; otherwise LSCS is to be done.

Third stage: Injection oxytocin must be given (10 unit IM).

Duration of trial labor: Each patient should be judged according to her own merit and there is no hard and fast rule. Fetal risk is obviously increased in case of prolonged labor. Trial labor should never be allowed to reach the stage of obstruction and impending rupture.

Q. Indications of termination of trial labor.

Ans. Maternal distress, fetal distress, prolonged labor and in-coordinate uterine contraction, cord prolapse.

Q. What are the values of trial of labor?

Ans.
 a. It reduces elective CS
 b. Eliminate injudicious premature termination
 c. Better obstetric future
 d. Maternal pelvis is tested for the size of the baby.

Q. Which type of pelvis is good for trial labor?

Ans. Flat and gynecoid pelvis.

Q. What type of pelvis is bad for trial labor?

Ans. Android pelvis is bad for trial labor.

Q. When do you say trial labor is unsuccessful?

Ans. The trial of labor is considered unsuccessful when the fetus is dead or needs craniotomy or rupture of uterus occurs.

> **Note**
> Fetal head is the best pelvimeter at term.

Q. What are the contraindications of trial of labor?

Ans.
 a. True conjugate ≤9 cm
 b. Elderly primigravida
 c. Occiput posterior
 d. Outlet contraction unless symphysiotomy is done
 e. Cesarean or myomectomy scar
 f. Malpresentation or breech
 g. Pre-eclampsia or hypertension
 h. Cardiopulmonary disease
 i. Previous stillbirth or spastic disease
 j. Previous failed trial of labor.

A CASE OF MULTIPLE PREGNANCY

Summary: Mrs X aged 22 years, married for 2 years G1 P0 + 0 admitted at 36 weeks of pregnancy with the complain of excessive distension of abdomen for last 3 months and cardiorespiratory embarrassment for last 2 days. She was treated by ovulating agents (clomiphene citrate) as a case of primary infertility for the last 6 months. She had no history of multiple pregnancies on her maternal side. No personal and family history of diabetes noted. She has mild pallor, edema on feet and lower legs of both sides and hypertension (mild, 150/108 mm of Hg) on the day of examination. Hypertension was detected after 28 weeks and she is taking antihypertensive drug gravidol (labetalol) 100 mg tds/day and it is continuing. On obstetrical examination, uterine size is greater than period of amenorrhea and fundal height and abdominal girth is greater than expected. Identification of two fetal head and three fetal poles and fetal heart sounds are audible at two different sites with a gap in-between with different rates differing from each other by >10 beats/minute as heard by two different doctors at the same time.

Provisional diagnosis: Multiple pregnancy at 36 weeks (D/Ds—wrong date, hydramnios, big baby, associated uterine fibroid and ovarian tumor, ascites with pregnancy).

To be differentiated by history, clinical examination and ultrasonography (USG).

Q. What is multiple pregnancy?

Ans. Development of two/or more fetuses in pregnant uterus.

Q. What is fecundability and fecundity?

Ans. Fecundability is the conception rate per month but fecundity means birth rate per month.

Q. What is Hellin's rule?

Ans. Twin—1 in 80
Triplet—1 in 80^2
Quadruplets—1 in 80^3
Quintuplets—1 in 80^4

Q. What are the different presentations in twin pregnancy?

Ans. VV—Vertex$_1$ Vertex$_2$—45%
VB—Vertex$_1$ Breech$_2$—25%
BV—Breech$_1$ Vertex$_2$—10%
BB—Breech$_1$ Breech$_2$—10%
Both transverse.

Q. What are the different types of twin pregnancy?

Ans. a. Uniovular (monozygotic).
b. Multiovular (dizygotic).

Q. How do you assess chorionicity? (For Postgraduates)

Ans. Chorionicity detection should be done in first trimester for better management of twin pregnancy.

Before 10 weeks of GA chorionicity is assessed by:
a. *Number of gestational sac*: The presence of 2 separate sacs indicates dichorionic (DC) pregnancy.
b. *Number of amniotic sacs*: It is very difficult to demonstrate separate amniotic sacs in early pregnancy, but if these are seen, then a diamniotic pregnancy can be determined.
c. *Number of yolk sacs*: A single yolk sac when there are two embryos should warrant a follow-up at 11–13 weeks scan to identify chorionicity or amnionicity.

In 11–14 weeks/second trimester scan indicates chorionicity by:
a. *Number of placental masses*: Separate placental mass indicates dichorionicity (DC) but a single placental mass does not necessarily indicates monochorionicity (MC), because of separate placental mass may fuse as they are close to each other.
b. *Twin peak or lambda sign (see USG) indicates dichorionicity*: As pregnancy advances chorionic frondosum regresses to chorionic leave and twin peak sign disappears at 16–20 weeks. A triangular portion of placenta is seen insinuating between the amniochorion layers. So absence of twin peak sign in 2nd or 3rd trimester cannot exclude dichorionicity.
c. *Membrane thickness*: The membrane of dichorionic (DC) pregnancy contains 2-amnions, and 2-chorions and is thicker (>2 mm). In 2nd trimester, the number of membranes, if counted and >2 suggest dichorionicity. Absence of dividing membrane suggests monochorionicity and it should be confirmed at 12–15 hours apart before stamping monoamniotic.
d. *Gender*: Different fetal genders signifies dizygosity and hence always dichorionic but same gender does not exclude dichorionicity (this is not routinely reported by Indian law).

Q. How do you differentiate the two?

Ans. Examination of babies
Examination of placenta
Examination of partition wall between the two amniotic sacs.

	Monozygotic	*Dizygotic*
Examination of babies		
Look	Mirror image	Fraternal resemblance
Sex	Same	Same/or different
Hair and iris	Color are always same	May or may not same
Dominant blood group	Same	May or may not same
Study of histocompatibility antigen	Identical	Always different pattern (important)
Examination of placenta		
Placenta	One	Two (more often fused)
Communicating vessels	Present	Absent
Examination of partition wall	2 (amnions only)	4 (2 amnions, 2 chorions)

Obstetric Cases

Q. If a mother delivers twin babies once, what is the possibility of twin in her subsequent pregnancies?

Ans. The possibility of twining is increased, if the first is dizygotic; however with the history of monozygotic (identical) twin in the first pregnancy, its chance of recurrence is very rare, and it has a fixed incidence of 30% in spontaneous twin.

> **Note**
> Predisposing factors of monozygotic twins are:
> i. Advanced maternal age,
> ii. ART (ICSI).

Q. Enumerate the causes of dizygotic twin (fraternal twin).

Ans. a. It is more common in multiparous woman and occurs more frequently in older women due to reduced gonadal-hypothalamic feedback with increase of FSH level
b. It is more common in negroes and less amongst Caucasians.
c. It is more common, if there is family history of twin pregnancy.
d. Induction of ovulation increases the incidence of twin pregnancy
e. Maternal obesity
f. It is also influenced by age and parity
g. Incidence is >90% in ART.

> **Note**
> *Superfetation*—Fertilization of two ova by two separate spermatozoa during two subsequent ovulation (frequency unknown)
> *Superfecundation*—Fertilization of two ova resulting from the same period of ovulation within a short time by spermatozoa from separate act of coitus.

Q. What are the types of monozygotic twins in relation to the number of placenta, amnion and chorion?

Ans. *Diamniotic-Monochorionic:* Here the zygote divides within 4–8 days, following fertilization (formation of inner cell mass). It is a common variety (single placenta).

Diamniotic-Dichorionic: Here the division of zygote occurs within 72 hours after fertilization (two separate placenta or fused placenta).

Monoamniotic-Monochorionic: Here zygote divides in 8–13 days following fertilization (Single placenta), rare about 1%.

Conjoined twin: If the division of zygote occurs after development of embryonic disc, i.e. after 13 days to 15 days of fertilization, conjoined twins of different types develops. Beyond the 15th day of fertilization twining does not occur.

Determination of zygosity (Figure 10.17).

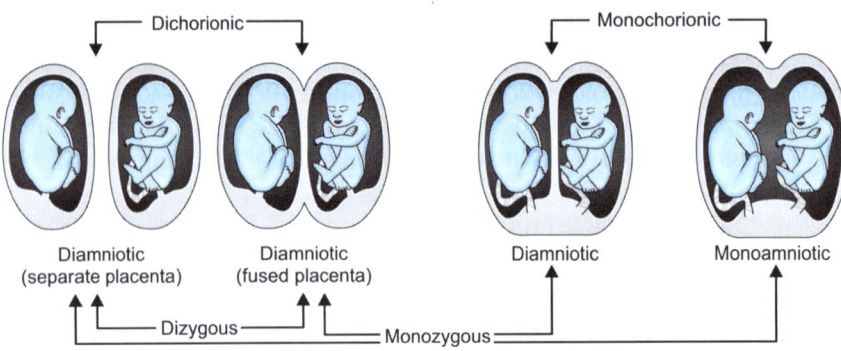

Figure 10.17: Different types of twin
(Dizygotic or monozygotic in relation to amnion, chorion and placenta)

> **Note**
> *Chorionicity is the most important factor than zygosity for fetal prognosis in multiple pregnancies.*

Q. What are the different types of conjoined twins?
Ans. Incidence is 1 in 200 monozygotic twins. Types are:
Thoracopagus (most common), pyopagus, ischiopagus, and craniopagus (least common).

Q. How do you diagnose conjoined twin?
Ans. By X-ray (best), or by USG (3D).

Q. How can you diagnose a twin pregnancy?
Ans. History of multipara, age > 35 years, twin pregnancy in family, previous twin, dyspnea, palpitation, excess vomiting, features of PIH in second trimester, swollen feet, pain in abdomen in present pregnancy.
On examination (O/E): Pallor, edema, raised BP, evidence of varicose veins
P/A:
Inspection: Abdomen is unduly enlarged in 2nd trimester
Palpation: Fundal height is large for date by 4 cm or more after 22 weeks. Palpation of too many fetal parts. Two heads in different quadrants or three poles are palpable. If only one head is palpable the size of the head is smaller in comparison to the total volume of the uterus.
Tape measurement (abdominal girth at umbilicus is higher), (30 inch at 30 weeks and then increases 1 inch per week—normal).
Auscultation: Two fetal heart sounds at a difference of 10 beats/minute are audible by two different persons auscultated simultaneously and there should be an area of silence in between these two heart sounds (Aurnoux sign). Fetal heart sound (FHS) is auscultated at unusual position due to abnormal presentation and position.
Investigations: X-ray at later months of pregnancy, USG at 6 weeks can diagnose twins. USG is helpful for diagnosis and treatment of twin. May have elevated hCG, HPL (human placental lactogen), AFP levels.

Obstetric Cases

Q. Is X-ray helpful in later months of twin pregnancy?

Ans. Yes, due to following reasons:
1. Better idea regarding the presentation and position of twin pregnancy.
2. USG may miss the diagnosis in later months, if operator is not conscious of the possibility.
3. Cost factor is also important.
4. It may not be possible to get fetuses in the same frame by USG in later months.

Q. What are the complications of twin pregnancy?

Ans. I. Mother:
During pregnancy: abortion, anemia, PIH (20%), acute hydramnios in monozygotic twin, pressure symptoms like in varicose vein, piles, edema leg, preterm labor, premature rupture of membrane (PROM), malpresentation.
During labor: Uterine dysfunction, prolapse of umbilical cord, locked twin, increased operative interference for malpresentation
Puerperium: Postpartum hemorrhage (PPH), subinvolution, infection.
II. Fetus: Abortion, intrauterine growth restriction (IUGR), prematurity (80%), IUFD, congenital malformations (3 times higher), respiratory distress syndrome (RDS), Twin-twin transfusion syndrome (TTTS) (8%), large placental infarcts (8%), Twin reversed arterial perfusion (TRAP), conjoined twins.
III. Placenta: Large placental infarcts (8%).

Q. What is acute intertwin transfusion syndrome?

Ans. Following fetal demise in twin pregnancy, there is an acute transfusion into the dead fetus through the shared placenta. This hemorrhage into the dead fetus may cause fetal hypotension, hypoxic end organ injury and potentially fetal exanguination—acute intertwin syndrome.

Neurologic abnormalities among surviving twin include necrosis and cavitation of cerebral white matter, cerebellar necrosis, multicystic encephalomalacia, hydrocephalus, hydroanencephaly, microcephaly and hemorrhagic infarction. Other abnormalities are ischemic bowel lesion, intestinal atresia, renal cortical necrosis. In most cases of monochorionic twin the neurologic injury occur following death of the shibling in the third trimester. Cystic changes detected by MRI or USG may warrant termination of pregnancy.

> **Note**
> *Congenital malformation is more common in monozygotic (MZ) twin.*

Q. Why PPH is common following twin delivery?

Ans. a. Placenta is large, separation time is higher.
b. Atonicity of uterus.
c. Implantation of a part of placenta in lower uterine segment, which is less retractile.

d. Injury of soft tissue due to operative delivery.
e. Retained bits of placenta.

Q. What is locking of twin?
Ans. Fetus or some parts of fetus obstruct the delivery of both fetuses. Incidence is very rare (0.1%)
Locking:
a. First breech and second vertex
b. Both head enter the pelvis at a time in cephalic presentation
c. First vertex or breech, second transverse.

Q. What are the causes of locked twin?
Ans. Uterine hypertonicity, scanty liquor, extension of head, absence of amnion.

Q. How do you manage a case of locked twin?
Ans. Incidence is 1 in 8,000 and common in primigravida and in smaller babies. Cesarean delivery is recommended when the potential for locking is identified.
 a. Where aftercoming head of first twin gets entangled with forecoming head of co-twins—cesarean delivery is preferable or follow the procedure below:
   - Push the head of second twin upward out of the pelvis under general anesthesia and permit the delivery of first twin.
   - Decapitation of 1st twin, if the baby is dead, push the decapitated head upward out of the pelvis followed by delivery of 2nd baby and lastly delivery of the decapitated head.
 b. Both head enters the pelvis at a time—disengagement can be tried under general anesthesia, and if fails LSCS should be done.
 c. If first baby is longitudinal and second is transverse or oblique, interlocking may occur and difficulty is encountered in delivery of first baby. LSCS is preferred in such cases.

Q. How do you manage labor in twin pregnancy?
Ans.
1. *First stage:* Rest in bed, IV line, monitoring of mother and fetal condition, progress of labor, if it delays syntocinon drip after exclusion of obstruction, two bottle of compatible and cross-matched blood should be ready at blood bank.
2. *Second stage:* PV examination to exclude the cord prolapse after rupture of membrane, episiotomy, forceps if necessary in vertex presentation, fetal distress or for delay of 2nd stage of labor. Clamping of cord at two places (8–10 cm of the cord is left behind to the baby). Do not use syntocinon/IV Ergometrine after delivery of 1st baby.
   Delivery of second baby—delay of greater than 1–2 hours is not associated with adverse outcome for the second twin when CTG is employed for continuous monitoring.
   Remove the gloves of hand and check presentation, position and heart sound of second twin per abdomen after delivery of first baby. A vaginal examination is also to be done to confirm any abnormal finding and to exclude the cord prolapse.

Obstetric Cases

    a. If the lie is longitudinal (presentation is either vertex or breech)
       i. Wait for 15–30 minutes for onset of spontaneous uterine contraction.
      ii. If no contraction appears, ARM is to be done after fixing the presenting part and do PV examination to exclude the cord prolapse, FHS is noted again abdominally.
     iii. If there is a tendency to delay, augment the labor with oxytocin
     iv. Spontaneous delivery usually occurs (Second baby is usually delivered within 30 minutes of the birth of first baby).
      v. If there is still delay in spontaneous labor or fetal distress or cord prolapse appear:
- Head low down—forceps delivery or LSCS according to clinical judgement
- If head is high up—CPD and hydrocephalus should be ruled out and internal version under general anesthesia is performed or delivery should be conducted by LSCS

Breech: The delivery should be completed by breech extraction for fetal distress or placental abruption, otherwise assisted breech delivery is performed.

Transverse lie: ECV is done to make the presentation cephalic, if fails, podalic. If ECV fails, go for internal podalic version (IPV) and breech extraction under general anesthesia.

> **Note**
> *Internal podalic version (IPV) is only indicated in second twin in present day obstetric practice.*

If vaginal delivery is not possible or fails, go for CS.

3. *Third stage:* Injection syntocinon (10 units IM, by WHO) after delivery of second baby (rule out triplet pregnancy before application), or injection ergometrine after the delivery of anterior shoulder of the second twin, if mother is not hypertensive (not a common practice nowadays).
   - Syntocinon infusion is to be continued for 2 hours after delivery
   - The placenta is to be delivered by controlled cord traction
   - The patient is to be watched for two hours following delivery.

> **Note**
> *Apply one clamp to maternal side for first baby, and two clamps for the second baby to recognize the cords of different twins.*

4. *Fourth stage of labor:* Monitor the following every 10 minutes for first 30 minutes, then every 15 minutes for next 30 minutes, and then every 30 minutes for next 2 hours by noting:
   - BP/P/T
   - Vaginal bleeding
   - Uterus contracted or not.

Q. When do you hurry for delivery in second twin?

Ans. a. If there is excessive bleeding PV following delivery of 1st twin
b. Presence of fetal distress
c. Hand prolapse or cord prolapse following spontaneous or artificial rupture of membrane
d. Accidental use of injection oxytocics following delivery of first baby
e. If delivery is conducted under general anesthesia.

Q. What are the indications of CS in second twin?

Ans. 1. If second baby is bigger and cervix fails to dilate.
2. Fetal distress, where safe and quick vaginal delivery is impossible.
3. Transverse lie—ECV and internal podalic version fails.
4. Trapped 2nd twin in case of IV methergine after delivery of 1st twin.
5. Prompt closure of cervix after delivery of first baby.

> **Note**
> Condition of second twin is comparatively better in twin pregnancy with HIV infection.

Q. What are the effects of one twin on the other?

Ans. 1. Vanishing twin: When one fetus aborts or gets absorbed within 10 weeks of gestation
2. *Fetus papyraceus*: When fetal death occurs in second trimester, it becomes compressed and become flattened by survivor
3. Prematurity or FGR
4. *Acardius fetus*: Heart is absent in affected fetus
5. *Twin transfusion syndrome*: Occur in monozygotic monochorionic twins.
After birth, one baby is anemic and small and other baby is plethoric and bigger. The plethoric baby is risky in perinatal period for polycythemia, cardiac overloading and hyperbilirubinemia
6. Conjoined twin
7. Congenital defect of baby
8. Intrauterine fetal death (IUFD).

FOR POSTGRADUATES

Monochorionic diamniotic twins (MCDA) multiple pregnancies are at risk of a number of other complications such as: (a) Isolated discordant growth, (b) TTTs (c) TRAP sequence (d) TAPS and (e) Discordant structural and karyotype anomalies.

Q. Can you diagnose twin-twin transfusion (TTT) syndrome in pregnancy? What is the treatment?

Ans. Yes. Placental arteriovenous vascular anastomosis is implicated resulting in discordance in fetal size and amniotic fluid volume. The "donor" twin is usually growth retarded, anemic, and oligohydramniotic. When there is reduction of amniotic fluid in one twin TTT sequence should be considered. Recipient twin shows hypervolemic, hyperviscous, hypertensive cardiac insufficiency and hydrops. Polycythemia, hyperbilirubinemia and kernicterus are common in recipients. Hence recipient twin is at higher risk than donor twin in this case.

Investigations:
a. USG criterias:
   i. Marked size disparity in fetuses of same sex
   ii. Disparity in the size between the two amniotic sacs
   iii. Disparity in the size of the umbilical cord
   iv. A single placenta
   v. Evidences of hydrops in either fetuses (volume overload of the recipient and high output failure of donor)
   vi. Finding of congestive heart failure in the recipient.
b. Doppler study to evaluate the fetal blood flow in suspected cases: Absent or reversal end diastolic flow in the umbilical artery, reversed flow in the ductus venosus or pulsatile flow in the umbilical vein in either twin is very suggestive of fetal hypoxia.

The diagnosis of TTS based on USG (summary):

Recipient	**Donor**
• Polyhydramnios	oligohydramnios
• A distended (polyuric) bladder	small bladder
• Evidence of circulatory overload (cardiac hypertrophy, cardiomegaly systolic dysfunction, atrioventricular regurgitation, or frank hydrops)	UmA wave form abnormalities (absent or reversed end diastolic flow)

c. Fetal echocardiography: To evaluate cardiac function [Myocardial performance index (MPI) or Tei index: It is a Doppler index of ventricular function calculated for each ventricle].

Incidence is 4–35% of pregnancies.

Quientero Staging System of TTTs

- *Stage I:* Discordant amniotic fluid volume (hydramnios: largest vertical pocket is > 8 cm in one twin and oligohydramnios, largest vertical pocket is <2 cm in other twin), but urine is still visible sonographically within the donor twin's bladder.
- *Stage II*: Criteria of stage 1, but urine is not visible within the donor's bladder
- *Stage III*: Criteria of stage II and abnormal Doppler studies of the UmA, ductus venosus, or umbilical vein
- *Stage IV*: Ascites or frank hydrops in either twin
- *Stage V*: Demise of either fetus.

Treatment

a. Elective delivery is recommended as soon as fetus survives outside in level III NICU.
b. Ablation of anastomotic vessels by LASER photocoagulation.
c. Repeated amniotic fluid aspiration (Serial amnioreduction) from recipient twin and administration of digitalis to the mother.
d. Intrauterine umbilical cord ligation (in experimental stage).

e. Septostomy: Deliberate puncture of intertwin amniotic membrane to cause leak, not a good method of treatment as cord entanglement may occur.
f. Selective feticide.

Q. What is twin anemia polycythemia sequence (TAPS)?

Ans. TAPS is charecterized by chronic fetofetal transfusion resulting significant hemoglobin differences in donor and recipient twins without any discrepancy of amniotic fluid volume typical to TTTs. It is diagnosed by MCA-PSV >1.5 MoM in antenatal period in the donor twin and <1.0 MoM in the recipient twin. It can occur in 3–5% of cases in monochorionic twin spontaneously but it occurs in 13% of cases, 5 weeks after photocoagulation. Spontaneous TAPs occur after 26 weeks.

Treatment: Intrauterine transfusion for the anemic twin and selective laser coagulation of the anastomitic vessels.

> **Note**
> Selective intrauterine growth restriction (SIUGR), TTTs and TAPS may not always be mutually exclusive conditions and may coexist in a patient.

Q. What is twin reversed arterial perfusion (TRAP)?

Ans. TRAP sequence is a rare anomaly (1%) in monozygotic twin. Circulatory failure occurs in one of the twin between 8–12 weeks. The donor twin is usually normal morphologically and the risk of aneuploidy is 9%. The mortality is 100% for the perfused twin. In TRAP there is a normally formed donor twin with features of heart failure, and a recipient twin having no heart (acardius).

TRAP sequence is due to direct arterial-to-arterial anastomosis or often venous–venous anastomosis without any arterial–venous connection in the monozygotic twin placenta. Within the single placenta, arterial perfusion pressure of the donor twin exceeds that in the recipient twin, who thus receives reverse blood flow of deoxygenated arterial blood from its co-twin through umbilical artery. The used arterial blood flow that reaches the recipient twin preferentially goes to iliac vessels and perfuses only the lower body, thus disrupts the growth and development of upper body resulting in failure of head growth, or head is poorly developed with identifiable limbs.

USG of acardia also include absence of normal cardiac structure and cardiac movement and variable structural abnormalities (acardiac twin or perfused twin or recipient twin) and the other twin is normal (pump twin) which supports its own circulation and pumps its blood to acardiac recipient.

The principal perinatal problems of normal donor twin (pump twin) are cardiac hypertrophy, congestive heart failure, fetal hydrops with maternal polyhydramnios and preterm delivery. The mortality rate of donor twin ranges from 50–75% without treatment.

Obstetric Cases

Q. How do you manage TRAP?

Ans. *Management*: Expectant—if acardiac volume is less or the flow velocity in the vessels is very low.

Mode and timing of delivery depends upon the presence of fetal compromise and presentation, with the potential for the grossly enlarged acardiac twin to obstruct labor.

Active management: The use of any technique to occlude the vascular supply of acardiac twin
a. Bipolar cord occlusion
b. Radiofrequency ablation to cauterize umbilical vessels in the malformed recipient twin so as to terminate the blood flow from donor
c. Interstitial laser,
d. Embolization of the vessels in the acardiac twin by platinum microcoils.

Q. Indications of CS in twin pregnancy.

Ans. a. Both transverse lie.
b. First baby is transverse or breech.
c. Conjoined twin, collision of two babies at pelvic brim.
d. Pregnancy with obstetric complications—contracted pelvis, placenta previa, severe PIH, post-CS pregnancy.
e. Cord prolapse of first baby.

Q. What is stuck twin syndrome?

Ans. The fetus in amniotic sac is oligohydramniotic and is adherent to the uterine wall sometime. It may occur in twin-twin transfusion syndrome, but may also be found in dichorionic twin. The outcome of such gestation is poor. In the recent times, therapeutic amniocentesis is advocated to reduce the volume of fluid in nonoligohydramniotic sac.

Q. What are the different preterm birth risk refinement techniques in multiple pregnancy?

Ans. The available techniques are:
  i. Calculation of cervical score.
  ii. Measurement of transvaginal cervical length (TVCL) by USG.
  iii. Cervical/vaginal fetal fibronectin level (FFL) in late second and third trimester is associated with increased risk of preterm birth.

Q. What is the importance of cervical score (CS)?

Ans. Antepartum digital cervical examination is done specially in late second and third trimesters:
CS = Cervical length (cm)—cervical dilatation at internal os (IOS) level (cm), e.g. If cervix = 2 cm long with a closed IOS; then CS = +2
If cervix = 1 cm long and IOS diameter = 1cm; CS = 1–1= 0
If cervix = 1 cm and IOS diameter = 3 cm; CS = 1–3= – 2
A CS < 0 on any single examination, the chances of preterm delivery within 14 days is very high.

Q. What is the importance of TVCL (transvaginal cervical length)?

Ans. 1. A TVCL measured by USG if < 25 mm at 24 weeks of gestational age is the best predictor of preterm birth before 32 weeks (27%), 35 weeks (54%) and 37 weeks (73%).
2. If TVCL is > 35 mm between 24–26 weeks, only 3% risks of delivery in <34 weeks of gestational age.

> **Note**
> TVCL of <15 mm at a previable gestation have remarkably poor outcome. However, the encirclage operation in a TVCL of < 25 mm or <15 mm is doubtful.

Q. What are the non-benificial interventions in antenatal management of multiple pregnancies?

Ans. a. Prophylactic circlage
b. Prophylactic tocolysis by beta-mimetics or progesterone therapy
c. Routine hospitalization can not prevent stillbirth, neonatal death or preterm birth in many cases.

Q. What is the role of USG in multiple pregnancies?

Ans. a. It can differentiate accurately dichorionicity [thick dividing membrane composed of 4 layers (2-Amnion and 2-Chorion) and twin peak or lambda sign (see USG in obstetrics)] from monochorionicity which is important for antepartum management. Determination of chorionicity is most accurate in the first trimester, as pregnancy advances the membrane progressively thins and the likelihood of placental fusion increases.
b. Identification of fetal lie, presentation, attitude of fetus, localization of placenta, number of placentas, placental anomalies, number of amniotic sacs, evidence of twin-to-twin transfusion syndrome, evaluation of fetal growth and congenital anomalies, amniotic fluid volume and fetal BPP.

Q. How do you manage monoamniotic monochromic twin?

Ans. a. Confirm monoamnionicity and exclude stuck twin syndrome
b. USG at 18–20 weeks to exclude the congenital defect and conjoined twin
c. Serial USG for assessment of fetal growth (TTTs)
d. DFMC from 26 weeks of gestation
e. NST three times in a week from 26 weeks of GA
f. Antenatal glucocorticoid administration
g. Amniocentesis at 32 weeks for assessment of lung maturity
h. Elective delivery at 34–35 weeks, if fetal lung maturity is not confirmed previously
i. CS is recommended for intrapartum fetal distress related to the tightening of the umbilical cord entanglement.

> **Note**
> Monoamniotic twin is rare, 1% of Monozygotic (MZ) twin. Monoamniotic pregnancies are at higher risk of IUGR, growth discordance, congenital anomalies, IUFD.

Q. What are the possible outcome of monozygotic twin?

Ans. Symmetrical
   a. Separate baby
   b. Conjoint twin

   Asymetrical
   a. External acardiac (TRAP)
   b. External parasitic
   c. Internal fetus in feto

> **Note**
> See also the questions and answers of X-ray (multiple pregnancies) and USG.

POSTDATED PREGNANCY

Summary: Mrs Z, 20-years-old, married for 1 year residing at Burdwan sadar, G2P 1 + 0, admitted in our hospital with 7 days post dated of her expected date of delivery with less fetal movement. Her LMP was on 2nd January, 2010 and EDD is on 9th October, 2010. Her past obstetrical history was normal. She stopped OCP 2 months before present pregnancy. She has mild pallor, BP (normal: 130/80 mm of Hg). Obstetrical examination shows uterus is of term size, longitudinal lie with head presentation and head feels hard and not engaged. The amount of liquor is scanty and the uterus is full of fetus as the fetal parts are easily palpable. FHR is normal and there is no evidence of CPD by abdominal examination.

P/V (not for undergraduate): Os is closed, cervix is tubular head high up, Bishop score is poor.

Provisional diagnosis: Postdated pregnancy of 7 days in a case of second gravida.

Q. What is post-dated pregnancy and prolonged or post-term pregnancy?

Ans. Postdated pregnancy implies pregnancy beyond the estimated due date at 40 weeks (i.e. EDD).

Prolonged or post-term pregnancy is one that is used to denote a pregnancy that has gone beyond 42 weeks or 294 days from the first date of last menstrual period (LMP) in a woman with regular menstrual cycle of 28 days.

Q. What is postmaturity?

Ans. Postmaturity is reserved for pathological syndrome, in which fetus experiences placental insufficiency and resultant IUGR.

Q. What is the incidence of postdated pregnancy?

Ans. 5–10%.

Q. When the expected date of delivery needs correction?

Ans.
a. If the date of LMP is wrong.
b. There is history of irregular or prolonged cycle. In case with prolonged cycle, the number of days beyond 28 days is added to the EDD to get corrected EDD.
In case with irregular cycle for determination of corrected EDD (see the following answer).
c. If the woman conceives in lactational amenorrhea period.

Q. How will you diagnose exact expected date of delivery (EDD)?

Ans. *Menstrual History:*
a. First day of LMP
b. *Regular cycle*: Patient has stopped oral contraceptive pill at least 2 months before conception.
In irregular cycle or if patient is not confident on her LMP (establishment of EDD), then diagnose:
- Date of positive pregnancy test just after missed period, if available
- *Date of quickening*: Primi earliest at 18 weeks, multi at 16 weeks (e.g. if date of quickening is ascertained at 18 weeks, add 22 weeks to get EDD)
- *Date of fruitful single intercourse*: If the women conceives by single fruitful coitus, add 266 days (266+14 = 280 days) to get EDC (Expected date of confinement)
- *Examination of the antenatal card*: If the first visit is within 12 weeks, estimation is more reliable [e.g if uterine size is 7 weeks, add 33 weeks to get EDD (40 weeks)]
- *Weight chart of mother*: Progressive loss of weight or stable weight is common in postdated pregnancy
- *Fundal height*: Serial clinical estimation of fundal height help in determination of GA Mc Donald's formula (see the case 'normal pregnancy at term')
- *Girth of the abdomen at the level of the umbilicus*: At 40 weeks it is about 40 inch
- *Obstetric palpation*: Height of the uterus, size of the fetus and hardness of skull bones and as the amniotic fluid is diminished, the abdomen is 'full of fetus'.
  Fetal heart auscultation by stethoscope (18-20 weeks) add 20 weeks to get EDD
- *PV examination:*
  i. Ripe cervix
  ii. Unripe cervix does not exclude maturity
  iii. Hard skull bones through the cervix usually suggest maturity.

> **Note**
> Quickening: Fluttering sensation felt by mother for active fetal movement for the first time.

Investigation
a. *Ultrasonography*
   Ultrasonography at early pregnancy (9–11 weeks) is helpful for establishment of EDD. Besides serial estimation of BPD, FL, head and abdominal circumference, placental grading, liquor volume measurement are important. BPD –9.8 cm signifies term baby and 10.1 cm is diagnosed as postmaturity.
b. *Straight X-ray of abdomen*: Ossification center appears at cuboid and upper end of tibia at 40 weeks and lower end of femur at 36 weeks.
c. *Amniocentesis*:
   i. Lesithin and sphyngomyelin (L/S) ratio is >2
   ii. Presence of phosphatidylglycerol
   iii. Positive shake test with increased dilution
   iv. Creatinine level is 2 mg% or more
       All the above-mentioned points indicate fetal maturity
   v. Presence of orange colored cells of more than 50% when stained with 0.1%. Nile blue sulfate is suggestive of postmaturity.

Q. What are the causes of post-term pregnancy?

Ans. Exact cause is unknown, but common in previous prolonged pregnancy, primigravida and elderly pregnant mother in particular with sedentary habit, higher socioeconomic status and familial tendency.
It is also found in:
a. Anencephaly.
b. Placental sulfatase deficiency with male fetus with low estriol level.
c. Extrauterine pregnancy.

Q. What are the complications of post-term baby?

Ans. a. *Macrosomia*: Relates with birth trauma
   Birth weight (BW) greater than 4.5 kg has been reported in 2.5% to 5.8% of post-term infants, so there will be an increased risk of shoulder dystocia and birth trauma. Incidence of CS delivery is high.
b. *Oligohydramnios*: Causes birth asphyxia
   Amniotic fluid index (AFI) increases steadily in first half of pregnancy reaching a plateau of 12 cm in third trimester. Between 40–42 weeks, it declines to 30%. So, meconium stained amniotic fluid, cesarean section for fetal distress, low Apgar score and umbilical pH value, increases the rate of fetal asphyxia, meconium aspiration syndrome (MAS). Umbilical cord compression leading to variable FHR decelerations are noted frequently.
c. *Meconium*: It causes MAS and bronchial dysplasia and fetal lung injury by partial obstruction of air ways, inflammation, sepsis, complement activation, inhibition of surfactant synthesis and function, apoptosis of epithelial cells, and increased pulmonary vascular resistance. Thick, undiluted meconium in diminished amniotic fluid volume causes MAS. The incidence of MAS in meconium stained liquor is 2–4.5%. MAS causes abnormal FHR pattern.

d. *Postmaturity (10–20%):* Causes systemic complications. Reduced subcutaneous fat, dry wrinkled and meconium-stained skin, hypothermia, hypoglycemia and hyperviscosity syndrome are common in babies. Placental insufficiency leads to nutritional deprivation, fetal wasting, decreased fat and glycogen stores and chronic hypoxia with compensatory hematopoiesis. A few long-term neurological sequels are also found.

Q. What are the conditions, where pregnancy should not be allowed beyond term?

Ans. a. Elderly primigravida
b. Any medical disorder with pregnancy such as hypertension, diabetes
c. Any other complicated pregnancy such as PIH, eclampsia, APH, IUGR, multiple pregnancy and Rh-negative mother.
d. Bad obstetric history (BOH) due to other causes.

Q. How do you manage a case of postdated pregnancy?

Ans. Antepartum fetal surveillance to identify the fetal risk is to be done twice, weekly after 41 weeks.
a. Daily fetal movement count (DFMC).
b. Amniotic fluid volume—AFI < 5 cm or vertical amniotic fluid pocket less or equal to 1 cm is vulnerable.
c. Clinical fetal heart rate or CTG monitoring— normal/bradycardia/tachycardia may be noted, NST and CST are to be done to determine the fetal status.
d. Modified biophysical profile (MBPP)—utilize the non-stress test (NST) as a short-term marker of fetal status and AFI as a marker of long-term placental function.
e. Doppler velocimetry—measured in umbilical artery, middle cerebral artery and descending aorta and its role in managing post-term pregnancy is limited as most practitioners induce labor at 41 weeks.

Q. What are the treatment?

Ans. a. If the maternal and fetal condition demands immediate delivery, CS is the right option.
   Indication of CS
   1. Fetal distress, amniotic fluid pocket <1cm
   2. Cervix remains extremely unfavorable
   3. Big baby
   4. Failure of induction.
b. When the indication is less emergent and there is no contraindication of vaginal delivery—induction of labor is preferable. If first induction fails, second induction is preferable within 2–3 days.

Q. When induction of labor is considered?

Ans. a. The pregnancy is passed beyond 7–10 days from EDD (practically)
b. No evidence of fetal hypoxia and macrosomia
c. If cervix is favorable, i.e. 50% effaced and more than 3 cm dilated or Bishop's score is ≥6, then,

Obstetric Cases

Induction must be carried out in one of the following ways:
- Medical—by syntocinon drip in escalating dose
- Surgical—low rupture of membrane (if liquor is meconium stained and fetal distress is detected—CS)
- Combined—ARM + syntocinon drip

d. If cervix is unfavorable—Cerviprime gel (0.5 mg) of dinoprostone in 2.5 mL of gel is injected in the cervical canal. Minimum of 2/3 insertions are required at 6–12 hours interval. If oxytocin is required, it should be started 6 hours later. Recently oral misoprostol (100 µg 6 hourly × 4 doses) or vaginal misoprostol (25–50 mcg 4 hourly for 4 doses) is as effective as PGE_2 gel; the major potential complication is hyperstimulation with/without fetal distress and meconium-stained liquor. So, hourly fetal and maternal monitoring is essential.

Q. What is intrapartum risk of post-term pregnancy? How do you manage it?

Ans. Risk depends on sonographic estimation of fetal weight and amniotic fluid volume.
- If estimated fetal weight (EFW) is more than 4,500 g, risks of macrosomia, including shoulder dystocia, birth trauma, so elective CS is considered.
- If EFW is equal to 4000–4500 g—the decision to attempt vaginal delivery include obstetrical history, clinical pelvimetry, diabetes and obesity.

In the intrapartum period, the post-term fetus is at high-risk for the sequel of uteroplacental insufficiency including meconium passage, oligohydramnios, umbilical cord compression. So continuous FHR monitoring is required for detection of fetal distress.

In the presence of oligohydramnios, intrapartum saline infusion may reduce the incidence of:
a. Variable deceleration
b. Fetal distress
c. Fetal acidemia
d. CS rate
e. Meconium aspiration syndrome (MAS).

Infusion of 250 mL of normal saline (by intrauterine catheter) increases AFI by 4 cm and AFI of more than 10 cm is desirable.

Q. What is the urgent neonatal care for post-term baby just after delivery?

Ans.
a. Suction of mouth, throat (oro-pharynx—4 cm) and nostril.
b. Oxygen inhalation
c. In presence of thick meconium tracheal suction by direct laryngo-scopy
d. Prevention of hypothermia
e. Management of hypoglycemia.

The baby should be monitored in the next 48 hours to detect the signs of meconium aspiration syndrome.

> **Note**
>
> *The common obstetric practice of suction of mouth and throat after delivery of head of the baby does not decrease the incidence of MAS by different multicentric randomized prospective study even in high risk babies, on the contrary it may lead to complications such as bradycardia, desquamation, and increased incidence of pneumothrax of newborn babies.*

Q. What is the time of maximum amniotic fluid during pregnancy?

Ans. At 36–38 weeks of gestational age (Volume: 1,000 mL).

Q. What is the volume of amniotic fluid at 41 weeks?

Ans. 500 mL.

Q. What is amniotic fluid index (AFI)?

Ans. It is the sum of the measurements of the deepest, vertical and cord-free pockets in each of four uterine quadrants (see the Chapter of USG).

Q. What is the measurement of AFI at term and at 40–42 weeks?

Ans. AFI increases steadily in first trimester and reaching a plateau of 12 cm during the third trimester and declines by 30% between 40–42 weeks.

Q. Define oligohydramnios.

Ans. Largest single pocket measurement is < 2 cm or AFI is < 5 cm.

Q. What are the effects of oligohydramnios?

Ans.
a. Meconium passage leading to MAS
b. Increased CS rate for fetal distress
c. Lower apgar score
d. Lower umbilical artery pH
e. Increased rate of intrapartum fetal distress
f. Umbilical cord compression
g. FHR deceleration.

Q. What is intrapartum amnioinfusion?

Ans. It is the procedure by which fluid is infused through an intrauterine catheter into the amniotic cavity to restore normal amniotic fluid volume.

Q. How do you perform it?

Ans. At normal temperature (37°C), normal saline is infused into the amniotic cavity. 500 mL is infused first at 20 to 30 minutes. The infusion is discontinued if uterine hyperstimulation or FHR abnormality is encountered. AFI is reassessed within 4 hours (or sooner if deceleration persists or reappears). Repeat infusion of 250–500 mL are performed to maintain an AFI to at least 10 cm. Infusion of 250 mL will increase the AFI by 4 cm and 500 mL will raise the AFI by 8 cm.

Q. What is the benefit of amnioinfusion?

Ans.
a. Relieves umbilical cord compression that results variable deceleration and transient fetal hypoxemia.

b. To dilute thick meconium to prevent MAS.
c. Prophylaxis for oligohydramnios as in prolonged rupture of membrane.
d. Significantly reduces the cesarean section rate for fetal distress and MAS.

Q. What are the criteria for intrapartum amnioinfusion?

Ans. a. Ruptured membrane
b. Singleton pregnancy
c. Cephalic presentation
d. Oligohydramnios: AFI lesser than or equal to 5 cm, thick meconium and prolonged and repetitive variable deceleration.

Q. What are the contraindications of amnioinfusion?

Ans. a. Multiple pregnancy
b. Malpresentation
c. Uterine anomalies
d. Active bleeding
e. Acute fetal distress.

Q. What are the complications of amnioinfusion?

Ans. a. Hypertonicity of uterus
b. Abnormal FHR
c. Chrioamnionitis
d. Cord prolapse
e. Uterine rupture
f. Placental abruption.

PUERPERIUM

(Do not say gravida during history taking as the patient is delivered)

Name: Mrs MS
Age: 20 years
Address: Burdwan
Parity: P 3 + 0
Religion: Hindu
Date of admission: 1-2-2008
Date of examination: 2-2-2008
(Day: 2nd day of puerperium).

Chief Complaints

- Vaginal discharge (Lochia)
- Pain abdomen (after pain), perineal pain for episiotomy or perineal tear repair
- Urinary problems—frequency, dysuria
- Bowel problem—constipation or diarrhea

- Fever
- Trouble on breastfeeding of newborn baby.

Obstetrical History

a. Previous pregnancy
b. Present pregnancy—antenatal check-up
   1. Duration and complication of pregnancy—Pre-eclampsia, APH, PROM
   2. Time and date of delivery
   3. Mode of delivery—ND with or without episiotomy, forceps or ventouse delivery, CS
   4. Third stage—normal or any PPH.

   Baby—alive or dead, if alive feeding habits and status of immunization, cried afterbirth or not, sex, detection of any congenital defect, jaundice, cyanosis, weight, height, head and chest circumferences, different reflexes, palmar and plantar creases and breast nodules. If dead—cause and time of death.

> **Note**
> *Other points in history taking as in antenatal case.*

Examination

- Consciousness and mental alertness of mother
- Pallor, jaundice, BP, systemic examination—chest for any evidence of infection
- Cardiovascular system (CVS).

Obstetrical Examination

Abdomen and Perineum

Inspection: Striae, scar, fullness of lower abdomen exclude retention of urine.

Palpation: Involution—measure from upper border of symphysis pubis to fundus, any tenderness of lower abdomen.

Examination of perineum: Inspection of vulva, episiotomy wound, if present, inspection of character of lochia from diaper, character of lochia–color, consistency, smell, any abnormality (blood clot, retained beats of placenta and membrane).

Breast

Engorged breast, nipple—retracted/flat, fissured, cracked, localized lump or tenderness of breast.

Baby—alive or dead, weight and color of baby on the date of examination if alive, reflexes, premature or not, breast nodule, planter crease, condition of skin for jaundice, any congenital defect, oral mucous membrane for thrush, condition of the umbilical cord, breastfeeding, urinary or bowel motion or any abnormality.

Obstetric Cases

Summary
The patient aged 25 years, third para (do not say gravida as the patient is delivered), delivered normally on 1.2.2008 at 10:15 am without any abnormality in general health and obstetrical condition. The patient is on 2nd day of puerperium (as the patient is examined on 2nd day after delivery) and the baby is matured, delivered at term, alive without any problem of breastfeeding.

Diagnosis
Normal puerperium on second day with normal baby

Q. Why do you say that the puerperium is normal?

Ans. The patient's complain is insignificant and on examination P/R/T/BP and breast are normal, involution of uterus and lochia are also normal.

Q. What is puerperium?

Ans. Puerperium is the 6 weeks period following delivery during which the body tissues especially the genital organs and the uterus revert back to non-pregnant state both anatomically and physiologically. Lactation is established during this period.
Immediate: First 24 hours; *Early*: Up to 7 days; *Remote*: Up to 6 weeks.

Q. What is involution of uterus?

Ans. Gradual diminution of the size of uterus to its prepregnant state.

Q. How do you measure the uterine involution?

Ans. *Prerequisites*:
- Bladder and bowel should be empty
- If deviation of uterus is on the right or left side, it should be replaced in the midline
- Height of the uterus is marked by color skin marking pencil
- Blood clots in the uterus should be removed by massaging the uterus before measuring height of fundus.
- Then the measurement from the upper border of symphysis pubis up to the mark on fundus is taken in inch or cm by measuring tape (thighs should be extended) at the same time by same observer. The symphysio-fundal height (SFH) measurement is usually 13.5 cm at the beginning.

Q. What is normal involution of uterus?

Ans. It is the diminution of the size of the uterus following delivery at the rate of 1.25 cm (1/2 inch per day) from 2nd day till the end of 2nd week. During first 24 hours, there is no involution.

Q. How involution occurs?

Ans. *Mechanism*: Autolysis of proteins of muscle fibers by proteolytic enzymes, so that peptone and creatinine is excreted. Blood vessels become thrombosed and new blood vessels grows in the thrombi, and hyaline and fibrous tissue of old blood vessels degenerate and phagocytosed. Reduction of myometrical cell size, but not the number is evident in involution.

Q. What is subinvolution?

Ans. When the process of involution becomes impaired. It is identified by:
   i. Delay of decrease in uterine size
   ii. Prolongation of lochial discharge (unhealthy)
   iii. Abnormal uterine bleeding
   iv. Fever
   v. Abdominal cramp.

   Causes
   1. Overstretching of uterus during pregnancy—twin, hydramnios, big baby.
   2. Others—retained beats of placenta, fibroid, puerperal sepsis, lochiametra, retroversion, blood clot with sepsis.

Q. How do you treat subinvolution?

Ans. Slight subinvolution does not require any treatment unless associated with infection or foul smelling lochia
   1. Early ambulation
   2. Sepsis by antibiotics
   3. Uterine exploration under general anesthesia to remove the placental products under antibiotic cover
   4. Retroversion—Hodge-Smith pessary.

Q. What is lochia?

Ans. Physiological postpartum discharge of blood and necrotic deciduas in first 3 weeks of puerperium following delivery.

Rubra—first 3-4 days, (Composition: RBC, deciduas, vernix, lanugo hair, meconium).

Serosa—next 5-9 days following lochia rubra (Composition: Less RBC, more leukocytes, mucus from the cervix, microorganism [non-pathological]).

Alba—next 10-15 days (Composition: Decidual cells, leukocytes, mucus, cholestrin crystals).

Amount—250 mL for first 5-6 days.

> **Note**
> When lochia is infected, it becomes foul smelling and profuse in amount (always check vagina for any forgotten swab, placed at the time of delivery or repair of episiotomy wound).

Q. What is colostrum?

Ans. Yellowish fluid, which appears in the breast after labor for 2-3 days and contains huge amount of protein, and fat and antibodies than breast milk. It contains fat globules, colostrums corpuscles and acinar epithelium cells.

Advantage: It improves immunity of baby and helps in expulsion of meconium from the gut of baby by its laxative action.

Obstetric Cases

Q. When will you start breastfeeding?

Ans. As early as possible in normal delivery and even after LSCS if the operation was performed by regional anesthesia. When general anesthesia is given, breastfeeding should be started when anesthetic effect is over.

Frank milk comes from breast from 4th day onwards after delivery. No galactagogue is necessary for milk secretion. Only the repeated suckling reflex by baby is necessary for effective milk secretion. First day milk production is 100 mL, 4th day 400 mL.

> **Note**
>
> Hind milk is very much important for baby's growth as it is reach in fat and calorie-dense which comes from later part of suckling (duration of suckling is 20 minutes in each breast).

Q. Say percentage composition of colostrums and breast milk?

Ans. See Table 10.2

Table 10.2: Composition of colostrums and breast milk per 100 mL

	Protein (g)	Fat (g)	Carbohydrate (g)	Water (%)
Colostrum	2.7	2.3	3.2	86
Breast milk	1.2	3.2	7.5	87

Q. What is the advantage of colostrum feeding?

Ans. a. Immunity of the baby is very high for colostrums ingestion due to the presence of antibody, which combats infection of newborn.
b. Helps in passage of meconium (Laxative action due to presence of fat globules).

Q. How do you suppress lactation?

Ans. a. Absence of suckling reflex by baby is the natural way of suppression of lactation.
b. Use of the drug bromocriptine/cabergoline (1 mg) (which may cause early ovulation) also suppress lactation.
c. Tab pyridoxine 50–100 mg twice daily for 7–10 days.

Q. What are the important care in puerperium?

Ans. 2D—diet, drug (iron, calcium, antibiotic if necessary)
7B—bed rest (no, early ambulation), bladder care, bowel care (constipation—Laxative, adequate intake of water), belly (involution of uterus), blood (Lochia), breast (wash nipple and areola by water in between feeding), and baby.

Q. What is the principle of management of normal puerperium?

Ans. Acronym **'BRIC'**
B—Breast care and breast milk promotion to baby
R—Restoration of health of mother
I—Infection prevention to mother and babies and immunization
C—Contraception.

> **Note**
>
> *Return of menstruation and ovulation: Ovulation occurs as early as 27 days (mean 70–75 days) after delivery with return of menstruation by 6th week in non lactating mothers. The risk of ovulation in exclusively breastfeeding women within first 6 months is 1–5%.*

Q. What are the parameters of normal term baby?

Ans. *Weight*—normal, 2.5–3 kg.

Height—50 cm, body is straight, legs straight, feet at right angle to the legs and toes are upward. Head to heel length is measured.

Head circumference—35 cm (measure by a tape passing over the more prominent part of the occiput and forehead above supraorbital ridges).

Chest circumference—32 cm, measured at the level of nipples midway between the inspiration and expiration.

Reflexes

Suckling reflex: The full term infant sucks vigorously. Stimulation of upper and lower lips produces movement of the lip and tongue in the direction of stimulus.

Rooting reflex: When the breast is brought in contact with the infant's cheek, it seeks nipple.

Moro reflex: The supine infant's head is generally raised above the bed and then released suddenly. A positive response means sudden abduction followed by adduction of both the arms. Hands open out and fingers remain flexed. In preterm babies, after 28 weeks, it can be elicited, but abduction component is weak. It disappears after 12 weeks.

Glabellar tap: When the glabellar region is tapped by finger, both eyelids of the neonate blink.

> **Note**
>
> *Injection Vitamin–K (0.5 mg–1 mg) is given to the infant soon after birth to prevent hemorrhagic disease of newborn. Breast milk is lacking of Vitamin K, D and iron.*

Q. What contraceptive advice do you suggest in puerperium?

Ans. **Permanent contraception**: Tubal ligation or vasectomy (nonscalpel vasectomy-NSV) for husband.

Temporary—minipill (It does not interfere the lactation, does not change the composition of breast milk and baby's growth), low dose pill [combined oral contraceptive pill (COCP)] following 6 months as it causes suppression of milk.

LARC (Long-acting reversible contraception): Injection depot medroxyprogesterone acetate (DMPA)—150 mg deep IM every 3 months.

Intrauterine contraceptive device (IUCD) after 6 weeks (as expulsion rate is less), or LNG IUS:

Others:
- LAM—Lactational amenorrhea (not a good method)—for high success rate answer of 3 questions must be 'yes' which are:
  a. No menstruation
  b. Exclusive breastfeeding
  c. If baby's age is less than 6 months.

  This is mainly due to high prolactin level following childbirth and low GnRH secretion. FSH is low resulting less folliculogenesis and low serum LH prevents LH surge and there will be no ovulation
- Postpartum IUCD (PPIUCD) may be inserted after 10 minutes to 48 hours of normal delivery or post placental (within 10 minutes of placental delivery) and after LSCS following delivery of placenta but before closure of incision. The absolute contraindication of PPIUCD is rare like chorioamnionitis, PPH. Expulsion rate is very low.

> **Note**
>
> *Contraception should be started after 3 weeks in nonlactating mothers and at 3 months in lactating mothers as ovulation may start before menstruation.*

Q. What is afterpain?

Ans. Lower abdominal colicky pain due to irregular uterine ischemic spasm. It is common in multipara, particularly during breastfeeding. It occurs in first few puerperal days (2-3 days) in well-retracted empty uterus. But blood clot and placental membrane inside the uterus may cause after pain in primi mother as uterus contracts to expel these out.

Treatment: Analgesics.

Q. What is milk fever?

Ans. Puerperial fever is due to breast engorgement and before breastfeeding. The fever ranged from 37.8°–39°C and seldom persists for 4–16 hours. Other causes of fever should be excluded.

Q. What is rooming in?

Ans. Baby should be kept in the same room and preferably by the side of the mother on the same bed.

Advantage: Cross infection of baby is less, breastfeeding is easy and the baby gives emotional and psychological support of mother and helps to build a bond between the mother and the baby.

Q. What are the complications of puerperium?

Ans. Complications of puerperium are:
1. *Puerperal pyrexia*: Puerperal sepsis
2. Deep vein thrombosis (DVT)
3. Secondary PPH
4. Breast complications
5. Subinvolution.
6. Puerperal psychosis.

Q. What is puerperal pyrexia? What are the different causes? Predisposing factors? How will you treat puerperal sepsis?

Ans. Rise of temperature of ≥38.4°C or 100.4°F on two separate occasions at 24 hours apart within first 10 days of delivery excepting first 24 hours is called puerperal pyrexia.

Practically, there should be no time limit and a number of factors can cause fever in the puerperium.

Features: Fever, chills, lower abdominal pain, foul-smelling vaginal discharge, tender uterus, hot vagina, septicemia, peritonitis, pelvic abscess.

Pelvic abscess is characterized by lower abdominal pain and distension, persistent spiking fever, tender swelling in fornices/POD.

Causes of puerperal pyrexia:
Causes of puerperal sepsis are genital infections—most common, urinary tract infection (UTI), breast complications, TB, malaria, respiratory tract infections (RTI), thrombophlebitis, infection of episiotomy and abdominal incision.

Factors:
a. *Antepartum*:
    i. Anemia
    ii. Poor nutrition
    iii. Sexual intercourse
    iv. PROM (silent chorioamnionitis)
b. *Intrapartum*: Bacterial contamination, trauma, blood loss
   Pathogens:
   1. Aerobes:
      Gram-positive—Gr A, B, D streptococci, *Enterococcus, Staphylococcus aureus*
      Gram-negative—*E. coli, Klebsiella, Proteus*
      Gram-variable—*Gardnerella vaginalis*
   2. Anaerobes: *Peptococcus, Bacteroides, Clostridium species, Fusobacterium species*
   3. Others: *Mycoplasma, hominis, Chlamydia trachomatis.*

Investigations:
Blood for Hb%, total leukocyte count (TLC), differential leukocyte count (DLC), malaria parasite (MP), blood culture
Urine—RE and C/S
Swab—high vaginal swab for C/S
USG—for detection of pelvic collection or subinvolution of uterus due to retained bits of placenta and MRI/CT

Management:
- Rest and analgesic
- Plenty of fluid to drink or IV fluid(RL)
- Proper antibiotics after investigations
- In severe cases (e.g. peritonitis) IV drip and IV antibiotics must be administered.
    a. *Ampicillin*—1–2 g IV 6 hourly
    b. *Gentamycin*—5 mg/kg IV OD
    c. *Metronidazole*—500 mg (100 mL) IV 8 hourly

d. Continue antibiotics for 7 days or at least 48 hours after the patient is afebrile, whichever is later.
- Pelvic abscess—Drain pus by culdotomy for poor response by antibiotics.

Q. What is parametrial phlegmon?

Ans. It is a parametrial cellulitis (unilateral) which is intensive and forms an area of induration within the leaves of broad ligament at its base following cesarean section. This type of infection should be considered when fever persists for more than 72 hours despite IV antibiotic therapy. Typically fever resolves in 5–7 days, but in some cases it persists longer. Absorption of induration takes several days to weeks.

In some cases severe cellulitis of uterine incision may lead to peritonitis and intra-abdominal abscess. Surgical debridement and hysterectomy is needed with preservation of ovary.

Q. What is cracked nipple? How do you treat it?

Ans. It is a painful condition of nipple due to faulty technique of breastfeeding to baby.

Preventive: If the child sucks breast milk with the whole of the nipple and areola in his mouth.

Curative:
a. The nipple is kept clean and the last part of breast milk which is rich in fat can be applied on cracked nipple for healing.
b. Application of emollients or lanolin cream on cracked nipple after feeding is complete.
c. Use of nipple shield can provide rest to the nipple.

Q. What is retracted nipple? How do you treat the condition?

Ans. There is no protrusion of nipple, rather it is retracted in breast tissue making breastfeeding difficult.

Treatment:
a. Advice to mother to role the nipple in between fingers several times/day.
b. The nipple can be lifted by making a vacuum in a 10 mL syringe.

Use of syringe:
i. The syringe is cut at the needle end
ii. The plunger is inserted in the cut end and the normal end is placed on the retracted nipple
iii. Mother pulls gently the plunger to create vacuum several times per day before feeding
iv. Before removing the suringe hold the breast for air entry and remove it.

Q. How do you manage a case of mastitis and breast abscess?

Ans. *Diagnosis of mastitis:*
- Time of occurrence—2nd to 3rd week.
- Systemic manifestation—fever, malaise may be present. Breast pain may also be present.

- Local—wedge-shaped, hot, swollen, red, tender skin overlying breast tissue.
- *Complication*: If not treated, breast abscess may form.

Treatment
- Adequate hydration, hot/cold compression, sedative and analgesic, antibiotics—ampicillin + cloxacillin, encourage breastfeeding or expressed breast milk (EBM) to baby several times. Support the breast with breast binder.
- Antibiotic treatment should be continued for 10–14 days.
- Breast pump can be used when areola is harder to grip.
- Suckling is to be started on the uninvolved breast to allow let down to commence before moving to the tender breast.

Breast Abscess is caused by Staphylococcus aureus
Diagnosis
- Brawny edema of skin overlying the breast tissue, marked tenderness with fluctuations, swinging temperature.
- USG is helpful for diagnosis.

Treatment
a. Incision and drainage under general anesthesia is followed by antibiotics. The cavity is loosely packed with gauze which should be replaced after 24 hours by smaller pack.
b. Less invasive technique sonographic guided needle aspiration under local analgesia gives also good result.

Encourage the mother for following:
a. Breastfeeding as soon as possible, from infected breast after 2 to 3 days.
b. Support the breast with breast binder.
c. Cold compression between the feeds to reduce the swelling and pain.

Q. How do you treat engorged breast?

Ans. Breast engorgement occurs due to exaggeration of lymphatic and venous engorgement before lactation—3rd day. The treatment comprises of the following:
Support of breast; manual expression of milk; if painful use breast pump; continuous suckling by baby, use of both breasts at each feeding; if baby cannot suck, EBM is to be used for feeding the newborn baby. Apply warm compression to the breasts just before breastfeeding and cold compression in between feeding and use analgesics, if required.

Q. Puerperal thrombophlebitis and phlebothrombosis.

Ans. Thrombophlebitis: It is infective in origin.
Diagnosis: The legs are swollen, hot and painful, usually occurs in the superficial veins and the veins become cord like.
Prevention: Early ambulation.
Treatment: Antibiotics, analgesics along with stockings.

Phlebothrombosis (DVT):

Here infection is absent. This has increased risk of pulmonary embolism. There may be swollen, tender, calf muscles; however this may be completely asymptomatic.

Predisposing factors of DVT: 1. Maternal anemia, 2. Immobilization, 3. Inadequate fluid intake, 4. Obesity

Diagnosis: Clinical
- Homan's sign is positive— in frak cases of DVT
Pain on calf muscle on dorsiflexion of ankle joint.
Investigations: Doppler USG, venography.
Treatment:
Preventive—early ambulation, deep breathing, SC heparin 5,000 IU, 12 hourly.
Curative—SC low molecular weight heparin (LOMOH)—0.6 mL. SC BD or injection heparin 6,000 IU SC, 6 hourly. A physician should always be consulted for management of such case.

> **Note**
> Antidote of heparin is Protamine sulphate (dose 10 mL 1%, IV).

Q. What are the causes of retention of urine during puerperium?

Ans. The recumbent position, stitches on perineum (pain), bruising and edema of tissues at bladder neck, reduced bladder tone, lack of privacy or by operative vaginal delivery.

Q. How do you treat this condition?

Ans. Ensure privacy, application of hot and cold bottle on lower abdomen, pain relief, drink of adequate amount of liquid and water, get out of bed, catheterization lastly. If a woman can not pass urine 4-6 hours after delivery she should be catheterized and urine volume should be measured. If urine volume is >200 mL, self retaining catheter should be kept in situ for another 24–72 hours or until the blader tone is regained. If less than 200 mL of urine is obtained, then catheter is removed and recheck after 4 hours.

Q. Which examinations are urgent at the time of discharge after vaginal delivery?

Ans.
a. Note whether the patient is passing stool and urine normally
b. Rule out anemia and jaundice (Hb estimation in doubt)
c. Abdomen is examined for the state of uterine involution
d. Breast examination for retracted nipple, cracked nipple
e. Color, amount and type of lochia
f. Condition of the episiotomy wound if present
g. Pelvic examination is not needed
h. Examine for calf tenderness.

Q. Postnatal advices to the mother.

Ans. Following uncomplicated vaginal delivery most of the patient are discharged from hospital after 48 hours but can be kept longer for any maternal and newborn problem.

Postnatal advices are as follows:
1. *Food and nutrition*: Balanced diet should be prescribed with 3,000 kcal/day. Iron supplementation (100 mg elemental iron), calcium (1200 mg) are to be continued for further 3–5 months.
2. Personal hygiene, care of vulva and baby care.
3. *Breastfeeding*: Exclusive breastfeeding on demand of baby for both maternal and fetal benefit.
4. *Postnatal exercise*: To strengthen the abdominal and perineal muscles. Exercise should be continued for atleast 3 months.
5. Child immunization.
6. Urgent report to hospital, if fever persists, lochia is heavy or having foul smell or severe backache.
7. *Postnatal check-up*: Before discharge of the patient form hospital and at the end of 6 weeks.
8. *Family planning*: Condom, progestogen-only pill, injection (depot medroxyprogesterone acetate [DMPA]), ligation, Cu-T insertion (PPIUCD or late after 6 weeks).
9. Sexual activity is to be resumed by 6 months or less according to desire of patient and it is unpleasant for hypoestrogenic state following delivery.

> **Note**
>
> For postnatal advice, remember 'ABCD'—(A) Abdominal exercise, (B) Breastfeeding, (C-2) Contraception and child immunization, (D-3) Balanced diet, Drugs (iron +folic acid, calcium) and management of pre-existing diseases like diabetes, hypertension, heart disease, thyroid problem, etc.

Q. What is baby friendly hospital initiative (BFHI)?
Ans. The BFHI is a global effort with hospitals and families to protect, promote and support breastfeeding.

Q. What are the 10 steps of successful breastfeeding?
Ans. By United Nations Children's Fund (UNICEF) and World Health Organization (WHO)
1. Have a written breastfeeding policy.
2. Train all health staff to implement this policy.
3. Inform all pregnant mothers about the benefits of breastfeeding.
4. Help mothers to initiate breastfeeding within half an hour.
5. Show mothers the best way of breastfeed.
6. Give newborn infants no food or drink other than breast milk, unless medically prescribed.
7. Practice rooming in by allowing mothers and babies to remain together 24 hours a day.
8. Encourage breastfeeding on demand.
9. Give no artificial teats, pacifiers, dummies or soothers.
10. Help to start breastfeeding support groups and refers mother to them.

Q. What are the benefits of breastfeeding?
Ans. Baby:
  a. Nutrition

Obstetric Cases

    b. Prevents infection due to presence of immunologic and antimicrobial factors.
    c. Reduces sudden infant death syndrome, diabetes, lymphoma, over weight and obesity.
    d. Potential increase of cognitive development.

Mother:
a. Reduction of PPH
b. Involution of uterus is earlier
c. Longer inter pregnancy interval
d. Reduction of incidence of breast cancer and ovarian cancer
e. Mother baby bonding
f. Contraceptive effect—if exclusive breastfeeding.

> **Note**
> a. A breastfeed baby may not pass stool for several days. This is not constipation. It is a sign that breast milk is perfect food for baby. A breastfeed baby may pass 8 or more very soft stool a day. It is not diarrhea.
> b. Breast milk can be preserved for 8 hours at room temperature and 24 hours in refrigerator.
> c. Lactobacillus bifidus and lactoferrin in breast milk prevents infection in baby.

Q. How do you know that breastfeeding is adequate to the baby?

Ans. Breastfeeding is considered adequate, if the baby:
a. Passes urine 6–8 times per day
b. Sleeps 2–3 hours after feeding
c. Gains weight adequately (10–15 g/kg/day)
d. Crosses birth weight by 7–10 days.

Q. What are the contraindications of breastfeeding?

Ans. It is contraindicated in:
a. Infants with galactosemia, who can not metabolize lactose due to galactose-1-phosphate uridyl-transferase deficiency causing accumulation of metabolites in the blood resulting diarrhea, vomiting, jaundice, hepatomegaly, splenomegaly, cataract and mental retardation.
b. Mother who are HIV positive (not strictly contraindicated in poor resource countries like India as per recent guideline of NACO-2014).
c. Active untreated tuberculosis [not strictly contraindicated as patient may give breast milk by wearing a facemask, but separation of baby is required in mother with multidrug resistant tuberculosis (MDR-TB)].
d. Treatment with radioactive isotopes, cytotoxic drugs and lithium as these substances are secreted in milk.
e. Uncontrolled alcohol intake by mother.
f. Marked immature and grossly ill baby.

> **Note**
> Breastfeeding is not contraindicated in hepatititis-B infection (if newborn receives immunoglobulin), hepatitis C, active herpes simplex (not involving breast tissue) and CMV infection.

Q. What is the physiology of lactation?

Ans. *The basis of lactation is:*
   a. *Preparation of breast*: Which occurs during pregnancy by estrogen, progesterone and growth hormones.
   b. *Synthesis and secretion from breast alveoli*: After delivery the level of prolactin hormone is high due to less secretion of prolactin inhibitory factors from hypothalamus and begins milk secretion in absence of estrogen and progesterone which are remarkably high during pregnancy. During pregnancy, high level of these two hormones prevent the action of prolactin hormone on breast tissue for secretion of milk.
   c. *Ejection of milk*: Suckling of breast by baby send afferent impulse via dorsal nerve roots to supraoptic and paraventricular nucleus of hypothalamus and produce oxytocin which reaches to posterior pituitary by circulation and stored there. The posterior pituitary secretes oxytocin in pulsatile fashion. Contraction of myoepithelial cells (basket cells) around alveoli and small milk ducts by oxytocin from posterior pituitary, helps in ejection of milk from alveoli to lactiferous duct and sinus where from milk is sucked by infant—milk let down reflex.
   d. *Maintenance of lactation*: By prolactin hormone and continuous suckling reflex by baby.

> **Note**
> The reflex may be provoked by infant cry and can be inhibited by anxiety, stress and worry.

Q. What is the protocol of immunization of newborn upto 16 years?

Ans. See Table 10.3.

Table 10.3: Immunization schedule

Number	Time	Immunization
1.	Birth to 24 hours	BCG, OPV(0), HBV(0)
2.	1½ months (6 weeks)	Pentavalent vaccine* (1), OPV(1)
3.	2½ months (10 weeks)	Pentavalent vaccine* (2), OPV(2)
4.	3½ months (14 weeks)	Pentavalent vaccine* (3), OPV (3)
5.	9 months	Measles(1)/MR(1), JE**(1), Vitamine A(1)^
6.	16–24 months	Measles(2)/MR(2), JE**(2), Vitamin A(2)^
		DPT (booster-1), OPV(4)
7.	5–6 years	DPT (booster-2),
8.	10 years	TT (booster-1)
9.	16 years	TT (booster-2)

HBV-Hepatitis vaccine, OPV: Oral polio vaccine; MR: Mumps, rubella; (0): Birth dose, (1): First dose; (2): Second dose; (3): Third dose, (4): Fourth dose
* **Pentavalent vaccine**— vaccine against Diphtheria + Pertusis + Tetanus (DPT) + HepB(hepatitis B virus) + Hib (Hemophillus influenzae B virus), (advantages—It prevents 5 killer diseases and needle prick is least)
** JE (Japanese encephalitis)—in selected district, where encephalitis is prevalent
^ Vit A doses upto 60 months at 6 months interval from 24 months

Obstetric Cases

Q. What are puerperal emergencies?

Ans. a. *Immediate:* PPH, shock due to hypovolemia (hemorrhage), postpartum eclampsia, uterine inversion and embolism (amniotic fluid embolism).
b. *Early (within 7 days):* Secondary PPH, thromboembolism, sepsis (septic shock), renal failure, pulmonary complications.
c. *Late (after 7 days):* Postpartum cardiomyopathy, psychosis, thyroiditis.

Q. What is postpartum blue? How do you treat it?

Ans. Transient mental depression which may appear in puerperal mother 4–5 days after delivery and persists for a few days. It is manifested by insomnia, depression, anxiety, restlessness and apathy to baby.
Treatment: Psychitric consultation, psychological support and re-assurance of mother. Some time antidepressant drugs may be required.

A CASE OF ANEMIA IN PREGNANCY

Summary: Mrs Y, aged 25 years of poor socioeconomic status with G4 P2 + 1, having pregnancy of 34 weeks admitted in the hospital with the c/o palpitation, breathlessness on exertion for last 15 days. She had no positive history of excessive blood loss before pregnancy or during present pregnancy. She has severe pallor as examined by multiple sites with edema on feet and lower extremities, vulva and abdomen without jaundice. Her blood pressure was normal (120/80 mm of Hg). Systemic examination revealed ejection systolic murmur at the base of the heart with no evidence of congestive cardiac failure.

Obstetrical examination shows single fetus, longitudinal lie, cephalic presentation, good liquor volume, FHS being present (130 beats/minute, regular). Per vaginal examination is mandatory for postgraduates at term. Blood for Hb% is 5 g%.

Provisional diagnosis: Severe anemia in pregnancy at 34 weeks of pregnancy.

Q. What is anemia in relation to pregnancy?

Ans. If Hb level is less than 10 g% (WHO <11 g%) during pregnancy and immediately postpartum period. Hematocrit value of less than 0.33 (WHO) is considered as anemia.

Q. What is the time of estimation of Hb during pregnancy?

Ans. Estimate the Hb level at the very initial antenatal visit again at 28 weeks. The initial Hb level will serve as a baseline, compare with the later result at 28–30 weeks. Repeat Hb level at 28, 32 and 36 weeks.

Q. Which factors are required for erythropoiesis?

Ans. 1. Protein (for globin moiety)
2. Hormones:
   - Erythropoietin (HPL and progesterone stimulate its secretion)
   - Thyroxin and androgens
3. Mineral and trace elements—Iron (for hem), zinc, copper, cobalt, 4 vitamins—folic acid, vitamin C, B6 and A.

Q. What are the different causes of anemia?

Ans. a. Lack of iron—iron-deficiency anemia
 b. Lack of folic acid—megaloblastic anemia
 c. Lack of both—dimorphic anemia
 d. Lack of vitamin B_{12}—rare in pregnancy
 e. Lack of protein—reduced formation of Hb, iron-deficiency anemia
 f. Anemia due to hemoglobinopathies—thalassemias, sickle cell disease
 g. Anemia due to blood loss.

Q. What are the reasons of hematinic deficiency?

Ans. a. Diminished intake
 b. Diminished absorption (chronic diarrhea, dysentery, malabsorption syndrome and tropical sprue)
 c. Reduced storage
 d. Abnormal utilization
 e. Abnormal demand.

Q. What are the important factors of anemia?

Ans. Poor diet, multiparity, abnormal bleeding due to menorrhagia, gastrointestinal (GIT) bleeding (bleeding from varices and piles), hookworm infestation, hemorrhagic diathesis and pregnancy disorders like APH, PPH.

Q. What are the fallacies for clinical diagnosis of anemia?

Ans. a. Lethargy and tiredness are common in pregnancy and many women consider these as normal and make no complain suggestive of anemia.
 b. Peripheral vasodilatation in pregnancy makes pallor less common and clinical diagnosis is very difficult.

Q. What are the important dietary sources of iron? Which one is the best?

Ans. *Animal source*—egg, meat, liver
Vegetable source—green leafy vegetables, mustard leaves, spinach, lentiles, fruits, jaggery, turnip green, cereals and sprouted peas, soyabeans
Heme iron (Source—shellfish, red meat, poultry products and fish) is the best, as non heme iron (source—plant food, green leafy vegetables, whole grain cereals, nuts and dried fruits) absorption is hindered by phytate and oxalate.
High bioavailable diet—diet reaches in meat, poultry, and fish.
Intermediate bioavailable diet—cereals, roots, tubers with ascorbic acid
Low bioavailable diet—vegetarian diet with low in ascorbic acid with excess of phytate, cereals, root, tubers, maize, rice, beans, whole wheat flour.

Q. How do you diagnose anemia?

Ans. *History*
 a. Age and parity—common in teen age and elderly pregnancy, grand multipara are more common

Obstetric Cases

b. History of menorrhagia and repeated pregnancy at short interval
c. Non-specific symptoms such as lethargy, palpitation, weakness, lack of concentration depends upon severity of anemia.
d. History of chronic illness—TB, renal disease, chronic diarrhea, worm infestation, chronic blood loss.
e. Family history of hemoglobinopathies is present or not.
f. Personal history regarding diet, socioeconomic status, use of contraception, nuclear and joint family and any addiction.

Examination
Pallor, edema—localized or generalized, ejection systolic murmur is best heard in pulmonary area, any evidence of heart failure in severe anemia, with obstetric detection of fetal growth restriction (FGR).

Investigations
Routine investigations:

a. *Hb percent and blood film*: RBC character is microcytic and hypochromic in iron-deficiency anemia, malaria parasite should be noted in endemic zone.
   Others: Packed cell volume [PCV (low in iron-deficiency anemia)], hematocrit(normal 32–36%) is reduced(<30%), reticulocyte slightly increases in iron-deficiency anemia
   Blood Indices: Mean corpuscular volume (MCV), mean corpuscular hemoglobin (MCH), mean corpuscular hemoglobin concentration (MCHC) should also be done when Hb% is low. RDW is >14 in IDA and <14 in thalassemia.
b. *Urine*: RE and microscopy (pus cells, cast, albumin) for detection of UTI and cases with chronic renal disease.
c. Stool for consecutive 3 days for ova, cyst and parasite (OPC) or any evidence of occult or frank blood.

Special investigations:

a. Automated blood counting for mean red cell volume, mean red cell Hb%.
b. In iron-deficiency anemia (IDA), serum ferritin is less than 12 µg/dl [N = 15–300 µg/dL], besides vitamin B_{12} and folic acid assay for detection of other types of anemia.
c. In IDA, serum iron is less than 40 µg/dL (N = 60–120 µg/dL); TIBC is more than 350 µg/dL and transferrin saturation less than 15% indicates IDA in pregnancy.
d. Serum soluble transferrin receptor (sTfR)appears to be specific and sensitive marker of IDA and levels >4.4 mg/L suggest iron-deficiency in tissues.
e. Bone marrow examination is necessary—where there is no response to iron therapy after 4 weeks or diagnosis of kala-azar or aplastic anemia.
f. Sputum examination and chest X-ray in pulmonary TB (abdominal shielding should be done).
g. Renal function tests and Hb electrophoresis.

Q. What is the amount of iron requirement during pregnancy?

Ans. *Drainage of iron by:*

Fetus	= 300 mg
Placenta	= 50 mg
Expanded RBC mass	= 450 mg*
Total	= 800 mg
Daily loss of Fe (1 mg/day)	= 280 mg for 280 days

Total 1, 080 mg/280 days is equal 3.9 mg daily requirement (pregnancy = 280 days), only 10% of iron is absorbed, so 39–40 mg of iron can meet 3.9 mg iron requirement.

(*expansion of blood volume by approximately 35% a 1.2 L [expansion from 3.5 L to 4.7 L] × 110 [Hb in g/L] × 3.4 [mg of Fe/g of Hb] = 448 mg).

Q. Mention the severity of anemia according to Hb level (ICMR).

Ans. See Table 10.4.

Table 10.4: Severity of anemia according to Hb level

Anemia	Hb (g/dL)
Mild	10.1–10.9
Moderate	7.1–10
Severe	4.1–7
Very severe	<4

(Hb concentration of <11 g% is considered as anemia according to WHO, but in our country Hb of 10 g% is considered to be anemic).

Q. What are the complications of anemia during pregnancy?

Ans. *Maternal complications:* Sepsis, heart failure, preterm labor, puerperal infection, subinvolution of uterus, PPH, obstetric shock.

Fetal complications: Low birth weight (preterm, IUGR), stillbirth (uncommon), baby is anemic at birth.

Q. How will you prevent anemia?

Ans. a. Prophylaxis of iron in non-pregnant women to build up iron store.
b. Iron supplementation during pregnancy (IFA-tab, 100 mg of elemental iron and 0.5 mg of folic acids) once daily for 100 days starting after first trimester.
c. High protein diet of 3,000 cal should be consumed daily along with iron supplementation and improvement of dietary habits and bioavailability of foods.
d. Treatment of women by antihelminthic (mebendazole—100 mg BD × 3 days, albendazole—400 mg stat dose to all anemic mothers after first trimester of pregnancy).
e. Social service: Proper sanitation, safe water supply, personal hygiene and better education.
f. Food fortification.

Obstetric Cases

Q. What are MCV, MCH and MCHC?

Ans. Mean corpuscular volume (MCV)

MCV= PCV × 10/RBC per cubic mm of blood (N = 75–96 fl)
(*In IDA it is reduced but in thalassemia it is very much reduced*)

Mean corpuscular Hb (MCH)

MCH = Hb × 10/RBC per cubic mm of blood (N = 27–33 pg)
(*In IDA it is reduced, but in thalassemia it is very much reduced*)

Mean corpuscular Hb concentration (MCHC)

MCHC = Hb × 100/PCV (N = 32–35%)
(*In IDA it is reduced, but in thalassemia it is normal or slightly reduced*)

Q. What is Red cell Distribution Width (RDW)? Advantages?

Ans. **RDW** is the coefficient of variation of red cell volume in a specimen of blood, e.g. fragmented red cells have tiny size, while the macrocytes and reticulocytes have large size.

RDW-SD is the standard deviation of the distribution curve of red cell volume.

The wider the curve is spread by erythrocytes of different sizes, there will be higher RDW-SD value.

RDW-CV is a percentage co-efficient of variation and is calculated from the following formula.

$$RDW\text{-}CV = \frac{\text{Standard deviation of the distribution curve of the erythrocyte MCV} \times 100\%}{MCV}$$

Advantages of having RDW
1. Recognizes RBC abnormality from CBC
2. Assists in differential diagnosis (Thalassemia and IDA)
3. Follow the course of a disease
4. RDW–CV tends to magnify variations in cell size in patients with microcytosis.

Q. What are the different oral iron preparations? What is the composition of its dose? When it is used?

Ans. Different oral iron preparations are ferrous sulfate, ferrous fumerate, ferrous gluconate, carbonyl iron, Ferrus ascorbate etc.

One tablet of ferrous sulfate (200 mg) contains 60 mg of elemental iron. The therapeutic dose of elemental iron is about 200 mg/day. So, one tablet, three times a day, is advised.

It is used in the following conditions:
In iron-deficiency anemia,
  a. Mild anemia presenting before 34 weeks of gestation
  b. Moderate anemia before 28 weeks of gestation.

Q. What is the rate of absorption of oral iron?

Ans. The rate of absorption of oral iron is 10% but the rate of absorption may be increased to 30–40% depending upon the severity of anemia.

Q. What are the side-effects of oral iron?
Ans. Nausea, vomiting, diarrhea, constipation, abdominal cramp and it is dose-related.

Q. How do you improve patient's compliance of oral iron?
Ans.
a. Iron should be given after 16 weeks of pregnancy
b. Build up the dose slowly and after meal, later in between meals
c. Ferrous sulfate is least expensive; if it is not tolerated, ferrous gluconate and ferrous fumerate and ferrous ascorbate should be given.

Q. How do you follow-up the patient with oral iron?
Ans. After initiation of iron supplementation, there is a latent period of 1 week before the Hb concentration starts rising. Hematologically, there is reticulocyte response in 5–10 days of start of oral therapy of 180 mg of elemental iron per day and Hb rises 0.3 to 1 g/week. If there is no improvement clinically and hematologically within 3 weeks, re-evaluation is needed.

Q. What is the advantage of parenteral iron therapy? When it is used?
Ans. It has no advantage over oral iron when the later is well-tolerated, but the main advantage of parenteral therapy is the certainty of its administration to correct the Hb deficit and to buildup iron stores. It is used in patients when oral iron is not absorbed or patient is non-compliant or develop serious side-effect, which cannot be corrected by simple means.

The rise of Hb concentration is as like oral iron (up to 1 g/week).

Q. What are different injectable iron preparations?
Ans.
a. Iron dextran (Imferon) for IM and IV route
b. Iron sorbitol citrate (Jectofer) can be used only by IM
c. Iron sucrose only by IV or IV infusion.
d. *Ferric carboxy maltose*: IV infusion within 15 minutes, not used in pregnancy at present (especially in 1st trimester), but may be used to treat anemia in puerperium.

Q. What is TDI?
Ans. Elemental iron (mg) =
(Normal Hb—patient's Hb) × weight (kg) × 2.21 + 1, 000
If the calculated dose is more than 2, 500 mg, give it in two divided doses or iron (mg) =
Weight × (Target Hb—Actual Hb g/L) × 0.24 + 500 mg.
For example, 60 kg × 40 g/L × 0.24 + 500 = 576 + 500 mg.

Q. What is 0.24 in the above calculation?
Ans. Blood volume—7% of body weight
- Hb contains 3.4 mg Fe/g
- 3.4 × 0.07 = 0.24.

Obstetric Cases

Q. What are the side-effects of TDI?

Ans. The side effects are chest pain, rigor, chills, fall in BP, dyspnea, hemolysis and anaphylactic reaction. If any such reaction occurs, stop transfusion and administer antihistaminics, corticosteroids and epinephrine.

Q. What are the indications of blood transfusion?

Ans. *Indications*:
   a. Severe anemia beyond 36 weeks
   b. Associated infection
   c. To replenish blood loss in APH and PPH
   d. Patient not responding to oral and parenteral iron
   e. In cases with hemoglobinopathies.

> **Note**
>
> ACOG recommends blood transfusion for a Hb of <6 g/dL and RCOG recommends that if the Hb is <7 g/dL, but clinically transfusion is offered to any women with symptoms attributable to hypotension or postural changes in vital signs, even with a Hb over 7 g/dL.
>
> Recombinant human erythropoietin (rHuEPO) is an alternative when patient refuses donor blood and can be used antenatally and postpartum in women without end stage renal disease without any adverse maternal, fetal and neonatal effects.

Q. What fractions of blood are preferred?

Ans. Transfusion of packed cells is very much preferred.

Q. What are the side effects of blood transfusion?

Ans. a. Transfusion reaction
   b. Precipitated preterm labor
   c. Overloading of heart, if whole blood is transfused.

Q. Management of severe anemia in pregnancy?

Ans. Figure 10.18.

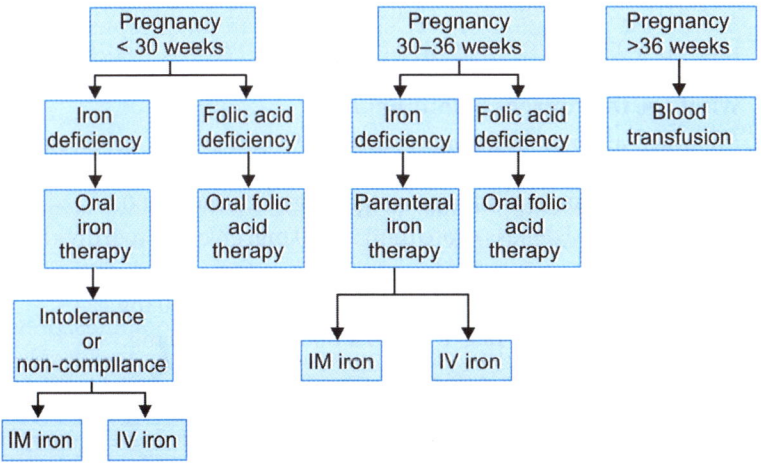

Figure 10.18: Management of severe anemia

Q. How do you manage anemic patient in labor?

Ans. *First stage*
1. Comfortable position
2. Pain relief
3. Oxygen, to be kept ready and is given in dyspnea
4. In case of preterm labor, β-mimetics and steroids (caution of pulmonary edema)
5. Antibiotic prophylaxis
6. Aim is vaginal delivery
7. Urine output should be monitored.
8. Continuous catheterization is generally not required for fear of infection.

Second stage

Prophylactic forceps as chance of heart failure is high.

Third stage
1. Active management of third stage of labor by syntocinon, except in very severe anemia for fear of heart failure
2. PPH, if occurs must be energetically treated by oxytocics or blood transfusion.
    Puerperium: Rest, iron and folic acid for 3 to 6 months, infection must be treated.
    Contraception: Barrier contraception is the method of choice. IUCD or sterilization should be used after improving anemia. Progesterone only pill can be used.

Q. Why folic acid is necessary during pregnancy?

Ans. As the store of folic acid is limited in the body. It is necessary for maturation of RBCs, intermediary in metabolism of amino acids, role of cell division, prevent fetal neural defects (NTDs), preterm labor, PROM, IUGR and improve vascular endothelial function and prevent hyperhomocystnemia.

Dose of folic acid is 5 mg for prevention of hyperhomocystneimia which may cause cardiovascular disease and pregnancy problem and 500 μg for prevention of NTDs (common are anencephaly and spina bifida).

Q. What are the sources of folic acid?

Ans. Potatoes, spinach, broccoli, asparagus, bananas, dark-green vegetables. The bioavailability of natural folate is not good as cooking or processing destroys these compounds. Synthetic L-methyl folate is more bio-available than regular folic acid.

Q. When its requirement increases?

Ans. Multiple pregnancies, pregnancy with hemoglobinopathies, pregnancy with anticonvulsant drugs treatment for epilepsy, cervical dysplasia (10 mg/day) and in neuropsychiatric conditions (50 mg/day).

Q. Why periconceptional supplementation of folate is necessary?

Ans. To achieve optimal folate status before conception and in first trimester of pregnancy which:

- Prevents congenital malformations of the heart, limbs, urinary system and orofacial clefts of fetus and NTDs
- Increases blood folate levels and prevent megaloblastic anemia
- Decreases homocysteine in blood and fluid
- Decreases the risk of anovulatory infertility
- Lowers incidence of miscarriages.

Q. Investigations of megaloblastic anemia.
Ans.
a. MCV—110 to 140 cubic microns (>110 fl)
b. MCH—33-38 pg (> 33 pg)
c. MCHC—30-35% (normal value)
d. Peripheral smear—macrocytic and hypersegmented neutrophil (> 5 lobes)
e. Serum folate—less than 3 ng/mL (N = 2.8 to 8 ng/mL)
f. RBC folate—(< 80 mg/mL)
g. Serum B_{12}— less than 50 pg/mL is indicative of B_{12} deficiency.

Q. What is Schilling test?
Ans. It is used for detection of intrinsic factors and to measure vitamin B_{12} absorption in vitamin B_{12} deficiency anemia, but is contraindicated in pregnancy secondary to use of radioactive cobalt. It is done safely in puerperium.

Q. How do you treat vitamin B_{12} deficiency anemia?
Ans. Treatment is Vitamin B_{12} 1 mg IM daily for 1 week, then every week for 4–8 weeks and continue at monthly interval for indefinitely.

Q. What is FIGLU test?
Ans. FIGLU is a breakdown product of histidine. Tetrahydrofolic acid (active form of folic acid) combines with FIGLU to form N5.
In severe folic acid deficiency this reaction is impaired. After histidine load, FIGLU accumulates in blood and its excretion in urine increases.

Q. How do you confirm that the patient is taking oral iron?
Ans.
a. Color of the stool may become black.
b. Biochemical—one drop of concentrated thioglycolic acid and one drop of 2, 2-dipyridyl in 60% acetic acid are added to fecal smear. An immediate red reaction indicates presence of iron and no color change indicates its absence.

Q. How do you use IV infusion of iron sucrose?
Ans. 2.5 mL of iron (Fe) sucrose (2 ampules) diluted in a maximum of 100 mL of 0.9% of NaCl, immediately prior to infusion. The infusion must be at a rate of 100 mg/15 minute. 100 mg IV, three times, weekly (Day-1, Day-3 and Day-5) (2.5 mL = 50 mg of Fe).

Q. How do you use erythropoietin?
Ans. Intravenous iron sucrose on day 2, 4, 6 and injection erythropoietin in doses of 50–150 U/kg S/C on day 1, 3, 5 for improvement of severe anemia (especially anemia with renal disease) instead of blood transfusion.

Normal Values

Hb	=	12–16% g
Serum iron	=	60–150 µg/dL
Serum TIBC	=	259–388 µg/dL
Serum ferritin	=	120 mg/mL
Soluble transferrin receptors	=	0.3–2.9 mg/mL
sTfR -F index	=	0.16–1.80
Transferrin saturation	=	20–45%

(**Note**: *TIBC—Total iron binding capacity; sTfR-F—Soluble transferrin receptors-ferritin*)

Q. Stages of iron deficiency?

Ans. See Table 10.5.

Table 10.5: Stages of iron deficiency

Parameters	Blood levels	Amount	Cut-offs
Iron depletion			
Reduction of iron stores	Serum ferritin	Decreased	<12 µg/L
	TIBC	Increased	360 µg/dL
Iron-deficient erythropoiesis			
Exhaustion of Fe-store	Serum iron	Decreased	<60 µg/dL
	Transferrin saturation	Decreased	<15%
	Free erythrocyte protoporphyrin (FEP)	Increased	>70 mmol FEP/mol heme
	Serum transferrin receptor (sTfR) conc	Increased	≥ 8.5 mg/L
Iron-deficient anemia	Hb	Decreased	<11 g/dL
	Hematocrit	Decreased	33%

POST-CESAREAN SECTION PREGNANCY

Summary: Mrs C, 22 years old, Gravida 2; Para 1 + 0 came to the hospital with the c/o pain on lower abdomen with the history of previous cesarean section delivery of a living female baby at term for premature rupture of membrane with induction failure and there was uneventful recovery. In the present, pregnancy she has mild pallor, BP normal and on obstetrical examination the pregnancy is of 38 weeks, longitudinal lie, with engaged cephalic presentation, normal fetal heart rate with no evidence of uterine contraction and scar tenderness.

P/V (not for undergraduate)—cervix is 80% effaced, Os—2 cm, membrane present and station is +1 cm, LOA and no evidence of cephalopelvic disproportion.

Provisional diagnosis: Post-cesarean section pregnancy at 38 weeks of gestation.

Treatment: Admission in Hospital and trial of vaginal delivery is advised.

Obstetric Cases

Q. Why is it included in high-risk pregnancy?

Ans. It is included in high-risk pregnancy, because of risk of scar rupture and subsequent risk of maternal and fetal complications.

Q. Which points are to be noted in Post-cesarean section pregnancy during history taking?

Ans. Details of last cesarean delivery:
   a. Indication of previous section
   b. Place of previous section or any technical difficulty
   c. Technique of closure-one/two layers closure
   d. Emergency/elective
   e. Type of cesarean section—Classical/LSCS
   f. Postoperative complications, if any—history of blood transfusion
   g. History of any infection or stay in hospital
   h. Outcome of child
   i. Expertise of the surgeon.

Past history of vaginal delivery:
Vaginal delivery following cesarean section may weaken the scar.

Factors in present pregnancy:
   a. Interval of present pregnancy from previous cesarean delivery (if interval is below 18 months chances of scar dehiscence is high).
   b. Twin, hydramnios and big baby may stretch the scar.
   c. Placenta over the scar may weaken the scar.
   d. Obesity.

Q. How do you assess the integrity of previous cesarean section scar?

Ans. Non-pregnant condition
- USG—Scar thickness of < 4 mm is usually regarded as a weak scar
- A wedge depression of >5 mm following HSG performed 6 months after cesarean delivery signifies a weak scar
- Hysteroscopy may be used to see the scar depression.

During pregnancy
USG can be used to localize the thickness and integrity of uterine scar in pregnancy. If myometrial thickness at scar region is 3.5 mm, it is considered as normal and scar thickness of <3.5 mm, chances of scar dehience is less. USG can also diagnose placental localization and adherent placenta when subplacental sonoluscent area representing decidua basalis and Nitabuch's layer are absent.

Q. What are the different types of cesarean section?

Ans. Classical or lower segment cesarean section.

Q. What are the effects of cesarean section in present pregnancy and labor?

Ans.
1. Miscarriage
2. Preterm labor
3. Pain abdomen
4. Placental previa and morbidly adherent placenta
5. Increased chances of repeat cesarean section
6. Retained placenta

7. PPH
8. Increased chances of peripartum hysterectomy.

Q. What are the dangers of post-CS pregnancy?

Ans. Scar dehiscence and scar rupture (when all layers of uterine wall including fetal membrane at scar are involved and unscarred tissue may also be involved leaing to bleeding from the margins).

> **Note**
> Scar rupture is less common, if pregnancy occurs after 16–18 months following previous CS.

Q. How do you diagnose scar dehiscence?

Ans. Incomplete uterine scar rupture (intact visceral peritoneum) or partial separation along the line of previous scar is called scar dehiscence.

Symptoms:
a. Suprapubic pain
b. Mild vaginal bleeding
c. Bladder tenesmus.

Signs:
a. Unexplained tachycardia
b. Low BP
c. Fetal heart sound (altered)
d. Tenderness over uterine scar
e. Failure of progress of labor
f. Ballooning of the lower uterine segment.

Q. Scar rupture is common in which type of scarred uterus? Why?

Ans. Scar rupture is more common in classical type of CS and it may occur in antenatal period because:
1. The apposition is not good.
2. Imperfect healing due to uterine contraction and relaxation.
3. The scar is stretched at right angle.
4. The placenta is adherent to the scar and trophoblast make the scar weaker in future pregnancy.

Q. How do you diagnose scar rupture?

Ans. Patient complaining of cessation of labor pain following a prolonged time of vigorous labor pain.

On examination (O/E): Features of shock, uterine contour could not be palpated properly; no contraction of uterus felt, no fetal heart sound is audible.

Per vagina (PV): Bleeding ++, presenting part goes high up, and cervix may hang like a curtain.

> **Note**
> The risk of scar rupture depends on: i. Type of previous uterine incision, ii. Number of previous cesarean section, iii. Other factors: (a) Post-operative convalescence in previous pregnancy; (b) Interval between previous CS and conception; (c) Use of oxytocics for induction and augmentation of present pregnancy.

Q. What is the incidence of scar rupture?

Ans. Incidence of lower segment scar rupture during labor is 1–2%. Incidence of scar rupture in classical CS is 5–10 times more.

Q. The patient underwent LSCS for fetal distress (non-recurrent cause) in previous pregnancy.
a. When do you admit this patient?
b. What will be the mode of delivery?

Ans. Patient with lower segment cesarean section in the past should be admitted at 37 weeks only if there is no other obstetrical problem. Urgent admission is needed, if patient goes into labor, appearance of symptoms and signs of scar dehiscence or rupture or any associated medical or obstetrical complications.

Overall assessment is to be done in relation to previous and present pregnancy, and if there is no contraindication of vaginal delivery, go for vaginal delivery which is called vaginal birth after cesarean section (VBAC) under strict supervision on:
1. Progress of labor
2. Maternal and fetal condition
3. Behavior of uterine scar.
   - Induction and augmentation is to be done under strict supervision
   - If any symptoms or signs of scar dehiscence appear, go for CS
   - In second stage, prophylactic forceps is to be applied to cut down second stage of labor
   - After placental delivery watch for bleeding per vagina and routine exploration of lower segment is controversial
   - Retained placenta and PPH are the possible complications, which should be kept in mind.

> **Note**
> *Timing of elective cesarean section: Elective CS is generally done in India at the gestational age (GA) of 37 weeks completed (38 weeks), which is documented by urine pregnancy test (UPT), fetal heart sound, or USG findings in first trimester. Best perinatal outcome is noted at 38 completed weeks (39 weeks).*
> *If the GA is not confirmed wait for spontaneous onset of labor.*

Q. What is repeat cesarean section pregnancy?

Ans. A repeat cesarean section pregnancy is defined as pregnancy following two cesarean sections.

Q. How do you manage a case of repeat CS pregnancy?

Ans. An elective CS should be performed at and following cares are taken during operation:
1. During opening of parietal peritoneum, care should be taken to prevent gut injury.
2. Bladder should be catheterized to prevent bladder injury and parietal peritoneum should be opened as high as possible.

3. Blood for grouping and cross-matching for management of PPH and retained placenta.
4. Extraperitoneal CS when anterior wall of uterus is grossly adherent with parietal peritoneum.

Q. How do you manage a case of postclassical CS pregnant mother?
Ans. The mother should be admitted at 34–36 weeks and elective CS is to be done at 37 weeks or before.

Q. What is the indication of classical cesarean section?
Ans.
1. Bladder is strictly adherent to the lower segment
2. Placenta previa
3. Impacted shoulder in the lower segment of uterus with drained liquor
4. Fibroid in lower segment of uterus
5. Carcinoma cervix.

Q. What is vaginal birth after cesarean section (VBAC)?
Ans. It is the vaginal birth after cesarean section. A trial of labor after cesarean section (TOLAC) is an acceptable alternative to repeat abdominal birth in the majority of woman with previous CS.

> **Note**
> Induction of labor may be an option for those women undergoing TOLAC, but the use of cervical ripening agent or misoprostol should be discouraged for increased risk of uterine rupture. Oxytocin may be allowed for augmentation of labor.

Q. What are the benefits of VBAC?
Ans. The principal benefits of VBAC is the avoidance of the morbidity, mortality and cost of major abdominal operation.

Q. When do you go for vaginal delivery in Post-CS pregnancy?
Ans.
a. Uncomplicated pregnancy
b. Average sized baby
c. Tall mother more than 5 ft 2 inches
d. Clinical pelvimetry shows adequate pelvis
e. Preferably cephalic presentation with engaged head
f. Previous CS was due to non-recurrent cause, not present in this pregnancy
g. In the absence of contraindications, a woman with previous low transverse incision without any postoperative complications should be encouraged to attempt labor in the current pregnancy.
h. When specific data on risks are lacking decisions regarding a trial of labor after cesarean (TOLAC) section must be made on individual basis.

> **Note**
> Once CS is not always CS in non-recurrent cases.
> Once CS is always CS in recurrent cases and repeat CS.

Obstetric Cases

Q. What are the contraindications of VBAC?

Ans.
a. Prior classical or T-shaped incision on uterus
b. Contracted pelvis or CPD
c. Medical or obstetrical complications that preclude vaginal delivery (malpresentation, placenta previa)
d. Patient refusal to undergo TOLAC
e. Inability for immediate surgery
f. Previous two LSCS without a vaginal delivery.

Questions on cesarean section (see the questions and answers on CS) and questions on rupture uterus (see the specimen of ruptured uterus)

Q. Mode of delivery depends upon which factors?

Ans. It depends upon all the points mentioned in history taking (see above) along with miscelleneous factors which needs LSCS
a. Pelvic inadequacy
b. Age of patient (>30 years)
c. Bishop score (poor)
d. Fetal weight (4 kg or more)
e. Twin pregnancy (combined weight of fetus is >4 kg) and polyhydramnios
f. Maternal obesity
g. Gestational age is >40 weeks.

Q. How do you elicit scar tenderness in post CS pregnancy? What are the factors in favor of scar tenderness?

Ans. Do not press the scar line on the skin. Gentle and deep pressure is applied on the lower uterine segment by ulnar border of right hand downwards and backwards, just above the symphysis pubis, where the scar of the previous section lies.

If patient complains of pain, scar tenderness is positive. It has no marked clinical significance in practice as pain sensation varies from person to person, but it gains clinical importance when the scar tenderness is associated with unexplained tachycardia, low BP, mild vaginal bleeding and bladder tenesmus.

> **Note**
> *Integrity of scar can also be seen by USG-see above. The upper margin of LUS is about the level of upper border of symphysis pubis in late pregnancy.*

Q. What are the risks of VBAC to mother and fetus?

Ans.
a. **Mother**: i. Increased rate of maternal morbidity; ii. Risk of uterine rupture; iii. Risks associated with failed VBAC (delivery by emergency CS, requirement of blood transfusion, endometritis); iv. Long-term complications of VBAC—vaginal birth may have adverse effect on pelvic floor, and may cause urinary incontinence.
b. **Infant**: (i) Antepartum still birth; (ii) Delivery related perinatal death; (iii) Non-asphyxial morbidity like intracranial hemorrhage, cerebral palsy (10%).

Q. What are the maternal and infant risks of planned repeat cesarean delivery (PRCD)?

Ans. *Mother:*
   a. Overall rate of morbidity increased due to: i. Complications of CS; ii. Primary infection, iii. Blood transfusion hazards
   b. Risks of placental problem in future pregnancy—placenta previa, morbid adhesion of placenta
   c. Future surgical problem—bladder trauma during hysterectomy, multiple cesarean delivery is a relative contraindication of vaginal delivery
   d. Subfertility and early pregnancy loss.

Infant:
   a. Transient tachypnea of newborn (TTN)
   b. RDS and persistent pulmonary hypertension.

Q. What is TTN?

Ans.
- A condition seen in babies following LSCS
- This is due to delayed clearance of lung fields due to less squeeze effect than vaginal delivery
- The baby looks normal
- Hurried respiration occurs within a few hours after birth, respiration rate (RR) is 60-80 may be as high ass 100/minute with mild chest retraction
- The condition gradually subsides within a few days of birth.

Q. How do you counsel women with a history of three or more cesarean deliveries?

Ans.
   a. Trial of labor after cesarean (TOLAC) section is not recommended after three or more cesarean deliveries (CD)
   b. Location of placenta in relation to cervix should be documented before CD
   c. Risks of placenta previa and accreta are high
   d. Even if a repeat CD is planned, the woman's obstetric history provides the basis for determining the optimal timing of delivery
   e. Type of surgery may be discussed, if there is anticipation of significant adhesion or distortion of anatomy
   f. If a difficult surgery is anticipated consultation with anesthetist and surgeon may be considered
   g. Need of blood transfusion and hysterectomy should be discussed and documented
   h. Maternal morbidity is high.

Q. How do you diagnose and manage bladder injury during cesarean section in a case of repeat or post CS pregnancy?

Ans. Diagnosis of bladder injury:
   a. During surgery, a gush of fluid in the operation field

b. Retrograde instillation of mytheline blue/gentian violet through Foley catheter into the bladder shows leakage of dye
c. In a bigger injury, bulb of Foley catheter can be seen from abdominal cavity

Management:
a. Primary repair is essential to prevent VVF after completion of uterine closure
b. Dissect the bladder from the lower uterine segment with fine scissors or with a sponge on a clamp to free the bladder tissue around the tear for easy mobilization and suturing without tension
c. *Repair:*
   i. Repair in two layers with 3-0 absorbable/delayed absorbable suture
   ii. Suture the bladder mocosa and bladder muscle
   iii. Invert the outer layer over the first layer of suture by reapproximation of bladder muscularis
   iv. Test of repair by introducing sterile color dye in the Foley's catheter into the bladder
   v. Continuous bladder drainage for 7–10 days.

ANTEPARTUM HEMORRHAGE (APH)

Placenta Previa

Q. What are the causes of APH?

Ans. Causes of APH are:
a. Placenta previa
b. Abruptio placentae
c. Marginal
d. Cervicitis
e. Trauma
f. Vulvovaginal varicosities
g. Genital tumor
h. Hematuria (Misdiagnosis)
i. Vasa previa.

Q. What is APH?

Ans. APH is bleeding per vagina or into the vagina after 20 weeks of gestation, but prior to the birth of baby.

Q. What is placenta previa?

Ans. Placenta that is inserted, at least in part, in the lower uterine segment is called placenta previa.

Q. What are the causes of placenta previa?

Ans. Exact cause is not known. Factors responsible for placenta previa are:
a. Age—old age
b. Parity—multiparous

c. Dropping down theory—fertilized ovum implants in LUS instead of UUS
d. Defective decidual basalis due to manual removal of placenta, endometrial ablation, previous D and C, or MTP
e. Big placenta
f. Previous scar for LSCS
g. Uterine anomalies
h. Fetal malpresentation.

Q. What are the types/grades?

Ans. *Types/Grades*:
a. I: Placenta is in the lower uterine segment, but the edge does not encroach on the internal cervical orifice of the uterus (os).
b. II: The placental edge reaches, but does not cover the internal os. It may Type II anterior or type II posterior.
c. III: The placenta partially or asymmetrically covers the internal os.
d. IV: The placenta covers wholly the internal os.

Q. What are the clinical prospects of placenta previa?

Ans. *Symptoms*: Painless, causeless, recurrent and bright red bleeding per vagina in late 2nd/3rd trimester.

> **Note**
> Bleeding is due to disruption of placenta at the implantation site in the lower uterine segment as it gradually thins in preparation of onset of labor and uterus is unable to contract adequately to stop flow of blood from the open vessels.

Signs:
a. Soft, non-tender, uterus
b. Easy to feel fetus—often high head, breech or transverse lie
c. No fetal distress.

Do not go for P/V examination in ward and double set-up examination is made in operation theater (OT) keeping everything ready for cesarean section. A gentle speculum examination when the patient is inpatient to exclude the causes of local bleeding—cervicitis, polyp, trauma or cervical malignancy.

> **Note**
> Indications of double set-up vaginal examination: (i) USG facilities not available; (ii) USG shows type I and IIA placenta previa; (iii) Inconclusive USG report
> Contraindications of vaginal examination: Profuse bleeding, major degree of placenta previa, contracted pelvis, post CS pregnancy, malpresentation which are indications of cesarean section.

Q. What are the maternal and fetal complications?

Ans. *Maternal*:
a. Hemorrhage—antepartum, intrapartum, postpartum
b. Shock
c. Sepsis

d. Postpartum hemorrhage (PPH):
   i. Non-contractile lower segment
   ii. Placenta accreta
   iii. Partially separated and retained placenta
   iv. Embolism
e. Postoperative morbidity
f. Hazards—due to blood transfusion
g. Postanesthetic complication, as CS rate is high.

Fetal:
Prematurity, anemia of fetus, hypoxia, abnormal fetal presentation, congenital anomalies, respiratory distress syndrome (RDS) due to prematurity (lungs immature) and anemia.

Q. What are the risk factors of placenta previa?

Ans.
a. Previous CS
b. Multiparity
c. Advanced maternal age
d. Multiple fetuses
e. Erythroblastosis
f. Cigarette smoking
g. Elevated prenatal maternal serum alfa-feto protein (MSAFP) level is at increased risk of previa, and if this level is ≥2.0 MoM at 16 weeks, more chances of late pregnancy bleeding and preterm birth.

Q. How bleeding in placenta previa is controlled spontaneously?

Ans.
a. Thrombosis of open sinus
b. Placental infarction
c. Mechanical pressure by presenting par
d. Uterine muscle acts as ligature.

Q. How do you diagnose placenta previa?

Ans. *Clinical*: As stated before

PV examination (under double setup) in OT: If cervix is partially dilated and placental tissue is felt, which is firm, tough and gritty while blood clot feels soft and friable.

If cervix is not dilated—spongy tissue felt through vaginal fornices. If firm fetal head is felt, rule out placenta previa.

Ultrasonography: By abdominal route, in suspicious cases careful transvaginal approach does not appear to increase the hemorrhage in placenta previa. It can also detect 'placenta free window' of entry during cesarean section of anterior placenta previa.

USG—False positives (5–7%)
a. Dates—be wary in first half of pregnancy. In 63–93% of cases will have normal implantation at term for placental migration/rotation
b. Overfilled urinary bladder induces compression leading to apposition of the lower anterior + posterior uterine walls (cervical length >3.5–4 cm) simulating placenta previa
c. Focal myometrial contraction (myometrial thickness >1.5 cm) in the region of lower uterine segment.

USG—False negative (2%)
a. Obscuring fetal head—remedied by trendelenburg position/gentle upward traction on fetal head
b. Lateral position of placenta previa, remedied by obtaining oblique scan
c. Blood in the region of internal os is mistaken for amniotic fluid.

MRI may also be used with some success in identifying morbidly adherent placenta.

Q. Management (placenta previa without bleeding).

Ans. Placenta previa diagnosed at 2nd trimester is managed expectantly as follows:
a. Assurance of spontaneous resolution occur at 90% of cases in later part of gestation
b. Placental location should be reevaluated at 28–36 weeks
c. Prevention of coital activity
d. If placenta previa persists at 32–34 weeks, resolution is uncommon, it persists up to term
e. In the asymptomatic patient, amniocentesis at 34– 36 weeks to assess fetal maturity, if fetus is mature delivery is indicated.

If there is fetal lung immaturity, steroid should be given and delivery timing must be individualized by taking the obstetrical history, GA, lecithin sphingomyelin (L/S) ratio, phosphatidylglycerol, AFI and uterine activity. Beyond 36 weeks, expectant management should not be anticipated to get much benefit for the fetus and mother.

Q. A primigravida admitted at less than or equal to 34 weeks with painless vaginal bleeding per vagina. How do you manage the case?

Ans. Hospital admission is mandatory as the patient bleeds per vagina
1. History and quick examination
2. General examination—pallor, pulse/respiration/blood pressure (BP) measurement
3. Per abdomen (P/A): Height of fundus, presentation of fetus, size of baby, FHS (present or not)
4. Inspection of vagina to note amount of bleeding, examination of under-garments. Passage of clots, blood trickling up to the toe along the lower limb signifies heavy bleeding (No PV examination in the ward).

If vaginal bleeding is more:
a. Start IV line with Ringer's lactate (RL)/normal saline (NS)
b. Grouping and cross matching of blood and arrangement for blood
c. Mark the height of the uterus
d. Maintain intake and output chart
e. Hb% and urine for albumin is tested.

Then assess:
a. General condition of the patient
b. Presence of severity of bleeding
c. Duration of pregnancy
d. Condition of the fetus

Obstetric Cases

Conservative management:
a. If bleeding is less or diminished
b. Condition of the fetus is good
c. Duration is less than 34 weeks (as mentioned in the question) (Two doses of injection betamethasone 12 (mg) at 24 hours interval for fetal lung maturity).
d. Patient is not in labor
e. Hb is greater than 8 g%.

Active management:
a. Bleeding is heavy, profuse and continuous
b. Condition of mother is deteriorating
c. Fetus is dead or fetal distress in a viable fetus
d. Active bleeding starts during the course of conservative management
e. Gestational age is greater than or equal to 34 weeks.

Q. What is expectant management in placenta previa?

Ans. Expectant management by McAfee-Johnson's regime is now universally accepted to prolong pregnancy and when bleeding is not excessive or there is significant risk of prematurity of fetus.

Indications
a. Good maternal condition (Hb is >10 g%).
b. Gestational age is <37 weeks.
c. Patient is not in labor.
d. No active per vaginal bleeding.
e. Fetus is in good condition clinically or by USG.

Conduction of expectant management
1. Rest in bed until bleeding stops, i.e. physical activity should be restricted.
2. Watch the pad daily to assess per vaginal bleeding.
3. Correction anemia by oral iron or blood transfusion, if necessary to maintain the Hb level ≥10 gm/dL and PCV ≥30%.
4. Blood should be kept ready in blood bank (four bottles).
5. Per vaginal examination usually not done.
6. Gentle speculum examination per vagina 7 days after stoppage of bleeding.
7. DFMC, FHR monitoring, GA, fetal weight (FW), localization of placenta by USG and MRI to exclude the invasion of placental villi to the uterine musculature.
8. Wait and watch policy, even by tocolytics (nifedipine is preferable) with caution.
9. Pregnancy is to be continued up to 37 weeks for better prognosis of baby provided, there is no recurrence of bleeding, if recurrence of bleeding is severe, terminate pregnancy.
10. Steroid therapy, if gestational age is <34 weeks to prevent RDS in newborn.

> **Note**
> Conservative management is discontinued if: (i) recurrent bleeding and blood loss is >500 mL, (ii) Fetal distress or IUFD, (iii) Suspicion of IUGR, (iv) PPROM, (v) Pregnancy has been reached to term or in labor.

Q. How do you do active management?

Ans.
a. Vaginal examination should be done under double set-up condition in OT keeping everything ready for CS, but in severe bleeding, no PV examination is required and go for LSCS directly.
b. Type I or II anterior (mild degree)—ARM with or without syntocinon
c. Type III, IV and II posterior (major degree)—delivery by LSCS.
d. When there is profuse bleeding in minor degree placenta previa inspite of amniotomy with fetal distress.

> **Note**
> In placenta, previa maternal bleeding occurs.

Q. When fetus loses blood?

Ans. In rupture of vasa previa, commonly at the time of delivery or ARM.

> **Note**
> It is very common in pregnancies due to in vitro fertilization and multiple pregnancies.

Q. How do you confirm fetal blood?

Ans.
a. Fetal RBCs—Nucleated on stain
b. Resistant to alkali denaturation (Singer's test—blood become cherry red color) is noted to identify fetal hemoglobin. Apt test may be used to determine maternal and fetal source of bleeding [Mix the vaginal blood with equal parts of 0.25% sodium hydroxide. Fetal blood remains red (Hbf is resistant to alkali); maternal blood turns brown due to alkali hemaglobin].

> **Note**
> In general, fetal bleeding is apparent on fetal heart rate tracing and intervention should not be delayed for APT testing.

Q. How do you diagnose vasa previa?

Ans. It is diagnosed by transvaginal scanning with color Doppler.

Q. What are the risks of vasa previa?

Ans.
a. Bleeding from the fetal vessels (intrapartum and after ARM)
b. Cord compression by presenting part during labor
c. Cord prolapse.

Q. What is the management in case of vasa previa?

Ans. If CTG evidence of fetal compromise is found, immediate CS.

Q. What is dangerous placenta previa?

Ans. Type II posterior placenta previa is the dangerous one.

Q. Why is it dangerous?

Ans.
a. It is difficult to control bleeding. The placenta occupies the hollow of the sacrum. Separation of the placenta occurs at its lower edge.

Obstetric Cases

The presenting part cannot become engaged, so it cannot press the opened maternal sinuses to stop bleeding.

b. Cord compression and cord prolapse may cause fetal Jeopardy.

FOR POSTGRADUATES

Q. What is placenta accreta? Increta? Percreta?

Ans. Abnormal firm attachment of placental villi to the uterine wall with the absence of normal intervening decidua basalis and fibrinoid layer of Nitabuch's membrane. It may be total (involving the total placenta), partial (involving one or more cotyledons) and focal (involving part of single cotyledon).
Increta—Villi invades upto myometrium;
Percreta—Villi penetrate myometrium and perforate serosa.

> **Note**
> *If central placenta previa does not bleed during pregnancy, think of adherent placenta*

Q. Risk factors of placenta accreta.

Ans. Placenta previa, previous CS, advanced maternal age, placental location with respect to uterine scar, multiparity, previous uterine curettage, and previous myomectomy, manual removal of placenta, adenomyosis, increasing parity.

Q. What are the sonographic findings of placenta accreta?

Ans.
a. Loss of the normal retroplacental hypoechoic zone.
b. Thinning or the disruption of the hyperechoic interface between the uterine serosa and the bladder.
c. Intraplacental vascular lacunae are irregularly spaced.
d. Loss of normal venous flow pattern of the peripheral placental margin and turbulent blood flow through the placental lacunae in Doppler.

Q. Describe management of placenta accreta.

Ans. If single cotyledon is involved it may be torn from the uterine wall and bleeding can be controlled by oxytocics. When large part of placenta is involved the safest treatment is hysterectomy.

Conservative approach:
Maintenance of IV line with RL or blood transfusion according to the conditions:

a. Ligation of the uterine and ovarian arteries and separate the placenta.
b. Angiographic embolization of pelvic arteries with gelatin sponge particles or sponge coil provide another option (in a very sophisticated hospital).
c. Placenta if left *in situ*, systemic methotrexate therapy. This approach is preferable for those who want:
  i. Future fertility

ii. Hemodynamically stable patient
   iii. Understand and accept the risk of delayed hemorrhage and infection.
  d. Bilateral internal iliac artery ligation (BIL) can also be tried before hysterectomy.

Definitive approach:

Hysterectomy/cesarean hysterectomy is the procedure of choice (90%) in uncontrolled hemorrhage and during or after surgery following measures are taken.
  a. Blood product replacement should be guided by hematocrit value, platelet count, coagulation study.
  b. Packed red blood cell (PRBC), when hematocrit is lesser than 25%, ideally hematocrit value of greater than 30% should be maintained.
  c. Massive hemorrhage coupled with aggressive blood and fluid replacement may deplete platelet and clotting factors which may cause (DIC).
  d. Fresh frozen plasma (FFP) transfusion when fibrinogen level is less than 100 mg%.
  e. Platelet transfusion when platelet count is less than 50,000/cubic mm.

Q. What are the sequelae of retained or adherent placenta?

Ans.
  a. Puerperial infection
  b. Subinvolution of uterus
  c. Secondary PPH
  d. Formation of placental polyp.

Q. What are the parameters for diagnosis of placenta previa by transvaginal sonography (TVS)?

Ans. TVS gives following information:
  a. Placental edge less than 10 mm from undilated cervical os at the time of delivery needs cesarean section as they are commonly found in placenta previa.
  b. Placenta greater than 20 mm from the undilated cervical os considered to have normal placenta and is not previa (routine classical management).
  c. Placenta within 10–20 mm from the internal os, however, remains in gray zone. This patient will be benefited from either double set-up examination or close observation and attempt for vaginal delivery (trial of labor), if there is no bleeding.

Q. Which difficulties are encountered during cesarean section in placenta previa?

Ans.
  a. Lower segment is not well fromed before term
  b. May require low uterine vertical incision
  c. Some prefer classical cesarean section which is difficult to repair
  d. Majority prefer lower segment cesarean section
  e. If placenta lies anteriorly:
    i. Ligation of the large dilated vessels by vicryl, if noted

ii. Cut through the placenta and deliver the baby and clamp the cord quickly to prevent fetal salvage
iii. Approach above the margin of placenta to deliver the baby.
f. If placental bed bleeds profusely:
i. Apply hot pack, bed sutures, balloon device, injection ergometrine, intrauterine packing to stop bleeding
ii. Uterine or internal iliac artery ligation can also be tried
iii. Pelvic artery embolization gives good success.
g. If atonicity appears use oxytocics or uterine compression sutures
h. If all measures fail or in cases of placenta acreta hysterectomy should be done.

ABRUPTIO PLACENTAE

Q. What is abruptio placenta?
Ans. Bleeding per vagina or into the vagina after premature detachment of normally situated placenta after 20 weeks of gestational age (GA), but before the delivery of baby.

Q. Causes of abruptio placentae.
Ans. Causes are as follows:
a. Hypertension—chronic or PIH
b. Trauma
c. Preterm labor, PROM, chorioamnionitis
d. Short cord
e. Uterine leiomyoma
f. Sudden uterine decompression due to the delivery of one twin or rupture of membrane of polyhydramnios and thrombophilias
g. Hyperhomocystinemia—Elevated level of homocysteine can cause vascular damage resulting placental abruption.

> **Note**
> 1. Risk factors of accidental hemorrhage—'**VASCULAR**'
>   **V**–Vascular disease+hypertension, **A**–Abruption (previous history), **S**–Smoking, **C**–Cocaine, **U**–Unknown, **L**–Leiomyoma, **A**–Anomaly (fetal malformation), **R**–Reckless driving
> 2. *Indeterminate bleeding (2–5%):* When diagnosis of placenta previa or accidental hemorrhage or any local lesions are not confident to account for per vaginal bleeding. The possible causes of bleeding are: (i) Marginal sinus hemorrhage, (ii) Circumvallate placenta, (iii) Excessive show there is higher incidence of preterm delivery.

Q. What are the different grade of accidental hemorrhage?
Ans. *Grade I:* Normal vaginal bleeding and uterine activity. Normal BP and fibrinogen level, normal FHR.
Grade II: Moderate vaginal bleeding and uterine activity, tetanic contraction may be present, normal maternal BP, elevated PR (pulse rate), fibrinogen level 150–250 mg%. FHR shows fetal distress.

Grade III: Severe vaginal bleeding and concealed hemorrhage, tetanic contraction and uterine pain is present, maternal hypotension, fibrinogen level less than 150 mg%, fetal death and evidence of DIC.

> **Note**
>
> Types: (a) Concealed—retroplacental clot, (b) Revealed—blood escapes through the vagina and blood-stained liquor is revealed, (c) Mixed type—combination of the two.

Q. How do you diagnose accidental hemorrhage?

Ans. Clinical:
   a. Placental bleeding, tender, rigid uterus
   b. Contractions are frequent, tetanic and intense
   c. Baseline uterine tone is elevated
   d. Severe hypertension—PIH or eclampsia
   e. Features of shock may be present
   f. Fetal death in 15% of cases
   g. If fetus is alive—fetal monitoring shows fetal tachycardia, loss of variability, late deceleration
   h. Height of the uterus increases in concealed accidental hemorrhage
   i. Dark amniotic fluid and blood may be observed on amniotomy
   j. USG shows retroplacental hematoma.

Laboratory evaluation:
   a. Anemia (Hb estimation, peripheral blood smear)
   b. Thrombocytopenia (platelet count)
   c. Decreased fibrinogen level
   d. Increased lactate dehydrogenase (LDH) level and MSAFP
   e. Prolonged prothrombin time (PT), activated partial thromboplastinime (aPTT)
   f. Significant proteinuria may be present
   e. Elevated serum transaminase may indicate severe pre-eclampsia and hemolysis, elevated liver enzymes and low platelet count (HELLP) syndrome.

Echogenicity of hemorrhage by USG (poorly sensitive in diagnosis)
- Hyperechoic/isoechoic hematoma (initially is difficult to distinguish from placenta
- Abnormally thick + heterogenous placenta (if blood is isoechoic)
- Hypoechoic/complex collection between uterine wall + placenta in 50% within 1 week (hematoma/placental infarction)
- Anechoic collection within 2 weeks.

> **Note**
>
> A normal USG can not rule out abruption if (a) separation occurs without hematoma, (b) hematoma isoechoic to placenta.

Q. What are the complications?

Ans. Maternal complications are:
   a. Hemorrhagic shock
   b. DIC: low fibrinogen < 300 mg/dL, prolonged PT and aPTT

Obstetric Cases

   c. Renal failure or oliguria—measure urine output by Foley's catheter (N: 30 mL/hr)
   d. PPH: Due to uterine atony or coagulopathy especially with fetal demise
   e. Puerperal sepsis
   f. Maternal death.

Fetal complications are:
   a. Asphyxia due to placental seperation
   b. Intrauterine fetal demise (IUFD) due to prematurity and asphyxia.

Q. Describe management of abruptio placenta.

Ans.
   a. Assess the maternal and fetal condition.
   b. Mother—if features of shock, management of shock.
   c. Rest in bed.
   d. To mark the height of fundus.
   e. IV drip with crystalloid.
   f. Pulse oximetry, if oxygen saturation (SpO_2) is less than 90%, oxygen is administered
   g. Arrange for blood
   h. Blood for Hb%, bleeding time (BT), clotting time (CT), platelet count, fibrinogen, bedside clot observation test, blood for gr and Rh, LFT, and urine for albumin.
   i. *Mild accidental hemorrhage:*
      1. Patient is in labor—ARM with or without syntocinon. If bleeding continues or fetal distress starts—LSCS.
      2. If patient is not in labor—conservative management, if fetus is premature or mother is stable. Perinatal outcome may be improved by delaying delivery 24–48 hours by steroid.
      3. Close observation of mother and careful fetal fetal monitoring by CTG.
      4. If tocolysis is necessary for a short period of 24–48 hours use injection $MgSO_4$.
      5. Adrenergic agonist is contraindicated for:
         i. Fetal tachycardia
         ii. Masking the clinical signs of hypovolemia and anemia.

> **Note**
> *Tocolysis is not strictly contraindicated, tocolytics should be used for a short course in patients with bleeding and uterine contraction provided the patient is stable, the abruption appears to be limited, fetal well-being is stabilized, gestational age is preterm and also for a full course of steroid.*

Tocolysis is contraindicated:
   i. If there is deterioration of hemodynamic condition
   ii. Persistent hemorrhage
   iii. Gestational age greater than 34 weeks
   iv. Estimated fetal weight (EFW) greater than or equal to 2,500 g
   v. *Fetal death and fetal distress*: In severe abruption, expedite the delivery.

a. *If cervix is fully dilated*: Forceps or vacuum
b. If vaginal delivery is not imminent go for LSCS
c. In case of intrauterine death (IUD), vaginal delivery is preferable, but not always possible.
d. If maternal status is unstable—correct hypovolemia by NS or blood to maintain adequate perfusion and hematocrit atleast 30% and urine output of at least 30 mL/hour.
e. If vaginal delivery is not possible within a reasonable time (6–8 hours), cesarean section is necessary to avoid coagulopathy. If coagulopathy starts before surgery correct it first and then go for surgery.

In many cases, acute blood loss may lead to coagulopathy which can be prevented, if blood volume is restored promptly by NS or RL, blood and plasma (fresh frozen).

Use of blood or blood product is helpful:
a. Give whole blood to replace clotting factors and RBCs
b. Fresh-frozen plasma to replace clotting factors (15 mL/kg BW)
c. Packed red cells to replace red cells.
d. Platelet transfusion, if platelet count is less than $20,000/mm^3$.

> **Note**
> - GA> 34 weeks, patient is in labor–delivery by ARM and syntocinon drip If not contraindicated
> - If patient is not in labor:
>   – Pregnancy is 34 weeks or more—delivery by induction of labor
>   – Pregnancy <34 weeks
>   - Bleeding moderate to severe and continuing- terminate pregnancy
>   - Bleeding mild or stopped—conservative management upto 34 weeks and then terminate pregnancy.

Q. What are the indications of CS in abruptio placentae?

Ans.
a. Fetal distress (matured fetus) without imminent vaginal delivery.
b. Severe abruption threatening the life mother.
c. Failed inuction of labor.
d. Urine output is consistently decreasing.
e. Hemodynamicaly unstable.

> **Note**
> General anesthesia is required for hypotension and coagulopathy, but when coagulation profile is corrected regional anesthesia may be used.

Q. What is Couvelaire uterus and what is the management?

Ans. It is diagnosed during CS. Uterus is dark, port-wine color, which may be patchy or diffuse. Subperitoneal petechial hemorrhage is found under the visceral peritoneum. There may be free blood in the peritoneal cavity or broad-ligament hematoma. The myometrial hematoma rarely interferes to the uterine contraction and this is not an indication of cesarean hysterectomy. It is managed by conservative management.

Obstetric Cases

Q. What are the postoperative complications related to mother?

Ans. Acute renal failure (ARF), acute respiratory distress syndrome (ARDS), severe hypotension causes infarction to anterior pituitary (Sheehan's syndrome), infection and PPH.

Q. What are the causes of DIC?

Ans.
a. Massive hemorrhage and massive blood transfusion (dilutional coagulopathy)
b. Abruptio placentae, IUFD
c. Septic abortion or sepsis
d. Missed abortion
e. Pre-eclampsia/HELLP not associated with thrombocytopenia
f. Amniotic fluid embolism.

Q. What is the mechanism of DIC?

Ans. Activation of coagulation cascade by the presence of large amount of tissue phospholipid is the most common stimulus for DIC. The basal phospholipids contribute to the utilization of large amount of clotting factors and lead to consumption coagulopathy. Once the wide coagulation has taken place the lysis process starts. The degradation of fibrin produces fibrin split products or fibrin degradation products (FDPs). FDPs when present in large amount contribute to bleeding by inhibiting fibrin cross–linking and produce platelet dysfunction.

Q. How do you diagnose DIC?

Ans. *Clinical:*
a. Bleeding from incision site or mucus membrane and from other site also
b. Profuse vaginal bleeding and firm uterus
c. Shock may be out of proportion to blood loss.

Investigation: Blood (Table 10.6)

Table 10.6: Investigation of blood for DIC	
Increased	**Decreased**
FDP, D-dimer	Fibrinogen
PT/INR, BT	Antithrombin III
APTT occasionally	Hematocrit and Hb%, Platelets
Bilirubin	
Peripheral smear: Schistocytes, non-clotting blood.	
Notes: The risk of developing fetal hemorrhage is dependent on factors known as 'triad of death' in trauma literature: Coagulopathy (International Normalized Ratio [INR'] >1.5), acidosis (pH ≤7.2), and hypothermia (T°<35°C)	

$$INR = \left\{ \frac{PT_{pt}}{PT_{ref}} \right\}^{ISI}$$

INR: International normalized ratio
PT_{pt}: Prothrombin time of patient
PT_{ref}: Prothrombin time of reference sample
ISI: International sensitivity Index.

Q. What are the treatment of DIC?

Ans.
- Massive hemorrhage—treatment of the underlying cause (uterotonic agents, repair of lacerations)
- Placental abruption—delivery, vaginal route is preferred
- PIH/HELLP—delivery
- Acute fatty liver—delivery
- Amniotic fluid embolism—CVS support and steroid (CVS-Cardiovascular system)
- Sepsis—broad-spectrum antibiotics
- Retained dead fetus—delivery vaginally and antibiotics.

Blood component therapy:
1. Fresh frozen plasma (FFP)— volume 250 cc to correct activated partial thromboplastin time (APTT), PT and fibrinogen level.)
2. Cryoprecipitate—(35–40 cc), if fibrinogen level is less than 100 mg/dL
3. Platelet—transfusion, if platelet count is less than 20,000/mm^3 without bleeding or platelet is less than 50, 000/mm^3 in the presence of bleeding.
4. Packed RBCs—increases oxygen carrying capacity, increases hematocrit greater than 25%, less reaction, less volume overload.
5. Discorded therapies—1. Fibrinogen, 2. Epsilon Amino Caproi Acid (EACA), 3. Heparin, 4. RBC concentrate.

FOR POSTGRADUATES

Q. What is thrombophilia?

Ans. A number of conditions that predisposes to vascular thrombosis. It includes both inherited and acquired disorders of hemostasis. Universal screening for thrombophilia is not recommended, unless there is personal and family history of venous thromboembolism (VTE).

Q. What are the different causes of thrombophilia?

Ans. Inherited thrombophilia:
 a. Protein C and S deficiency
 b. Anti-thrombin III deficiency
 c. Leiden mutation
 d. Prothrombin gene G 20210A variant
 e. Homocystinuria
 f. Hyperhomocystinemia.

Acquired thrombophilia:
 a. APLAS
 b. Myeloproliferative disease
 c. Malignancy
 d. Paroxysmal nocturnal hemoglobinuria
 e. Nephrotic syndrome.

Obstetric Cases

Q. What are the risk factors of thrombophilia?

Ans.
a. Parity >4
b. Maternal age >35 years
c. Prolonged immobility
d. Pre-eclampsia
e. Operative or difficult instrumental delivery
f. Previous thromboembolism.

Q. Which factors are to be noted for thrombophilias?

Ans. Anticardiolipin antibodies, lupus anticoagulant, protein C and S deficiency, antithrombin-III deficiency and the genetic cause (factor V Leiden mutation), also known as activated protein C resistance (APCR), methylene tetrahydrofolate reductase (MTHFR) mutation and the prothrombin 20210A gene mutation as well as the rare congenital dysfibrinogenemia.

Q. How hyperhomocysteinemia causes thrombophilia?

Ans. Homocysteine is metabolized from methionine and again remethylated by MTHFR to methionine. The enzyme MTHFR converts 5,10 -MTHF to 5-MTHF which donates its methyl group to cobalamine (B_{12}) forming methyl cobalamine. Methionine synthetase catalyzes the donation of a methyl group from methylcobalamin to homocysteine, converting it to methionine (Figure 10.19).

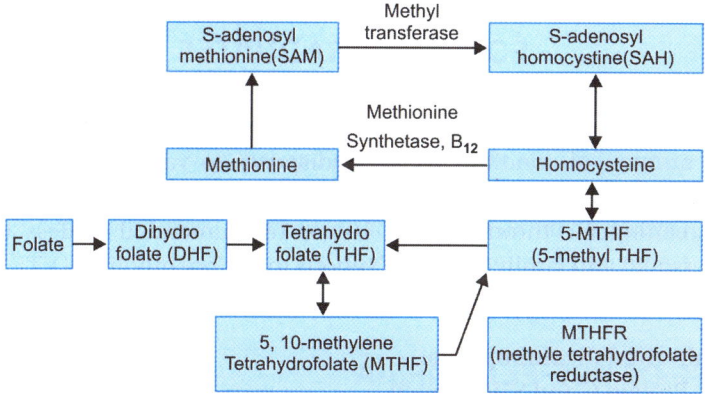

Figure 10.19: Mutation of MTHFR

Mutation of MTHFR gene prevents normal remethylation, which leads to increased levels of homocysteine, and causes vascular damage of endothelium. In placental abruption, when definite cause is not known, this factor should be considered and investigated.

Four fundamental mechanisms of vascular disease are:
a. Thrombosis
b. Oxidative stress
c. Apoptosis (genetically based programmed cell death)
d. Cellular proliferation.

Q. What is Virchow's triad for thrombosis?

Ans.
a. Venous stasis
b. Hypercoagulable state
c. Vascular inhury.

Q. How do you treat hyperhomocysteinemia?

Ans. This condition is treated by L-methyl folate and vitamin B_{12}.

Q. What are the effects of thrombophilia in pregnancy?

Ans. It causes placental abruption, IUFD, Fetal growth restriction (FGR), recurrent miscarriage.

Q. How do you treat a case of thrombophilia?

Ans. It is treated by unfractionated heparin (UFH), low molecular weight heparin (LMWH), aspirin, folic acid and vitamin B_{12}. LMWH is good, as it has less side effect than UFH and follow-up is not strictly needed as in UFH (Table 10.7).

Table 10.7: LMW heparin dose schedule		
LMWH	**Therapeutic dose**	**Prophylactic dose**
Dalteparin	100 U/kg twice daily	5000 U daily
Enoxaparin	1 mg/kg twice daily	40 mg daily
Tinzaparin	175 IU/kg daily	75 IU/kg daily

Q. What are the advantages of LMWH?

Ans.
- Greater bioavailability
- More predictable dose-response profile
- Longer half-life allowing dosing once or twice daily
- No necessity to monitor anticoagulant effect with aPTT
- Decreased incidence of heparin-induced thrombocytopenia
- Decreased incidence of hemorrhagic complications
- Decreased incidence of heparin resistance.

A CASE OF PRE-ECLAMPSIA

(Relevant questions of eclampsia are included)
(Recording of BP and urine protein detection are very essential to establish pre-eclampsia in the examination)

Summary

A primigravida aged 25 years with no complaints at the present pregnancy of 9 months. She is a unbooked case.

O/E: Pallor (+), edema ++, BP 160/100 mm of Hg, urine albumin (+) and obstetrically gestational age is 36 weeks, cephalic presentation, FHS +, adequate amount of liquor.

Per vaginal examination should be done for postgraduate examination.

Diagnosis

A case of 36 weeks of pregnancy with a live baby in mild pre-eclampsia.

> **Note**
> If BP is raised (≥140/90 mm of Hg); and protein is absent in urine, diagnosis should be hypertensive disorderes of pregnancy (HDP).

Case Discussion

Q. What is pre-eclampsia?
Ans. It is a syndrome characterized by hypertension (BP 140/90 mm of Hg or greater on two occasions 4 hours apart) with edema (not essential feature) and proteinuria in pregnancy after 20 weeks of gestation in previously normotensive women.

Features:
BP≥140/90 mm of Hg; urinary excreation of protein of 0.3 g or more in 24 hours urine specimen or 1+ (0.3 g/L) on urine dipstick; or a protein/creatinine ratio (PCR) is ≥0.3 mg/dL.

> **Note**
> In the absence of proteinuria, new onset hypertension with thrombocytopenia (less than 100,000 platelets/mL) or renal sufficiency (serum creatinine concentration >1.1 mg/dL) or impaired liver function (transminase twice the upper limit of normal concentration) constitute diagnostic criteria of pre-eclampsia.

Q. What are the conditions where pre-eclampsia starts early?
Ans. Hydatidiform mole, multiple pregnancies, hydramnios.

Q. What are the predisposing factors of pre-eclampsia?
Ans. Predisposing factors of pre-eclampsia are as follows:
   a. Elderly primigravida
   b. Grand multipara
   c. Pregnancy complications like hydatidiform mole, multiple pregnancies, acute hydramnios, Rh-incompatibility
   d. Medical diseases—hypertension, diabetes, malnutrition, obesity, thyroid disease, presence of antiphospholipid antibody (SLE), thrombophilia, hyperhomocysteinemia, chronic renal diseases.

Q. What is the most constant feature of pre-eclampsia?
Ans. Hypertension is the most constant feature of pre-eclampsia.

Q. What is significant proteinuria?
Ans. Presence of protein in the 24 hours urine of more than 300 mg (0.3 g) or more than 0.3 g/L in 2 or more specimen obtained 6 hours apart. ACOG (2013) gives least importance to proteinuria and showed that maternal and perinatal outcome and delivery decession do not depend upon the amount or change in amount of protein in urine.

Q. How do you predict pre-eclampsia?

Ans. *Clinical tests*

a. Mean arterial blood pressure (MABP) = $\dfrac{SBP + (DBP \times 2)}{3}$

   If MABP is greater than 90 mm of Hg in second trimester, it is predictive.
b. *Roll over test*: Blood pressure is measured in left lateral and supine position at 28–32 weeks. If the difference of diastolic reading is greater than 20 mm of Hg, it is considered as positive.
c. *Hand grip test*: This involves holding of blood pressure cuff in hand to measure BP at 200 mm of Hg for 3 minute and then reassess the DBP. If the rise is greater than 20 mm of Hg, it is taken as positive.

Biochemical tests

a. *Microalbuminuria*: Urinary albumin excretion of more than 30 mg/24 hours at 18 weeks.
b. Hypocalciuria: Reduced calcium excretion in urine less than 195 mg in 24 hours urine collection is a good predictor of pre-eclampsia in later pregnancy.
c. *Calcium-creatinine ratio*: False positive rate is 33% and false negative rate is 4%.
d. *Plasma fibronectin*: It is found to be elevated in both pre-eclampsia and eclampsia in 1st trimester.

Renal tests

a. *Uric acid*: Serum uric acid is raised in pre-eclampsia. In mild variety, it ranges from 4.5–5.0 mg/dL while in severe pre-eclampsia it varies from 4.8–7.8 mg/dL and raised uric acid level in last trimester is a poor indicator of fetal outcome.

   It results from diminished glomerular infiltration, increased tubular reabsorption and decreased secretion
b. *Urea and creatinine levels*: Raised plasma urea and creatinine in presence of normal uric acid indicates renal impairment.
c. *Urinary Kallikrein and creatinine ratio*: This ratio at a random urine sample between 16 and 20 weeks of GA is of predictive value for the diagnosis of pre-eclampsia.

Hematological tests

Hb percent, hematocrit, RBC morphology, platelet count and coagulation profile were tested, but hyperferritinemia in PIH could be a reflection of placental damage.

USG tests

Umbilical artery systolic/diastolic (S/D) ratio and diastolic notch have proved to be useful for PIH. Diastolic notch at 20–24 weeks in uterine artery is presently the most helpful test.

Hormone tests

Higher level of prolactin is found.

Cytokines

Oxidative stress markers such as glutathione peroxidase (GPx), superoxide dismutase (SOD), malondialdehyde (MDA) plays a significant role in the pathophysiology of pre-eclampsia.

Obstetric Cases

New markers

Inhibin-A, Activin-A, β-HCG, PlGF, VEGF increases 5 weeks before the clinical onset of disease. Using multivariate analysis, it is seen that the best predictor of preterm and term pre-eclampsia are soluble endoglin + soluble fims like-tyrosine kinase-1 (S-endoglin +sFlt-1) which inactivate circulating free placental growth factor (PlGF) and vascular endothelial growth factor (VEGF) concentrations leading to endothelial dysfunction.

> **Note**
>
> For screening of pre-eclampsia
> **Pro-angiogenic factors:**
> - Vascular endothelial growth factor (VEGF)
> - Placental growth factor (PlGF)
>
> **Anti-angiogenic factors:**
> - Soluble fims like tyrosine kinase-1 (sFlt-1)
> - Soluble endoglin (sEng)
>
> **Remodelling of spiral arteries:**

Q. What is gestational hypertension?

Ans. Hypertension of 140/90 mm of Hg or more on two occasions 4 or more hours apart after 20 weeks of GA or during the first 24 hours postpartum without protenuria or other signs of pre-eclampsia. The BP should come down within 12 weeks following delivery.

Q. How do you differentiate pre-eclampsia and gestational hypertension?

Ans. Comparision of gestational hypertension and pre-eclampsia (see below).

Features	Pre-eclampsia	Gestational hypertension
Development	After 20 weeks	After 20 weeks
Duration	Upto 4–6 weeks postpartum	Disappears within 12 weeks of postpartum period
Diagnosis	Antepartum	Final diagnosis is made 12 weeks after postpartum
Proteinuria	• Present (300 mg or more in 24 hours or persistent) • 1+ or more on dipstick random sample	Absent

Q. What is 'white coat' hypertension?

Ans. Blood pressure is elevated in the office but outside record are normal. Forty percent of such cases will progress to gestational hypertension later in pregnancy and proteinuric pre-eclampsia in 8% of cases.

Q. What is gestational edema?

Ans. Demonstrable pitting edema over the ankle greater than 1+ after 12 hours of bed rest or gaining weight of 2 kg or more in a week due to pregnancy.

Q. What are the causes of swelling of feet?

Ans. a. Physiological
b. *Pathological*: Pre-eclampsia, eclampsia, severe anemia, CCF, nephrotic syndrome, severe malnutrition, hypoproteinemia, orthostatic edema.

Q. How do you classify the edema?

Ans. a. Minimal edema of pedal or pretibial area (+)
b. Marked edema of lower extremities (++)
c. Edema of face, hand, lower abdomen and sacrum (+++)
d. Anasarca with ascites (++++).

Q. What is gestational proteinuria?

Ans. It is the presence of protein > 0.3 g in 24 hours urine during or under the influence of pregnancy in absence of hypertension, edema or renal infection.

Q. Why proteinuria occurs in pre-eclampsia?

Ans. Spasm of afferent glomerular arterioles leading to anoxic damage of endothelium of glomerular tuft increases capillary permeability, and leakage of protein. Tubular reabsorption is simultaneously decreased. Glomerular filtration rate is also decreased.

> **Note**
> In glomerular capillary endotheliosis, the endothelial cells are swollen and their fenestrate narrowed and the pedicles emanting from podocytes are narrowly spaced causing protenuria.

Q. How do you test protein in urine?

Ans. a. *Heat acetic acid test*: Two-third of the test tube is filled with urine. The upper part of urine is heated and becomes turbid. Then add 5–10% of acetic acid and if turbidity is dissolved then it is due to the presence of phosphate and if turbidity persists and reappears, then it is due to protein.
b. *Albustix test (Reagent strips)*: It is dipped in urine. Wait for 1 minute and color is matched against the standard to determine the presence of albumin (+, ++, +++).
c. *Measurement of proteinuria*: Dipstick is used for screening of proteinuria
   1. *Negative*: 0 mg/dL
   2. *1+*: 30–100 mg/dL
   3. *2+*: 100–300 mg/dL
   4. *3+*: 300–1000 mg/dL
   5. *4+*: >1000 mg/dL.
   When urinary dipstick proteinuria ≥ 2+ and, even if tests 1+ it needs to be evaluated completely.
d. *Esbach's test*: For quantitative estimation of protein in urine.
Methods: If urine is alkaline, render it acdic by acetic acid, filter if hazy, and dilute urine, if specific gravidity is high (>1024). The result obtained with diluted urine should be multiplied by dilutional factor (2) to obtain the actual value in undiluted urine.

Obstetric Cases

Fill the Esbach's albuminometer tube with urine upto mark 'U', pour the reagent (Esbach's reagent) upto 'R'. Put the rubber cork at open end and invert it several times to ensure through mixture. It is then kept in vertical position at room temperature for 24 hours and then read the level of precipitate. Graduation at the end of albuminometer represents dry albumin in g/L of urine.

(*Esbach's reagent*: Boiling picric acid—1 g; Citric acid—2 g in 20 mL of diluted water, cool and make upto volume 100 mL).

> **Note**
> *Protein: Creatinine ratio (PCR) is a better test than 24 hour urine measurement.*

Q. Classify hypertension in pregnancy.

Ans. **I. Pregnancy-induced hypertension (PIH):**
  a. *With edema and or proteinuria*:
    1. Pre-eclampsia
    2. Eclampsia
  b. *Without edema and proteinuria*: Gestational hypertension.

II. Chronic hypertension in pregnancy:
  a. Essential hypertension
  b. Renal hypertension
  c. Coarctation of aorta
  d. Pheochromocytoma
  e. Thyrotoxicosis.

III. Hypertension worsened by pregnancy:
  a. Superimposed pre-eclampsia: Exacerbation of hypertension and new onset of proteinuria as symptoms of headache, epigastric pain and elevated liver enzyme appears
  b. Superimposed eclampsia.

> **Note**
> *Hypertension in pregnancy is diagnosed as chronic, if present before conception, or prior to 20 weeks gestation, or if it persists longer than 12 weeks after delivery [SBP is ≥ 140 mm of Hg; DBP ≥90 mm of Hg measured on two different occasions].*

Q. What is clinical classification of pre-eclampsia (PE)?

Ans. Clinical classification of easily onset and late onset pre-eclampsia are as follow:

	Early onset PE (<34 weeks)	Late onset PE (>34 weeks
1	Fetal disorder associated with placental dysfunction	Maternal disorder due to underlying maternal constitutional factors
2	Placental volume reduced	Normal or larger placental volume
3	IUGR	Normal fetal growth
4	Abnormal uterine and UmA Doppler	Normal uterine and UmA Doppler
5	LBW	Normal birth weight
6	Adverse maternal or neonatal outcome	More favorable maternal and neonatal outcome

Q. What is mild pre-eclampsia?

Ans. It is characterized by:
  a. BP >140/90 mm of Hg but <160/110 mm of Hg
  b. Proteinuria >300 mg/24 hours urine but <5 g/24 hours
  c. Asymptomatic.

Q. What is severe pre-eclampsia?

Ans.
  a. BP ≥ 160/110 mm of Hg
  b. Proteinuria > 5 g/24 hours
  c. Oliguria < 400 mL/24 hours
  d. Thrombocytopenia (Platelet is < 100,000/cu mm)
  e. HELLP syndrome
  f. Pulmonary edema
  g. Persistent headache, altered mental status, right upper quadrant pain, epigastric pain, blurred vision.
  h. Progressive renal insufficiency (creatinine level is >1.1 mg/dL or 2-fold increase in creatinine level in absence of underlying renal disease.

Q. Etiopathology of PIH.

Ans. Figure 10.20.

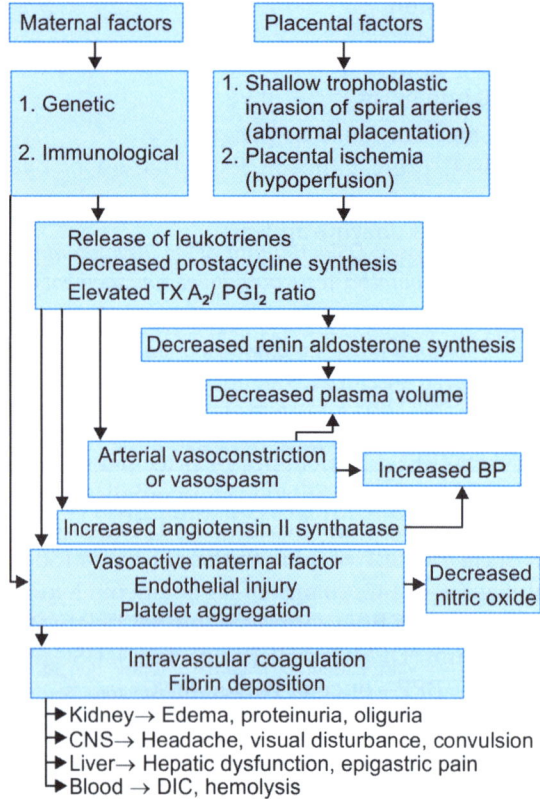

Figure 10.20: Etiopathology of pregnancy-induced hypertension
Abbreviations: TXA2 = Thromboxane A2; BP = Blood pressure; CNS = Central nervous system; DIC = Disseminated interavascular coagulation; PGI_2 = Prostacyclin 2

Obstetric Cases

Q. What is the principle of management of pre-eclampsia?

Ans.
  a. Severity of the disease process (History: persistent headache, visual disturbances, right upper quadrant abdominal or epigastric pain)
  b. Maternal condition:
   - *Physical evaluation*: BP measurement, weight measurement daily
   - *Laboratory evaluation*: CBC (Hematocrit and platelet count, TLC, DLC), LFT (SGOT, SGPT, LDH), 24 hours urine collection at diagnosis for total protein excreation and creatinine clearance or protein/creatinine ratio, coagulation profile like PT (INR), aPTT (if thrombocytopenia), serum uric acid.
  c. Fetal condition—DFMC, NST, BPP, if NST is non reactive and USG for amniotic fluid assessment and Doppler study of umbilical artery, MCA and DV.
  d. Fetal gestational age and fetal growth—by clinical or by USG biometry.
  e. Presence of labor or rupture of membrane.
  f. Antihypertensives and anticonvulsant.
  g. Mode of delivery—vaginal or LSCS.

Q. A primigravida aged 25 years at 34 weeks of pregnancy show a BP of 150/96 mm of Hg with severe degree of edema and 2+ albumins in urine. Outline the management.

Ans. Assess:
  a. DBP 90–110 mm of Hg
  b. Proteinuria ++
  c. No convulsion.

> **Note**
> In carefully selected cases, DBP<100 mm of Hg, asymptomatic with minimal proteinuria, normal laboratory tests, outpatient management is followed.

Management:
  a. Rest and normal diet
  b. No salt restriction
  c. Monitor BP and urinary protein (BP 4 hourly, protein—everyday) and laboratory test (LFT, Platelet once or twice per week), hematocrit.
  d. Do not use sedative, tranquilizers, anticonvulsants and diuretics
  e. Prescribe Methyldopa or labetalol if DBP is greater than or equal to 100 mm of Hg and SBP of more than or equal to 150 mm of Hg. Goal is to stabilize BP to 140/90 mm of Hg and avoid hypotension.
  f. Monitor fetal status by—symphysis-fundal height (SFH), daily fetal movement count (DFMC), FHS (twice daily), USG (3–4 weeks), CTG (twice weekly). BPP—once or twice/week.
  g. Follow-up every 7–10 days regarding laboratory and clinical evaluation
  h. *Plan of delivery*:
   - DBP is controlled to 90 mm of Hg, continue GA upto 37–40 weeks and do not go for postdated pregnancy [Some prefer for continuation of pregnancy upto 37 weeks but not more than that as uteroplacental blood flow is suboptimal after 37 weeks].

- Earlier if, proteinuria worsen? significant IUGR, BP control is unsatisfactory and appearance of fresh symptoms such as frontal/occipital headache, visual disturbances, right upper quadrant abdominal or epigastric pain

i. *Method of termination*:
- Assess for Bishop's score, if the score is favorable (>6) go for induction by ARM and ARM + oxytocin in escalating dose
- If cervix is unfavorable (<6) insert cerviprime gel intracervically, if required two insertions at 12 hours interval
- *Monitoring during labor*:
   - *Progress of labor (POL)*: Descent of the head with uterine contraction
   - Maternal condition is to be noted by appropriate hydration, measuring BP and antihypertensive medication, vigilance for eclampsia, HELLP and abruption
   - Fetal condition by FHS and CTG
   - Second stage of labor is curtailed by forceps, but this traditional concept is no longer true in HDP (hypertensive disorder in pregnancy)
   - No IV injection. Methergine for active management of labor, instead injection oxytocin 5 units IM should be used
- *During puerperium*: Continuous antihypertensive drugs until the DBP < 90 mm of Hg.

Q. How do you manage a case of severe pre-eclampsia?

Ans. All cases of severe pre-eclampsia should be managed actively and symptoms and signs of impending eclampsia (blurring of vision, nausea, vomiting, epigastric pain, hyper-reflexia) should also be managed actively. No scope of expectant management, if maternal and fetal complications are severe (see the answer of the next question) or maternal or fetal condition deteriorates in initial 24–48 hours of observation. Delivery is the only cure by induction of labor (IOL) or LSCS according to the clinical condition.

Assess:
a. DBP greater than 110 mm of Hg
b. Proteinuria^{+++}
c. Reduced urine output
d. Headache, blurring of vision

Management can be done as follows:
a. Hospitalization of the patient
b. Acute BP control by antihypertensive (hydralazine, labetalol, nifedipine, if DBP ≥ 110 mm of Hg) to achieve BP 130–140/90–100 mm of Hg to maintain fetal perfusion
c. $MgSO_4$ for prevention in eclampsia (MAGPIE)
d. Watch for HELLP syndrome
e. *Maternal examination*: Monitor BP, urine output (UOP), cerebral edema, or any impending signs of eclampsia, platelet count, LFT, creatinine level, urine albumin
f. *Fetal evaluation*: Clinically, DFMC, CTG(NST), BPP including liquor volume and UA, MCA Doppler Study

Obstetric Cases

g. If maternal distress, non-reassuring fetal status or PROM and GA greater than 34 weeks—Injection MgSO$_4$ and delivery
h. In case of severe IUGR, give steroid to the mother and delivery
i. • In non-viable fetus if BP is not controlled and GA is <24 or 24–28 weeks—termination of pregnancy (TOP) by prostaglandins (PGs) or oxytocin
   • If GA is 30–32 weeks—counseling is recommended on risks and benefits of prolongation of pregnancy:
      i. Injection of steroid should be given to the mother
      ii. Antihypertensives
      iii. Daily evaluation of maternal and fetal condition–if there is no maternal and fetal jeopardy delivery at 34 weeks.
   • If GA is at 33–34 weeks, give injection of steroid and delivery.
j. Manage actively the IIIrd stage of labor with oxytocin 10 units IM (never methergin)
k. The patient is kept under close observation following delivery:
   • Note for HELLP syndrome after delivery and continue injection MgSO$_4$ for 24 hours as in eclampsia, and PPH if occurs should be managed actively by oxytocin, injection PGF$_2$ alpha and misoprostol due to less intravascular volume
   • If hypertension persists after delivery, continue antihypertensive drugs even after discharge and patient should be seen every week or two as outpatients until they become normotensive (DBP is ≤90 mm of Hg)
   • If hypertension persists after 12 weeks, the diagnosis of chronic hypertension should be considered.
   • Counseling with respect to future pregnancies (next pregnancy should only be allowed if renal functional status is normal and BP is under control).
   • POP, Cu-T, PPIUCD, Injection DMPA may be used to avoid next pregnancy.

> **Note**
> Strict fluid balance (1 mL/kg/hr) is maintained as fluid over load may *cause pulmonary edema and Adult respiratory distress syndrome (ARDS).*

Q. When expectant treatment is indicated in severe pre-eclampsia?

Ans. Expectant management is considered when GA is <34 weeks and there is no evidence of organ involvement, thrombocytopenia, HELLP, symptoms of cerebral irritation, labor, abruption and immediate danger of fetus recorded by NST.

Q. Indications of expedient delivery in severe pre-eclampsia (within 72 hours).

Ans.
a. Hypertension not controlled by two antihypertensive drugs.
b. No growth of fetus within 3 weeks.
c. Absent/or Reversal of diastolic flow on Doppler of UmA
d. Abruptio placentae.
e. Poor BPP (<4 on two occassions at 4 hours interval).

f. HELLP syndrome
g. IUFD
h. Severe IUGR at 34 weeks
i. Convulsion
j. Oligohydramnios and organ involvement
k. Pulmonary edema
l. Deterioration of renal function or oliguria (<0.5 mL/kg/hour) that does not resolve with fluid intake.

Q. Why do you manage hypertension?

Ans. Antihypertensives are used to protect cerebrovascular hemorrhage, hypertensive encephalopathy, eclamptic convulsion and severe pre-eclampsia, if uncontrolled. Other complications such as hypertensive afterload congestive heart failure, placental abruption, and HELLP syndrome can also be minimized by antihypertensive drugs. Current recommendations from NICE guideline (2011) suggests maintaining of blood pressure 130–150/90–100 mm of Hg, but not lowering DBP below 80 mm of Hg. Drugs used for treatment of hypertension (Tables 10.8 and 10.9).

Table 10.8: Medication for severe pre-eclampsia/eclampsia

Medication	Onset of action	Dose
a. Hydralazine (vasodilatation)	10–20 minute	5–10 mg IV every 20 minutes to a maximum dose of 30 mg
b. Labetalol (combined α_1 and β blockers)*	10–15 minute	10–20 mg IV, then 40–80 mg every 10 minutes to a maximum dose of 300 mg or continuous infusion at 1–2 mg/minute
c. Nifedipine (Calcium-channel blockers)	5–10 minute	10 mg PO repeated in 30 minutes, then 10–20 mg every 4–6 hours up to a maximum 240 mg/24 hours

Notes:
*Contraindications: a. Bronchial asthma, b. COPD, c. Severe bradycardia, d. heart block (2° or 3°)
- Advantage of labetalol—enhances fetal lung maturity
- Hydralazine causes tachycardia and palpitation, whereas labetalol causes bradycardia and hypotension but both drugs have been associated with a reduced frequency of fetal heart rate acceleration
- Nifedipine sublingually is no longer recommended as it causes sudden hypotension and may precipitate myocardial infraction.

Q. What are the drugs used for long-term treatment of hypertension?

Ans. See Table 10.9.

Table 10.9: Drugs for treatment for hypertension

Drugs	Starting dose	Maximum dose	Remarks
1. Methyldopa	250 mg bid	4 g/day	Rarely indicated
2. Labetalol	100 mg bid	2400 mg/day	First choice
3. Atenolol	50 mg qd	100 mg/day	Associated IUGR
4. Propranolol	40 mg bid	640 mg/day	To be used with associated thyroid disease
5. Nifedipine	10 mg bid	240 mg/day	Second choice
6. Thiazide diuretics	12.5 mg	50 mg/day	Use only in CCF, not used in PIH for fear of IUGR
7. ACE-inhibitors	Never		

Obstetric Cases

Q. How do you prevent eclampsia?

Ans. Regimen widely used nowadays Inj MgSO$_4$ ['Rule of Four' due to low BW (body weight) of average Indian women].

Loading dose
a. Injection MgSO$_4$, 20% solution 4 g (= 8 mL) over 4 minutes (12 mL normal saline + 8 mL Injection 50% MgSO$_4$ = 20 mL) IV.
b. 8 g Inj MgSO$_4$ solution (4 g in each buttock, deep IM), 50% solution
c. If convulsion occurs after 15 minutes (recurrence of convulsion) then 2 g of Injection MgSO$_4$ (20% solution) IV over 10 minutes (MgSO$_4$, 4 mL of 50% MgSO$_4$ + 6 mL of saline).

Maintenance dose
a. 4 g Injection MgSO$_4$ (50% solution) every 4 hours into alternate buttocks
b. Continue treatment with MgSO$_4$ for 24 hours after delivery or the last convulsion, whichever occurs last Or
c. IV infusion of MgSO$_4$ 1 g/hr [6 g (12 mL) of 50% MgSO$_4$ in 500 mL RL at 20 drops/min (80 mL/hr)].

Before repeat administration of Injection MgSO$_4$, ensure
a. RR is at least 16/minute
b. Patellar reflex (PR) is present, if absent lower Injection MgSO$_4$
c. Urine output is at least 30 mL/hour over 4 hours (Mg^{++} excretes through kidney).

> **Note**
> For Pritchard regime, Zuspan regime, see Chapter 2 (Drugs in obsteteics, magnesium sulfate)

Q. What are the features of Injection MgSO$_4$ toxicity and how do you manage it?

Ans. Clinical:
a. If RR (respiration rate) falls below 16/minute
b. Patellar reflex is absent
c. Urine output <30 mL/hour over 4 hours plasma Mg^{++} level.

Biochemical: Plasma Mg^{++} level and plasma creatinine level (>1.0 mg/mL, adjust MgSO$_4$ infusion rate).

d. Magnesium level and signs of toxicity are as follows:

Plasma level of magnesium (mEq/L)	Signs of toxicity
4–7	Required level of prevention of eclampsia
8–10	Uterine relaxation
>10	Patellar reflex disappears
10–12	Respiratory depression (breathing weakened)
>12	Respiratory paralysis

Management of MgSO$_4$ toxicity
a. Discontinue Injection MgSO$_4$ and obtain serum Mg^{++} level
b. In case of respiratory arrest—assist ventilation by mask and ambu bag and O$_2$ inhalation (Cardiopulmonary resuscitation)

c. Give calcium gluconate 1 g (10 mL 10% solution) IV slowly and repeat the dose, if necessary. It should be given slowly to avoid hypotension, bradycardia and vomiting.
d. Injection calcium chloride 1 g may also be used instead of calcium gluconate.

Note: Contraindication of Injection $MgSO_4$
   a. Renal disorders (Serum creatinine level >1 mg%)
   b. Myasthethenia gravis (Alternate regime: Phenytoin sodium, Diazepam).

> **Note**
> Neonatal side effect of injection magnesium sulfate: hypotension, hypotonia, respiratory depression, lethargy and decreased sucking reflex. Calcium gluconate may be administered to neonate with pediatric consultation, if there is magnesium sulfate toxicity to baby.

Q. How do you deliver the baby in case of severe pre-eclampsia?

Ans. In women with severe pre-eclampsia vaginal delivery is the preferred approach, instead of routine cesarean section. Prophylactic forceps is to be applied to cut short second stage of labor for prevention of maternal exhaustion and intrapartum eclampsia, but this traditional concept is no longer true in hypertensive disorder in pregnancy (HDP) in recent years.

Steps
a. *Assess the Bishop score*: If cervix is favorable (soft, thin, partly dilated), ARM should be done and induce labor by oxytocin.
b. If vaginal delivery is not anticipated within 24 hours for severe pre-eclampsia, CS is the choice.
c. To avoid pulmonary edema, total IV fluid (RL), such as maximum 2.5 L/24 hours (1 mL/kg/hour).
d. If the fetal heart rate (< 100/minute) is abnormal—LSCS.
e. If cervix is unfavorable (firm, thick, os is closed) ripen the cervix by PGE_2 gel or misoprostol; if all measures fail—cesarean section.

> **Note**
> ARM is to be done early to reduce induction-delivery interval. Indications of cesarean sectionin hypertension: a. Severe FGR or reversed end-diastolic flow in Umbilical artery on color Doppler, b. Any obstetrical contraindication of vaginal delivery.

Q. If CS is performed in pre-eclampsia what precautions must be taken?

Ans. a. Coagulopathy is to be ruled out
    b. General anesthesia is helpful but may increase BP during intubation or extubation; if spinal anesthesia is used it may cause hypotension, but safe. So prehydration (IV crystalloid fluid 500–1,000 mL infused by wide bore needle) is essential prior to administration of spinal anesthesia. Vigorus intravenous infusion may develop cerebral edema or pharyngolaryngeal edema.

Obstetric Cases

> **Note**
> Do not use ketamine in pre-eclampsia and eclampsia as it increases blood pressure. Regional anesthesia is safe and has dual benefit—i. Effective analgesia, ii. BP stabilizing effect.

Q. What are the complications of pregnancy-induced hypertension?

Ans. *Maternal complications*:
a. Eclampsia (1–2%)
b. Accidental hemorrhage
c. Renal failure, pulmonary edema
d. DIC, HELLP syndrome
e. Cerebral hemorrhage
f. PPH and shock, maternal death.
Delayed—chronic hypertension (1/3 cases), recurrent pre-eclampsia (25%), renal failure, and impaired cognitive function
Fetal complications:
IUFD, IUGR, asphyxia, prematurity, perinatal death.

Q. If examiner asks you, how do you manage severe pre-eclampsia at ≥36 weeks of gestation?

Ans. No wait and watch policy as the GA is 36 weeks or more. Termination of pregnancy is only the treatment of choice but before that stabilization of the patient is necessary.
a. IV hydration (1mL/kg/hour) to prevent pulmonary edema
b. Urine output is measured by continuous Foley's catheter
c. Use antihypertensive—discussed before
d. Start magnesium sulfate for prevention in eclampsia (MAGPIE) discussed above
e. Blood for CBC (hematocrit and platelet count, TLC, DLC), LFT (SGOT, SGPT, LDH), RFT, coagulation profile like PT (INR), aPTT (if thrombocytopenia) and serum uric acid
f. In coagulopathy, correction of coagulation factors by blood, FFP and platelet concentrates
g. Expedite the delivery by close fetal and maternal monitoring
h. Aim is vaginal delivery—spontaneous or induction of labor by amniotomy or syntocinon or intracervical PGE2 gel (in poor Bishop score)
i. LSCS may be needed in obstetrical indications, uncontrolled BP, induction failure, and fetal distress
j. Maternal monitoring in puerperium.

Q. What is eclampsia?

Ans. Development of convulsion and unexplained coma during pregnancy and postpartum period in patients with signs and symptoms of pre-eclampsia.

> **Note**
> Eclampsia before 20th week of gestation or more than 48 hours postpartum is called atypical eclampsia.

Q. What are the components of typical eclamptic fits?

Ans. a. *Premonitory phase*: Patient is unconscious, twitching of the muscles of face, tongue and eyeballs roll and fixed to one side and duration is 30 seconds.
b. *Tonic stage*: The whole body goes on tonic spasm (duration 30–60 seconds).
c. *Clonic stage*: All voluntary muscles go on alternate contraction and relaxation and duration is 1–4 minutes.
d. *Stage of coma*.

Q. What are the reasons of convulsion in eclampsia?

Ans. a. Cerebral anoxia due to arteriolar spasm
b. Cerebral edema and infarction
c. Cerebral dysrhythmia
d. DIC in cerebral microcirculation.

> **Note**
> *Radiological studies may show evidence of cerebral hemorrhage and edema particularly in posterior hemispheres which may explain the visual disturbances (Figure 10.21).*

Q. Differential diagnosis of eclampsia.

Ans. a. Epilepsy (past history and normal BP)
b. Hysteria
c. Cerebrovascular accident (CVA)
d. Meningitis—stiff neck and fever
e. Brain tumor
f. Metastatic gestational trophoblastic disease
g. Thrombotic thrombocytopenic purpura
h. Cerebral malaria (confimed diagnosis)
i. Other poisioning.

Q. What are the bad signs of eclampsia?

Ans. a. Deep coma
b. Number of fits are greater than 10/day
c. PR greater than 120/minute
d. SBP greater than 200 mm of Hg
e. Temperature greater than 103°F
f. Appearance of jaundice
g. Urine solid on boiling
h. Blurred vision or blindness.

Q. When MRI is indicated in eclampsia?

Ans. Cerebral imaging finding is eclampsia, are similar to that found in pregnancy with hypertensive encephalopathy and it is not necessary for management of eclampsia.
a. Cerebral imaging is necessary in total neurologic deficits or prolonged coma.

b. In atypical presentation of coma:
   1. Onset less than 20 weeks of GA
   2. More than 48 hours of delivery
   3. Eclampsia refractory to MgSO$_4$ therapy.

> **Note**
>
> In MRI, posterior reverse encephalopathy syndrome (PRES) in subcortical and cortical regions of the parietal and occipital lobes is seen frequently in ECl-mothers, but less frequently in pre-eclampsia. It also involves basal ganglia, brain stem and cerebellum.

Q. How do you manage a case of eclampsia?

Ans. Always Institutional management.

Quick history taking/referral card assessment, BP measurement and urine albumin examination and confirm diagnosis within a minute and prompt intervention.

I. General:

First priority of management is to prevent maternal injury and support respiratory and CVS functions, which can be done with the following steps:

1. Assess estimation of airway patency and start IV line with necessary drugs (RL at 60 drops/minute)
2. Ensure maternal oxygenation—4–6 L/minute
3. Bedside rail should be elevated
4. Padded tongue blade in between teeth
5. Aspiration is minimized by keeping the patient in left lateral position and vomits and oral secretion are suctioned as needed
6. Continuous blader drainage by self-retaining catheter.
7. Check for pulmonary edema (basal crepitations) and other complications

Quick investigations: CBC, LFT, RFT, platelet count, serum electrolytes and prothrombin time (PT) and aPTT are essential.

II. Convulsive episodes:

Hypoventilation and respiratory acidosis occurs:

1. In initial seizure—oxygen administration by face musk 8–10 L/minute
2. Transcutaneous pulse oximetry to monitor oxygenation in all eclamptic mothers.
3. Arterial blood gas analysis is required, if the pulse oximetry results are abnormal (O_2 saturation at or below 92%).

Management of convulsion and recurrent convulsion:

Injection MgSO$_4$ therapy

a. Pitchard's regimen
b. Zuspan regime

(See Chapter 2 –Magnesium sulfate)

Management of BP: Nifedipine, labetalol to maintain BP in 140–150/90–100 mm of Hg and BP is assessed every 15 minutes. Lower the BP promptly and slowly.

III. Mode of delivery:

Maternal hypoxemia and hypercarbia causes FHR changes (bradycardia, transient late deceleration, decreased beat-to-beat variability and compensatory tachycardia) and uterine activity include increased frequency and tone.

These changes usually resolve in 3–10 minutes after convulsion and correction of hypoxemia.

The patient should not be rushed for LSCS with this condition, however if bradycardia and late deceleration persists between 10 to 15 minutes despite all resuscitative efforts then a diagnosis of abruptio placentae or non-reassuring fetal status should be considered.

> **Note**
> *Depending on the various parameters, the following options for delivery can be considered:*
> *a. Cesarean section < 34 weeks and patient not in labor and Bishop's score less than 5.*
> *b. Patient's having labor or rupture of membrane is allowed to deliver vaginally in the absence of any obstetric complications.*

When labor is indicated it is initiated by oxytocin infusion or PGs (intracervical gel or misoprostol) with GA > 34 weeks irrespective of Bishop's score and prophylactic forceps during second stage of labor and no injection of methergine should be administered in IV route. Vaginal delivery should be completed by 12 hours of starting convulsion. Actively manage IIIrd stage of labor with 10 units of syntocinon IM within 1 minute of delivery of baby by ensuring the fact that there is no second baby inside the uterus.

IV. Puerperium:

a. After delivery, patient with eclampsia should be watched for vital signs, fluid intake and output and symptoms for 48 hours.
b. Mobilization of extracellular fluid leads to increase intravascular volume, pulmonary edema and exacerbation of hypertension.
c. Injection of $MgSO_4$ should be continued for 24 hours after delivery or 24 hours after last convulsion.
d. If the patient has oliguria (100 mL/4 hours) injection of $MgSO_4$ and rate of fluid administration should be reduced.
e. Labetalol and nifedipine should be used to keep SBP less than 155 mm of Hg and DBP, 100 mm of Hg [Labetalol 200 mg × 8 hourly (maximum dose 2,400 mg/day) and nifedipine 10 mg orally every 6 hours (maximum 240 mg/day)].
f. Instructions for contraception—POP, Inj DMPA, Cu-T to delay next pregnancy.

> **Note**
> *Proteinuria and eye problem ordinarily disappears within 2–3 weeks. Patient is discharged after normal laboratory values and control of hypertension and to return in 1 week for out patient evaluation and counselling of future pregnancy.*

Obstetric Cases

Q. What are the indications of cesarean section in eclampsia?

Ans.
a. A deeply unconscious patient (unless delivery is imminent)
b. All uncooperative patients due to restlessness
c. If vaginal delivery is not possible within 12 hours on the onset of first eclamptic seizure
d. Obstetric indications of cesarean section
e. Fetal distress.

Q. What are the common causes of maternal death in eclampsia?

Ans. Cerebral hemorrhage with hyperpyrexia and coma, pulmonary edema with heart failure, renal failure, DIC, HELLP syndrome, asphyxia due to inhalation of vomits (ARDS), postpartum shock.

Q. Common causes of fetal death in eclampsia.

Ans.
a. Fetal hypoxia due to placental insufficiency
b. Prematurity and its complications
c. FGR
d. Fetal death: Trauma due to instrumental delivery.

Q. Management of HELLP syndrome.

Ans. See the case discussion of jaundice in pregnancy.

Q. How do you manage status eclampticus?

Ans. If repeated convulsion occurs after $MgSO_4$ injection, thiopentone sodium (0.5 g dissolved in 20 mL of 5% dextrose) is given slowly IV in collaboration with anesthetist. If it fails, patient should be shifted to CCU for muscle relaxation and assisted ventilation.

FOR POSTGRADUATES

Q. How do you follow-up and counsel hypertensive disorders of pregnant (HDP) mothers after delivery? What preventive measure do you take for HDP in the next pregnancy?

Ans. Follow-up

Women diagnosed with pre-eclampsia, should receive close follow-up
a. Postpartum care should induce blood pressure surveillance (treatment may need adjusting).
b. Follow-up every week or two as outpatient until the blood pressure normalizes.
c. Patient with hypertension (persisting beyond 6 weeks post delivery), warrant referral to physician and should be designated as chronic hypertension if hypertension persists beyond 12 weeks.
d. *Contraceptive advice*: Better to avoid estrogen containing OCPs in hypertensive and breastfeeding phases. Other contraceptions like POP, Cu-T or long acting reversible contraceptives (LARC) such as, Injection DMPA and implantable progesterone, LNG-IUS, may be used safely but if family completed ligation or vasectomy should be considered.

Counseling
a. 39% of patients with hostory of early onset of severe pre-eclampsia may develop chronic hypertension.
b. Patient with pre-eclampsia are at increased risk of developing pre-eclampsia during subsequent gestation and the risk depends upon the severity of pre-eclampsia as well as gestational age at the onset of index pregnancy.
c. The recurrence rate is 65%, if pre-eclampsia develops in the mid trimester and 20%, if develops at term.
d. The recurrence rate of pre-eclampsia in normotensive group is 19% and the risk of recurrence of HELLP is 3%. Even HELLP may not recur in subsequent pregnancies, but there is high incidence of pre-term delivery, FGR, placental abruption and cesarean delivery.
e. The rate of recurrence of eclampsia is 1–2%.
f. Women with severe pre-eclampsia remote from term may have underlying renal disease for which they should be evaluated after delivery [*Investigations*: Blood–urea, creatinine; *Urine*: Routine and *Microscopy*: Specific gravity, pus cells, albumin, cast, RFT (creatinine clearance test), ultrasound Doppler of kidney and renal artery, *Back-up investigation*: Ophthalmoscopy, antiphospholipid antibodies, anticardiolipin antibodies, lupus cells, LFT]. Also pregnancy when RFT and BP become normal.

Prevention of hypertensive disorder in next pregnancy:
a. Prophylactic low dose aspirin started early in next pregnancy is effective in reducing the frequency pre-eclampsia and is contra-indicted by recent NICE guideline in hypertensive disorder in pregnancy (HDP) (see below).
b. If patient is normotensive following PIH of Index pregnancy, umbilical artery Doppler study is essential for detection of pre-eclampsia in the next pregnancy. Diastolic notching at 23–24 weeks is a good predictor of pre-eclampsia in high-risk women.
c. Proper antenatal check-up and use of drugs such as calcium supplementation, administration of fish oil and evening primrose oil, antioxidant therapy may be tried for prevention of PIH, but not hopeful as the etiology of disease is unknown.

Q. What is the role of aspirin in prevention of pre-eclampsia?

Ans. Low dose aspirin (50–150 mg/day) corrects the prostacyclin/thromboxane A_2 imbalance in pre-eclampsia. Current guidance NICE (National Institute for Health and Care) recommends that low dose aspirin is reserved for high-risk patients who meet selected criteria. If a patient has two moderate risk factors or one major risk factor, clinicians are advised to use 75 mg aspirin from 12 weeks gestation until delivery.

High-risk factors	Moderate risk
Hypertensive disease in previous pregnancy	Primigravida
Chronic kidney disease (CKD)	Age >40 years
Autoimmune disease, e.g. APLAS	Pregnancy interval >10 years
Diabetes mellitus	Family history of preeclampsia
Chronic hypertension	Multiple pregnancy
	BMI>35 kg/m² at booking

Obstetric Cases

Q. What is WHO guideline for prevention of pre-eclampsia by calcium supplementation?

Ans.
- Dosage: 1.5–2.0 g elemental calcium/day
- Frequency: Daily, with the total daily dosage divided into three doses (preferably taken at meal time)
- Duration: From 20 weeks of gestation until the end of pregnancy
- Target groups: All pregnant women, particularly those at higher risk of gestational hypertension
- Settings: Areas with low calcium intake.

Q. What are the changes in fundus occuli in PIH?

Ans. Grade 0—normal fundus
Grade 1—minimal constriction and irregularity of arterioles
Grade 2—arterio-venous nipping, venous narrowing and spasm—the stage of angiospasm
Grade 3—above with edema, hemorrhage and exudates—Retinopathy
Grade 4 — papilledema.

> **Note**
> *Retinal detachment may occur in eclampsia or in chronic hypertensive cases. Blindness from retinal lesions caused by retinal ischemia or infarction is also called Purtscher retinopathy. Permanent blindness is due to a combination of infarctions in the retina and lateral geniculate nucleus bilaterally.*

FOR POSTGRADUATES

Posterior Reversible Encephalopathy Syndrome (PRES)

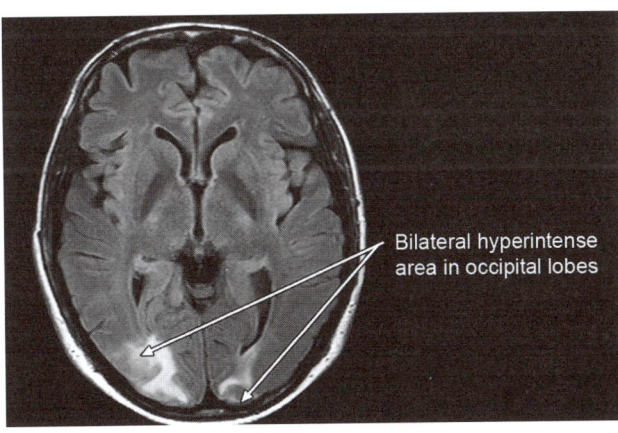

Figure 10.21: MRI showing bilateral hyperintense areas in occipital region

Q. What is PRES?

Ans. PRES is a clinicopathological condition that is characterized by neuro-imaging and non-specific symptoms such as headache, confusion, visual disturbances and seizures.

Q. What is the pathophysiology of PRES?

Ans. It is due to vesogenic edema predominantly in the posterior cerebral hemisphere and reversible with appropriate management.

Q. How do you diagnose PRES?

Ans. Clinicopathological—PRES is common in eclampsia. So BP, ophthalmoscopy, RFT, LFT, serum electrolytes and serum calcium levels measurement are important.

MRI: The typical findings are hyperintensity of FLAIR images in the parieto-occipital and posterior-frontal cortical and subcortical white matters. Less commonly brain stem, basal gangalia and cerebellum are involved. MRI shows bilateral hyperintense areas in occipital region (Figure 10.21).

Prognosis: can good, but irreversible liver damage may occur due to late recognition and incorrect treatment.

Q. How do you treat this condition?

Ans. Acute treatment for cerebral vasospasm is essential

Calcium antagonists
a. Nimodipine reduces cerebral vasospasm and infarction
b. Injection Magnesium sulfate (Pritchard regimes) for 24 hours also reduces cerebral vasospasm

Others:
a. Injection levetriacetum 1 g IV bid for 24 hours
b. Injection Mannitol 100 mL infusion tds for 24–72 hours.

Chronic Hypertension

Q. How do you define chronic hypertension?

Ans. Hypertension occurring before 20 weeks of GA or by hypertension persisting beyond 6 weeks postpartum and SBP of atleast 140 mm of Hg and DBP of atleast 90 mm of Hg on two occasions at least 4 hours apart is called chronic hypertension. The pregnant woman whose prepregnancy BP is not known, the diagnosis of chronic hypertension is very difficult and is based on the presence of sustained hypertension.

> **Note**
>
> *Dilemma of diagnosis: Hypertension occurring before 20 weeks may be the first manifestation of pre-eclampsia and physiologic decrease of blood pressure in healthy pregnant women may occur in first and second trimesters in many patients with chronic hypertension. These patients are erroneously diagnosed as transient hypertension and pre-eclampsia.*

Q. What is the etiology and classification?

Ans. It is a complex disease with genetic predisposition interacting with multiple environmental factors:
a. Primary/idiopathic (90%)

Obstetric Cases

b. Secondary hypertension (10%)
   i. *Renal disease:* Glomerulonephritis, interstitial nephritis, nephropathy, polycystic kidneys, renal artery stenosis, and renal transplant
   ii. *Collagen vascular disease:* SLE and scleroderma
   iii. *Endocrine disease:* Diabetes, pheochromocytoma hyperaldosteronism and throtoxicosis
   iv. *Vascular disease:* Aortic coarctation.

> **Note**
> A SBP of 160 mm of Hg or greater with or without DBP (Korotkoff phase V) of 110 mm of Hg or higher constitute severe chronic hypertension.

Q. What is high-risk chronic hypertension?

Ans. Severe hypertension (SBP ≥160 mm of Hg and/or DBP ≥110 mm of Hg) alone or mild hypertension (SBP ≥ 140 mm of Hg and/or DBP ≥90 mm of Hg) associated with any of the following conditions:
- Renal disease (all causes)
- Cardiomyopathy
- Coarctation of aorta
- Diabetes
- Previous perinatal loss
- Collagen vascular disease
- Previous pre-eclampsia
- Maternal age > 40 years
- Duration of hypertension ≥4 years.

> **Note**
> Pregnant women with chronic hypertension are considered to be at low risk of mild hypertension without any organ involvement.

Q. What are the maternal and perinatal risks?

Ans. Maternal: Abruptio placentae, superimposed pre-eclampsia, HELLP syndrome

Perinatal: Preterm deliveries, small–for–gestational age (SGA) and neonatal intraventricular hemorrhage (IVH).

Q. How do you manage choronic hypertension in pregnancy?

Ans. Management of chronic hypertension should begin before conception. Aim is to reduce pregnancy-related complications and maternal cerebral hemorrhage.
   i. Adverse antihypertensive drugs should be withdrawn before pregnancy.
   ii. History (poor obstetric history, if any) and clinical examination to divide high-risk and low-risk cases.
   iii. The physical examination includes measurement of BP at 4 hours interval, auscultation of any abdominal bruits, evaluation of retinopathy, left ventricular hypertrophy and renal disease.

iv. Investigations:
   a. Fundoscopy, EKG
   b. Blood—Hb%, suger, lupus cells
   c. Urine—proteinuria
   d. Urine collection over 24 hours for protein estimation and creatinine clearance.

> **Note**
>
> *A maternal serum creatinine >1.4 mg/dL at conception is another risk factor for increased fetal loss and progressive worsening of maternal renal disease.*

Categorize the patient in low-risk and high-risk group and manage accordingly.

Management:

Low-risk groups:
a. Complication of accidental hemorrhage and superimposed pre-eclampsia is less.
b. Periodic check-up to evaluate the high-risk factors as low-risk group may be converted into high-risk group during pregnancy
c. 24-hours urine for protein and creatinine clearance.
d. Fetal evaluation by USG for estimation of fetal weight, amniotic fluid volume based on clinical findings and a weekly fetal heart rate testing (NST, BPP), which can be started after 32 weeks.
e. Pregnancy may be continued upto term (41 weeks), if BP is controlled and there is no complications like superimposed pre-eclampsia or FGR.

High-risk groups:
a. Counseling of patients for complications of pregnancy such as accidental hemorrhage, superimposed pre-eclampsia and associated risks of renal insufficiency, diabetes, collagen vascular disease, cardiomyopathy and fetal risks such as SGA, IUD and prematurity.
b. Instruction to receive weight gain and nutrition during periodic check-up.
c. Avoid abuse of smoking, alcohol and caffine which worsens blood pressure.
d. Salt intake should be limited to 2 g.
e. 24 hours urine collection for protein and creatinine clearance in first trimester and later in pregnancy.
f. Fetal evaluation by USG by fetal biometry and amniotic fluid volume every 4 weeks from 26 weeks.
g. Fetal status by BPP, NST from 28 weeks of gestation—twice weekly and is instructed for DFMC.
h. Patient should be hospitalized for severe hypertension or superimposed pre-eclampsia.
i. The time of delivery must be individualized and should not be contimued beyond 40 weeks.
j. Mode of delivery depends upon clinical and obstetrics findings.

Obstetric Cases

Medications:
a. Use antihypertensive drugs when DBP is greater than 100 mm of Hg or higher in high-risk group.
b. In women with low-risk group antihypertensive therapy is recommended if DBP is 105 mm of Hg or higher.

> **Note**
> Antihypertensive drugs are already discussed in pre-eclampsia and it is not clear whether antihypertensive treatment improves maternal and fetal outcome in mild chronic hypertension.

Management in puerperium:
a. Women with high-risk chronic hypertension is more prone to postpartum complications such as pulmonary edema, hypertensive encephalopathy, or renal failure.
b. Complications in puerperium depends upon organ involvement, superimposed pre-eclampsia, abruptio placentae, obesity and long standing hypertension.
c. BP must be closely monitored for 48 hours after delivery.
d. IV labetalol/hydralazine may be used for severe hypertension otherwise oral antihypertensive preparations must be used.
e. Diuretics in association may be used for pulmonary congestion.
f. ACE inhibitors or beta-blockers may be used for sustained myocardial infarction and diabetic nephropathy, better should be avoided.
g. Breast milk is not contraindicated with any medication of hypertensive agents as they have no side effects to neonates.
h. ACE inhibitors and angiotensin receptors blockers should be avoided as they have effect on neonatal renal function though their concentration is low in breast milk.
i. For breastfeeding women with renal disease, calcium-channel blockers are ideal in chronic hypertension.
j. Contraception by POP, IUCD to delay pregnancy.

FOR POSTGRADUATE STUDENTS

A CASE OF HIV IN PREGNANCY

Human immunodeficiency virus (HIV) is a ribonucleic acid (RNA) retrovirus, which encodes an enzyme reverse transcriptase that allows DNA to be transcribed from RNA.

Q. What are the different types of HIV virus?

Ans. There are two different types: HIV-I and II. Type II HIV virus is less common.

Q. Pathogenesis of HIV.

Ans. HIV selectively infect CD4 cluster of differentiation antigens, such as T-lymphocytes and macrophages, which maintain the body's defense mechanism. Within $CD4^+$ cells, these viruses grow and kill them. In the process, these defensive cells rupture, leading to liberations of millions of viruses in the blood stream, which in turn infect first $CD4^+$ cells and kills them. As a result of progressive depletion of $CD4^+$ cells, the immune system is damaged and patient is susceptible to secondary infection by virus, bacteria and fungi.

Q. How HIV infects body?

Ans.
a. Through sexual intercourse
b. Through transmission of blood and blood products
c. By the use of contaminated syringe
d. From mother to infant
   i. Vertical transmission—through the placenta when the fetus is in utero
   ii. Horizontal transmission.

Q. What is the course of HIV infection?

Ans.
a. Progress of HIV is uncertain
b. Half of the patients do not develop serious infection or neoplasm up to 10 years
c. Chances of full blown acquired immune efficiency syndrome (AIDS) is related to:
   1. Duration of infection
   2. Age
   3. Nutritional status
d. $CD4^+$ cells in the peripheral blood as well as antigen testing may be useful in assessing progress.

Q. What is the time of HIV transmission during or after pregnancy?

Ans.
a. Prenatal mother (antenatal factor)
b. Labor and delivery (obstetrical factor)
c. Postpartum (neonatal feeding factor)
d. Infancy (infant feeding).

Q. How do you give antenatal care to HIV pregnant mother?

Ans.
a. Most of the patients are asymptomatic and have no major obstetric problem during pregnancy
b. No need to increase number of antenatal visit provided, there is no complications of the HIV infection
c. Counseling and mental support is an integral part of management
d. Unprotected coitus should be avoided in pregnancy.

Q. How do you examine and investigate HIV-infected mother in pregnancy?

Ans. Full physical examination in first visit:
a. HIV-related opportunistic infections such as TB, oral and vaginal thrush, lymphadenopathy, herpes zoster in a young woman, is an early sign of HIV
b. Other causes of coexistence of sexually transmitted diseases (STIs) such as syphilis increase the number of transmission of virus in vagina and cervical secretion

Obstetric Cases

c. Associated UTI and respiratory tract infection
d. Maternal weight should be monitored
e. Oropharynx should be examined for thrush
f. Clinical diagnosis of vaginitis and cervical inflammation or discharge or STIs should be a priority.

Laboratory Investigations:
1. Venereal disease research laboratory (VDRL) for syphilis, HBsAg for hepatitis B
2. Hb% and complete blood count (CBC) and T-cell subset investigations
3. Repeat Hb test as anemia is more common
4. Cervical smear
5. Colposcopy for abnormal cervical smear
6. CD4 count less than 200 indicates severely immunocompromised state (baseline CD4 count should be recorded before ART).

Investigation of HIV
1. Antibody detection; blood/plasma/serum
2. Antigen detection
3. Viral isolation
4. Other tests:
   a. Detection of p24 antigen (expensive)
   b. Polymerase chain reaction (PCR)
   c. Viral load assay (every 3–4 months).

Q. How do you diagnose HIV positive mother?

Ans. HIV screening is a routine screening during antenatal check-up.
   a. Antibody tests
   b. Screening tests are enzyme-linked immunosorbent assay (ELISA) and rapid test (E/R)
   c. Confirmatory or supplementary test—2nd/3rd E/R to confirm 1st E/R and western blot assay.

All tests are to be done in the same sample.

> **Note**
> Up to six months between infection and seroconversion is possible, although 2 months or less is typical. Patient undergoing screening must be informed of the "window period" and should have testing repeated in approximately 2 months if they had recent high-risk of exposure.

Q. How does baby is infected by vertical transmission?

Ans. Maternal anti-HIV IgG crosses the placenta and remains in neonatal circulation for 12–18 months and is not useful to diagnose in neonates. Testing of the neonates will identify HIV seropositive mothers and identify the infants at risk of HIV. HIV DNA PCR (antigen-based test) and viral culture are used to demonstrate HIV infection in neonates at 6 weeks of age.

Q. Management of HIV mother during pregnancy.

Ans. **I. General antenatal care:**

a. Early registration—8–10 weeks; 4 antenatal check-up (first within 12 weeks; 2nd at 14–26 weeks; 3rd at 28–32 weeks; 4th at 36–40 weeks). History, physical and abdominal examination:

b. Supportive measure

Supplementation of vitamin A
- Iron (100 mg) + Folic acid (0.5 mg) daily for 100 days after first trimester
- Albendazole to use in a case of high hookworm prevalent area
- Malaria causes high maternal and infant morbidity and mortality with increased risk of mother to child transmission of HIV. So antimalarial drug is highly effective in malaria endemic zone. This should be started from the second trimester and given at an interval of not more than one month.
- *Prophylactic treatment of opportunistic infection*
   - TB—ATT drug
   - *Pneumocystitis carinii* pneumonia (PCP)—Sulphmethoxazole/trimethoprim or pentamidine
   - Hepatitis vaccine or pneumococcal vaccine
   - Herpes—acyclovir can be used safely after first trimester
   - Local antifungal agents for any fungal infection.

c. Injection tetanus toxoid–first dose at early registration, 2nd dose after 4-6 weeks of the first dose

d. Blood for Hb%, blood grouping and Rh, VDRL, HbSAg, screen for diabetes mellitus (blood sugar) and USG. Urine routine is to be done in all visits and Hb% is to be rechecked at the third visit (28–32 weeks of gestation)

II. Special care considering her positive status

a. Screening for other genital tract infections in HIV positive mothers should include tests for *Chlamydia trachomatis, Neisseria gonorrhoeae* and bacterial vaginosis.

b. USG for fetal anomalies is important after first trimester exposure of highly active antiretroviral therapy (HAART) and folate antagonists used for prophylaxis of PCP.

c. Plasma viral load and CD4 T-lymphocytes measurement should be reviewed periodically and advice should be given as to the choice of ARV therapy.

III. Strategies to reduce the risks of transmission of HIV from mother to child

Antepartum, intrapartum and postpartum ARV therapy (TDF +3TC +EFV) to the mother till lifelong and postpartum ARV to the newborn after delivery, delivery by elective LSCS and avoidance of breastfeeding can reduce the HIV transmission from 30% to less than 2%, but these are not mandatory in Indian scenario.

Q. Guidelines for starting of ARV therapy during pregnancy (HAART).

Ans. Highly active antiretroviral therapy (HAART) consists of 3/4 drugs regime:

Obstetric Cases

British HIV Association (BHIVA)-2012 guidelines of HAART

1. It advises that women who conceives on HAART, the CD4 count should be measured at least at booking and at delivery.
2. In those who started HAART during pregnancy, a viral load (VL) should be performed at 36 weeks and at delivery. The aim is to keep VL undetectable (<50 copies/mL) at 36 weeks to achieve normal vaginal delivery. HAART should be started early in pregnancy usually after first trimester.
3. See Table 10.10

Table 10.10: British HIV Association (BHIVA)-2012 guidelines of HAART	
VL > 100,000 HIV copies/mL Or CD4 count is < 350 cells/mm³ Or Presence of other co-morbidities	Start immediately
VL > 30,000 copies/mL	Start by 14 weeks
VL >30 000 copies/mL	Start by 24 weeks

HIV resistance testing should be done before initiation of treatment and if a woman books late, this should not delay commencement of treatment.

4. Stavudine and Didanosine should be avoided as a nucleoside reverse transcriptase inhibitor (NRTI) backbone, whenever, possible in pregnancy. Efavirenz can be used safely in pregnancy. The adult prescribing guideline recommend a regimen based on two NRTIs (neucleoside reverse transcriptage inhibitors) plus an NNRTIs (non-nucleoside reverse transcriptase inhibitor) or boosted protease inhibitors to achieve maximum potency, durability, adherence and tolerability and to void long term toxicities and drug interactions.
   HAART in pregnancy are based on zidovudine/lamivudine backbone.
   Ritonavir boosted protease inhibitors (PI) may have risk of preterm delivery.
5. Most clinicians start HAART from below 24 weeks gestation and give neonate prophylaxis, along with advice of exclusive formula feed.

> **Note**
> HAART— Start, AZT + NVP + 3TC or if Hb is <7 g%; use NVP + d4T + 3TC

Q. What is PPTCT? What is the strategy of PPTCT?

Ans. It is the prevention of parent to child transmission of HIV infection. It has 4 prongs of care:
1. Primary prevention of HIV among men and women of child bearing age.
2. Prevention of unwanted pregnancy among HIV-positive women.
3. Prevention of HIV transmission from HIV-infected women to their infants.
4. Provision of treatment, care and support to HIV-infected women, their infant and families.

Q. What are the interventions to prevent transmission of HIV from mother to child?

Ans. Establish HIV status in pregnant women
1. Preconception care—known HIV-infected case and already receiving ART should continue ART as per guideline.
2. Obstetric interventions—In newly detected HIV infection, sent blood for CD4 count and initiate ART (TDF + 3TC + EFV) regardless of WHO staging and CD4 count result. If HIV test is negative in pregnancy—repeat HIV test according to risk factors and window period
   a. Antepartum interventions (continue ART as above)
   b. Intrapartum interventions (continue ART as above)
      i. *Institutional delivery*: It is important prevention for vertical transmission.
      ii. *Mode of delivery*: Elective LSCS is not a standard protocol for prevention of intrauterine transmission. This is because of risks of LSCS in HIV-infected women and wound infection, dehiscence and risk to healthcare workers. National AIDS Control Organization (NACO) recommends normal delivery unless the woman is obstetrically indicated for LSCS.
      iii. *ART therapy TDF + 3TC + EFV*
      iv. *Postpartum interventions*—ART interventions is to be continued as before and thereafter life long Indications of ART in infants: Daily Nevirapine (NVP) from birth until 6 weeks of age, then stop (irrespective of choice of infant feeding). Exclusive breastfeeding or exclusive replacement feed are recommended.

Q. ARV prophylaxis (monotherapy) in PPTCT.

Ans. *Two indications*:
   a. To improve the health of mother
   b. Prevention of HIV transmission.

Nevirapine (NVP) NACO guideline, GOI (Government of India): Previous protocol:

Mother—orally single dose, NVP—200 mg at the onset of labor or 4 hours before elective CS, if in any case the patient vomits within 30 minutes or baby is not delivered within 4 hours of the drug ingestion, the same dose is to be repeated for the second time.

Baby syrup—NVP 2 mg/kg should be given within 72 hours of delivery (single dose). This regimen was found to decrease the risks of transmission to 13.1% in women who breastfed their babies.

If the woman delivers within 2 hours of administering NVP, then baby needs syrup NVP 2 mg/kg soon after delivery and a second dose at 72 hours of age.

If the woman gets NVP and the labor turns out be false labor, there is need to repeat NVP, only if she does not deliver in the next 7 days.

However, the National guideline has been revised from 1st January, 2014 and it is recommended that:
   a. All HIV pregnant women should be initiated on ART (on triple ART) lifelong regardless on WHO clinical staging or CD4 cell count

b. ART should be initiated in ART centre and should not be delayed for want of CD4 cell count report. All HIV-infected pregnant women should start ART through pregnancy, delivery, breastfeeding period and thereafter lifelong. If the pregnant mother comes late (after 36 weeks of gestation, start ART promptly).
The first line of treatment is fixed dose combination.
Tenofovir (TDF)—300 mg + Lamivudine (3TC)—300 mg + Efavirenz (EFV)—600 mg, if there is no prior exposure to NNRTIs (NVP/EFV) at any gestational age.

Q. Regime, if the pregnant woman is unable to tolerate what will be the alternate of first line regime?

Ans. First line regimes and alternative regimes are as follows:

First line ART	Preferred first line regime	Alternate first line regime
HIV-positive Pregnant women	TDF + 3TC + EFV	AZT + 3TC +EFV AZT +3TC + NVP TDF + 3TC + NVP

Q. What is the safety of EFV?

Ans. It is evidence-based that EFV has been recommended for use in pregnant women in all trimester of pregnancy including first trimester without any major side effect to mother and fetus.

Q. Which ART regime you will choose for pregnant women having prior exposure to NNRTIs for PPTCT?

Ans. HIV-infected pregnant women who have standard exposure to NVP (EFV) for PPTCT prophylaxis in prior pregnancy, an NNRTI-based ART regimen like TDF+3TC+EFV may not be fully effective due to persistence of archived mutation of NNRTIs. Thus the women may require protease inhibitor-based ART regime.
TDF + 3TC +LPV/r(Lopinavir/ritonavir)
The dose will be TDF +3TC (1 tablet daily) + LPV (20 mg)/r (50 mg) (2 tablet BD)
- Baby syrup—AZT 2 mg/kg for 6 weeks.

Q. When will you start antiretroviral therapy and what is the regime?

Ans. Previous NACO guideline was:
- ART was indicated for maternal health with clinical stage 3 and 4 diseases.
- *Stage 3*: Persistent diarrhea, weight loss greater than 10%, fever, Kaposi's sarcoma (KS) alveolar pneumonia, labial or genital herpes, oral candidiasis, oral hairy leukoplakia, pulmonary TB.
- *Stage 4*: PCP, toxoplasmosis, KS

Mother:
- CD4 less than 250—AZT + 3TC (Lamivudine) + NVP (start any time)
- CD4 250 to 300—AZT + 3TC + EFV (Efavirenz) start after first trimester
- Baby—AZT syrup 2 mg/kg BW × 4 weeks

Regular clinical follow-up of mother and baby should be done with regular counseling.

According to NACO guideline, 2014, all HIV pregnant women should be initiated on ART (on triple ART as stated before) lifelong regardless on WHO clinical staging or CD4 cell count.

In pregnancy due to hemodilution, CD4 cell count decreases. After delivery body fluid change normalized to the nonpregnant state and CD4 level rises by 50–100 cells/UL.

So, a decrease in CD4 count in pregnancy receiving ART in comparison to CD4 cell values prior to pregnancy may not necessarily indicate immunologic decline and should be interpreted with caution.

However, it is important to obtain blood CD4 sample for baseline tests before initiating ART, but initiation of ART should never be delayed for want of CD4 test results.

Women who are found HIV positive during labor or just after delivery should get top priority for clinical management and CD4 assessment in ART center.

WHO clinical staging helps in monitoring the patient clinically, potential disease progression or treatment failure.

Q. What will you do, if pregnant women already receive ART?

Ans. Continue the ART regimen if the women gets ART for their own health and continue it through pregnancy, labor, puerperium and lifelong. There is no necessity to change EFV to NVP.

Q. What are the indications of prophylactic co-trimoxazole therapy in pregnancy?

Ans. When CD4 cell count is <250 cells/cu mm and this prophylaxis is helpful in reducing opportunistic infections such as *Pneumocystitis jirovecii* pneumonia (PCP), toxoplasmosis and diarrhea as well as other bacterial infections (dose–Double strength tablet—1 tab daily). Ensure that the pregnant women are taking folate supplements regularly.

Q. Care during labor and delivery.

Ans.
 a. Prolonged rupture should be avoided, if membrane is ruptured > 4 hours vertical transmission is increased
 b. ARM should not be undertaken, minimum PV examination, avoid prolonged labor
 c. Keep the viral load of the mother at 50 or less copies/mL at 36 weeks to vaginal delivery
 d. Avoid scalp electrode, fetal scalp sampling, operative vaginal delivery and episiotomy
 e. If assisted vaginal delivery is undertaken, forceps is preferable than ventouse as chances of micro laceration of the scalp are more in the vacuum cup
 f. Prophylactic antibiotics and steroid, if PPROM occurs at less than 34 weeks of GA
 g. ART (TDF+ 3TC +EFV) is to be continued.
 h. There is no increasing evidence that elective LSCS reduces transmission of HIV to baby, use forceps to hold needle instead of using fingers.

i. Infection of the attending doctor should be prohibited by proper dress designed for delivery of HIV +ve mother.
j. ARV should be given before operation, if patient is unbooked and admit in labor ward with labor pain.
k. Mode of delivery according to viral load (Table 10.11)

Table. 10.11: British HIV Association (BHIVA)-guideline for mode of delivery		
1. Viral load at 36 weeks	<50 copies/mL	Vaginal delivery
2. Viral load at 36 weeks	50–399 copies/mL	Prelabor CS (PLCS) taking account of viral load, length of treatment, compliance with medication, obstetric complications and mothers' views
3. Viral load at 36 weeks	>400 copies/mL	Elective LSCS

Note

Use Efavirenz safely from first trimester and cesarean section in HIV mother should be done only for obstetric indication.

Q. Describe the postpartum care of infected mother.

Ans.
a. Mother should take ART regularly
b. Infant should take ART prophylaxis immediately after birth
c. After delivery make skin-to-skin contact with baby to the mother
d. Human immunodeficiency virus (HIV) positive mother are more prone to postpartum infectious complications such as urinary tract infections (UTI), chest, episiotomy and cesarean section (CS) wound infections. Mother should give information on the early symptoms of infection.
e. Proper handling of lochia and blood-stained sanitary pad.
f. Recommendations (National guideline, 2011) of infant feeding of HIV- exposed and infected infants <6 months.
- Exclusive breastfeeding for last 6 months
- In conditions where breastfeeding is not possible (maternal death, severe maternal illness) or individual mother's choice (at her own risk), exclusive replacement feeding (ERF) may be considered. 'ERF' should be done when *AFASS* criteria is fulfilled. A-Affordable, F-Feasible, A-Acceptable, S-Sustainable, S-Safe

Note

- *Mixed feeding causes damage of intestinal mucosa resulting more chances of HIV infection to baby.*
- *The risk of mother having cracked nipple, mastitis increase the HIV infection rate to baby as blood being mixed with the breast milk.*

g. *Contraceptive advice*: Barrier method (male or female condom—for dual action) oral contraceptive pills (OCP), intrauterine contraceptive devise (IUCD), PP (postpartum)-IUD (Cu-T 380A) may be inserted within 48 hours of delivery, Injection DMPA, Non scalpel vasectomy (NSV) at 18 months to 2 years (when baby's survival has been ensured), male should use condom at every sexual exposure and even after vasectomy operation.

h. Psychological support of patient and family.

> **Note**
> Combined COCPs are not recommended with ritonavir (PI inhibitors) due decreased efficacy of contraception.

Q. Describe the care of HIV exposed infants?

Ans. NACO guideline, December, 2013

a. Baby should be handled carefully, until maternal blood and secretions are washed off
b. Anemia of baby should be treated
c. Exclusive breastfeeding (EBF) for first 6 months and no mixed feeding like fruit juice, water, cow's milk, formula feed) or exclusive replacement feeding (ERF) for first 6 months.
d. Start daily NVP immediately for minimum 6 weeks in EBF (or more indicated), use Syrup NVP prophylaxis from birth until 6 weeks in ERF.
e. Early infant diagnosis (EID) at 6 weeks, 6 months and 12 months (or after 6 weeks of stopping breastfeeds completely). Final diagnosis at 18 months (3 rapid tests, even if HIV-1 rapid test is negative). Do DBS at 6 weeks for all babies; if positive do WBS (whole blood sample), If WBS is positive, start pediatrics ART irrespective of CD4% for babies less than 2 years.

> **Note**
> No DBS/WBS (whole blood sample) (DNA PCR testing is to be done after 18 weeks).

f. Start CPT (co-trimoxazole prophylactic therapy) at 6 weeks and continue until baby is 18 months of age.
g. Do immunization—Start 1st dose of DPT/OPV/Hep-B vaccine (2nd dose) at 6 weeks.

Q. What is the dose and duration of NVP prophylaxis in infants?

Ans. NACO guideline, December, 2013.

BW	NVP daily dose (mg)	NVP daily dose (mL)	Duration
BW to 6 weeks			
<2000 g	2 mg/kg once daily	0.2 mL/kg once daily	Up to 6 weeks irrespective of whether exclusively breastfeed or exclusively replacement feed (may be extended to 12 weeks, if mother has not received ART for adequate duration, i.e. atleast 24 weeks.
2000–2500 g	10 mg once daily	1 mL once daily	
>2500 g	15 mg once daily	1.5 mL once daily	

Note: Considering the content of 10 mg Nevirapine in 1 mL suspension.

Q. Measures to reduce the risk of vertical transmission.

Ans. a. Keep the mother's viral load at 50 copies or less and allow vaginal delivery

Obstetric Cases

b. Elective CS for women with viral load of 499 or more at 38 weeks
c. Maximize the chance of delivery
  i. Reduce maternal smoking to prevent preterm rupture of membrane (PROM)
  ii. Reduce ingestion of alcohol
  iii. Treat maternal infection
d. Treat vitamin A deficiency
e. Avoid invasive fetal procedure—chorionic villus sampling (CVS), amniocentesis
f. Avoid scalp electrode, fetal sampling, artificial rupture of membranes (ARM), operative vaginal delivery
g. Avoid episiotomy
h. Wash the infant with antimicrobial bath as soon as possible
i. Continue ART in pregnancy and labor and thereafter lifelong.

Q. Prevention of perinatal transmission by zidovudin.

Ans. a. *Antenatal period*: World Health Organization (WHO) regimes: Zidovudin (ZDV or AZT) 300 mg twice daily, since 14 weeks should continue it during labor with addition of 150 mg of lamivudine (3TC) and single dose nevirapine 200 mg at the onset of labor and continuation of ZDV and 3TC for 7 days postpartum to prevent development of resistance to NVP.

b. *Intrapartum*: Zidovudin [PACTG 076] 2 mg/kg intravenously (IV) for 1 hour as a loading dose followed by 1 mg/kg/hour until delivery.
No doubt, it is very effective option for Prevention of Parent to Child Transmission (PPTCT) but neither cost-effective nor available in resource poor settings.

c. *Newborn*: Zidovudin, 2 mg/kg every 6 hours beginning 8–12 hours after birth and continued for 6 weeks. [In examination say NACO approved TDF +3TC +EFV regime (updated guidelines, December, 2013 by NACO, implemented on January, 2014)].

Q. Will pregnancy accelerates the disease prognosis?

Ans. Pregnancy does not make HIV infection worse though pregnancy is a relatively immunocompromised state.

Q. How do you treat Pregnancy with HIV-2 infection?

Ans.
- HIV-2 treatment consists of 2NRTIs + LPV/r
- Prophylaxis NVP with AZT (instead of syr NVP) is to be given to babies in mother with HIV-2
- Dose of AZT for infant with HIV-2 infection—WHO guideline. Administration of AZT according to birth weight and duration are as follows:

Birth weight (gm)	AZT daily (in mg)	AZT daily (in ml)	Duration
<2000	5 mg/dose twice daily	0.5 mL twice daily	6 weeks
<2500	10 mg/dose twice daily	1 mL twice daily	6 weeks
2500 and greater	15 mg/dose twice daily	1.5 mL twice daily	6 weeks

> **Note**
>
> If pregnant women is infected with both HIV/I and 2, she should receive standard first ART regimen (TDF+3TC+EFV) recommended for women with HIV-1 infection.

Q. Classes of antiretrovirals (ART).

Ans.
a. *Nucleoside reverse transcriptase inhibitors (NRTI)*: AZT, lamivudine (3TC), stavudine (d4T), didanosine (DDI), abacavir (ABC), tenofovir (TFV), Zalcitabine (ddC), Emtricitabine (ETC)
b. *Non-nucleoside reverse transcriptase inhibitors (NNRTI)*: Nevirapine (NVP), efavirenz (EFV), delaviridine (DLV)
c. *Protease inhibitors (PI)*: Indinavir (IDV), nelfinavir (NFV), saquinavir (SQV), Ritonavir (RTV), Amprenavir (APV), Fosamprenavir, Lopinavir (LPV), Atazanavir
d. *Fusion inhibitors*: T-20.

The drugs, which are available in NACO programs—AZT, 3TC, D4T, NVP, EFV, Tenofovir, Lopinavir/Ritonavir.

> **Note**
>
> Glucose tolerance test (GTT) is required at 26–28 weeks of pregnancy as anti-retroviral medications such as protease inhibitors (PI) and reverse transcriptase inhibitors can induce type II diabetes mellitus.

Q. Side effects of some important ART.

Ans.
a. Zidovudine—Anemia, nausea, headache, bone marrow suppression, pigmentation of nails.
b. Lamivudine—Hypersensitivity, rarely pancreatitis (in children)
c. Stavudine—Neuropathy, pancreatitis
d. Nevirapine—Skin rash, hepatitis, Stevens-Jhonson syndrome.
e. Tenofovir Disoproxil Fumarate (TDF)—Nephrotoxicity, hypophosphatemia
f. Efavirenz (EFV)—Neuropsychiatric symptoms such as hallucination, suicidal ideas, nightmares, vivid dreams
g. Lopinavir/Ritonavir (LPV/r)—GIT disturbances, glucose intolerance, lipodystrophy and hyperlipidemia.

Q. How do you follow-up pregnant women receiving ART?

Ans. Clinical evaluation including weight measurement every month is important. Laboratory follows up like Hb%, LFT (ALT), urine analysis, RFT. CD4 count (baseline and every 6 months) HBV and HCV screening, VDRL, blood sugar and lipid profile (especially for LPV/r-based regime) should be performed at intervals. Blood urea and creatinine should be undertaken before starting Tenofovir based regimen. All the investigations should be undertaken at baseline and at regular interval.

Obstetric Cases

> **Note**
> Follow-up of HIV-infected pregnant women apart from ART and Pre-ART care:
> - Pap smear or trichloroaceticacid screening of cervix should be done annually for all HIV-infected pregnant women
> - Family planning and birth spacing
> - Contraception—condom for dual protection is the best one, other are mentioned before, NVP, EFV, AZT, and TDF can be used safely with COCPs without loss of contraceptive efficacy.

Q. Estimated risk factors of PPTCT.

Ans. *Timing Risks*:
- During pregnancy 5–10%
- During labor 10–15%
- During breastfeeding 5–20%
- Overall with breastfeeding to 6 months 20–35%.

Q. Maternal risk factors influencing PPTCT.

Ans.
a. High viral load (VL of ≥100,000 HIV RNA copies/mL, risk of transmission is 40%, but the rate drops to 1% at <50 HIV-1 RNA copies/mL)
b. HIV subtype
c. Resistant strains
d. Advanced clinical stage
e. Recurrent infection
f. Viral, bacterial and parasite infestation (malaria)
g. Malnutrition.

Q. Infant risk factors of PPTCT.

Ans.
a. Baby premature
b. Low-birth weight (LBW) less than 2.5 kg
c. First infant of multiple births
d. Altered skin integrity
e. Immature gastrointestinal (GI) tract
f. Genetic susceptibility [human leukocyte antigen (HLA) genotype]
g. Immature immune system—preterm baby.

Q. How do you use ART in pregnant women?

Ans. See Figure 10.22A.

Q. Protocol for treatment for unbooked cases?

Ans. See Figure 10.22B.

Q. What are the steps of postexposure management?

Ans.
a. Manage the wound wash skin with soap and water or flush mucus membrane with water or saline
b. Report exposure
c. Assess infection risk
d. Conduct appropriate treatment as early as possible, follow-up and counseling.

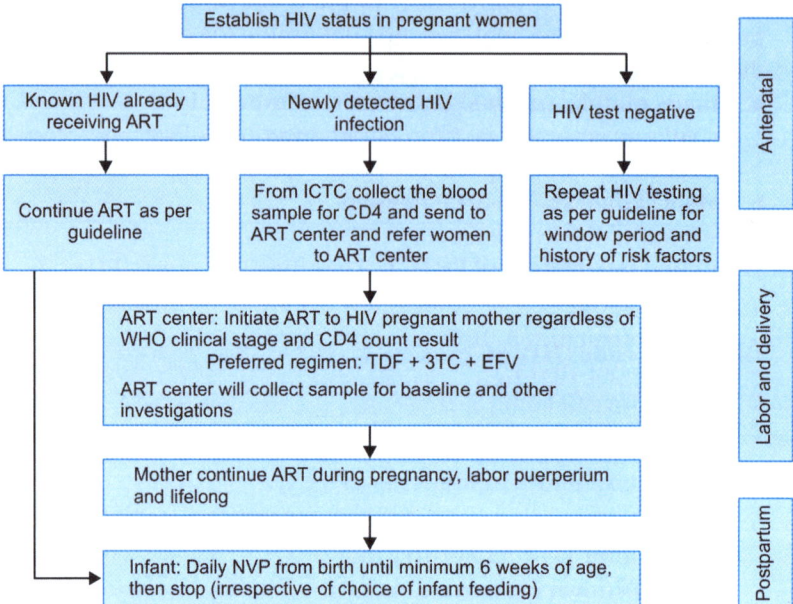

Figure 10.22A: Algorithm for ART use in pregnant women

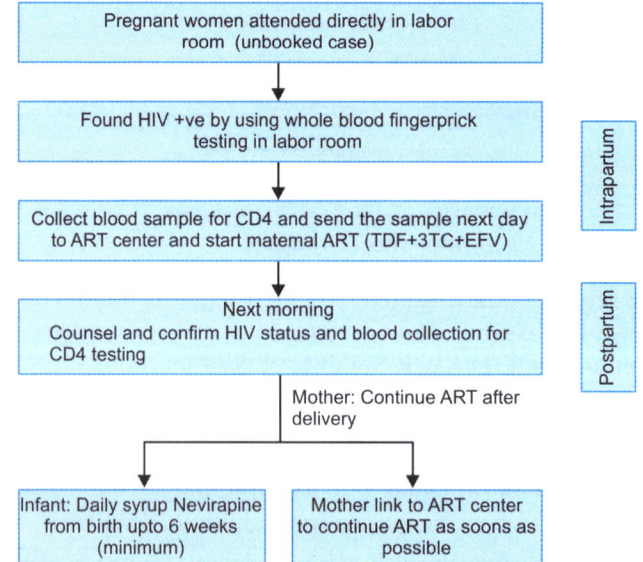

Figure 10.22B: Algorithm for ART use in pregnant women directly in labor (Unbooked case)

Obstetric Cases

Q. How do you determine the postexposure infection risk by HIV?

Ans. For post-exposure prophylaxis (PEP) of blood and body fluid or other potentially infectious material, first determine the exposure code (EC), then HIV status code (HIV SC). If exposure is on EC code:

a. Mucus membrane or skin integrity compromised
 1. Volume is small (few drops short duration)—EC1
 2. Large (several drops major blood splash, longer duration)—EC2

b. Intact skin only—No PEP needed

c. Percutaneous exposure
 1. Less severe (e.g. solid needle, superficial scratch)—EC2
 2. More severe (Large bore hollow needle, deep puncture)—EC3.

HIV status code (HIV SC):
a. *HIV negative*—No PEP needed
b. *HIV positive:*
 1. Lower the exposure (asymptomatic and high CD4 count)—HIV SC1
 2. Higher the exposure (advanced AIDS, primary HIV, high viral load, low CD4 count)—HIV SC2
c. Status unknown or source unknown—HIV SC.

Q. What is PEP recommendations?

Ans. PEP recommendations are as follows:

EC	HIV SC	PEP recommendation
1	1	PEP may not be warranted
1	2	Consider **basic regime**
2	1	Recommend **basic regime**
2	2	Recommended **expanded regime**
2/3	Unknown	If the source (unknown), the setting where the exposure occurred suggests a possible risk of HIV exposure and EC is 2/3, consider PEP **basic regime**

Basic regime—Zidovudine (300 mg) and Lamivudine (150 mg) twice daily for 4 weeks duration

Expanded regime—Basic regimen plus either indinavir, 800 mg every 8 hours or nelfinavir (750 mg) three times a day for 4 weeks.

Q. How do you immunize HIV infected baby?

Ans. HIV exposed or infected but asymptomatic child should receive all vaccine as per Immunization schedule discussed in the case discussion of puerperium. HIV infected children with immune suppression or symptoms should receive all vaccines except inj BCG, OPV and varicella.

FOR POSTGRADUATE STUDENTS

INTRAUTERINE GROWTH RESTRICTION (IUGR)

Summary: Mrs V, aged 21 years old married for 5 years G2P 1 + 0 came to the hospital with the c/o failure of adequate growth of gravid uterus noted by the patient and her relative for last two months. Her LMP was on 2-2-11 and EDD is on 9-11-11. Her previous baby was small and BW was 1.8 kg, living and delivered normally at term without any complication in labor and puerperium. She has no significant history of hypertension, heart disease, kidney disease or any addiction. In the present pregnancy on general examination, she has mild pallor, BP (normal), serial weight gain is poor (antenatal record). Systemic examination of lungs and heart show no abnormality. Obstetric examination reveals fundal height is lower (34 weeks) than the actual period of amenorrhea (38 weeks as noted by LMP), abdominal girth is decreased at the level of umbilicus, liquor volume is reduced and fetus is small, lie longitudinal, cephalic presentation and FHS is normal.

P/V (not for undergraduate)—Os closed, cervix tubular, head high up, pelvis roomy.

Provisional diagnosis: IUGR at term.

Case Discussion

Q. What is IUGR?

Ans. According to American College of Obstetricians and Gynecologists (ACOG), IUGR refers to a condition in which fetus is unable to achieve its genetically determined potential size. Infants born below 10th percentile of mean weight for their gestational maturity is called SGA. Infants in whom intrauterine growth has been restricted is of small for gestational age (SGA), but not all SGA fetuses are pathologically growth restricted, rather may be constitutionally small.

> **Note**
>
> Abdominal circumference (AC) less than 2SD for GA on USG is also suggestive of IUGR. IUGR is suspected when estimated fetal weight lies below 10th percentile or 2SD of the mean for GA on serial USG scan.
>
> [Notes: Appropriate for gestational age (AGA): Birth weight is between 10th and 90th percentile for infant's gestational age (GA); Large for gestational age (LGA)- Birth weight >90th percentile for GA].

Q. What are the different causes of IUGR?

Ans. a. *Group A (10%–40%), fetal growth failure:*
  1. Genetic anomalies
  2. Intrauterine infections
  3. Teratogenic effect
  4. Congenital malformation.
b. *Group B (5%–10%), combined maternal and fetal effects:*
  1. Severe malnutrition

Obstetric Cases

   2. Drugs
   3. Smoking
   4. Alcohol.
  c. *Group C (30%–35%), maternal disease and placental dysfunction:*
     1. Hypertensive pregnancies
     2. Renal diseases
     3. Cardiopulmonary diseases
     4. Severe anemia
     5. Placental infarcts, circumvallate placenta, vasculopathy and chorioangioma
     6. Multiple gestations.
  d. *Group D (40%), Unknown.*

Q. In which type of mother IUGR is more common?

Ans. a. In a woman with previous history of SGA babies
  b. Pregnancy loss in former pregnancy
  c. Poor maternal weight gain in current pregnancy
  d. Maternal complication affecting uterine and placental blood flow
  e. Maternal smoking.

Q. What are the different types of IUGR?

Ans. a. Symmetrical
  b. Asymmetrical.

Q. How do you differentiate between the symmetrical and asymmetrical IUGR?

Ans. *Symmetrical:*
  a. Small symmetrically—Both head and abdomen are small
  b. Ponderal index (PI)—[birth weight/crown-heel length]—normal
  c. Cause—genetic, infections such as toxoplasma, rubella, cytomegalovirus and herpes (TORCH)
  d. Ultrasonography (USG)—Normal
     i. Head-abdominal ratio(HC/AC)
     ii. Fl/AC
  e. Total cell number is reduced but cell size is normal
  f. Prognosis—complicated neonatal course.

  Asymmetrical:
  a. Head greater than abdomen
  b. PI is low
  c. Causes—placentovascular insufficiency
  d. USG—high head-abdominal ratio(HC/AC) and FL/AC
  e. Total cell number is normaln but cell size is reduced
  f. Prognosis—benign neonatal course, if complications are treated adequately.

Q. How do you diagnose IUGR?

Ans. **1. History:**
  a. Previous obstetrical history—previous IUGR babies, adverse fetal outcome and maternal medical problems

b. **Medical history**—heart disease, severe anemia, renal disease, malabsorption syndrome (acronym HARM), connective tissue disorder, thrombotic events, endocrine problem
c. **Drugs**—therapeutic and recreational
d. **Family history** of congenital abnormality and thrombophilia
e. **Antepartum hemorrhage (APH)**, pregnancy-induced hypertension (PIH), hypertension, history of recent viral illness.
f. **Estimation of GA by LMP.**

2. Weight gain: Decreased maternal weight gain in present pregnancy (< 3 kg throughout pregnancy, or 0–2 kg in second half of pregnancy). Assessing maternal weight gain is not a sensitive or specific method for detection of IUGR.

3. Symphysis-fundal height measurement (SFH): Low sensitivity and high false-positive rate (as it is an open error in pregnancy with too obese or too thin in multipara with flaccid abdominal wall and patients with transverse lie). Serial tape measurement from upper border of symphysis pubis (leg extended) to the top of the fundus in 'cm'. If the measurement shows less than 2 cm/week during 20 to 36 weeks of gestational age, it is a useful screening.

> **Note**
> It remains the most common method of screening for IUGR in low-risk patients.

4. Less liquor on abdominal palpation

5. USG scanning: Serial USG scanning for fetal biometry is important
   a. **Biometry**—Measurement of BPD, HC, AC, HC/AC, FL, FL/AC, EFW (Estimated fetal weight) and cerebellum [Transcerebellar diameter (TCR) remains unaffected in asymmetric IUGR]. TCR in 'mm' corresponds to the weeks of GA in second trimester.
   Growth profile of different fetal parameters in different gestational periods should be plotted on graph. If there is low profile curve—the interpretation is symmetrical IUGR and late flattening indicates asymmetrical IUGR.
   - FL/AC ratio—0.2 to 0.24 (normal), SGA fetus generally have ratio >0.24
   - In asymmetric IUGR, HC/AC is >1.08 at term [Normal HC/AC =< 1 at term and HC/AC is >1 in preterm fetus (before 36 weeks)]
   b. **Anatomy**—Structural abnormality may arise suspicion of chromosomal anomalies.
   c. **Liquor pocket**—Liquor pocket <1 cm or AFI <5 cm is associated with increased perinatal mortality.
   d. **BPP (biophysical profile)**—see USG (Chapter 8)
   e. **Doppler wave form** (Second line of investigations for management purpose)- Postcardiac: 1. UmA; 2. MCA.
      1. **Umbilical artery (UmA) Figure 10.23A** blood flow indicates fetoplacental status in utero and in normal study RI is between 0.5–0.7; S/D ratio <3 (normal). Abnormal fetoplacental blood

Obstetric Cases

flow is characterized by (a) absent end diastolic velocity, (b) S/D ratio (due to increased low resistance velocity) is going to stay in elevated range (>3), (c) PI increased. Decreased diastolic flow (RI >0.7) indicates early placental insufficiency, absent end diastolic flow indicates the fetal acidosis and when there is reversal of flow, it may require clinical emergency because most of the fetus dies within 1–2 weeks *in utero*.

2. **Middle cerebral artery (MCA) Figure 10.23B** indicates fetal status in utero—initially flow in MCA is normal and PI value is also normal (Normal RI of MCA >0.7 and PI >1.3 [50% normal reference value RI 0.65–0.8; PI =1.2–1.9]). Fetus with mild hypoxia (decreased umbilical arterial blood flow velocity) causes centralization of blood flow and will dilate the cerebral vessels as a compensatory brain sparing effect (RI <0.7) seen in asymmetrical IUGR, resulting in increased diastolic flow; so PI is decreased in MCA in initial phase of hypoxia. But later with fetal acidosis and before death of fetus with failing heart the diastolic blood flow is decreased, and there can again be increased PI. (So S/D ratio of umbilical artery (normal =<3; if >3 compromised fetus; PI of MCA/UmA (umbilical artery), Normal >1, if the ratio is < 1, hypoxic fetus, needs quick delivery).

Precardiac (precordial and venous): 1. Ductus venosus (DV), 2. Hepatic veins, 3. IVC, 4. Hepatic and amniotic cavity umbilical vein.

DV wave (M-pattern) Figure 10.24:
[What is ductus venosus (DV)? Embryological channel connecting fetal umbilical vein (UV) with inferior vena cava (IVC), and hence the right heart. In the fetus it carries most of the blood from the umbilical vein to the right atrium. DV arises at the junction of UV and right branch of portal vein angling posteriorly and cephaled towards IVC by making an angle of 45°–60°].

a. First peak (S-wave) corresponding with right atrial filling during ventricular systole. Ventricular systole induces the greatest pressure gradient between the right atrium and the precordial vein during cardiac cycle.

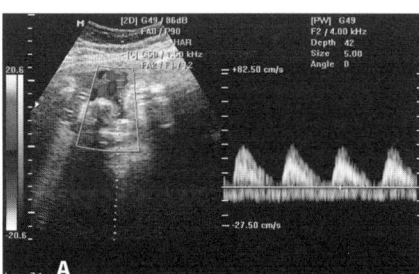
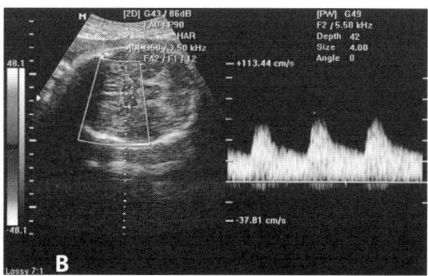

Figures 10.23A and B: (A) UmA—Absent end diastolic flow (IUGR), (B) MCA increased diastolic flow (IUGR) *(For color version, see Plate 4)*

b. Second peak (D-wave) during passive ventricular filling during early diastole (ventricular diastole).
c. The a-wave is the trough which represents atrial contraction (kick), the point at which forward flow towards the heart is normally slowest in late diastole. Under normal condition, the a-wave in the DV remains in a positive direction, i.e. blood continues to move towards the heart even during the phase of lowest pressure gradient during atrial contraction. Abnormalities of the DV are characterized by a decrease in velocity of the a-wave. If the fetus continues to deteriorate, a-wave shows absent or reversed flow velocity which needs quick delivery of fetus.

> **Note**
> Anoxia causes hypoxic cardiomyopathy leading to fall in cardiac function and hence rise in central venous pressure (CVP) causing reversed flow in DV.

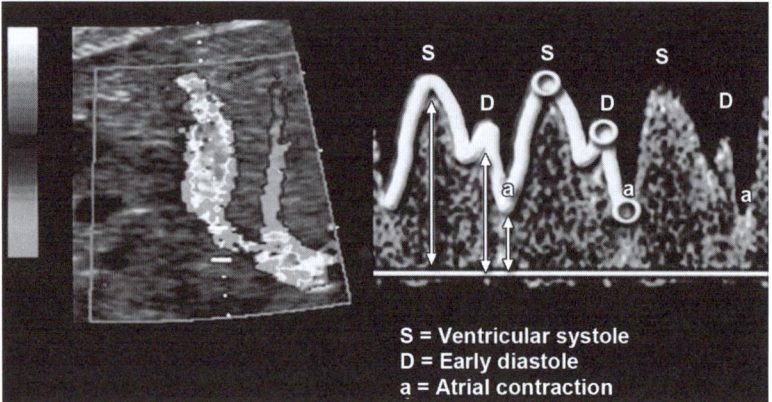

Figure 10.24: Normal Doppler study in ductus venosus (DV)
(For color version, see Plate 4)

> **Note**
> 1. DV wave provides more detailed information on the fetal heart and fetal acid-base balance.
> 2. In about 90% of cases the DV-Doppler becomes abnormal only 48–72 hours before BPP change.
> 3. When the end diastolic flow of the UmA is absent or reversed, urgent evaluation of color flow Doppler in the DV is necessary and if a-wave is absent or reversed, emergency and quick delivery of the compromised fetus, otherwise the baby will die in utero. If the a-wave is normal along with the absent end diastolic flow of UmA, wait for delivery for a couple of days with steroid to the mother for fetal lung maturity if the GA is at 32–33 weeks.

f. Ponderal Index (PI): USG criteria for diagnosis of fetal malnutrition in utero

Obstetric Cases

$$PI = \frac{EFW \text{ (Estimated Fetal Weight)}}{FL^3 \text{ (Femur Length)}}$$

EFW and femur length is measured by USG.
Normal value = 8.325 ± 2.5 (2SD)
EFW = 94.583 × HC + 34.227 × AC − 2134.616 (Weiner and Associates for GA 24–32 weeks)
EFW = Estimated fetal weight
HC = Head circumference, AC = Abdominal Circumference
Shepard and Associates at 32 weeks
Log EFW (g) = 0.02597 × AC + 0.2161 × BPD − 0.199 × AC × BPD2/1000 + 1.2659
BPD = Parietal diameter.
Hadlock's formula when the fetus is expected to be very small.
Log 10EFW (g) = 1.3596 − 0.00386 (AC × FL) + 0.0064 (HC) + 0.00061 (BPD × AC) + 0.0425 (AC) + 0.174 (FL).

Q. Antepartum management of IUGR.

Ans. Management can be done in the following ways:
1. Diagnosis—On USG fetal weight is <10th percentile of GA.
2. Exclude—If symmetrical—rule out fetal anomalies, karyotype anomalies, congenital infection, if asymmetrical—rule out also fetal anomaly.
    a. IUGR for early fetal insult—no effective therapy
    b. IUGR of extrinsic growth failure because of placental disease or reduced placental flow—antepartum fetal monitoring and timely delivery
3. Treatment—Rest in left lateral position, increased fluid intake, stop smoking, continuous maternal oxygen therapy.
4. Fetal surveillance:
    a. Clinical examination, fetal kicks chart, serial growth scan (every 3 weeks), biophysical testing, doppler velocimetry and non-stress test (NST).
    b. Antepartum evaluation: USG—for fetal biophysical profile (BPP)—every 2 weeks (BPP <4 carries a 60–70% risk of fetal acidemia), or moified BPP—NST + measurement of amniotic fluid volume is also a useful tool.
        - NST twice a week/daily testing
        - Doppler as indicated (UA-weekly)
    c. If all are normal, delivery should be done at 37–39 weeks.

> **Note**
> *If oligohydramnios is present hospitalization and delivery should be considered. Vaginal delivery is not safe in low prelabor BPP score points and non-reassuring fetal status, as fetal hypoxia and acedemia may progress in labor.*

Q. Timing of delivery.

Ans. It is often a critical management issue. The crux of the management is to balance the hazards of prematurity with the threat of intrauterine demise, which can be done with the following steps:

a. *Amniocentesis*: Important adjunct for decision making process:
   - Lecithin/sphingomyelin (L/S) for pulmonary maturity and dating of pregnancy
   - Low L/S ratio suggest earlier GA than fetal growth rate (FGR)
   - Late amniocentesis for fetal karyotyping for symmetrical IUGR
b. *When biophysical test*: NST, contraction-stress test (CST), BPP, USG-Doppler and end diastolic flow is normal—delay delivery up to 37 weeks
c. When end-diastolic flow of UA is absent or reversed, admission, close surveillance and administration of steroid if GA of fetus is <34 weeks. If other surveillance results (BPP, venous Doppler) are abnormal, delivery is indicated. If GA greater than 34 weeks, even if other results are normal, delivery is considered
d. Corticosteroid is offered to all women who may need delivery between 24–34 weeks and counseling on fetal morbidity or mortality is necessary
e. Delivery should be done in a unit, where optimal neonatal experts and facilities are available.

Q. Intrapartum management.

Ans.
a. Intrapartum monitoring with cardiotocography (CTG)—fetal heart rate (FHR) abnormalities are associated with a degree of asphyxia greater than in normally growth fetus
b. A skilled resuscitator should attend birth, regardless of the modality of delivery
c. Amnioinfusion—in nonreassuring FHR, meconium stained liquor and low AFI.

Q. Termination of pregnancy.

Ans. It depends on GA, fetal presentation, and maternal complications
a. If the cervix is favorable, liquor volume is good (Bishop score >6), induction of delivery by ARM and syntocinon drip
b. When cervix is unfavorable (Bishop Score <5), prostaglandin (PG) gel is placed endocervically to ripen the cervix, followed by ARM + syntocinon drip
c. Use of ventouse or forceps to minimize 2nd stage of labor.

Q. When CS is indicated?

Ans.
a. Fetal distress
b. Liquor pocket less than 1 cm
c. Malpresentation
d. Failed induction
e. Arrest of progress of labor
f. Previous CS
g. Fetal compromise—poor BPP, late deceleration and reduced variability
h. Abnormal UmA Doppler—Absent or reversed end diastolic flow
i. Abnormal ductus venosus Doppler and fetal scalp pH acidosis.

Q. Delivery management in IUGR pregnancy.

Ans. Figure 10.25.

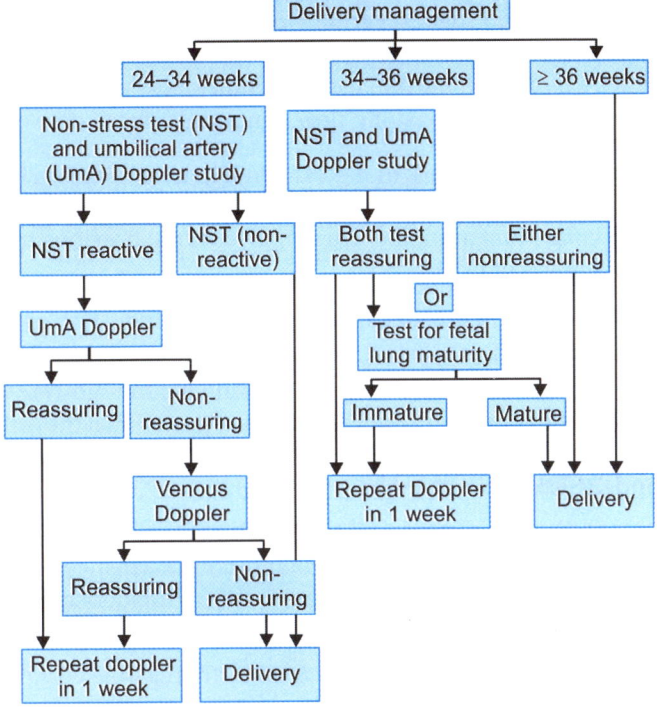

Figure 10.25: Delivery management of IUGR fetus; *Abbreviations:* NST—Non-stress test; UmA—Umbilical artery

Q. What are the neonatal complications?

Ans.
a. Meconium aspiration syndrome (MAS).
b. Hypoxic ischemic encephalopathy (HIE)—convulsion, irritability, twitching and apnea.
c. Hypoglycemia—blood sugar less than 30 mg/dL for less glycogen in liver and muscle, deficient hepatic gluconeogenic enzyme.
d. Hypocalcemia—serum calcium less than 8 mg/dL in mature IUGR, and less than 7 mg/dL in premature baby.
e. Polycythemia—increased production of red blood cells (RBCs) in response to intrauterine hypoxia.
f. Hypothermia—decreased amount of stored body fat.
g. Congenital anomalies—10% of IUGR babies trisomy 18 and 21, NTDs (neural tube defects) and Potter's syndrome. Long-term effects—Type-2 diabetes and hypertension, hyperlipidemia, and therefore increased incidence of cardiovascular disease.

> **Note**
> *Doppler velocimetry of the venous circulation may be the best way to assess the timing of delivery in preterm growth related fetus. Umbilical vein—Pulsatile flow in severely hypoxic fetus.*

FOR POSTGRADUATE STUDENTS

A CASE OF PREGNANCY WITH DIABETES

Q. What is gestational diabetes mellitus (GDM)?

Ans. Glucose intolerance first diagnosed during current pregnancy.

Q. What are the high-risk factors of GDM?

Ans. Obesity (BMI >30 kg/m^2), diabetes in first degree relatives, h/o glucose intolerance or prior gestational diabetes, past h/o unexplained stillbirth or congenital anomaly, current glycosuria, previous macrosomic baby, diagnosis of PCOS.

Q. What is the time of screening of low-risk and high-risk mothers?

Ans. Average or low-risk mothers should be screened at 24–28 weeks of gestation. Early screening at first prenatal visit in high-risk cases. The test is repeated between 24 and 28 weeks of gestation if the initial screen was normal (first screening: 12–16 weeks or at the time of first visit; second: 24–28 weeks; third 32–34 weeks).

Q. Is screening mandatory in all cases of pregnancy?

Ans. It is mandatory in all cases of pregnant mother irrespective of low and high-risk groups particularly in India where incidence of diabetes is very high.

Q. What are the criteria of low-risk group?

Ans.
a. Normal pregnancy weight and normal weight gain during pregnancy
b. No diabetes in first degree relatives
c. No H/O glucose intolerance
d. No H/O macrosomia
e. No H/O unexplained still birth and congenital defect of babies
f. Less than 25 years of age.

Q. How do you screen and diagnose GDM?

Ans.
a. Oral glucose challenge test (OGCT)—The two-step method 50 g of glucose is ingested without diet preparation at any time of day with a venous plasma glucose level measured 1 hour later. A positive screening test is most commonly seen if plasma glucose level > 140 mg/dL, which necessitate a follow-up of oral GTT by 100 g of glucose (see below).
b. The second method eliminates the 50 OGCT. The one step approach uses a 75 g of glucose solution and venous blood is taken at fasting, 1 hour, 2 hours. The criteria for the diagnosis of GDM are the same as the 2 hours GTT (see the GTT Table 10.12).

Table 10.12: Oral GTT (Diagnostic criteria of GDM)

	100 g OGTT	*75 g OGTT*
Fasting	95 mg/dL (5.2 mmol/L)	95 mg/dL (5.2 mmol/L)
1 hours	180 mg/dL (10 mmol/L)	180 mg/dL (10 mmol/L)
2 hours	155 mg/dL (8.6 mmol/L)	155 mg/dL (8.6 mmol/L)
3 hours	140 mg/dL (8.1 mmol/L)	

Obstetric Cases

c. Diabetes in pregnancy study group in India (DIPSI)—safe, one step, economical and feasible procedure. GCT— with 75 g oral glucose.

Principle: Screening of all pregnant mothers between 24–28 weeks of gestation, but recent concept is to screen at first trimester, if negative repeat at 24–28 weeks and finally around 32–34 weeks.

Procedure: DIPSI recommends in the antenatal clinic, a pregnant woman after undergoing preliminary examination should take a 75 g oral glucose load, without regard to the time of last meal. A venous blood sample is collected at 2 hours for estimating plasma glucose by GOD-POD method.

Results: ≥ 200 mg/dL—Overt diabetes; 140–199 mg/dL—GDM; 120–140 mg/dL—Gestational glucose intolerance; <120 mg/dL— normal.

Advantages of one step screening:
a. Fasting is not required
b. Helps in both screening and diagnosis
c. Routine daily activities are not hampered
d. Patient will not come on second day.

Q. Is oral GTT mandatory in all cases of pregnancy?

Ans. After overnight fasting, if the fasting blood glucose is greater than 126 mg/dL, or random glucose > 200 mg/dL further OGTT is not indicated as the patient has diagnosed or overt diabetes.

Q. How do you perform OGTT?

Ans. The oral glucose tolerance test (OGTT) is performed after an overnight fasting of 8 to 14 hours after 3 days of unrestricted carbohydrate diet intake (150 g/day). Then 100 g of glucose in 200 to 400 mL of water is taken by mouth over a period of 5 minutes to avoid vomiting. Venous plasma glucose level is measured at fasting (0 hour), 1 hour, 2 hours and 3 hours interval after drinking glucose solution (Table 10.12).

Interpretation
a. The diagnosis of GDM is made when one and or more values exceed or exceed the cut-off threshold
b. If any one value is abnormal, the test is considered normal
c. If all the values are border line, the test is to be repeated
d. If the test is negative, but there is high-risk of suspicion of diabetes, repeat it at 28–30 weeks.

> **Note**
> *Features of overt diabetes: If fasting blood glucose is ≥126 mg/dL, HbA1C ≥6.5%; Random plasma glucose 200 mg/dL (>11.1 mmol/L).*

Q. How do you evaluate a pregnant mother with diabetes?

Ans. *History*
a. If the patient is a case of known diabetic—previous obstetric history in details—prepregnancy control of diabetes and type of medications (insulin/oral antidiabetic agent) are to be noted.

b. In a known diabetic or potentially diabetic mother enquire about:
    i. Previous large baby (> 4 kg or more)
    ii. Previous unexplained death of baby in utero or any delivery of congenital defective baby
    iii. First degree family history of diabetes
    iv. Recurrent UTI.

Examination

A general physical examination—Height, weight, pallor, pulse, jaundice; jugular venous pressure, blood pressure and edema—as pre-eclampsia is more common in diabetes. Systemic examination—respiratory system and CVS.

Abdominal examination:

Height of fundus—Large for gestational age as hydramnios and big baby is more common in uncontrolled diabetes.

Investigations

- Completete hemogram—Hb%, TLC, DLC, Platelet
- Blood sugar—if fasting blood glucose is greater than 95 mg/dL and postprandial (PP-2 hours) blood glucose is greater than 155 mg/dL
- Hemoglobin (Hb)A1C—gives an idea of control of blood sugar during the previous 8–12 weeks
- Urine for routine examination (RE) and CS
- Fundoscopy and ophthalmoscopic examination
- Renal function test—assess every 4 weeks, a baseline level of creatinine greater than 0.8 mg/dL requires a full 24 hours creatinine clearance test.

> **Note**
> *Relation of serum creatinine and creatinine clearance by Cokroft-Gault method.*

$$Ccr = \frac{(140 - \text{age in years}) \times \text{weight in Kg}}{72 \times \text{serum creatinine (mg/dL)}}$$

In female the derived creatinine clearance is multiplied by 0.85 [mL/min], in pregnancy the value is 140–160/minute.

- Hepatic function test
- Electrocardiography (ECG)
- USG:
    a. Exact dating of pregnancy
    b. Detection of congenital malformation of baby
    c. Detection of liquor volume, size of baby, EFW and fetal biometry.
- Fetal evaluation: Kick test, NST, BPP, Doppler velocimetry, fetal echo.

Q. What is the risk of congenital defect of baby in pregnancy with diabetes?

Ans. The risk of congenital defect is increased with poor glycemic control (6–12%) in frank diabetes with pregnancy but less in GDM. The magnitude of risk correlates well with fasting blood glucose (FBG) and HBA_{1C} (HbA_{1C} level should be kept ≤ 6% before pregnancy).

Obstetric Cases

Defects
a. *Heart*: Transposition of great vessels, atrial septal defect (ASD), ventricular septal defect (VSD), coarctation of aorta.
b. *Central nervous system (CNS) and vertebral*: Caudal regression syndrome (caudal dysplasia and sacral agenesis), spina bifida, hydrocephalus, anencephaly, meningomyelocele, vertebral dysplasia, holoprosencephaly.
c. *Genitourinary system*: Renal agenesis, cystic kidney, ureteric duplex.

> **Note**
> Formation of free radicals and different expression of Pax-3 gene by an embryo exposed to hyperglycemia has been indicated as a possible mechanism of congenital defect.)

Q. What is HbA_{1C} and what is its importance?

Ans. Hemoglobin (Hb) combines with glucose at its β-terminal valine residue to form HbA_{1C}, when exposed to glucose for a long-time. It should be around ≤ 6%, if the level is greater than 7% or more, it indicates poor glycemic control in previous 8–12 weeks. If poor glycemic control coincides with the period of organogenesis, there is an increased risk of fetal anomalies. The mean glucose represented by HbA_{1C} level can be calculated using 'rule of 8S'.
A value of 8% = 180 mg/dL and each 1% increase or decrease represents ± 30 mg/dL. It is not helpful as a screening or diagnostic tool.

Q. Why oral antidiabetic agent is not preferred for management of diabetes in pregnancy?

Ans. It is not teratogenic, but it can cross the placenta and reach the fetus and produce hyperinsulinism and also produce fetal hyperbilirubinemia. Insulin cannot cross the placenta.

Q. What is total calorie intake in GDM?

Ans. Normal pregnancy weight [body mass index (BMI) < 26 kg/m²]—30 kCal/kg body weight (BW)/day
Overweight pregnancy (BMI > 29 kg/m²)—25 kCal/kg BW/day
Minimum—1,800 cal/day
Maximum—2,500 cal/day
Distribution of calories (% of total calories):
Carbohydrate: 60–65%; Protein: 15–20%; Fat: 15–25%.
In mild cases carbohydrate restriction is sufficient to control blood sugar. The carbohydrate is restricted to 150 g/day; 2 g of protein/kg BW is advised and the rest of the calories should come from fat.

> **Note**
> - Cut-off glucose level in diabetes: Venous plasma sugar (Fasting <95 mg/dL and 2 hours PP < 120 mg/dL, chances of macrosomia is low)
> - Whole blood values are 15% less than plasma.
> - Values can be converted into mmol/L by multiplying mg/dL by a factor 0.055.

Q. What are the effects of pregnancy on diabetes?

Ans. a. Pregnancy is a diabetogenic state due to increased production of cortisol, estrogen and progesterone, insulin resistance, increased lipolysis and fetus uses alanine and other amino acids and deprive mother of a major glucogenic source.
b. GDM may appear during pregnancy.
c. In pregnancy with insulin-dependent diabetes mellitus (IDDM)—glycosuria, ketonuria, ketoacidosis may occur.
d. Renal glycosuria—when glucose is detected in second fasting urine specimen voided 1/2 an hour after the first, it becomes significant, this is because the FBG is lowered in pregnancy and this glucose excretion on the basis of lowered renal threshold alone is difficult to explain, raising the suspicion of diabetes.
e. Effects on fetus and mother—discussed later.

Q. When do you start insulin?

Ans. 1. All IDDM patients
2. GDM—When diet and exercise for 30 minutes fail to maintain euglycemia within 1 week time
   a. FPG>/= 105 mg/dL in two consecutive check-up
   b. 1 hour postprandial plasma glucose (PPPG)>/=140 mg/dL
   c. Two hours postprandial plasma glucose >120 mg/dL
   d. History of requiring insulin in previous pregnancy
   e. History of unexplained fetal death
   f. Noninsulin-dependent diabetes mellitus (NIDDM) with poor glycemic control
   g. Oral hypoglycemic agents are usually be avoided during pregnancy though no apparent complications are seen in metformin and glyburide.

Q. What is the principle of insulin schedule?

Ans. Insulin schedule:
- If two hours PPPG is >120 mg/dL, advise intermediate acting insulin (premixed insulin 30/70, 4 units, 30 minutes before breakfast)
- Repeat 2 hours PPBG after 2 weeks. If the plasma glucose is within normal limits (<120 mg/dL), same dose is continued
- Change in dose are made in small amounts of 2–4 units at a time and should be adjusted once in 15 days after testing 2-h PPPG
- Usually a combination of regular or isophane insulin is given. The morning dose is determined by glucose level 2-h after breakfast, while evening dose is determined by blood sugar level after evening meal or bed time. The morning dose reflects the blood sugar after lunch and before dinner, while evening dose is reflected in fasting morning blood sugar or presence or absence of nocturnal hypoglycemia
- Repeat the blood sugar after 15 days and titrate the dose to achieve the PPPG between 110–120 mg/dL
- If the total insulin dose is ≥20 units/day, split dose of insulin is recommended. The total dose of insulin is divided into 2/3rd morning dose (14 U) and rest 1/3rd (6U) is given at night with regular

Obstetric Cases

monitoring of plasma glucose, fasting and PPPG every 15 days (to detect proportion of intermediate and short acting insulin, see Table 10.14 and the example below).

Q. What is glycemic index (GI)?

Ans. The increase in blood glucose after a test dose of carbohydrate compared with that after an equivalent amount of glucose (as glucose or from a reference starchy food) is known as glycemic index (GI). Foods with low GI are considered to be beneficial since they cause less fluctuation of insulin secretion (for details see Appendix 1).

Q. What is the euglycemic goal of diabetes in pregnancy?

Ans.
Timing of day	Capillary glucose (mg/dL)
Fasting	60–95
Before lunch, dinner, bed time snack	60–95
PP	
2 hours PP	< 120
1 hour PP	< 140
2 AM to 6 AM (Nocturnal)	60–135.

Q. Why human insulin is used?

Ans. Less allergic and decreased risk of antibody formation and has quicker absorption rate than animal based insulin.

Q. Name the different 'human insulin' and duration of action?

Ans. See Table 10.13.

Table 10.13: Onset, action and duration of human insulin

Insulin type	Onset (h)	Peak action (h)	Duration (h)
Rapid-acting (Lispro, Aspart, Glulisine)	5–15 min	1–2	4–6
Short-acting (regular)	0.5–1	2–4	6–10
Intermediate–acting (NPH)	1–2	4–8	10–18
Long-acting (Glargine, Detemir)	1–2	Peak less	Up to 24 hours

> **Note**
> A common insulin regime is rapid-acting or short-acting insulin before breakfast and dinner, or before each meal and intermediate-acting before breakfast and at bedtime. Intermediate-acting insulin is not usually injected before dinner because of possible nocturnal hypoglycemia.

Q. What are the starting doses of insulin therapy?

Ans. Table 10.14.

Table 10.14: Trimester dose of insulin

Trimester	Total units of Insulin (unit/kg actual body weight per day)	Twice daily	Split dose
1st	0.6 – 0.7	AM: 2/3rd of total dose	2:1 ratio of NPH and regular insulin—AM dose
2nd	0.7 – 0.8		
3rd	0.8 – 0.9	PM:1/3rd of total dose	PM dose: 1:1 ratio of NPH and regular insulin

Example: Insulin requirement: 0.8 unit × 60 (Kg) = 48 unit in 24 hours
Total daily insulin dose (TDD) = 48 unit

Split dose path way:

AM (Prebreakfast) 2/3 × 48 = 32   2/3 as NPH = 21 unit of NPH 1/3 as regular = 11 unit of regular

PM (Pre-dinner) 1/3 × 48 =16   1/2 as NPH = 8 units of NPH (**pre-bed time**)

1/2 as regular = 8units regular (rapid acting insulin) (**pre-dinner time**)

- Regular blood sugar monitoring is essential

Basal-bolus insulin regimen:

TDD= 48 unit as above

1/2 TDD basal insulin 1/2 × 48 = 24 units*

Long acting Lantus/levemir

*Use single dose at bedtime or split 1/2 in the AM and PM doses
(*Splitting the dose in 1/2 is recommended if total basal insulin is >40 units)

1/2 TDD prandial bolus insulin (rapid acting insulin)

1/2 × 48 = 24 units

Prebreakfast 1/3 × 24 = 8 unit

Pre-lunch 1/3 × 24 = 8 unit

Pre-dinner 1/3 × 24 = 8 unit

Insulin correction using supplemental rapid-acting insulin scale (SRAIS):

The insulin sensitivity factor:

How much of a reduction in blood glucose should you expect for each 1.0 unit of insulin delivered to the patient?

The 1500 rule:

Insulin sensitivity factor = 1500/Total daily insulin

If the patient receives a total daily insulin of 50 units

1500/50 = 30 mg/dL blood glucose drop per 1.0 unit of insulin

To correct a patient's blood glucose to 100 mg/day:

$$\frac{\text{Patient's blood glucose} - 100}{30} = \text{Supplemental units of insulin}$$

Additional insulin is rapid-acting insulin.

Q. What is the pharmacokinetics of other insulin preparation given sub-cutaneously?

Ans. Table 10.15.

Table 10.15: Pharmacokinetic of semilente and lente insulin

Type of insulin	Onset of action (hr)	Peak action (hr)	Duration of action (hr)
1. Semilente (IZS-amorphous insulin)	1/2	4–6	12–16
2. Lente (IZS insulin amorphous–3 parts + 7 parts crystalline)	3	8–12	18–28

Insulin zinc suspension (IZS)—The rate of release of this insulin from the tissue is related to the size of the insulin particles which are suspended in acetate buffer.

Ultralente—IZS crystalline insulin is slower in action than IZS amorphous (Semilente).

> **Note**
> 1. a. Regular insulin and NPH can be drawn in the same syringe
>   b. Intermediate acting insulin causes more delayed hypoglycemia. So rapid-acting insulin is preferred nowadays which provide better control of blood sugar with improved maternal and fetal outcome.
> 2. Regular insulin half lives
>   a. IV regular insulin—5 minutes half life
>   b. IM regular insulin—2 hours half life
>   c. S/C regular insulin—4 hours half life.

Q. How many times do you measure blood glucose?

Ans. At least four times a day (Fasting and 1–2 hours after meal) in women with GDM and 5–7 times a day in women with preexisting disease. (7 point—prebreakfast, lunch, dinner (30 minutes before each meal) and postbreakfast, lunch and dinner (performed 2 hours after meal) and late night super).

Q. How do you monitor a case of diabetes in pregnancy?

Ans. Mother:
a. Blood glucose estimation 4–7 times a day
b. HbA_{1C}
c. Urinary ketones is useful to detect inadequate calorie and carbohydrate intake
d. Measurement of blood pressure (BP)
e. Ophthalmoscopic examination and renal status
f. Insulin treated pregnant women are generally admitted at any time if blood sugar is not properly controlled at home or after 34 weeks of gestational age to investigate stabilization of diabetic controll and fetal heart rate (FHR) is monitored three times each week by CTG and to decide the mode and timing of delivery.

Fetal:
a. Clinical examination to assess fetal growth, liquor volume and FHS
b. Daily fetal kick chart
c. Weekly NST and BPP
d. USG and fetal echocardiogram
e. Fetal Doppler of UmA, MCA and DUC has venosus.

Q. How do you manage a case of diabetes?

Ans. a. *Diet*: As mentioned above
b. *Obstetric care*: Patient should be checked very frequently and if there is any complication, it should be detected very early
c. *Insulin*: If mother is diabetic and diet fails to maintain euglycemia within 1 week time

I. Fasting plasma glucose (FPG) less than 95 mg/dL—exercise + diet to maintain fasting glucose 60–90 mg%—weekly follow-up of sugar
    a. Weekly FPG less than 95 (+/- 2H-PP <120)—continue weekly monitoring—antepartum testing at 38–40 weeks (antepartum testing—twice weekly NST and AFI).
    b. Weekly FPG ≥95 or +/- 2H-PP ≥120—start SMBG (self-monitoring blood glucose 4–7 times/day) [2 H-PP: Two hours postprandial blood glucose].
II. If FPG 95–120 mg/dL—diet, exercise + SMBG, if mean FPG less than 95 mg/dL and mean 2H-PP ≤120 mg/dL—continue daily SMBG and antepartum testing at 38–40 weeks.
    If mean FPG ≥95 mg/dL and mean 2H-PP ≥ 120 mg/dL, start insulin and titrate insulin and antepartum monitoring at 32–34 weeks.
III. FPG greater than 120 mg/dL → diet + exercise + SMBG and Insulin—titrate insulin to achieve euglycemia—antepartum test at 32 to 34 weeks.

> **Note**
> SMBG is to be done 4–7 times per day. Capillary blood glucose (CBG) which is tested by glucometer are plasma glucose calibrated.

Q. When do you deliver the baby (Timing and mode of delivery)?

Ans. GDM is not an indication of CS. Delivery may be delayed upto term or the onset of spontaneous labor if:
a. Tight glycemic control (Fetal lung development is normal and less chance of RDS)
b. Estimated fetal weight is good
c. Facilities for measuring good fetal surveillance at regular interval is available. But if there is medical, obstetrical and fetal complications, deliver it at 38 weeks.

> **Note**
> We should not deliver after 40 weeks for fear of macrosomia and stillbirth. If there is no spontaneous labor, induction is necessary.

Q. What are the indications of cesarean section?

Ans.
a. Macrosomia (>4000–4500 g)
b. Failed induction of labor
c. Severe PIH
d. Uncontrolled diabetes
e. Abruptio placentae
f. Bad obstetric history (BOH)
g. Malpresentation
h. Elderly primi mother
i. Fetal distress
j. Post CS pregnancy.

Q. What are the indications of elective delivery?

Ans.
a. Poor metabolic control
b. Worsening hypertensive disorder
c. Fetal macrosomia
d. Growth retardation
e. Polyhydramnios.

In all these conditions elective delivery is planned for fear of fetal death after lung maturity has been confirmed. If elective delivery is planned in < 38 weeks of gestational age, amniocentesis should be done for confirmation of fetal lung maturity (measure phosphatidylglycerol than L/S ratio).

Q. How do you monitor GDM in labor?

Ans. 1. Monitoring of intrapartum glycemic control:
a. Induction of labor/CS is best started in early morning
b. AM insulin dose is omitted as diet is stopped
c. Continuous IV fluid D5/lactate ringer solution (125 mL/hour) to avoid ketonemia
d. The mean plasma glucose is maintained at 100 mg/dL
e. If the plasma glucose is, 70 mg/dL then IV solution should be changed to 5D given at the rate of 2.5 mg/kg/minute
f. Blood glucose is measured hourly and ketone level 4 hourly.

Table 10.16: Doses regimen of intrapartum insulin infusion

Capillary blood glucose (CBG) (mg/dL)	Insulin dosage (U/hour)	Fluid rate (125 mL/hour)
< 100	0	D5/lactated Ringer's solution
100–140	1.0	D5/lactated Ringer's solution
141–180	1.5	Normal saline (NS)
181–220	2.0	NS
> 220	2.5	NS

Dilution: 50 units in 500 mL of normal saline (equals to 1 unit/10 mL), insulin 0.5-1 unit for every 40 mg/dL of glucose increase with target glycemic control 100-119 mg/dL. Capillary blood glucose (CBG) level performed hourly and if marked hyperglycemia is present (>180 mg/dL), an IV bolus of regular insulin of 2-4 units is given every hour so that the blood glucose level is >120 mg/dL (Table 10.16).

> **Note**
> Usual starting dose of insulin 1 unit/hour (= 10 mL/hour = 150 drops/60 min = 3 drops/minute).

2. Monitoring of labor and fetal well-being by CTG and partogram:

> **Note**
> Shoulder dystocia may occur during the delivery of big baby in GDM if uncontrolled.

Q. How do you manage the case during puerperium?

Ans.
a. Plasma glucose 150–200 mg/dL is acceptable in the puerperium. Generally, insulin can be restarted between 2 and 5 days after delivery in type-1 diabetic mother (0.5–0.6 µ/kg).

Requirement of insulin is less. The use of oral antidiabetic agent is contraindicated with breastfeeding (type-2 diabetes); if overt hyperglycemia is there, start insulin therapy when the patient takes diet orally.

b. Puerperal infection should be managed properly
c. Family planning advice
d. Breastfeeding: Lactation may improve glucose control, mobilize fat stores, promote weight loss and protect against further risk of developing diabetes. Weight loss (1–2 kg/month) is acceptable.

> **Note**
>
> Women with GDM should be tested in the postpartum period (4–12 weeks) for their glycemic status. GDM will have a more than 50% risk of developing diabetes within 10–20 years. If OGTT is normal at 6–12 weeks postpartum the woman should be reassessed every 3 years, but Impaired glucose tolerance (IGT) needs the test annually.
>
> Factors that increase the risk of GDM in subsequent pregnancy are hip to waist ratio (> 0.84), weight gain > 11 lbs (5.0 kg) between pregnancies, and a fat intake > 40% of the total cloric intake.

Q. What are the effects of hyperglycemia in pregnancy, labor and puerperium?

Ans. Pregnancy:
a. Spontaneous abortion
b. Polyhydramnios (20%) [due to osmotic diuresis associated with fetal hyperglycemia]
c. PIH (10–25%)
d. Infection—recurrent UTI and candidal vulvovaginitis.
e. Preterm labor
f. PROM
g. Diabetic ketoacidosis

Labor:
a. Prolonged labor
b. Shoulder dystocia in a big baby
c. Operative delivery.

Puerperium: Sepsis.

Medical complications: Hyperglycemic coma, nephropathy, neuropathy, hypoglycemia at night (1:00 am–6:00 am) that results in rebound hyperglycemia and an elevated prebreakfast glucose value (Somogyi phenomenon) and hyperglycemia in the early morning (4:00 am–7:00 am) due to insulin resistance (Dawn phenomenon) with prebreakfast fasting hyperglycemia. It is probably caused by exaggerated growth hormone, or cortisol effect or conjunction with morning waking process.

Obstetric Cases

Q. Which oral hypoglycemic agents (OHAS) are used to maintain blood sugar in GDM?

Ans. a. Glyburide (Glibenclamide)—Second generation sulphonyl urea that lowers blood glucose level by enhancing the release of insulin from β cells in pancreas, and may cause hypoglycemia in mother but transplacental transfer is minimal and no fetal complications have been reported. Dose—Minimum dose 2.5 mg/day, maximum recommended dose is 10 mg twice daily (total 20 mg/d), beyond which insulin is started.

b. Metformin—A insulin sensitizer increases peripheral utilization and decreases the hepatogluconeogenesis. It is safe and effective for the treatment of GDM. The recommended starting dose of metformin is 500–1000 mg in divided doses, maximum daily dose is up to 2,550 mg. It does not cause hypoglycemia or weight gain as there is no stimulation of insulin secretion from pancreas. It can be continued safely during pregnancy if metformin is used in PCOS.

Q. What are the long-term consequences of OHAS?

Ans. Glyburide improves glycemic control by increasing β-cell insulin secretion and repeated use may cause β-cell exhaustion which may lead to early development of type-2 diabetes in later life. Metformin has no effect on β-cell but the transplacental transfer of metformin helps in decreasing the fetal insulin resistance, but its transplacental transfer causes alteration of fetal gene expression. It may induce lactic acidosis which may cause fetal distress. So OHAS should be used cautiously till long-term effect of these drugs on babies are documented (a long trial is necessary).

Q. What are the fetal complications?

Ans. Immediate
a. Congenital malformations (6–12%).
b. Respiratory distress syndrome (RDS)—Fetal lung maturity is delayed for hyperinsulinemia and hyperglycemia.
c. Fetal death—cause due to hyperglycemia, hypoglycemia (over dose of insulin), congenital defect, hyperviscosity syndrome, placental insufficiency, SLE and APLAs when associated.
d. Macrosomia and birth trauma—maternal hyperglycemia—fetal hyperglycemia—fetal hyperinsulinemia converts fetal blood sugar into fatty substance, which are deposited in the subcutaneous tissue causing large baby. Fetal macrosomia may be due to increased insulin like growth factor (IGF I and II), epidermal growth factor, leptin, adiponectin and maternal obesity.
e. Hypoglycemia (blood glucose < 30 mg/dL) interm baby and 25 mg/dL in preterm baby.
f. Hypocalcemia—due to transitional fractional neonatal hyperparathyroidism (Ca^{++} < 7 mg/dL).

> **Note**
> C-peptide level (measurement of by-product created during insulin production) >90th percentile in cord blood is found in almost a third of newborn in the highest glucose categories.

g. Polycythemia—due to hypoxia renal erythropoietin and increased turn over of heme in polycythemic neonates
h. Hyperbilirubinemia.
i. IUGR (10%) due to vasculopathy of retinal, renal or hypertension and may result from compromised uteroplacental blood flow
j. Shoulder dystocia
k. Cardiomyopathy.

Late complications: Obesity of child, neurophysiologic deficit and diabetes.

Q. Contraception in diabetes.

Ans.
a. Barrier method is safe
b. Oral contraceptive or combined oral contraceptive pill (COCP) has high-risk for thromboembolism, myocardial infarction and cerebrovascular accident (CVA).
c. IUCD: Infection rate is very high, glucose precipitates with copper and reduces its efficacy.
d. Permanent: Ligation or vasectomy of husband.

Q. What is white classification for pregnant women with diabetes mellitus?

Ans.

Class	Criteria
A_1	GDM not requiring insulin or oral agents
A_2	GDM requiring insulin or oral agents
B	Onset ≥20 years of age or duration of < 10 years
C	Onset at 10–19 years of age or duration of 10–19 years
D	Onset <10 years of age or duration of ≥20 years or any onset/duration but with background retinopathy or hypertension
F	Nephropathy (≥500 mg proteinuria per day at <20 weeks of pregnancy)
H	Aterosclerotic heart disease, clinically evident
R	Proliferative retinopathy or vitreous hemorrhage
T	Prior renal transplantation.

FOR POSTGRADUATE STUDENTS

A CASE OF HEART DISEASE IN PREGNANCY

History and Examination of Heart Disease in Pregnancy

Patient aged 24 years G2P0 + 1 admitted with shortness of breath, palpitation, dizziness, edema and intolerance to exercise and edema of feet for 15 days.

Obstetric Cases

(Sometime patient may have no complaints or any of the complains above fit to the patient should be considered). Her LMP is on d/m/y and EDD is on d/m/y. H/O rheumatic fever in child hood is suggestive of rheumatic valvular heart disease. Cardiac failure in previous pregnancy is the high-risk factor for failure in the present pregnancy. Presence of anemia, hypertension, infective endocarditis, atrial fibrillation and thyrotoxicosis in present pregnancy can lead to heart failure in presence of organic heart lesion. Grading of heart disease by American Heart Association should be done. Any suggestive history of congenital heart disease is present or not. If patient undergoes cardiac surgery, details of the operation should be noted including valve replacement if any, use of prophylactic antibiotics and anticoagulants should be asked carefully and to be continued in the present pregnancy.

Other drug therapy like digitalis, diuretic, antihypertensives should be enquired and to be continued accordingly.

General survey—Pallor, edema, cyanosis, condition of the thyroid and jugular venous distension with prominent pulsation should be noted and neck vein is examined by reclining the patient at an angle of about 45° with support to the neck to make the neck muscles relaxed. Arterial pulse (rate, rhythm, character, volume, condition of the vessel wall the presence or absence of delay of the femoral pulse with the radials), respiration, temperature, BP, liver (enlarged in CCF) and Spleen (enlarged in infective carditis) respiratory system—Whether any basal rales, wheeze and ronchi.

Cardiovascular System

Inspection: To inspect the precordium for any brisk and diffuse apex pulsation in lying straight position the normal position of apex beat is 9 cm from the mid line or 1cm internal to the midclavicular line in the fifth intercostal space and right ventricular impulse and to note also the pulsation on suprasternal notch, neck veins, and epigastrium.

Palpation: Palpate the apex beat, right ventricular lift over the precordium just lateral to the sternum, a palpable murmur which is called thrill and transmit to the hand a sensation just like the purring of a cat.

Auscultation: Auscultate the different areas on precordium as mentioned below. First heart sound in mitral (S1M increased and widely split-normally) area, second heart sound in pulmonary area (S2 P increased, S2 splitted-normally), presence of third heart sound occasionally or any abnormal sound like murmur in mitral, aortic, tricuspid and pulmonary area should be noted carefully. If murmur is present, note the points—

  i. Time of occurrence, i.e. systolic, diastolic or continuous through systole or diastole
  ii. Behavior of murmur during respiration
  iii. Point of maximum intensity and direction of selective propagation
  iv. Character of murmur. Continuous venous hum at the root of the neck is normal.

> **Note**
> Mitral area—which corresponds to the apex beat; Tricuspid area—Lies just left to the lower end of sternum; Aortic area—right to the sternum in 2nd IC space; Pulmonary area—left to the sternum in 2nd IC space; at the onset of ventricular systole mitral and tricuspid valve close almost simultaneously producing first heart sound. The closure of the aortic and pulmonary valves give rise the two components of second heart sound

Obstetric examination—See history taking and examination in obstetrics to rule out IUGR

Investigations—ECG, echocardiography, chest x-ray (with shielding of abdomen), Holter for assessment of cardiac status. Others like Hb%, TLC, DLC serum electrolytes, uric acid in PIH and USG are also important.

Q. What is the incidence of heart disease in pregnancy?
Ans. 1 percent.

Q. What special points are to be noted in history and examination?
Ans. Any previous cardiac surgery, problem in previous pregnancy like heart failure, H/O rheumatic fever, or monthly prophylaxis of antibiotic, drug and alcohol abuse, functional class assessment. Examination: Height, weight, cyanosis, clubbing, edema, pulse, BP, chest, scar, rales; heart thrill and murmur and varicose veins.

Q. What are the different types of heart disease?
Ans.
a. Rheumatic valvular heart disease (90%), mitral stenosis (80%), mitral regurgitation may be combined
b. Congenital heart disease (discussed later)
c. Cardiomyopathy.

> **Note**
> Stenotic valvular lesions are at high risk in pregnancy. Regurgitant lesions like mitral and aortic regurgitation improve due to decreased systemic vascular resistance in pregnancy.

Q. What is normal cardiac physiology in pregnancy?
Ans.
a. Heart is enlarged slightly.
b. Heart has to work more due to extra volume of blood (40% during pregnancy)—rise in blood volume started from 3rd month and peak at 32 weeks and then a plateau till term.
c. Pulse rate is increased by 10 beats/minute.
d. Cardiac output (COP)—increases due to increase in stroke volume and heart rate (HR). COP increases in pregnancy (30–40%); during labor (40%) and immediately after delivery (30–60%) due to extra 500 mL of blood is thrown into circulation by contracted uterus.

Q. Cause of death in heart disease in pregnancy.
Ans.
a. Pulmonary edema
b. Congestive cardiac failure (CCF)
c. Active rheumatic carditis

Obstetric Cases

d. Subacute bacterial endocarditis (SABE)
e. Pulmonary embolism.

Q. What are the predictors of adverse maternal events?

Ans. Acronym 'NOPE-CM'
a. New York Heart Association (NYHA) functional class II
b. Obstruction of left heart
c. Prior cardiovascular events
d. Ejection fraction of ventricle is <40%
e. Cyanosis (SaO_2 <90%)
f. Marfan's and dilated aortic root > 4 cm diameter.

Q. What are the indications of pregnancy termination?

Ans.
a. Primary pulmonary hypertension (systolic pulmonary arterial pressure is > 50 mm of Hg) due to ASD, sever VSD, DDA
b. Eisenmenger's complex (central right → left shunt)
c. Marfan syndrome with CVS involved (dilated aortic root if > 4 cm increases the risk of dissection and aneurysm formation)
d. Any uncorrectable cardiac lesion in functional class III and IV refractory to medical management
e. Severe left heart obstructive lesion
f. Systemic ventricular dysfunction (due to cardiomyopathy), ejection fraction <20%.

Q. Grading of heart disease?

Ans. New York Heart Association (NYHA)
Class I   Symptomatic with extraordinary physical work
Class II   Symptoms with ordinary physical activity
Class III Symptom with less than ordinary activity
Class IV   Symptom at rest

Q. How do you evaluate known or suspected cardiac disease during pregnancy?

Ans. History:
Previous surgery, previous pregnancy outcome, H/O rheumatic fever or of monthly prophylactic antibiotic injection, medications, feature of anemia and thyrotoxicosis, functional class assessment.

Physical examination:
Height, weight, facies, cyanosis, evaluation of pulse in all extremities, BP, presence of precordial thrill, auscultation of heart (character of S1, S2, rate, rhythm, murmur) and supraclavicular and infraclavicular region, thoracic auscultation (rales), fundal height and fetal heart tone, vaginal examination.

Ancillary tests:
1. Complete blood count, Hb%, PT, aPTT, urine analysis, LFT, RFT
2. ECG, echocardiography, holter exercise testing (in selected cases), chest radiograph (in selected cases with abdominal shield) and if indicated cardiac catheterization or MRI are recommended in moderate and high-risk cases.
3. Obstetric ultrasound.

Q. How do you provide antenatal care in pregnant patient with heart disease?

Ans. a. *Antenatal care*: In uncomplicated cardiac disease, care should be taken once in a month up to 28–30 weeks and then every 2 weeks, until 36 weeks and finally weekly until delivery.

b. A constant vigilance of symptoms like hemoptysis, cough, severe dyspnea and sign (weight gain, tachycardia, and distension of neck vein, rales, wheezes and newly palpable liver).

Advice given:
1. Limit the physical activity
2. High protein and low-salt diet (2 g/day)
3. Vitamin and minerals supplement
4. Avoid cigarette and alcohol
5. Anemia is to be corrected
6. Avoidance of infection like UTI and reproductive tract infection (RTI)
7. Injection of Benzathine penicillin IM at 3 weeks interval is to be continued
8. Follow-up of fetal growth—by clinical and USG.
9. Discussion of anticoagulating agents for fetal teratogenicity (or ICH)
10. Fetal echo at 18–20 weeks of GA.

Q. When do you admit the patient?

Ans. Elective admission

Grade 1 at 38 weeks; Grade II at 28 weeks; Grade III and IV as soon as diagnosis is made and the patient is kept in hospital throughout pregnancy.

Emergency admission
1. Deterioration of functional grading
2. Appearance of dyspnea, basal crepitations and rising pulse rates
3. Appearance of complications like anemia, PIH, abnormal weight gain.

Q. How do you manage the case during labor?

Ans. First stage
1. Semi-recumbent position, avoid supine position
2. Oxygen inhalation if dyspnea
3. Oral fluid only, IV fluid is to be avoided
4. Analgesia
5. Monitoring of maternal pulse, BP and cardiac failure
6. Prophylactic antibiotic—Injection of ampicillin, 2 g IV + injection of gentamicin, 80 mg IV, 30 minutes before delivery, at 8 hours and after 24 hours of delivery
7. Intensive fetal monitoring.

Second stage
1. Cut-short second stage by prophylactic forceps or ventouse, difficult forceps is to be avoided.
2. IV methergine is to be avoided after delivery of anterior shoulder to prevent overloading of heart (Q. Why methergine is contraindicated? Ans. After injecting methergine, sustained contraction can lead to

Obstetric Cases

addition of 500 mL of blood into the maternal circulation, thereby increasing the left atrial pressure up to 10 mm of Hg, which can lead to frank pulmonary edema).

> **Note**
> Epidural anesthesia may be used except in (CAT PIE)-Coarctation of aorta, Aortic stenosis, Tetralogy of Fallot (uncorrected), Pulmonary hypertension, Idiopathic hypertrophic subaortic stenosis, Eisenmenger's syndrome (CAT-PIE).

Third stage

After delivery, uterine bleeding should be managed by uterine massage and IV/IM administration of oxytocin. A rapid IV injection of oxytocin should not be given because it can cause significant hypotension, additionally in pregnant woman with prolonged QT interval (measure between the Q-wave and T-wave in the heart's electrical cycle), and may also cause ventricular tachycardia.

Puerperium

1. The patient is to be observed closely in first 24 hours—pulse, respiration and signs of cardiac failure
2. The patient should be kept in hospital for 2 weeks
3. Puerperal pyrexia if any is to be managed energetically
4. Prophylactic antibiotics
5. Breastfeeding, if there is no heart failure.

> **Note**
> For fluid maintenance during labor 5% dextrose at 50 mL/h is preferable over NaCl containing solution.

Q. What are the fetal risks?

Ans. IUGR, prematurity, fetal loss, recurrence of congenital heart disease in the offspring.

Q. What are the indications of CS in heart disease with pregnancy?

Ans. Cephalopelvic disproportion (CPD), malpresentation, placenta previa, prolonged labor, severe IUGR.

Q. How do you manage a heart failure case? When heart failure is common?

Ans.
a. Injection of morphine, 15 mg IM/sedation
b. Propped up position
c. Oxygen (O_2) inhalation and monitoring of P/RR (P = Pulse, RR-Respiration rate), BP
d. Salt-restricted diet
e. Digitalization—0.5 mg IV followed by 0.25 mg every 6 hours
f. Diuretics—40–60 mg IV.

> **Note**
> Management of pulmonary edema—alphabets "LMNOP": **L**asix (diuresis); **M**orphine (to dilate air ways); **N**a⁺ and water restriction; **O**xygen; and **P**osition of patient upright.

Heart failure is common:
1. At 30–32 weeks of GA (highest blood volume).
2. 2nd stage of labor.
3. Just after delivery (most common time).

Q. Which investigations are important in heart disease?

Ans. Echocardiography—gives information regarding structural heart disease, valve area, valve gradient, myocardial contractility and ejection fraction (EF).

EF= stroke volume (SV)/end-diastolic volume = (EDV− ESV)/EDV
Stroke volume = end-diastolic volume (EDV)−End-systolic volume (ESV).
It is a sensitive indicator of left ventricle

Left ventricle (LV)

Normal value	50–65% (5%variation)
Definitely abnormal	<50%
Hypertrophic myocardium	>65%

Peak exercise LVEF (left ventricular ejection fraction) is an indepenent predictor of coronary artery disease

Right ventricle (RV)

Mean normal value	>45%

RVEF is smaller than for LV because RV has greater EDV than LV, but the same stroke volume. ECG is most effective for diagnosis of arrhythmia, e.g. atrial fibrillation.

Q. Can you induce a patient with heart disease in pregnancy?

Ans. Many patients with heart disease go into spontaneous labor, and women especially in higher functional classes need cervical ripening before oxytocin induction. Cervical dilatation may be done by Foley's catheter or misoprostol or dinoprostol gel. The Foley's catheter is the method of choice in higher functional classes and patient with cyanotic heart disease. Antibiotic is required for women who are at risk for bacterial endocarditis. Prostaglandins are required for lower functional classes without tachycardia and H/O asthma.

Q. What is the normal mitral valve area?

Ans. 4–6 cm^2
Critical mitral stenosis—valve area is less than 1 cm^2
Moderate stenosis—1.5 cm^2–1 cm^2
Mild stenosis—< 4 cm^2 but >1.5 cm^2.

Q. What are the indications of mitral valvotomy in pregnancy? What is the best time of operation?

Ans.
a. Tight mitral stenosis—failure to medical management
b. Pulmonary edema not responding to treatment (refractory pulmonary edema)
c. Recurrent and refractory hemoptysis: 16–28 weeks of pregnancy is the best time of operation.

Obstetric Cases

Q. What is the choice of contraception in woman with heart disease?

Ans. Temporary (WHO)
1. Barrier contraception—nirodh (best)
2. COCP—not advised for complicated valvular heart disease
3. IUCD—can be used for complicated and uncomplicated valvular heart disease
4. POP, injection DMPA can be used safely in any type of valvular heart disease.

Permanent
1. Ligation is the best method
2. Vasectomy of husband is advised, if the heart of the patient is not well-compensated.

Q. What is the role of anticoagulants? How do you administer it?

Ans. Administration of anticoagulant is necessary in patients with congenital heart disease, pulmonary hypertension, artificial valve replacement and atrial fibrillation. When pregnancy is diagnosed if the patient receives warfarin before pregnancy should be stopped immediately and women with low-risk profile (no h/o thromboembolism, newer low profile prosthesis) might be managed with s/c unfractioned or low molecular weight heparin at 12 hours interval until the 14 weeks of GA, after which oral anticoagulant is started. Again patient is readmitted 4 weeks before EDD and heparin reinstituted, so that infant free of coumarin anticoagulant may be delivered. Patient is advised to with held heparin during labor. If the patient needs for anticoagulant for a long-time warfarin can be started the day after delivery with an overlap with the heparin for 1-2 days more as warfarin precedes its antithrombotic effect by 24 hours and during that period a transient hypercoagulable state persists due to rapid reduction of protein level. In absence of significant bleeding heparin can be resumed 4-6 hours after delivery and warfarin begun orally.

Patient having high-risk profile (a h/o thromboembolism, or any older generation prosthetic valve) should be managed with unfractioned heparin during 1st trimester 6 hourly and activated partial thromboplastin time (aPTT) is 2-3 × control value. Warfarin is started thereafter.

Q. Why warfarin is stopped at 35–36 weeks of GA?

Ans. Warfarin is stopped as preterm delivery occurs in 36% of cases in pregnancy with heart disease.

Q. If the patient goes on labor on warfarin therapy, what will be the line of management?

Ans. If the patient on warfarin therapy goes on labor cesarean section is recommended to avoid certain risks of fetal cerebral hemorrhage due to trauma in vaginal delivery and mother should receive 2-4 units of fresh frozen plasma and vitamin K, but vitamin K is slow-acting, therefore should not be given alone.

Q. What is low-molecular-weight heparin (LMWH)? What are its advantages?

Ans. Low-moleculor-weight heparin (LMWH) are fractions of standard heparin, obtained by chemical and enzymatic depolymerization, so that the size becomes 1/3rd to 1/4th of the size of unfractionated heparin. Dose 0.5–1 mg/kg subcutaneous (SC) should be given every 12 hours for prophylaxis. The side-effects like osteoporosis, thrombocytopenia is very much less.

Q. How do you monitor a case of LMWH therapy?

Ans. Laboratory monitoring is not usually recommended. Antifactor Xa level is measured once after the first 2–3 days of initiation of treatment and the level should be minimum of 1.0 U/mL to decrease the incidence of thromboembolic events.

> **Note**
> 8.6% of cases of LMWH therapy may have valve thrombosis. So higher doses may be required than the dose required for prevention of vein thrombosis.

Q. How do you monitor anticoagulant therapy?

Ans. Warfarin treatment is monitored by prothrombin time and expressed in international normalized ratio (INR) and kept at 2–3 times control. An INR higher than 3, increases the risk of bleeding. Besides, heparin is monitored by Activated partial thromboplastin time (APTT) 2.5 times control. The partial thromboplastin time (PTT) is checked 6 hours after SC injection.

> **Note**
> When the patient is under anticoagulant therapy, INR value is to be maintained between the levels of 2 and 2.5.

Q. Does coumarin group of drugs cross placenta?

Ans. Yes, it can cross. So, it should be withheld in first trimester of pregnancy as it causes congenital defect of baby. Heparin cannot pass through the placenta.

> **Note**
> When valve replacement is required, tissue valve rather than artificial valve is recommended, so anticoagulant is not needed.

Q. If mother is on warfarin, can she continue breastfeeding?

Ans. Breastfeeding is safe in this case and it does not go into the breast milk, because it is highly bound to plasma protein and not lipid soluble in ionized form.

Q. Classify the congenital heart disease.

Ans. a. *Venous overload*: Acyanotic (Left-to-right shunt) ASD, VSD, PDA
b. *Cyanotic heart disease*: (Right-to-left shunt) tetralogy of Fallot, Eisenmenger's syndrome (Right sided pressure is > left side,

reversal of shunt leads to cyanosis)—a congenital communication exists between systemic and pulmonary circulation, with resultant pulmonary arterial hypertension (PAH) and reversal of flow through the defect.
c. *Other congenital heart diseases*: Coarction of aorta, primary pulmonary hypertension, Marfan's syndrome
d. Cardiomyopathy.

Tetralogy of Fallot:
a. VSD
b. Right ventricular outflow obstruction (Subvalvular pulmonary stenosis)
c. Right ventricular hypertrophy
d. Overriding of arch of aorta.

Poor prognostic indicators are hematocrit >65%, syncope, CCF, right ventricular hypertrophy or peripheral oxygen saturation <90%. Avoid hypotension, bradycardia and myocardial depressant drugs.

Eisenmenger syndrome:
The syndrome develops when pulmonary vascular resistance exceeds systemic resistance. It is the reversal of left to right shunt (ASD, VSD, PDA) due to progressive pulmonary hypertension. Right to left shunt causes cyanosis and the degree is determined by the extent of pulmonary vascular obstructive disese. Termination of pregnancy is advisable due to worsening hypoxia and maternal death and fetal loss are high.

Atrial septal defects (ASD): Secundum type of defect is most common. Systolic ejection murmur at left sternal border and wide fixed split of second heart sound are generally noted. Patient with large defect may cause atrial arrhythmia (atrial fibrillation) and congestive heart failure in pregnancy. Thromboembolism may occur which needs attention of DVT prophylaxis and compression stocking during pregnancy.

Venticular septal defects (VSD): Pregnancy is well-tolerated. The defect closes spontaneously during childhood in 90% of cases. Large defect may be associated with arrhythmia, CCF, and may lead to pulmonary hypertension, causing reversal of shunt (right to left), cyanosis and Eisenmenger syndrome. When this develops maternal mortality is high. Prophylactic antimicrobials are required for bacterial endocarditis.

Coarction of aorta: It is a stenosis of aortic arch usually at or distal to the ductus arteriosus. Rare in pregnancy and is a rare cause of secondary hypertension. Needs surgical repair at childhood. It may be associated with bicuspid aortic valve and berry aneurysm of the circle of Willis. The pressure is lower distal to coartation. The risk of aortic dissection and rupture is small. This may compromise placental perfusion and fetal growth should be monitoried. Prophylaxis of bacterial endocarditis is necessary.

Patent ductus arteriosus (PDA): Ductus connects the proximal left pulmonary artery to the descending aorta just distal to the left subclavian artery. Functional closure occurs just after birth. Not common in pregnancy. Common in childhood and is corrected in childhood. Tolerance of small PDA is well during pregnancy. However pulmonary hypertension, heart failure and cyanosis develops if systemic blood pressure falls and leads to shunt reversal from pulmonary artery to the aorta (Eisenmenger syndrome). A drop of systemic blood pressure may cause fatal collapse. Prophylaxis of bacterial endocarditis is needed.

Q. What is the effect of pulmonary hypertension?

Ans. Pulmonary hypertension secondary to fixed pulmonary vascular resistance, a right-to-left shunt is associated increased maternal and perinatal mortality rate. If pulmonary hypertension is noted on cardiac catheterization in early pregnancy and not reactive to oxygen administration, therapeutic abortion is needed.

Q. What are the high-risk and low-risk cardiac lesions having associated maternal risk during pregnancy?

Ans. High-risk:
a. Cyanotic heart disease
b. Severe pulmonary hypertension
c. Severe aortic stenosis (AS)
d. NYHA class III and IV cardiac lesion with any valvular or myocardial lesion
e. Severe LV dysfunction (EF<35%)
f. Peripartum cardiomyopathy
g. Marfan's syndrome—Autosomal dominant, having aortic root dilatation and valvular (commonly mitral valve) prolapse and regurgitation can occur.

Aortic root diameter < 3.7 cm does not show obstetric complications, but when this diameter is > 4 cm increased risk of aortic rupture during pregnancy.

Management: Beta blocker to reduce the heart rate <90 bpm, endocarditis prophylaxis and echocardiography (serial assessment). Vaginal delivery with regional analgesia and assisted second stage is safe with an aortic root diameter of <4 cm. When the aortic root is 4–5 cm or greater, elective cesarean section is recommended with consideration of postpartum replacement of proximal aorta with a prosthetic graft.

Low-risk:
a. ASD/VSD/PDA with normal LV function and no PAH
b. Chronic MR/AR/NYHA I or II with normal LV function
c. Mild or moderate MS/AS/or PS
d. Postoperative cases of acyanotic heart disease.

Q. What are the benefits of prosthetic valve types?

Ans. Bioprosthetic valve
a. Low-risk of thromboembolism
b. No need for anticoagulation
c. Increased rate of structural valve degeneration.

Obstetric Cases

Mechanical prosthetic valve
a. Excellent durability
b. Superior hemodynamic profile
c. High-risk of thromboembolism
d. Anticoagulant required
e. Associated with fetal and neonatal complications.

Q. Which cardiac drugs are avoided or used with caution?

Ans. Avoid:
a. ACE inhibitors or angiotensin II receptor antagonists due to risk of renal impairment of fetus
b. Amiodarone (anti-arrhythmic drug causes neonatal hypothyroidism)

Use with caution:
a. Warfarin (< 5 mg dose is less teratogenic)
b. Spironolactone
c. Anti-arrhythmic drug (Sotalol)—can be associated with FGR, so monitoring of fetal growth is necessary.

Q. What are the causes of elective CS in heart disease?

Ans. a. On warfarin and not switched to heparin 2 weeks before labor (as warfarin crosses placenta and may cause fetal ICH during vaginal delivery)
b. Aortic dissection
c. Marfan syndrome with dilated aortic root
d. Severe pulmonary hypertension
e. Coarctation of aorta
f. Severe aortic stenosis.

Q. High-risk patients required for IE (infective endocarditis) prophylaxis?

Ans. a. Valvular stenosis and regurgitation
b. Prosthetic heart valve
c. Structural congenital heart disease (except uncomplicated ASD, fully repaired VSD and PDA, cardiomyopathy, Marfan's without aortic insufficiency)
d. Previous infective endocarditis
e. Hypertrophic cardiomyopathy.

> **Note**
> *Current recommendation of antibiotic prophylaxis is 2 g of amoxicillin and 1.5 mg/kg of gentamicin IV/IM 30 minutes before the procedure followed by amoxicillin 1.5 g orally 6 hours after the initial dose, alternatively parenteral regimen may be repeated once 8 hours after the initial dose.*

Q. What is rheumatic fever (RF)? What are the major and minor criterias of RF?

Ans. Rheumatic fever generally appears 2–3 weeks after streptococcal pharyngitis in children of 5–15 years.

WHO criteria (2004) based on revised Jone's criteria
A. Major criteria: 1. carditis, 2. polyarthritis, 3. chorea (Sydenham's), 4. erythema marginatum, 5. subcutaneous nodules
B. 1. Fever, 2. arthralgia, 3. previous history of rheumatic fever, 4. laboratory findings—reactive protein and leukocytosis, elevated ESR, 5. ECG—Prolonged PR interval.

> **Note**
>
> *Rheumatic heart disease accounts for 90% of cardiac disorder in pregnancy. Cardiac valves affected in order of frequency are mitral, aortic, tricuspid and pulmonic (Marry and Tomy Play).*

Mitral stenosis: Most common valvular lesion in pregnancy. Stenosis of mitral valve (normal valve surface area is 4.0 cm^2, symptoms usually develops when the surface area is <2.5 cm^2) impedes flow of blood from left atrium to left ventricle resulting elevated left arterial and pulmonaty pressure. It causes arrhythmia (atrial fibrillation), thromboembolism which can cause stroke, pulmonary edeme, pulmonary hypertension and right heart failure. Diuretic and beta-blocker are the mainstay of therapy. Therapeutic anticoagulation with heparin is needed with persistent fibrillation. Anticoagulants are also recommended for sinus rhythms. Patient not responding to medical therapy should be considered for mitral valvotomy and valve replacement.

Caution: Avoid tachycardia, as it shortens ventricular diastolic filling (tocolytic agents that cause tachycardia are contraindicated), fluid overload, hypotension and increase in pulmonary vascular resistance. Shorten second stage of labor and epidural anesthesia for labor is ideal.

Aortic stenosis: Aortic stenosis in younger age group (<30 years) is congenital. The patient is symptomatic when valve orifice is reduced to 1cm^2 from its normal size 3–4 cm^2. It leds to decreased fixed cardiac output. The three cardinal symptoms are, i. exertional dyspnea (decrease in pulmonary capillary pressure), ii. chest pain (due to decrease in coronary artery perfusion in hypertrophied myocardial mass), iii. syncope (decrease in cerebral perfusion). Appearance of arrhythmia may cause sudden death. Limitation of physical activity and prompt treatment of infection is advisable during pregnancy. If symptoms persists inspite of bed rest, valve replacement or valvotomy using cardiopulmonary bypass is considered. Avoid hypotension and bradycardia which may reduce artery perfusion and cause sudden death. Cut short the second stage of labor and epidural anesthesia is contraindicated. Narcotic epidural may be used.

JAUNDICE IN PREGNANCY

Q. What is jaundice?

Ans. Yellowish discoloration of sclera, mucous membrane and or skin due to high concentration of bilirubin in the body fluid and when the plasma bilirubin level is greater than 2 mg/dL [Latent jaundice means plasma bilirubin level is 1 mg/dL – 1.9 mg/dL].

Q. Etiology of jaundice in first and second trimester.

Ans. More common to least common causes are:
  a. Viral hepatitis
  b. Cholestasis of pregnancy
  c. Hyperemesis gravidarum
  d. Gallstone.

Q. Etiology of jaundice in 3rd trimester.

Ans. a. Pre-eclampsia
  b. Cholestasis of pregnancy
  c. Viral hepatitis
  d. Acute fatty liver
  e. Gallstone.

Cholestasis of Pregnancy

Q. What is this disease?

Ans. It is a form of intrahepatic cholestasis that is associated with severe pruritus and usually, occurs in third trimester of pregnancy.

Q. What is the character of pruritus?

Ans. The pruritus is most severe at night and on palm and soles.

Q. What is the obstetric outcome?

Ans. There is an increased incidence of frequency of fetal distress and stillbirth and need for preterm delivery and neonatal care.

Q. How do you diagnose the condition?

Ans. a. Prominent symptoms of pruritus
  b. Aspartate aminotransferase (AST) and alanine aminotransferase (ALT)—2–10 times normal
  c. Bile salt markedly increased—sometimes 100 times normal.

Q. What are the ICP (intrahepatic cholestasis of pregnancy) associated disorders?

Ans. a. Benign recurrent intrahepatic cholestasis of pregnancy (ICP)
  b. Cholelithiasis and increased risk of fatty liver
  c. May present as primary biliary cirrhosis
  d. Increased risk of acute fatty liver.

Q. What is the recurrence rate?

Ans. About 60–70% of patients affected in their initial pregnancy have a recurrence.

Q. Precautions and monitoring during jaundice.

Ans. a. *Serum bile acid testing*: In ICP, serum bile acid levels (>12–14 μmol/L) levels are determined weekly, until delivery and again afterwards in order to rule out underlying problems of liver.

Every pregnant woman with raised bile acids should be treated.

b. *Liver function tests (LFT)*: Level of AST, ALT and alkaline phosphatase (ALKP) are recommended twice, weekly.

c. CTG, Doppler and ultrasound surveillance should be done twice weekly, until delivery through the above mentioned parameter and will not totally eliminate the risk of still born.

d. *Prothrombin time (PT)*: Due to increased risk of vitamin K malabsorption, PT levels are high and it is monitored weekly, till delivery to prevent the risk of maternal hemorrhage and intracranial hemorrhage of infants.

Q. How do you treat pruritus?

Ans.
a. *Ursodeoxycholic acid (UDCA)*: It improves maternal liver function by replacing more toxic bile acids in blood stream. It also improves bile acid transport across the placenta, which may greatly reduce the risk of stillbirth. So, it down regulates bile acid synthesis and has been proposed to have antiapototic and antifibrotic properties as well. Dose of UDCA—500 mg BD until delivery. UDCA is present only in trace amount in human bile.

b. *S-adenosylmethionine (SAMe)*: Given IV (600–900 mg) also prevents preterm labor. Cholestasis reduces the fat soluble vitamin K absorption.

c. *Vitamin K*: Oral vitamin K reduces the risk of PPH. Vitamin K helps in synthesis of factors II, VII, IX and X.

d. *Steroids*: Dexamethasone, 12 mg orally × 7 days with a reducing dose of 3 days, will reduce the total bile acids and ALT. It also reduces the estrogen production by fetoplacental unit.

e. *Cholestyramine*: Chelating agent, mixed with water taken in a dose of 4 g, 2 to 3 times daily. It exacerbates vitamin K deficiency and associated with intracranial hemorrhage of child and maternal hemorrhage. It is not recommended for routine use.

Q. How do you prevent fetal death in ICP?

Ans. Fetal death in cholestasis of pregnancy is very high inspite of intense monitoring. All deaths occur in late pregnancy. So, labor is induced when the fetal lung is matured regardless of other parameters.

Liver Disease in Pre-eclampsia and HELLP Syndrome

Incidence: 3–10%.

Pre-eclampsia

Q. What are the criteria for diagnosis?

Ans. Sustained hypertension after 20 weeks of pregnancy with a BP of 140/90 mm Hg or high in a woman who was normotensive previously and proteinuria of 300 mg or greater in 24 hours urine testing or 1+ on dipstick test which corelates well with 30 mg/dL, or urinary protein: creatinine ratio is ≥0.3 mg/dL.

Obstetric Cases

Q. What are the clinical features (CF)?
Ans.
a. Occurs after 20 weeks of pregnancy in 5–10% of cases
b. Hypertension, protenuria, edema (not significant)
c. Severe disease leads to eclampsia and HELLP (stands for hemolysis [H] elevated liver enzymes [EL] and low platelet [LP] count) syndrome.

Q. What are the risk factors?
Ans.
a. Nulliparous and multiple gestations
b. Diabetes mellitus and hypertension
c. Extremes of maternal age.

Q. What is the pathophysiology?
Ans.
a. Features of uterine spiral arteries to lose their muscular media
b. Acute atherosis (fibrin deposition, lipid-laden macrophage)
c. Increased reactivity of angiotensin-II, decreased prostacyclin
d. Decreased glomerular filtration rate (GFR) (creatinine 0.9–1.2 mg/dL).

> **Note**
> See the Figure 10.20 in 'a case of pre-eclampsia'

Q. Differential diagnosis (D/D) of HELLP syndrome?
Ans.
1. Cholestasis
2. Acute fatty liver of pregnancy (AFLP)
3. Viral hepatitis (ALT > 1,500 IU/L, normal creatinine level)
4. Thrombotic thrombocytopenic purpura with normal liver function.
5. Others—SLE, APLAS, ITP, septic shock.

Q. How do you manage the patient?
Ans.
a. Hospitalization and manage hypertension
b. Delivery if GA greater than 36 weeks
c. Delivery at any gestational age of pregnancy if evidenced by impending eclampsia, HELLP syndrome and renal dysfunction.

HELLP

Q. What is HELLP syndrome?
Ans. Hemolysis, elevated liver enzyme and low platelet count.

Q. What are the criteria of HELLP syndrome? Classification.
Ans.
1. **Hemolysis:**
   a. Abnormal peripheral blood smear
   b. Increased bilirubin greater than 1.2 mg/dL
   c. Increased lactate dehydrogenase (LDH) greater than 600 IU/L
2. **Elevated liver enzyme:**
   a. Increased serum glutamic oxaloacetic transaminase (SGOT) > 72 IU/L
   b. Increased LDH greater than 600 IU/L.

3. **Thrombocytopenia:** Platelet count is less than 1,00,000/mm³.

> **Note**
> Life-threatening complication of HELLP is subcapsular liver hepatoma.

Classification

A. Tennessee classification:
a. *Partial HELLP*: One or two components of above abnormalities
b. *Full HELLP*: All the three abnormalities
   Full HELLP syndrome is more prone to DIC than partial HELLP. Candiadates with full HELLP is considered for delivery within 48 hours, whereas partial HELLP are the candidates for temporizing.

B. Mississippi or Martin classification:
Classified on platelet count
Class I: Platelet is <50,000/mm³
Class II: 50,000 to <100,000 mm³
Class III: 100,000 to 150,000 mm³.
Patients with Class I HELLP are at higher risk than Class II and III.

Q. Are HELLP syndrome and DIC same?
Ans. No. In HELLP syndrome coagulation parameter like PT, PTT, serum fibrinogen level are normal, but in disseminated intravascular coagulation (DIC), presence of thrombocytopenia, low-fibrinogen level (< 200 mg/dL, and high fibrin degradation products (FDP) > 40 mg/mL), a prolonged PT and a PTT.

Q. In which condition hematoma or hepatic rupture is common?
Ans. a. Pre-eclampsia—third trimester
b. HELLP syndrome (subcapsular hematoma)
c. Postpartum.

Q. What is the pathophysiology of hepatic rupture?
Ans. Hepatic rupture in pre-eclampsia is due to extravasations of blood, presumably from one or several microscopic areas of periportal hemorrhage under Glisson's capsule, as is typical of HELLP syndrome. When pressure under the capsule is excessive, it ruptures resulting hemoperitoneum.

Q. How do you diagnose hepatic rupture?
Ans. a. Hemoperitoneum—confirmed by paracentesis
b. Computerized tomography (CT) scan
c. USG and magnetic resonance imaging (MRI) of the ruptured liver.

Q. How do you manage ruptured liver?
Ans. Rapid delivery of the fetus and repair of liver. Correction of coagulopathy and massive product transfusion of blood is needed. Recent recommendation for treating rupture of subcapsular hematoma in pregnancy is packing and drainage. Maternal and fetal mortality is over 50%.

Obstetric Cases

Q. Management of HELLP syndrome.

Ans. Treatment is like severe pre-eclampsia by using antihypertensives, anticonvulsants and delivery of baby. Blood and blood products (FFP and platelets) may be used. Role of steroids in HELLP syndrome is controversial but can be used for fetal lung maturity (Figure 10.26).

> **Note**
> Some authors recommend administration of high dose of dexamethasone (12 mg 12 hourly) for patients with HELLP syndrome, but others do not.

Q. How do you deliver baby in HELLP syndrome?

Ans. Cesarean section is not mandatory in HELLP syndrome. If cervix is favorable go for induction of labor by oxytocin and if cervix is unfavorable LSCS is to be done. But before planned CS, correct platelet deficiency and appropriate replacement of blood and blood components like FFP to replenish fibrinogen.

Q. What are the risks of conservative or delayed management of HELLP syndrome?

Ans.
a. Abruptio placentae
b. Pulmonary edema
c. Adult respiratory distress syndrome (ARDS)
d. Rupture of liver hematoma
e. Acute renal failure (ARF)
f. DIC.

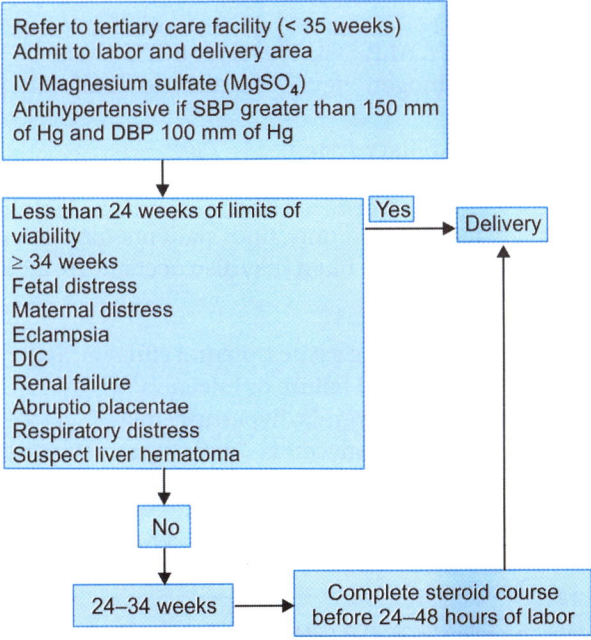

Figure 10.26: Management of HELLP syndrome

g. Eclampsia
h. Intracerebral hemorrhage and maternal death.
i. Perinatal mortality and morbidity is high.

> **Note**
> So delivery is preferable after 48 hours of glucocorticoid therapy to avoid maternal risk. The risk of recurrence of HELLP is low (3%–5%).

Q. What is the perioperative management of HELLP syndrome requiring CS?

Ans.
a. Control of BP by antihypertensive drugs
b. IV injection $MgSO_4$
c. Injection betamethasone (12 mg) at 24 hours apart (2 such) if GA is < 34 weeks
d. General anesthesia if platelet count is less than 75,000/cu mm
e. Platelet transfusion 5–10 unit before surgery if platelet count is less than 50,000/cu mm
f. Subfascial and subcutaneous drain
g. Postoperative transfusion of blood component if needed
h. Intense monitoring at least 48 hours after delivery regarding vital signs, fluid intake and output, laboratory values, pulse oximetry.

Acute fatty liver of pregnancy (AFLP), 1 in 13,000 (It is a true hepatic failure case with coagulopathy and encephalopathy).

Q. How do you diagnose this case?

Ans. *Symptoms*: Malaise, nausea, vomiting, epigastric pain.
Signs: Right upper quadrant tenderness, encephalopathy, jaundice
Investigations: LFT—
a. Increased PT, AST, ALP, SGOT level is >SGPT levels
b. Decreased fibrinogen level in second half of pregnancy—coagulopathy
c. USG of liver and biliary system.

Q. What is the pathophysiology?

Ans. Microvascular fatty infiltration and patients are affected late in pregnancy at 34–37 weeks, but it may also occur at 19–20 weeks of GA.

Q. What are the complications?

Ans.
a. Hepatic failure including ascites, pleural effusion, acute pancreatitis, respiratory failure, renal failure or infection
b. Coagulopathy, hypoglycemia, hyperuricemia
c. Encephalopathy—hypoglycemia and hyperammonemia causes altered mental state
d. Intrauterine fetal demise (IUFD)
e. Postpartum hemorrhage (PPH).

> **Note**
> Remember acronym 'PICKLE'–P-PPH, Pancreatitis; I: Infection, IUFD; C: Coagulopathy; K: Kidney failure; L: Liver failure; E: Edema (Pulmonary) or Encephalopathy.

Obstetric Cases

Q. What is the treatment of acute fatty liver of pregnancy (AFLP)?

Ans. Monitoring and supportive measurement in intensive care unit. Delivery of the fetus is the correct treatment, but hypoglycemia, coagulopathy and hypertension has to be controlled.

Q. What is the prognosis?

Ans. Spontaneous resolution after delivery and no recurrence, but CS may be associated with coagulation failure.

Q. Laboratory tests in women with viral hepatitis (VH), intrahepatic cholestasis of pregnancy (ICP) and acute fatty liver of pregnancy (AFLP).

Ans. See Table 10.17.

Table 10.17: Laboratory test (LFT) with difference liver diseases in women

Laboratory test	VH	ICP	AFLP
AST (N = 8–40 IU/L)	> 1,000	< 200	Usually < 500
ALP (N = 32–93 IU/L)	2–4 times higher than normal	2–5 times higher than normal	5–10 times higher than normal
Bilirubin (N = < 1.2 mg/dL)	1–30	< 5	3–40
Increase PT (N = 11–15 sec)	Rare	Common, respond to vitamin K	Common, often implies to DIC

ALP: Alkaline phosphatase, AST: Aspartate transaminase, DIC: Disseminated intravascular coagulation.

Q. What are the different types of viral hepatitis?

Ans. Viral hepatitis A, B, C, D, E (Table 10.18).

Table 10.18: Different types of viral hepatitis

	HAV	HBV	HCV	HDV	HEV
Genome	RNA	DNA	RNA	RNA	RNA
IP (weeks)	2–7	6–26	2–26	6–26	2–9
Transmission	Fecal-Oral	Blood saliva, STIs	Blood saliva	Blood saliva	Fecal oral
Acute attack	Depends on GA	Mild or severe	Usually mild	Mild or severe	Usually mild
Rash	Yes	Yes	Yes	Yes	Yes
Serology	IgM anti- HAV	IgM anti HBc, HBsAg, HBV-DNA	IgM anti- HCV, HCV-RNA	IgM anti- HDV	IgM anti- HEV
PEAK ALT (SGPT)	800–1,000 U/L	1,000–1,500 U/L	300–800 U/L	1,000–1,500 U/L	800–1,000 U/L
UP and down	No	No	Yes	Yes	No
Prevention	Vaccine	Vaccine	–	–	
Treatment	Symptomatic	Symptomatic	Symptomatic	Symptomatic	Symptomatic
			Antivirals	Antivirals	Antivirals

Source: Sherlock S, James Dooley. Disease of the liver and billiary system. The liver in pregnancy (10th ed.), Blackwell Scientific Publication. 1999; 265–75, 475–83.

Q. What is the risk of vertical transmission in hepatitis B virus and how do you prevent it in the newborn baby?

Ans. The vertical risk is 25% when the mother is HBsAg negative, but 80% to 100% when she is hepatitis B surface antigen (HBsAg) positive. When the mother is infected quantitative HBV DNA estimation is done now and in second trimester. If HBV DNA is > 10^8 IU/mL consider treatment with lamivudine or tenofovir in the third trimester, but if the level is below 10^8 IU/mL, no such treatment is required. The Indian Academy of Pediatrics recommends immunization of babies with hepatitis B vaccine at birth, 1 month and 6 months, irrespective of maternal hepatitis status. Neonates born in infected mother with hepatitis B should be given hepatitis B immunoglobulin (HBIG) and vaccine at birth (see below) and vaccine at 1 and 6 months.

This provides 90–95% protection rate to the neonates.

HBIG		Vaccine	
Dose	Timing	Dose	Timing
0.5 mL (250 IU)	Within 12 hours	5–10 µg IM	Within 12 hours

First dose is given concurrently with HBIG, but at different anatomical site and by IM route. Breastfeeding is not contraindicated in the baby who has commenced immunoprophylaxis and active immunization.

Q. Which type of mother needs vaccination?

Ans. Seronegativity for HBsAg, as well as negativity of hepatitis BsAB and hepatitis BcAB will identify those that remain susceptible and require vaccination to prevent future HBV infection. If both the antibodies mentioned above are positive, but HbsAg is negative, mother is immune to hepatitis B and does not require any hepatitis vaccination, but in both the cases hepatitis vaccine is given to baby at birth and ages of 1 and 6 months.

Q. What is the protocol of vaccine?

Ans. HB Vax or Engerix-B vaccine in three divided doses (3×20 µg adults) by deep IM into the deltoid or thigh (not buttock) at time 0, 1 and 6 months. It is safer when used in pregnant mother after first trimester of pregnancy. Active immunization (vaccine) should be considered along with HBIG, for effective pre-exposure and postexposure immunoprophylaxis in susceptible pregnant women. HBIG is given as a single dose (500 IU) by deep IM at a contralateral site of vaccine by using a new needle and syringe.

Q. How do you treat viral hepatitis in pregnancy?

Ans. There is no definitive treatment for jaundice due to viral hepatitis.
   a. Rest and restricted physical activity
   b. *Nutrition*: Glucose (oral or IV, 10% glucose)
   c. *Diet:* Well-balanced diet including high carbohydrate, low fatty diet

Obstetric Cases

d. *Drugs*:
  i. Hepatotoxic drugs should be avoided.
  ii. Bowel should be kept empty by laxative (duphalac syrup)
  iii. Oral neomycin, vitamin B complex and vitamin C
  iv. Control of pruritus by cholestyramine or ursodeoxycholic acid (300 mg bd/day)
  v. Inj vitamin K – 10 mg IM to mother
  vi. Vaginal delivery is preferred: Fetal scalp electrode is avoided
  vii. There is more chances of PPH (so, active management of third stage of labor is required) and blood and FFP should be kept ready for active management of PPH
  viii. Breastfeeding is allowed.

> **Note**
> All pregnant women should be screened for HbSAg, if positive, further tests should be performed: a. HbeAg, b. HbeAB, c. HBV DNA, d. LFTs, e. PT, f. USG of liver.

FOR POSTGRADUATES

RECURRENT PREGNANCY LOSS (RPL)

Q. How do you evaluate a patient with recurrent pregnancy loss?

Ans. History:
Determine pattern and trimester of pregnancy losses. The complete evaluation should be made regarding autoimmune disease, exposure to environmental toxins, infections, drugs, previous gynecologic disorder or surgery including D and C operation.

Physical:
Abnormalities of pelvic examination, abnormal cervix, uterine anomalies.

Investigations:
a. Evaluation of uterine shape by HSG, hysteroscopy, MRI in non pregnant condition.
b. Lupus anticoagulant (LAC) and anticardiolipin antibodies (ACAs) (moderate to high level of IgG-aCL antibody).
c. Parenteral chromosome analysis (father and mother).
d. Chromosome analysis of conceptus.
e. Other relevant tests related with history and physical examinations.

Q. Define recurrent miscarriage (RM).

Ans. The traditional definition includes three or more spontaneous, consecutive pregnancy loss. The couples with two or more consecutive spontaneous miscarriage warrant evaluating the causes of pregnancy loss.

Q. What are the causes of recurrent miscarriage?

Ans. a. **Genetic factors:** The most common chromosomal abnormality is a balanced translocation with abnormal genetic complement, other abnormalities are Robertsonian translocation, inversions, sex chromosomes aneuploidy and supernumerary chromosomes.

b. **Anatomic factors**:
   1. *Congenital*: Common abnormality associated with pregnancy loss is the septate uterus. Other abnormalities are bicornuate or unicornuate uterus.
   2. *Acquired*: Asherman's syndrome which interferes normal placentation. Similarly leiomyomas and polyps interfere placentation and cause pregnancy loss.

c. **Endocrine factors**:
   1. *Luteal phase defect*: Classical diagnosis was obtained after an endometrial biopsy on d26 or d27 of the cycle that was more than 2 days out of phase and more recently the use of midluteal progesterone concentration <10 ng/mL is suggestive for diagnosis. So, there is defect in progesterone receptors and abnormal expression of $\alpha V\beta 3$ biomarker of uterine receptivity which appears in the endometrial glands on cycle day 20–21 during 'the window of implantation'.
   2. Untreated hypothyroidism.
   3. *Insulin resistance*: Poorly controlled diabetes, PCOS
   4. *Elevated day 3 FSH*: Decreased pregnancy rate in women undergoing IVF.
   5. Hyperprolactinemia.

d. **Immunologic factors:** Antiphospholipid antibody syndrome-antiphospholipid antibodies (IgG-aCL, IgM-aCL), LE cells, antithyroid antibodies (antithyroid peroxidase and antithyroglobulin), antinuclear antibodies (ANA) and alloimmune factors.

e. **Infections**: Ureaplasma urealyticum, *mycoplasma, chlamydia*

f. **Thromboembolic factors**: Factor V-Leiden mutation, factor II prothrombin mutation (G20210A), hyperhomocysteinemia, Protein C and S deficiency and elevated factor VIII.

g. **Others:** Psychological and iatrogenic (tobacco, alcohol, exposure to toxins, chemicals).

Q. How do you diagnose and manage recurrent pregnancy loss?

Ans. Genetic: Diagnostic evaluation is by karyotype of partners. Treatment includes genetic counseling, amniocentesis, chorion villus sampling, donor gamets, or preimplantation genetic diagnosis.

Anatomic: Diagnosed by HSG, hysteroscopy, MRI, and laparoscopy. Treatment is by septum transaction by hysteroscopy, myomectomy when it encroach or distort uterine cavity and lysis of adhesion.

Endocrinologic: Diagnosed by hormone assay like midluteal progesterone, TSH, prolactin, fasting insulin: glucose, day-3 FSH and estradiol. Treatment is by 25 mg progesterone suppositories in vagina (morning and night) for 8–10 weeks of pregnancy, levothyroxine, bromocriptine, metformin and counseling.

Immunologic: Lupus anticoagulant and antiphospholipid antibodies (high level of IgG aCL) is treated by aspirin, heparin + aspirin.

Obstetric Cases

Infection is diagnosed by cervical cultures and treated by antibiotics thrombophilia is treated by aspirin + heparin or LMW heparin and hyperhomocysteinemia is treated by folic acid.

Q. What is antiphospholipid antibody syndrome (APLAS) or Hughes syndrome?

Ans. It is an autoimmune disorder defined by distinct clinical and laboratory features including the presence of antiphospholipid (aPL) antibodies. Definite APLAS is present if a patient meets at least one of the following clinical criteria and one of the laboratory criteria.

Criteria for diagnosis:

a. *Clinical criteria*
   1. *Vascular thrombosis*: One or more episodes of arterial, venous, or small vessel thrombosis in any tissue or organ confirmed by imaging, Doppler studies, or histopathology. Superficial venous thromboses are excluded.
   2. *Pregnancy morbidity*
      - One or more unexplained deaths of a morphologically normal fetus at or beyond the 10th week of gestation
      - One or more premature births of a morphologically normal neonate at or before the 34th week of gestation due to severe pre-eclampsia or IUGR
      - Three or more unexplained consecutive spontaneous abortions before the 10th week of gestation.

b. *Laboratory criteria*
   - *Anticardiolipin antibodies (aCL)*: aCL antibodies of IgG and/or IgM isotype in blood present in medium to high titer on two or more occasions at least 12 weeks apart. Titers must be measured by ELISA for beta-2 glycoprotein 1- dependent anticardiolipin antibodies:
      - Prolonged phospholipids–dependent coagulation on a screening test such as aPTT, kaolin clotting time, Russel viper venom time
      - Failure to correct prolonged coagulation time on the screening test by mixing with normal, platelet poor plasma
      - Shortening or correction of the prolonged coagulation time on a screening test by the addition of excess phospholipids
      - Exclusion of other coagulopathies such as factor VIII inhibitor, or heparin
   - *Lupus anticoagulant antibodies (LAC)*: It is present in plasma, on two or more occasions at least 12 weeks apart, detected according to the guidelines of the International Society on Thrombosis and Hemostasis
      - Antibeta-2 glycoprotein 1- dependent antibodies (IgG and IgM isotype).

Q. How do the antibodies cause adverse effects?

Ans. a. The antibodies are directed against an ionic phospholipids and phospholipids binding protein like GPI, prostacyclin, protein C,

annexin V and tissue factors expressed on the cell membrane and thus interfere with prothrombotic and antithrombotic mechanism.
b. The antibodies cause endothelial cell activation and oxidant mediated endothelial injury
c. They also lead to platelet and complement activation
d. APS related adverse pregnancy outcome is related to abnormal placentation, defective spiral artery formation, defective trophoblastic invasion, and defective trophoblastic hormone production.

Q. What is the incidence of recurrent miscarriage by APLAS?
Ans. Incidence of pregnancy loss is 5–20%.

> **Note**
> APLA are found 5–7% of healthy subjects and up to 35% of patients with SLE.

Q. How do you manage APLAS in pregnancy?
Ans. Before conception:
- Pregnancy counseling regarding the potential maternal and obstetrical complications like possibilities of risks of thrombosis and stroke as well as risks of miscarriage, preterm delivery, pre-eclampsia, abruption placenta and neonatal physical and mental handicap should be done.
- Assess for evidence of anemia, thrombocytopenia, underlying renal disease and associated SLE.
- Women with APLAS who had previous episodes of thrombosis and are on long-term warfarin will require change to conventional or low molecular weight heparin (LMWH) as warfarin is teratogenic between 6–12 weeks of gestation. It is desirable to change LMWH within 2 weeks of missed period.

Antenatal period:
- Early USG scan
- *USG Doppler*: If diastolic notch is present in uterine artery waveforms at 20–24 weeks, growth scan should be monitored closely (every 2–3 weeks) for detection of pre-eclampsia or FGR of placental origin. When there is no diastolic notch, assessment of growth and amniotic fluid should be done every 4 weeks.
- Serial Doppler flow of UmA and MCA is necessary to allow timely intervention when diastolic notch in the uterine artery persists with the evidence of IUGR.
- High–risk women require close surveillance of blood pressure and urine analysis to detect early onset pre-eclampsia.

Drugs to improve pregnancy outcome:
1. Aspirin: It inhibits thromboxane and reduces the risk of vascular thrombosis. Aspirin in a dose of 75 mg once daily has been used as soon as pregnancy is diagnosed and should be given up to 34 weeks.
2. Heparin: It is potentially helpful for the treatment at present. APLAS patients with no history of thromboembolic disease are treated with a unfractionated heparin 5,000 IU BD or LMWH (Enoxaparin 40 mg

Obstetric Cases

SC once daily or dalteparin 5000 IU SC once daily). Postpartum prophylactic warfarin and heparin is to be started 12 hours after vaginal delivery and 24 hours after cesarean section and continued till 6 weeks postpartum, patient with history of thrombosis should receive a dose of heparin that will provide full anticoagulation as soon as fetal heart is documented and given throughout pregnancy. LMWH (Enoxaparin 1 mg/kg 12 hourly or dalteparin 200 IU/kg 12 hourly). The goal of therapy is to maintain the activated partial thromboplastin time (aPTT) 1.5–2 times normal when unfractioned heparin is used either SC 3 times daily or continuous infusion. If using LMWH antifactor Xa levels should be checked every trimester in order to maintain levels 0.5–1.1 U/mL. LMW heparin is stopped 24 hours before induction or as soon as patient feels labor pain. If patient is at a very risk of thromboembolism then LMWH can be switched over to unfractioned heparin at 36 weeks. Unfractioned heparin is to be stopped when patient is in active labor. Postpartum therapeutic anticoagulation with heparin is to be started 6 hours after vaginal delivery or 12 hours of cesarean delivery and simultaneously warfarin should be started orally. Once the prothrombin time (PTINR) of 2–3 is achieved with warfarin, heparin should be discontinued and postpartum anticoagulation should be continued for atleast 6 weeks. Important side effects of unfractionated heparins include bleeding, thrombocytopenia and osteopenia.
3. **Warfarin:** It should be avoided in first trimester as it crosses the placenta and potentially teratogenic. It should be discontinued 2 weeks prior to planned delivery to allow clearance from maternal and fetal circulation and heparin or LMWH should be substituted.
4. **Steroid:** Steroids are not as efficient as heparin and aspirin and also carry a high rate of maternal complications. Steroids are useful in patients with SLE (secondary APLAS) and when APLAS is associated with thrombocytopenia.
5. **Immunoglobulin:** Efficacy is doubtful.

Postpartum

Thromboprophylaxis (or full anticoagulation) should be continued 6 weeks postpartum with warfarin which can be used during breastfeeding. Combined OCPs should be avoided for increased risk of thrombosis.

Q. What are the complications of APLAs?

Ans.
1. Thrombotic—arterial/venous thrombosis
2. Obstetrical
   a. Pre-eclampsia
   b. Recurrent pregnancy loss, fetal death
   c. Placental insufficiency—poor fetal growth and fetal distress.

Q. How do you diagnose SLE?

Ans.
a. *Clinical:* Malar rash, photosensitivity, arthritis, arthralgia, renal disease, cardiovascular disease
b. *Hematological:* Anemia, leukopenia, thrombocytopenia, creatinine

c. *Urine*: Proteinuria, cast
d. *Biochemical*: Positive antinuclear antibody (ANA) titer, anti-dsDNA (anti-double-stranded DNA) (increased), complement C3 and C4 (decreased), antibodies to the Smith (Sm) antigen, anti-SSA, anti-SSB, anti-RNP.

Q. What are the obstetric complications in SLE?

Ans. Risks of pre-eclampsia, eclampsia, IUGR, pregnancy loss, moderate to severe renal insufficiency (serum creatinine > 1.5 mg/dL) causes severe prematurity and fetal loss. Neonatal lupus erythematosus (NLE) is a rare condition of the fetus and neonate. NLE is manifested by congenital complete heart block (CCHB) due to inflammation mediated destruction of the conduction system in the A-V node, which is associated with anti-SSA (anti-Ro) and anti-SSB (anti-La) antibodies in the mother that crosses through placenta and reach to the fetus. (Diagnosis of CCHB—fixed bradycardia of fetus in second trimester 60–80 beats/minute and fetal echocardiography is necessary for its confirmation, treatment: Glucocorticoids, plasmapheresis, IVIG, digoxin may not be helpful, hydrops fetalis occurs in most severe cases). Such babies may require pacemaker in early pregnancy.

> **Note**
> Women without renal involvement and Ro/La and aPL antibodies have usually normal outcome.

Q. What are the medical complications of SLE in pregnancy?

Ans. Medical complications—Anemia, thrombocytopenia, thrombotic (stroke, pulmonary embolism, DVT), infection (sepsis, pneumonia).

Q. Obstetric management in SLE?

Ans.
a. Glucocorticoid: Prednisolone is very much useful but glucocorticoid with fluorine at 9a position (dexa or betamethasone may cause undesirable side-effects as they are not metabolized well by placenta). Prednisolone—dose 1–2 mg/kg/day. After the disease is controlled it is tapered to 10–15 mg/day. It may cause GDM.
b. Low dose aspirin can be used throughout gestation.
c. Antimalarial drugs like hydroxychloroquine may be used in pregnancy safely to avoid lupus flare.
d. Cytotoxic agents like methotrexate, cyclophosphamide are rarely used in pregnancy for teratogenecity but azathioprine is not human teratogen and may be associated with growth impairment and impaired neonatal immunity.
e. High dose of IVIG.
f. NSAID: Indomethacin for short-term is useful, but long-term use may cause neonatal renal insufficiency.
g. *Antihypertensive*: ACE inhibitors should be stopped when pregnancy is diagnosed for renal complications of fetus.

Obstetric Cases

Q. Which contraceptions are useful in SLE?

Ans.
a. COCP: Avoid in women who have nephritis, antiphospholipid antibodies, vascular disease.
b. Progestin only implant or injection provides effective contraception without lupus flare.
c. IUCD can also be used safely as it is evidence based that it it does not increase infection rate with immunosuppressive therapy.
d. Postpartum ligation or ligation in quiescent phase of the disease is also safe.

Q. What are the causes of recurrent mid trimester abortion?

Ans.
a. Cervical incompetence—Following D and C/D and E operation, trauma to the cervix due to operative delivery through undilated cervix, amputation of cervix/Fothergill's operation, cone biopsy
b. Uterine anomalies—septate, double uterus, fibroid uterus, synechiae
c. Infection—syphilis, toxoplasmosis
d. Maternal genetic, endocrinal, immunologic, systemic (hypertension, SLE, APLAS)
e. Fetal—chromosomal, structural
f. Placental causes—previa, abruption, chorioamnionitis
g. Idiopathic.

Q. How do you diagnose a case of cervical incompetence?

Ans. History:
Repeated mid-trimester abortion with painless expulsion of products of conception with watery discharge and rupture of membrane before painful contraction.
On examination—bulging of amniotic sac through the cervical canal on speculum examination.

Investigations:
1. Nonpregnant condition—passage of no. 8 Hegar dilator through internal os in premenstrual phase.
2. Premenstrual HSG shows funnel shaped shadow. Similar HSG shadow may be found if it is done in proliferative phase with cervical incompetence.

USG during pregnancy—cervical canal diameter is > 6 mm; length < 3 cm; width at internal os >1.5 cm at first trimester and > 2 cm at second trimester [Funneling of the cervix with the changes in forms TYVU (Trust your vaginal ultrasound) and bulging of membrane].

Q. How do you treat cervical incompetence?

Ans.
a. Improvement of general health, bed rest, adequate treatment of thyroid dysfunction, avoidance of sexual intercourse.
b. Cerclage operation.

Q. What is the exact time of cerclage operation and mention different types of cerclage operation?

Ans. It should be done at 14 weeks of gestation or two weeks before the lowest period of previous wastage as early as the tenth week during pregnancy.

1. McDonald operation (simpler and currently practiced)
2. Shirodkar's operation: A 1.5 cm long transverse incision is made on the anterior vaginal mucosa. Bladder is dissected away up to the level of internal os, a 1cm longitudinal incision is made on the mucosa at the junction of cervix and the vagina posteriorly and nonabsorbable suture (Mersilene tape or no. 2 black braided silk) is passed with the Shirodkar's needle submucously around the cervix. Both the ends are tied posteriorly and vaginal mucosa is closed over sutures. At the end of 38 weeks the stitch is removed by cutting the posterior mucosa. It is necessary when a repeat circlage operation is required in next pregnancy, the cervix is shortened or scarred and to gain adequate length of cervix, bladder mobilization is necessary to complete the procedure.

Other methods:
a. Benson: Done by abdominal route, done for short or excessively amputated cervix, and the mersilene tape suture is placed at the level of isthmus medial to the uterine vessels and between the uterosacral ligaments and the patient is delivered by cesarean section and the cerclage is kept undisturbed for next pregnancy, but in case of preterm labor the knot is cut by laparotomy.
b. Wurm operation: Two number three braided silk mattress suture 1cm wide are placed over the external os, at right angle each other, i.e. U or mattress suture and is used when minimal length of cervix is left.
c. Lash and lash operation: In nonpregnant condition a wedge-shaped tissue is taken from the anterior wall of cervicouterine junction after displacement of bladder downwards and the defect is repaired by interrupted delayed absorbable stitches.

Q. What are the preoperative considerations of encirclage operation?

Ans. a. Definite indication for circlage operation
  b. Gestational age at the time of presentation
  c. Exclusion of chorioamnionitis by:
    i. Measurement of maternal white blood cells count and C-reactive protein (CRP) which is a quick useful method to exclude subclinical chorioamnionitis
    ii. Amniocentesis for clinical suspicion of infection
    iii. Genital swab for exclusion of infection is not helpful as it takes several days for report
  d. USG to locate the site of placenta and cardiac activity of fetus.

Q. What are the contraindications of cerclage operation?

Ans. a. Uterine contraction or active preterm labor
  b. Unexplained vaginal bleeding
  c. Infection in vagina or uterus or chorioamnionitis
  d. Rupture of membrane
  e. Major fetal anomaly
  f. GA after 28 weeks
  g. Fetal compromise.

Obstetric Cases

> **Note**
> Sexual coitus is inhibited 1 week before and after surgery.

Q. What are the steps of McDonald stitch and mention its complications?

Ans.
    a. Consent of operation.
    b. Ask the patient to evacuate the bladder.
    c. The patient is placed in lithotomy position, antiseptic dressing and draping.
    d. General anesthesia.
    e. Introduce Sim's posterior vaginal speculum.
    f. The anterior and posterior lip is grasped by sponge holding forceps or Allis tissue forceps if there is prolapse of membrane it should be introduced into the cervical canal by Foley's catheter gently or by reducing membrane directly with wet swab or by applying sponge holding forceps circumferentially around the cervix to gently pull it over the bulging membrane.
    g. Number 2 black braided silk is passed at 10 o'clock at cervicovaginal junction in purse string fashion anticlockwise encircling the cervix under the mucosa till the end exits by the side of the entry point or at 2 o'clock position.
    h. The knot is placed anteriorly at 12 o'clock and it is tightened till only the little finger can enter.

> **Note**
> Anterior knot is difficult to remove and it may cause bladder irritation and erosion, so posterior (6 o'clock) or lateral knot is preferred.

Postoperative management
- Bedrest—48 hours
- Sedation
- Parenteral betamimetic (ritodrine 10 mg 8 hourly for 5–7 days)
- Antibiotics
- Patient is discharged on 7th PO day after confirmation of cardiac activity by USG with instructions to report if there is any vaginal bleeding, leaking or abdominal pain
- She should take regular antenatal check-up and avoid intercourse throughout pregnancy and the stitch is to be removed at 37 completed weeks (38 weeks) or earlier if labor pain starts
- Periodic USG for fetus and cervix
- Progesterone hormone is helpful for short cervix detected by TVS or for patient having history of preterm labor.

Complications
    a. *During operation*: Rupture of the membrane and hemorrhage, entrapment of bladder.
    b. *Immediately after operation*: Onset of threatened abortion and preterm labor, infection
    c. *Delayed*: Cutting the suture through the cervix and coming out through the cervical canal, Bucket-handle tear of the cervix if labor

contraction occurs with the stitch in place, uterine rupture if the suture *in situ* but no tear of cervix, cervical dystocia due to fibrosis.

d. Anterior knot in McDonald operation may cause bladder erosion in neglected condition where it is kept for a long time.

Q. What are the nonsurgical treatment of cervical insufficiency?

Ans. a. Use of progesterone along with rest and abstinence for 37 weeks
   i. Injection α-hydroxy progesterone caproate 500 mg IM weekly
   ii. Oral progesterone—200 mg bd
   iii. Natural micronized progesterone—100 mg bd per vagina

b. *Vaginal pessaries*: Hodge Smith pessary
   It alters cervical canal axis and weight of pregnant uterus is displaced away from cervix, posteriorly. It should be inserted at 12–14 weeks and removed at 37 weeks, but weekly removal and insertion is necessary for cleaning and size readjustment.

EPILEPSY IN PREGNANCY

Epilepsy is defined as ≥ 2 unprovoked seizures greater than 24 hours apart.

> **Note**
>
> *Recent American Academy of Neurological (AAN) guideline stated that prolactin measurement within 10–20 minutes after a generalized or complex partial seizure is a helpful in differentiating epileptic seizures from psychogenic nonepileptic seizures. However, serum prolactin elevation does not differentiate epileptic seizures from syncope.*

Special points to note
1. Type of seizure like partial or generalized
2. Taking new or old generation of AEDs (antiepileptic drugs) and whether it is mono or polytherapy
3. Folic acid is administered or not
4. Any convulsion in last 6 months before planned conception or any convulsion during pregnancy
5. Seizure associated with menstrual cycle- catamenial epilepsy
6. History of infertility as epilepsy or AEDs may cause infertility
7. Previous abortion or any congenital defective baby
8. Family history of epilepsy—Juvenile myoclonic epilepsy, partial epilepsy syndrome (benign rolandic epilepsy) are related to genomic makeup.
9. PCOS occurs in 10–25% with epilepsy, with some of this association possibly due to the use of valproic acid (VPA).

Q. What is the incidence of epilepsy in pregnancy?
Ans. 0.5–1%.

Q. What is the effect of pregnancy on epilepsy?
Ans. Pregnancy does not have any deleterious effect on the course of epilepsy except alteration of seizure rate which varies from person-to-person

or in the same patient with different pregnancies. Probable cause of increased seizure frequencies are:
   a. Physiologic or psychologic changes
   b. Changes in sex hormone concentration (estrogen)
   c. Changes in antiepileptic drug (AED) metabolism
   d. Sleep deprivation and new stress
   e. Non-compliance of the medication and altered pharmacokinetics of AED.

Q. What is gestational epilepsy?

Ans. In a few cases with no previous history of epilepsy, a chronic epileptic disease appears during pregnancy and disappears one or two months after delivery. The incidence of gestational epilepsy is 50 per 100,000 pregnant women.

Q. What is the effect of epilepsy on pregnancy?

Ans. Effects of epilepsy on pregnancy depend upon,
   i. Effects of epilepsy itself,
   ii. The effects of seizures,
   iii. The effect of AED (antiepileptic drugs).

A wide range of obstetric complications like spontaneous miscarriage, pre-eclampsia—eclampsia, preterm labor (9–11%), hyperemesis gravidarum, anemia, stillbirth and neonatal death, hemorrhagic disease of newborn, low Apgar scores, LBW babies. Genaralized tonic-clonic seizures (GTCSs) can cause maternal and fetal hypoxia and acidosis secondary to utero-placental circulation.

Many types of seizure can cause trauma, which can result in rupture of fetal membrane, with an increased risk of infection, preterm labor, fetal death, and abruptio placenta.

Weak uterine contraction are noted in women taking AEDs, which may account for the two-fold increase in use of interventions during labor and delivery, including induction, mechanical rupture of membrane, instrumental deliveries and cesarean section.

Q. Antiepileptic drugs (AEDs)—should these be used during pregnancy? What are the alterations of dose regimen? What are the adverse effects on fetus?

Ans. Most of the antiepileptic drugs are C or D and the risk of medication to the fetus must be considered. The women who are on AED before pregnancy and by the time they realizes that they become pregnant; it is too late to make medication adjustment to avoid malformations. Polytherapy of AED causes more malformation when compared to monotherapy. The rate of major malformation increased to 25% for those women taking 4/or more AEDs. The risk of fetal defects could be decreased by using monotherapy with lowest possible dose. Management of AEDs during pregnancy can be complex. Adjustment of dose, type of AEDs and the dose of AEDs should be altered on clinical grounds. Increase in seizure frequency is an indication of increased dosage and or addition of new AEDs.

> **Note**
>
> *Clearance of all the AEDs increases during pregnancy, resulting in decrease in serum concentration due to decreased albumin concentration and induction of the hepatic microsomal enzymes by the increased sex steroid hormones and distinctive metabolic pathway of glucuronidation.*

Adverse effects of AEDs on fetus:

Minor anomalies (6–20%)—distal digital and nail hypoplasia, midline craniofacial anomalies including broad nasal bridge, hypertelorism, epicanthal fold, altered lips and low hair line.

Major (1.25–11.5%)—congenital heart disease (ASD, VSD, PDA, pulmonary stenosis, coarctation of aorta, and tetralogy of Fallot), cleft lip and palate, urogenital defects (glandular hypospidias), neural tube defects (NTDs).

> **Note**
>
> *Open type of NTDs are caused by Valproic acid (VPA, 1–3%), or carbamazepine (CBZ, 0.5–1%). So valproic acid should be avoided before 8 weeks of gestation.*

Q. What are the possible mechanisms of drug teratogenecity?

Ans.
a. Antifolate effect of phenytoin, phenobarbital, carbamazepine, lamotrigine and valproate.
b. Reactive intermediates of AEDs include free radicals (via per oxidation) and oxidative metabolites, both of which may contribute AED teratogenesis. The metabolites may accumulate in the fetus due to low level of epoxide hydrolase which inhibit epoxide metabolism.
c. Alteration of embryonic pH, which is mainly found in valproate.

Q. Which drugs are used for epilepsy?

Ans. Commonly used drugs (first generation) are phenytoin sodium, carbamazepine, sodium valproate and phenobarbitone. All these drugs are more teratogenic and USFDA category of such drugs in pregnancy is 'D' (positive evidence of risk).

The newer generations (second generation) of AED are less teratogenic and they are oxcarbazepine (OXC), topiramate (TPM), gabapentin (GBP), tiagabine, levetiracetam (LEV), and Zonisamide (ZNS) and all these are included in pregnancy category 'C'(risk cannot be ruled out).

Q. How do you impart preconceptional care in a case of epilepsy?

Ans.
1. In preconception period if the patient has no convulsion for 2 years supervised withdrawal of AED at 6 months before planned conception or in case where drug withdrawal is inappropriate, use single drug regime with lowest possible dose.
2. Proper counseling of patient.
3. Folic acid supplement.
4. Review necessity of AEDs.

Obstetric Cases

5. Consider changing to an alternative to VPA (valproic acid) therapy if possible prior to conception.

> **Note**
>
> *Women having epilepsy and are treated with valproic acid or carbamazepine receive at least 0.4–5 mg/day of Folic acid (American College of Obstetricians and Gynecologists).*

Q. What is the approach of antenatal care in pregnancy with epilepsy?

Ans.
1. Pregnancy are managed with the consultation of neurologist especially when the convulsions are not controlled.
2. Control of nausea and vomiting for better action of the drugs.
3. Transvaginal USG at 16-20 weeks to exclude congenital defects of fetus.
4. NTD should be screened with a combination of alfafetoprotein at 15-22 weeks.
5. As the pregnancy progresses the dose of AED should be adjusted and the first adjustment should be at the end of first trimester when all major organs have already been developed.
6. Good nutrition and avoid sleep disturbance as sleep deprivation may provoke seizure
7. Vitamin K supplementation—Certain AEDs like carbamazepine, phenytoin, primidone, phenobarbitone causes hemorrhagic problems in the babies due deficiency of vitamin K dependent clotting factors (II, VII, IX, X) especially in the first 24 hours after birth. The abnormality is reversed with the oral administration of vitamin K1 to the mother from 36 weeks of gestational age until delivery and baby should receive vitamin K—1 mg IM at birth.
8. Higher dose of steroid (24 mg betamethasone at 12 hours apart) for management at risk of preterm delivery. Higher dose is required as steroid is metabolized by enzyme inducing AEDs.
9. AED level should be measured before each trimester and in last 4 weeks of pregnancy.

Q. How do you manage labor and delivery in epileptic pregnant mother?

Ans. Epilepsy is not an indication of cesarean section (CS), but CS may be needed for refractory seizures during labor.
1. During labor the chances of convulsion increases due to exhaustion.
2. No special treatment at delivery is required when seizure is well-controlled by AEDs during pregnancy.
3. Pain relief during labor or epidural analgesia is required for reduction of seizure occurrence because hyperventilation with pain may lead to respiratory alkalosis that could lower the seizure threshold.
4. Convulsive and repeated seizures during labor should be treated with parenteral lorazepam or diazepam (10-20 mg). Benzodiazepines can cause neonatal respiratory depression, decreased heart rate, and maternal apnea if given in large doses and these potential side effects should be monitored carefully.

5. Sometimes the newborn after delivery may be irritable or have mild seizures due to withdrawal of drugs which are taken by mothers during pregnancy.

Q. What is the postpartum care?

Ans.
1. Most of the AED levels gradually increases after delivery and plateau by 10 weeks postpartum. Lamotrigine (LTG) levels increase immediately and plateaus within 2–3 weeks postpartum (so adjustment of the dose is necessary in first few days after delivery).
2. Encourage breastfeeding though most anticonvulsants are excreted in breast milk but concentration is lower than maternal plasma.
3. Sleep disruption in puerperium may provoke seizure recurrence in women who have had previously controlled seizure.
4. Changing diaper and clothes are performed best on the floor; bathing should never be performed alone
5. Contraception:
   a. Epileptic mother who are not on AEDs can safely use any method of contraception like COCPs, monthly injectable, combined patch or vaginal ring, POPs, implants, Cu bearing IUCDs or LNG-IUS (WHO).
   b. Epilepsy with AEDs
      i. Use of methods not usually recommended (category 3, WHO) are COCPs, monthly injectable hormone, combined patch or combined vaginal ring, POPs.
      ii. Use methods in any circumstances (category 1, WHO)
         Injection DMPA, Cu bearing IUCD and LNG IUS.
6. Newborn has immature drug eliminating system and they should be observed for signs of drug intoxication like lethargy, poor feeding, irritability, etc.
7. Neonates exposed to enzyme induced antiepileptic drugs (EIAED) should be observed for clotting disorder.

Q. What are different types of malformation at different times of organogenesis?

Ans.

Tissues	Malformations	Postconceptional age
Central nervous system (CNS)	Neural tube defect (NTDs)	28 days
Heart	Ventricular septal defect (VSD)	42 days
Face	Cleft lip	36 days
Cleft maxillary palate		47–70 days

Q. Which drugs are commonly used in epilepsy?
Ans. Drugs of epilepsy is shown in Table 10.19.

Obstetric Cases

Table 10.19: Drugs of epilepsy

Drug	Dose	Side effects	Malformation rate (%)
Phenytoin	300–600 mg/day in divided doses	Anomalies in craniofacial, limb, neonatal growth, performance delays-fetal hydantoin syndrome	5–11%
Carbamazepine	200–1200 mg/d	All defects mentioned above with spina bifida	1–2%
Phenobarbital	60–240 mg/d	All defects mentioned above with congenital heart disease, orofacial clefting	
Valproic acid	10–15 mg/kg/d	Spina bifida, cardiac defects, orofacial clefting, genitourinary anomalies	2% with monotherapy, 8–16% with polytherapy
Clonazepam	1.5–20.0 mg/d		
Gabapentin	Newer drugs		
Lamotrigine	300–500 mg in two divide doses	Increased risk of cleftlip and palate	2.7%
Levetiracetam	1000–3000 mg in two divided doses		2.7%

Note

If convulsion continues ≥30 minutes or repeated seizures over a ≥30-minutes period without full recovery between attacks (status epilepticus)—Infuse phenytoin sodium 1 g (18 mg/kg body weight) in 50–100 mL of normal saline over 30 minutes (final concentration does not to exceed 10 mg/mL). Dextrose solution should be avoided as it causes crystallization of phenytoin sodium. Complete administration is within 1 hour of preparation. Infusion at a rate of >50 mg/minute causes irregular heart beat, hypotension and respiratory depression. So, BP and EKG monitoring are necessary, other drugs are midazolam 10 mg IM, fosphenytoin (not phenytoin)-20 mg/kg PE (phenytoin equivalent) IM or diazepam 20 mg per rectum. Other measures are ABC—airway, breathing, circulation: IV infusion, oxygen, cardiopulmonary resuscitation (CPR), and intubation if required.

THYROID DISORDER IN PREGNANCY

Q. What is the incidence of thyroid disorder irrespective of pregnancy?

Ans. Thyroid disease is present in 2–5% of women and 1–2% of women in the reproductive age group.

Q. What are the effects of pregnancy on thyroid function?

Ans. 1. High hCG during the first trimester of pregnancy can result in low TSH level, which return to normal by second trimester and are maintained throughout the pregnancy.
2. Estrogen during pregnancy increases the amount of TBG and increases the total thyroid hormones in the blood.

3. So free T4, free T3 and TSH should be measured to assess the thyroid function during pregnancy.
4. Physiological enlargement of thyroid gland (goiter) may occur in pregnancy due to increased fetal use of iodine and increased maternal clearance of iodide.

> **Note**
>
> ***Recommendations for management in pregnancy***
> *a. Go for universal thyroid screening in high endemic zones of India to protect lives of many more women and unborn babies suggested by Federation of Indian Chambers of Commerce and Industry (FICCI) and Frost & Sullivan, India (F & S), 2016*
> *b. Target TSH of mother*
>   *i. First trimester ≤2.5 mIU/L*
>   *ii. Second and third trimester ≤3 mIU/L*
> *c. In pre-existing hypothyroidism, increase thyroxin dose by 30% (2 additional tablet per week) once pregnancy is established to decrease the risk of hypothyroidism in the first trimester*
> *d. Free T4 and TSH levels should be tested every 6 weeks*
> *e. In neonates, screening of hypothyroidism atleast on 5th day/or days 2–4 of life is mandatory to prevent risk of mental retardation and other neurologic sequelae.*

Q. When do you screen for thyroid dysfunction in pregnancy?

Ans. Screening of thyroid disease should be done early in pregnancy to detect asymptomatic thyroid dysfunction, which can lead to serious adverse events for both the mother and child. Routine screening is not yet practised.

Conditions where screening is essential:
a. History of hyper or hypothyroid disease, postpartum thyroiditis, thyroid lobectomy
b. Family history of thyroid disease
c. Women with a goiter
d. Women older than age 30 years
e. Thyroid antibodies when known
f. Symptoms including thyroid overfunction or underfunction including anemia, elevated cholesterol and hyponatremia
g. Women with type-1 diabetes
h. Women with other autoimmune diseases
i. Women with previous therapeutic head neck irradiation
j. Women with history of miscarriage and preterm delivery.

HYPOTHYROIDISM

Q. What are the causes of hypothyroidism in pregnancy?

Ans. Approximately 2–3% women have raised TSH level during pregnancy.

Causes of Hypothyroidism

Primary thyroid dysfunction:
- Hashimoto's disease (chronic thyroiditis, chronic autoimmune thyroiditis), subacute thyroiditis
- Circulatory receptor blocking antibody

Hypothalamic dysfunction:
- Prior thyroid surgery
- Radioactive iodine therapy
- Iodine deficiency—Relative hypothyroidism and goitrogenesis.

Drugs: Lithium, amiodarone.

> **Note**
> Hashimoto's thyroiditis is the most common cause of hypothyroidism which is confirmed by demonstrating the presence of circulating antithyroglobulin and antimicrosomal antibodies.

Q. How do you diagnose hypothyroidism in pregnancy?

Ans. Most of the women with mild hypothyroidism have no major symptoms. Symptoms include excessive fatigue, dry skin, cold intolerance, constipation, bradycardia, and irritability. Myxedema is rare.

Laboratory investigations:
- Low free T4 and high TSH levels is the most sensitive indicator of primary hypothyroidism

Elevation of antithyroid antibodies like anti-thyroid peroxidase antibody (anti-TPOAb) and anti-thyroglobulin antibody (anti-TgAb) is associated with higher rate of miscarriage and preterm labor.
- Increased cholesterol is not a sensitive marker during pregnancy.
- Normocytic anemia, abnormal LFT (reversible).

Q. How do you treat hypothyroidism in pregnancy?

Ans. 1. Most of the patient who are treated for hypothyroidism during pregnancy are diagnosed before pregnancy and already are on replacement therapy. In these patients the dose should be checked to determine if it is adequate or not and the therapy should be followed throughout pregnancy. A patient also may develop hypothyroidism during pregnancy.

> **Note**
> Patient should strive for an euthyroid state prior to conception and immediately seek care to have thyroid function test when pregnancy is confirmed for optimal management.

2. Once the diagnosis of hypothyroidism is made full replacement doses of T4 should be instituted regardless the degree of thyroid function.
3. Therapy should be titrated rapidly in young pregnant women with no other comorbid conditions starting with 0.1 mg T4 daily for 3–5 weeks. Thereafter dosage adjustment can be made depending on the thyroid function test result.

4. Since, T4 has a long half-life it can be given once-a-day in empty stomach at bedtime or first thing in the morning.
5. If hypothyroidism is newly diagnosed in pregnancy L-thyroxin should be started at 1.5–2 mcg/kg.
6. The optimal goal of TSH during pregnancy is to maintain <2.5 mIU/L in the first trimester and <3.0 mIU/L in the second and third trimester.
   TSH should be measured at 4–6 weeks after each dose adjustment and each trimester once the optimal serum TSH levels have been reached.
   - TSH 4–10   Increase dose by 25–50 mcg daily
   - TSH 10–20   Increase dose by 50–75 mcg daily
   - TSH >20   Increased dose by 75–100 mcg daily
7. After delivery the prepregnancy dose of thyroxin should be given and TSH level is rechecked 6 weeks later.
8. Iron decreases the absorption of thyroxin from the gut, so it should not be given together. Calcium, antacid, sucralfate and caffeine can interfare its absorption.

> **Note**
> It is important to note that total T4 (TT4) and triiodothyronine (TT3) concentration in pregnancy is higher (1.5 times higher than the normal reference range for non-pregnant women) throughout pregnancy and the thyroid binding globulin (TBG) is the primary binding protein for T4 and T3 in plasma.
> Estrogen stimulation during pregnancy increases the serum TBG by 50%.
> So free T4 (fT4) and free T3 (fT3) are more accurate measure of thyroid status.

Q. What are the complications if the hypothyroidism is inadequately treated or unrecognized during pregnancy?

Ans. Chances of increased risks of miscarriage, pre-eclampsia, abruptio placentae, cardiac dysfunction, PPH, preterm baby, intrauterine fetal demise, low birth weight babies, impaired neurophysiological development and irreversible brain damage of the newborn are more common.

> **Note**
> The range of TSH in normal pregnancy is between 0.2–2.5 micron unit/mL.
> a. If the value is >2.5 micron unit/mL and antimicrosomal antibodies are positive, the patient should be treated irrespective of clinical condition and check TSH every 4 weeks.
> b. If the value is >2.5 micron unit/mL and antimicrosomal antibodies are absent, the patient should be monitored closely (repeat TSH after 4 weeks), if TSH is >3.5 micron unit/mL, start T4 replacement.
> c. Women with TSH <2.5 micron unit/mL and antibody negative, do not require further evaluation, and if the level of TSH >5 micron unit/mL start treatment irrespective of antibody status.

Q. Is neonatal thyroid screening necessary?

Ans. Many centers of India perform cord or baby's blood for TSH and T4 for detection of primary hypothyroid babies at birth. The confirmation should be done on day 3-4 of neonatal life which shows high cord blood TSH level (>50 μU/mL) with normal or low levels of serum T4 (<8 μg/dL).

Obstetric Cases

After 3rd day; the TSH level.>20 µU/mL is suggestive of congenital hypothyroidism.

> **Note**
>
> Within 30 minutes after birth cord blood T3, T4 and TSH is high and persists for >24 hours for birth stress or significant fall in the newborn's temperature. Following the burst of thyroid hormone, TSH declines exponentially within 48 hours due to negative feedback.

Q. How do you treat if hypothyroidism is detected in newborn baby?

Ans. In neonates the initial starting dose of L-thyroxin is 10–15 mcg/kg/day in the morning in empty stomach to ensure better absorption from the gut and to maintain T4 level between 8–12 microgram/dL. The thyroid function test should be performed at 2 and 4 weeks after starting treatment and then every 1–2 months in the first year, every 2–3 months between 1–3 years and 6 monthly thereafter.

Myxedema coma

It represents severe hypothyroidism and is considered as medical emergency with 20% mortality rate.

Q. What are the characteristic features of myxedema coma?

Ans. It is characterized by hypothermia, hypotension, hypoventilation, bradycardia, lethargy and fatigue, delayed deep tendon reflex, and constipation. Supporting laboratory evidences: Increased TSH, decreased T4 and free T4, presence of antithyroid antibodies, hyponatremia, elevated serum creatinine, hypoglycemia and elevated CPK (skeletal muscle usually).

EKG—sinus bradycardia, low amplitude QRS complexes, prolonged QT interval, flattened or inverted T wave.

Q. How do you manage myxedema coma?

Ans.
a. IV fluid and electrolyte and IV sodium should be needed if Na$^+$ is < 120 mEq/L.
b. Endotracheal intubation and ventilation
c. Warming by normal blanket
d. Cardiac monitoring—BP, EKG, troponin and CPK to rule out myocardial infarction
e. Corticosteroid—100 mg hydrocortisone every 8 hours
f. Levothyroxin sodium—slow bolus IV dose 300–500 µg, Daily IV dose 75–100 µg daily, oral dose 50–200 µg when the patient is ambulatory.
g. Liothyronine T3 replacement in young patient with low cardiovascular risk—10 µg IV every 8 hours
h. Antibiotics.

> **Note**
>
> In pregnancy, euthyroid is defined as normal TSH (0.2–2.5 µIU/L); Subclinical hypothyroid defined as high TSH (>2.5 µIU/L) and in the presence of normal level of free T4 (0.8-2.0 ng/dL); overt hypothyroid is defined as high TSH (>2.5 µIU/L) with low free T4 (<0.8 ng/dL).

HYPERTHYROIDISM IN PREGNANCY

Hyperthyroidism in pregnancy occurs in 0.2% of pregnancies.

Q. What are the different causes of hyperthyroidism during pregnancy?

Ans.
a. Graves' disease
b. Toxic nodular goiter
c. Acute (subacute) thyroiditis
d. Toxic adenomas
e. Hyperemesis gravidarum
f. Gestational trophoblastic disease
g. Exogenous thyroid hormones.

Q. What is the most common cause of hyperthyroidism?

Ans. Grave's disease—Autoantibody [thyroid-stimulating antibody (TSAb)- formerly known as Long acting thyroid stimulator (LATS)] against TSH receptors acts as a TSH agonist, thereby stimulating increased production of thyroid hormones.

Q. How do you diagnose hyperthyroidism in pregnancy clinically?

Ans. The diagnosis of mild hyperthyroidism is very difficult in pregnancy because the patient may report symptoms that are seen commonly in normal pregnancy. Fatigue, increased appetite, vomiting, palpitation, tachycardia, heat intolerance, increased urinary frequency insomnia and emotion liability may confuse the diagnosis. More specific symptoms highly suggestive of hyperthyroidism include tremor, nervousness, frequent stools, excessive vomiting, brisk reflexes, muscle weakness, goiter, hypertension, and weight loss.

Graves' ophthalmopathy like stare, lid lag and retraction, exophthalmos and dermography like localized or pretibial myxedema are diagnostic.

Laboratory evaluation confirms the diagnosis:
a. Free T4 level is high in hyperthyroid patient
b. Rarely (in 3–5% of cases), the free-T4 level may be normal and free T3 elevated
c. TSH is uniformly suppressed
d. Autoantibodies confirm the autoimmune nature of the disease and may have fetal implication.
e. Thyroid receptor antibodies (TRAB) are present in 90% of patients with Graves' disease.

Q. What are the maternal and fetal risks of untreated hyperthyroidism?

Ans. Maternal: Pre-eclampsia, maternal heart failure, infection, anemia and thyroid storm.
Fetal: Spontaneous abortion, prematurity, low birth weight, IUFD, fetal/neonatal thyrotoxicosis.

Q. What are the hemodynamic changes with hyperthyroidism?

Ans.
a. Increased stroke volume and cardiac output
b. Increased pulse rate
c. Reduced peripheral vascular resistance

Obstetric Cases

   d. Increased blood volume
   e. Impaired myometrial contractility
   f. ECG-changes,
      1. Left ventricular hypertrophy (15%)
      2. Atrial fibrillation (21%)
      3. Wolf-Parkinson-White syndrome—shortening of PR interval and slurring of QRS complex called a delta wave.

Q. What are the treatment options for hyperthyroidism?

Ans. a. *Observation*: It is a reasonable treatment plan for mild clinical disease without cardiovascular compromise.
   b. Antithyroid drugs
   c. Beta adrenergic blocking drugs
   d. Thyroid surgery.

Antithyroid drugs: Useful for overt disease (hyperthyroidism) when TSH is <0.1 μu/mL and TSHR-Ab positive and T4/T3 increased. Monitoring should be done every 4 weeks. If TSH is <0.1 μu/mL, TSHR-Ab is negative and T4 level is normal. Monitor TSH level and if TSH is <0.01 μu/mL, clinical decision should be taken.

1. Antithyroid drugs like methimazole and carbamizole blocks the intrathyroid hormone, crosses the placenta and impairs the baby's thyroid function and cause aplasia cutis in infancy. Methimamazole is given 10–20 mg every 12 hours. As symptoms improve and fT4 decreases, the dosing of ATD is reduced. In stable patient methimazole is given once daily. Embryopathy, primary aplasia cutis, and choanal or esophageal atresia are rare complications of methimazole.

2. Propylthiouracil (PTU) is the preferred drug (drug of choice) during pregnancy as it minimally crosses the placenta and also blocks peripheral conversion of T4 to T3 along with the blocking of intrathyroid hormone production. It also lowers the T4 levels faster than methimazole. The recommended dose of PTU is 300–450 mg initially, followed by 100 mg three times daily to control hyperthyroidism in 4–8 weeks. The goal of the treatment is to use the smallest dose that maintain the maternal free T4 level at or just above the upper limit of nonpregnant reference range. In a stable patient it should be given two to three times daily. Clinical and laboratory follow-up (TSH, free T4 and free T3) should be done every two to four weeks. Most symptoms (90%) improve within two-four weeks. Rapid improvement requires the lowering of the dose. Improvement commonly occurs in the second trimester, and as many as 40% of the mother discontinue the therapy. But continuation of the therapy in low dose is necessary to avoid the risk of fetal thyrotoxicosis imposed by transplacental passage of TSAb and to reduce the incidence of thyroid storm during labor.

3. Beta adrenergic blocker may be used as an adjunctive therapy to control the symptoms of tremor and palpitation until the thioamides decrease the thyroid hormone levels. Contraindication of beta blocker (Propranolol)—Obstructive lung disease, heart block, heart

failure and insulin use. Effects on fetus—bradycardia, FGR, and neonatal hypoglycemia.

> **Note**
> Although small amount of PTU and methimazole are found in breast milk, breastfeeding is considered with these medications.

Q. What are the side effects of the drug PTU?

Ans. Adverse reaction includes skin rash, bronchospasm, drug fever, hepatitis oral ulcer, sore throat, idiopathic agranulocytosis (0.5%) and neutropenia. So, baseline white blood cell count, LFT and differential count should be noted.

Q. What are the differences between PTU and carbimazole?

Ans.

PTU	Carbimazole
Dose to dose less potent	About 5 times more potent
Highly plasma protein bound	Less bound
Less transfer across placenta and in milk	Larger amount crosses in fetus and milk
Plasma t ½: 1–2 hours	6–10 hours
Single dose acts for 4–8 hours	12–24 hours
No active metabolite	Active metabolite-methimazole
Multiple doses (2–3/day) needed	Mostly single daily dose
Inhibits T4 to T3 conversion	Do not inhibit T4 to T3 peripherally conversion

Q. When thyroid surgery is needed in hyperthyroid patient in pregnancy?

Ans. Subtotal thyroidectomy is needed in patients with severe antithyroid drug side effects or failed medical suppression of thyroid function with the dose of PTU >300 mg daily. It should be done in second trimester.

Q. What precaution do you take before and after operation?

Ans. Preoperatively, the hyperthyroid mothers should be treated with antithyroid medications for 7-10 days, a beta adrenergic blocker (Propranolol 20 mg tds daily) and inorganic iodide (Lugol iodine, 3 drops twice daily) for 4-5 days. The later two can be discontinued 48 hours postoperatively. Iodide must be used cautiously to minimize the fetal risk of hypothyroidism and goiter.

> **Note**
> Radioactive iodine (Iodine-131) administration is contraindicated in pregnancy.

Thyroid storm

It is a hypermetabolic complication of hyperthyroidism.

Q. How do you diagnose thyroid storm?

Ans. a. *Hypermetabolism*: Fever above 100°F, perspiration
b. *CVS*: Tachycardia, atrial flutter, CCF

Obstetric Cases

  c. *CNS*: Irritability, agitation, tremor, delirium, psychosis, coma
  d. *GIT*: Nausea, vomiting, diarrhea, jaundice
  e. *Supportive laboratory evidence*: Leukocytosis, elevated liver function values, hypercalcemia, low TSH, high free T4 and/or T3.

Q. What are the common precipitating factors for thyroid storm?

Ans. Surgical trauma, infection, labor and delivery, severe anemia, induction of anesthesia, hypertension/pre-eclampsia, diabetic ketoacidosis and myocardial infarction.

Q. How do you treat thyroid storm?

Ans. a. *Propylthiouracil*: 600 mg PO (nasogastric tube) then 300 mg 6 hourly.
  b. *Sodium iodide*: 1 g in 500 mL of fluid qd.
  c. *Propranolol*: 40–60 mg every 4–6 hour.
  d. *Dexamethasone*: 1 mg IV or IM 6 hourly.
  e. *Supportive therapy*: Oxygen, actaminophen, fluid replacement.

> **Note**
> Subclinical hyperthyroid, defined as low serum TSH (<0.2 µIU/L) concentration with normal free T4 (0.8–2 ng/dL); Overt hyperthyroid, defined as high free T4 (>2.0 ng/dL) with decreased TSH (<0.2 µIU/L).

OBESITY AND PREGNANCY

Q. What is obesity?

Ans. Body mass index (BMI) is considered the gold standard for determining weight status of the individual. The BMI is not valid while pregnant and so, should be measured pre- and post-gestation. In the case where prepregnancy weight is not known the first weight measured at prenatal clinic is generally used to calculate prepregnancy BMI.

Pregestation and postpartum obesity is most commonly defined according to WHO.

BMI (Kg/m²)	Weight
<18.5	Underweight
18.5– 24.9	Normal weight
25–29.9	Overweight
>30	Obese
30–34.99	Obese (class 1)
35–39.99	Obese (class 2)
40	Obese (class 3)

> **Note**
> Ideal body weight of an adult:
> Female: 100 + (4 × {height in inch minus 60}) lbs
> Male: 120 + (4 × {height in inch minus 60}) lbs.

Q. What are the maternal complications associated with pregnancy obesity?

Ans. I. *Prior to pregnancy and early gestation*
   a. Infertility
   b. Miscarriage

II. *Late gestation*
   a. Hypertensive disorders—Pre-eclampsia or gestational hypertension due to endothelial dysfunction and or insulin resistance
   b. GDM
   c. Thromboembolic disease.
   d. Infection (UTI)

III. *Labor and delivery*
   a. Increased incidence of CS and anesthetic complication like intubations and respiratory problem in general anesthesia (GA) for shorter and fatter necks and location of physical reference point in vertebra is difficult for high subcutaneous fat during spinal and epidural anesthesia
   b. Increased incidence of preterm labor
   c. In mismanaged vaginal birth chances of complete perineal tear (CPT) is high.

IV. *Puerperium*
   a. Bleeding, infection (wound, endometritis) and urinary problem
   b. Poor lactation outcome due to additional source of progesterone from adipocytes which inhibit the activation of prolactin.
   c. PPH—To be prevented by active management of IIIrd stage of labor.

Q. What are the fetal/neonatal complications in pregnancy with obesity?

Ans. *Fetal*—miscarriage, neural tube defects, heart and craniospinal defects, ventral wall and intestinal defects, preterm birth, IUFD
Neonatal—Neonatal death, macrosomia, shoulder dystocia, birth trauma, SGA baby.

Q. What are the reasons for infertility in obese women?

Ans.
   a. Menstrual irregularities
   b. Hyperandrogenism
   c. Oligo/amenorrhea
   d. Chronic anovulation
   e. Decreased conception after assisted reproductive technology (ART)
   f. Increased risk of miscarriage.

Q. How do you manage a case of obesity with pregnancy?

Ans. Weight loss is not recommended during pregnancy however, overweight and obese she is.
   a. **Weight loss strategies for prepregnancy**
      For women with obesity or overweight, use low calorie diet (American Diet Association)

Obstetric Cases

Low calorie: 1000–1500 kcal/d, low fat (25–30% of energy), generous amount of protein (15–25% of energy) and regular exercise as a first line of approach. The rate of weight loss is recommended no more than 1.5–2 lbs per week which equals to calorie deficit 750–1000 kcal/day.

b. **Consideration of bariatric surgery**
Prepregnancy weight loss surgery—Roux-en-Y gastric bypass (RYGB), laparoscopic adjustable gastric band (LAGB), vertical banded gastroplasty (VBG), biliopancreatic diversion with duodenal switch (BPD-DS), or stomach stapling and sleeve gastrectomy (recently developed).

> **Note**
> 1. Side-effect of surgery: Vomiting, constipation and dumping syndrome (common in RYGB that consumption of simple surgery causes nausea, tachycardia, syncope and diarrhea).
> 2. Nutritional deficiencies after weight loss surgery—suboptimal maternal absorption of calcium, iron, folic acid and vitamin B_{12}. So vitamin and micronutrient supplementation during pregnancy is necessary.
> 3. In patients who have undergone BPD-DS, additional laboratory testing is recommended to screen the deficiencies of the fat soluble vitamins (A, D, E, K), folate trace elements and to screen the development of metabolic bone disease.
> 4. Surgery has positive impact on GDM and hypertensive disorders but case reports of IUGR, premature birth, and NTDs have been documented.
> 5. American College of Obstetrics and Gynaecology recommends that women delay pregnancy for 12–18 months after surgery to avoid pregnancy during the rapid weight loss phase.

c. **Improving compliance to IOM recommendations:** Weight gain within IOM recommendations range was associated with best outcome for mothers and fetus (optimize neonatal BW to between 3–4 kg and prevent morbidity and mortality associated with LBW). According to Food and Nutrition Board of the Institute of Medicine (IOM).

BMI Kg/m²	Weight for height status	Recommended weight gain
< 19.8	Underweight	28–40 lbs (12.5–18 kg)
19.8–26	Normal weight	25–35 lbs (11.5–16 kg)
26–29	Over weight	15–25 lbs (7–11.5 kg)
> 29	Obese	≤ 15 lbs (7 kg)

d. **Successful intervention:**
   1. Individual counseling on diet and physical activity during pregnancy could increase diet quality and leisure time physical activity and prevent excessive weight gain among healthy pregnant women.
   2. Screening of GDM – OGTT by 75 g glucose at 26–28 weeks. In women of high BMI (class 2 and 3) an early assessment for pre-existing diabetes should also be done.

3. Prevention of pre-eclampsia—by aspirin 75 mg/day from 12 weeks until birth of baby.
4. Thromboprophylaxis—The RCOG guideline recommends prophylactic low molecular weight heparin (LMWH) antenatally early in pregnancy for woman with BMI ≥30 who also has two or more additional risk factors for thromboembolism. All women receiving LMWH antenatally should continue prophylactic doses of LMWH until 6 weeks postpartum, but a postnatal risk assessment should be made.

e. **Assessment of comorbidity:**
   1. Cardiac risk assessment in class 3 obesity who have other risk factors like smoking and type 2 diabetes.
   2. Risk assessment of obstructive apnea.

f. **Management of complications if occur:**
   i. Pre-eclampsia—see the management of pre-eclampsia
   ii. GDM—see the management of GDM
   iii. Thromboembolic complications—The risk of thromboembolism is increased in 6-8 weeks following delivery especially after cesarean section. So, postpartum heparin or LMWH is recommended in patients with high-risks of venous thromboembolism. Early ambulation is needed.
   iv. Infection—prophylactic antibiotics.

Q. What are the long-term effects of maternal obesity in the mother and the infant?

Ans. a. Mother—Women with GDM have a higher risk of developing DM2 later in life and if obesity is also present chances of cardiovascular disease (CVD) is very high.

b. Infant—Children with GDM may have higher risk of developing DM in adolescent and CVD in adulthood. It is due to increased body fat at birth.

Q. Which contraceptives can be used in obesity?

Ans. The contraceptives which can be used safely are POP tablet, IUCD and barrier methods, but COCP, combined vaginal ring and DMPA may be used with caution. Chances of thromboembolism is high in COCP (containing 50 mcg estrogen) and chances of failure rate is high in low dose combined OCPs. Increased weight gain occurs in DMPA.

> **Note**
>
> *Thromboprophylaxis: For 7 days regardless of mode of delivery and the appropriate dose is weight dependent:*
>
> | Weight (kg) | Dose |
> |---|---|
> | 91–130 | 60 mg Enoxaparin, 7500 units Dalteparin, 7000 units Tinzaparin daily |
> | 131–170 | 80 mg Enoxaparin, 10,000 units Dalteparin, 9000 units Tinzaparin daily |
> | >170 | 0.6 mg/kg/day Enoxaparin, 75 units/kg/day Dalteparin 75 units/kg/day Tinzaparin. |

A CASE OF BETA THALASSEMIA AND PREGNANCY

Q. Classify hemoglobinopathy.

Ans. i. The structural hemoglobin variants, e.g. sickle cell disease (SCD).
ii. Inherited abnormalities of the synthesis of globin chains of hemoglobin, e.g. Thalassemias (Hemoglobinopathy—It means mutation in genes encoding Hb).

Q. Why screening is necessary?

Ans. The various hemoglobinopathies should be identified (probably before pregnancy) and offered genetic counseling and the availability of antenatal factor testing to the heterozygote (carriers) prevent birth of the affected child.

Q. What is thalassemia? Types.

Ans. Thalassemia is a group of recessive disorder characterized by a reduced synthesis of one or more globin chains of hemoglobin (Hb).
Based on globin chain deficiency: Two important types are:
a. *Alpha thalassemia*: Deficiency of Alpha chain
b. *Beta thalassemia*: Deficiency of Beta chain.

Q. What is β Thalassemia?

Ans. Mutation that affect synthesis of structural normal-globin due to diminished production of m-RNA.
β°—No Beta globin chain are produced by affected gene.
β+ —Globin chain are synthesized but at reduced rate.

Q. What are the effects of thalassemia on child-bearing woman and in pregnancy?

Ans. Thalassemia major:
a. Longevity of the victimized woman was low in the past
b. May become pregnant though infertility is the problem
c. Cardiac dysfunction, endocrine disorder like hypothyroidism and diabetes has a great impact on child-bearing.
d. Anemia worsens during pregnancy (β-thalassemia major and in HbH)[HbH— mutation of three of four alpha genes in hemoglobin-H disease].

Thalassemia minor: No significant effect on pregnancy outcome

β-Thalassemia minor with sickle cell disease: Maternal and fetal morbidity are increased

β-Thalassemia major and in HbH: Adverse outcome depends on severity of oxygen deprivation (If oxygen content is ≤70 mm of Hg)—
a. **Effect on mother:** Cardiovascular failure in early pregnancy
b. **Effect on fetus:** Abortion, IUGR, Preterm labor, SB (stillbirths).

Q. How do you prevent thalassemia in the population?

Ans. 1. **Health education**
   i. Population education

ii. Awareness campaign at schools and colleges
   iii. Information to be given
      a. Where the blood examination is done?
      b. When this should be done:
      c. Request of individuals for testing
   iv. Education of doctors controlling the community.
2. **Mass screening:**
   Premarital and newly married groups
   a. Peripheral blood smear
   b. *RBC indices*: MCV (decreased), MCH (decreased), MCHC (normal or decreased), RDW (N), HbF slightly elevated (2–3% and HbA2 elevated above 3.5% (usually 3.5%–7%) confirm the diagnosis.
   c. Mentzer Fractions—see below
   d. Nacked eye single tube red cell osmotic fragility test (NESTROFT)—shows increased resistance to hemolysis, i.e. decreased osmotic fragility.
   e. Confirmation by Hb electrophoresis, or gel electrophoresis or high performance liquid chromatography (HPLC).
3. **Genetic counseling:** Thalassemia minor should avoid marrying another minor, but it is not mandatory
   a. If two minors marry—Option for prenatal diagnosis
   b. One partner minor—There is no chance of them having Thalassemia major child but 50% chance of Thalassemia minor child, but gene study should be done in both the partners.

> **Note**
> Thalassemia should not be screened just after blood transfusion, as it may give erroneous result. Ideal time of testing is 4 weeks after blood transfusion.

Q. If both partners are carrier what will be the outcome of offspring?

Ans. Chances of thalassemia major are 25%, carrier 50%, normal child 25%.

Q. What is Mentzer index?

Ans. Mentzer developed a signified index using patients with hemoglobin above 9 g/dL.
Mentzer index = MCV/RBC count/cu mm
If fraction <11.5, BTT (β-Thalassemic trait) or >14 IDA (Iron-deficiency anemia).

> **Note**
> β-Thalassemic trait is confirmed by HbA_2 on electrophoresis.

Q. What is the rationality of screening?

Ans. Thalassemia of fetus can be diagnosed in utero; couple at risk can avoid having affected children without remaining childless, spared several months of anxiety awaiting the outcome of pregnancy.

> **Note**
> If both the partners are carrier they can go for prenatal diagnosis to detect affected children or may become pregnant by the use of intrauterine insemination of donor (normal person).

Q. How do you diagnose thalassemic fetus in utero?

Ans. Prenatal diagnosis is necessary when both the couples are beta-Thalassemic carrier
1. During antenatal period if the pregnant thalassemic women report within 8 weeks-chorionic villi biopsy (CVS) should be done at 9–11 weeks (Trophoblastic tissue 25–30 mg is taken). The risk of fetal loss is 1% and misdiagnosis is 1%.

> **Note**
> Diagnosis is available within 1 week by DNA analysis which is amplified enzymatically by PCR.

2. If the patient misses to come before 8 weeks, prenatal diagnosis at 15–17 weeks of pregnancy by following tests:
    a. Amniocentesis (15–20 mL of liquor for fetal cells)
    b. Cordocentesis (3 mL of fetal cord blood).
   DNA is prepared from amniocytes for study.

> **Note**
> Affected child: MTP, unaffected child: Thalassemia minor/trait—Continue pegnancy.

Q. How do you treat β-Thalassemia minor or trait during pregnancy?

Ans. Screen partner and consider counseling and prenatal diagnosis if trait or minor. Give folate, oral (not parenteral) iron when ferritin level is low, packed cell transfusion for severe anemia, induction of labor and pain relief is essential at labor, breastfeeding is not contraindicated following delivery.

Q. How do you treat β-Thalassemia major in pregnancy?

Ans. Pregnancy is a rare event, but possible
   a. Avoid iron
   b. Stop chelating agent (deferoxamine), vitamin C
      (Note: Deferoxamine has a teratogenic potential but may be used safely in 2nd and 3rd trimester without fetal compromise)
   c. Give folate
   d. Blood transfusion for anemia and assessment of cardiac status
   e. Screening of blood-borne diseases
   f. Fetal surveillance
   g. Chances of CS is high for short stature though induction of labor and vaginal delivery is encouraged.
   In puerperium—Breastfeeding is allowed and deferoxamine should be started within 7 days of the puerperium.

Q. What is sickling disorder?

Ans. It consists of Hb-S which differs from Hb-A by the substitution of valine for glutamic acid at position 6 in the beta chain. Homozygous state (genotype-SS) is called disease and heterozygotes (genotype-AS) is called trait. In anoxia sickle RBCs can not squeeze through microcirculation and causes microvascular obstruction resulting local hypoxia and tissue damage.

Q. How do you diagnose sickling disorder?

Ans.
a. By hemoglobin electrophoresis-pattern is characterized by predominantly Hb-S with a variable amount of Hb-F and the absence of Hb-A.
b. Bedside sickling test: Take a drop of blood and mix it with a drop of sodium metabisulfite, and place a cover slip over the mixture. Seal the edges with vaseline, and examine the slide for sickling after one hour.

Q. What factors precipitate sickling crisis?

Ans. Any pathologic state causing acidosis, dehydration, or hypoxemia can precipitate sickling, hemolysis, vasoconstriction, and infarction. Pregnancy also increases the sickling crisis.

Q. What are the complications of sickling disorder in pregnancy?

Ans.
a. Worsens anemia
b. Increases frequency of painful crisis—pain on bones, back pain, abdominal pain
c. Increases frequency of infection
   i. UTI
   ii. Pyelonephritis
   iii. Pneumonia
d. Precipitation of CCF by severe pre-eclampsia
e. Spontaneous abortion
f. IUGR
g. Proliferative retinopathy.

Q. How do you manage pregnancy with sickle cell disorder?

Ans. Management is by a team approach between obstetrician, hematologist and anesthesiologist especially in labor

I. Antenatal
a. Comprehensive assessment
b. Adequate hydration
c. Iron and folic acid supplementation
d. Blood transfusion
e. Routine urine analysis and serial USG for fetal assessment

II. Labor and delivery
a. Oxygen supplementation and optimal hydration
b. Avoid over sedation
c. Blood transfusion when necessary (acute painful crisis with rapidly developing anemia), rapid control of infection or stressors that could precipitate a crisis
d. Induction of labor and vaginal delivery should be encouraged but CS may be necessary for disproportion due to pelvic bone deformity.

III. Puerperium
a. Ambulation
b. Adequate hydration
c. Monitor the crisis
d. Infection should be controlled by antibiotics, and breastfeeding is allowed
e. Family planning (POP, progesterone only injection is very much suitable, but low dose COCP and Cu-T may be used).

Hemoglobin E trait: Common in Asia (India)
HbE—HbE is a common inherited condition caused by the production of abnormal hemoglobin protein. HbE is caused by change in beta globin chains.

HbE trait (AE): People with HbE trait have both normal hemoglobin and hemoglobin E in their red cells. Hemoglobin E trait means AE (one working beta globin gene (A) and one hemoglobin E gene). This is not a disease and does not affect health. The trait can cause the RBCs to be slightly smaller than usual and cause iron-deficiency anemia. The importance of identifying HbE trait helps to find couples whose children may be born with related blood disease.

Hb-EE (EE): People with HbE have two beta globin chains (Two hemoglobin E genes) without hemoglobin A. This makes the RBCs smaller than usual and does not cause any health problem. The importance of identifying Hb-EE is to help to find couples whose children could be born with related disease.

> **Note**
> Chorion villus sampling (CVS) is not required for detection of the affected child in utero as the problem is less in these conditions.

HbE-Beta thalassemia:
When one patient has Hb-E trait or Hb-EE and the other parent has a different blood trait (Beta thalassemia trait) they could have child with hemoglobin E-beta thalassemia disease. This disease needs lifelong regular blood transfusion and extensive medical care due to severe anemia. Repeated transfusion may cause problems of iron overloading. It is possible to test the developing baby for HbE-beta thalassemia disease as early as 10 weeks in pregnancy by chrionic villi sampling (CVS). If testing shows the baby has the disease parents can choose whether or not continue the pregnancy. One parent with Hb-E trait (AE) and other with beta-thalassemia trait (AB), each pregnancy has 25% chances of E-beta thalassemia disease (EB)[possibilities are: AA- no trait, AE-HbE Trait, AB- Beta thalassemia trait, EB (E-beta thalassemia disease)].

When one parent has Hb-EE and the other parent has beta-thalassemia trait (AB). There is 50% (1 in 2) chances of HbE-beta thalassemia disease in each pregnancy.

People can adopt or can consider assisted reproductive techniques (such as donor egg or donor sperm).

Chapter 11

Flying Questions

LIQUOR AMNII, HYDRAMNIOS AND OLIGOHYDRAMNIOS

Q. What is the origin of amniotic fluid?

Ans. Early pregnancy:
a. As an exudates from maternal plasma, amniotic membrane covering placenta and cord
b. Fluid passing through the fetal skin also contributes in the formation of liquor amnii.

Late pregnancy:
Kidney plays a major role [kidney starts functioning 12-14 weeks of gestational age (GA)]. Besides kidney, fetal lung skin and amniotic membrane also play an important role in its formation.

Q. How amniotic fluid volume is regulated?

Ans. Major inflows are:
1. Fetal urine 800–1200 mL
2. Lung field contributes 300–400 mL. So, 1000 mL flows in per day

Major outflows are:
1. Swallowing 500–1000 mL
2. Intramembranous contribution is 200–500 mL. So, 1000 mL daily flows out.

Q. What is the volume of amniotic fluid in different GA?

Ans. At 10 weeks 30 mL
20 weeks 300 mL
36 weeks 1000 mL
40 weeks 800 mL
42 weeks 200 mL.

Q. What are the functions of amniotic fluid?

Ans.
1. Provides a medium for fetal growth
2. Maintain an even temperature
3. Helps in lung maturity
4. Acts as a cushion against injury and trauma
5. Provides information against fetal health and maturity

6. Hydrostatic action helping dilatation of cervix in labor
7. Provides barrier against infection.

HYDRAMNIOS

Q. What is hydramnios?

Ans. It is a pregnancy state where liquor amnii exceeds 2000 mL.

> **Note**
>
> *Ultrasonically single pocket of amniotic fluid free of fetal parts is used to classify polyhydramnios into mild (8–11 cm), moderate (12–15 cm), and severe (≥16 cm). In most cases polyhydramnios arises in second and third trimester of pregnancy.*

Q. What is the etiology of hydramnios?

Ans.
a. Multiple pregnancies (monozygotic twin)
b. Fetal anomalies (20%): Anencephaly (50%), open spina bifida, esophageal and duodenal atresia
c. Maternal: Diabetes mellitus (30%), cardiac and renal disease
d. Placenta: Chrioangioma of placenta
e. Idiopathic.

> **Note**
>
> *Mnemonic: 'TARDI'*
> *T–Twins; A–Anomalies, fetal; R–Rh incompatibility; D–Diabetes; I– Idiopathic.*

Q. What are the different types of hydramnios?

Ans.
a. Acute type: Onset is sudden and occurs within 20 weeks. Common causes are uniovular twin and chorioangioma of placenta. It is seen in association with twin-to-twin transfusion syndrome.
b. Chronic type (common): Onset is insidious and takes weeks to appear.

Q. How do you diagnose a case of chronic hydramnios?

Ans. History of: Dyspnea, palpitation, edema leg, undue enlargement of abdomen
On examination: Features of pregnancy-induced hypertension (PIH), dyspnea, tachycardia
Per abdomen (P/A). Inspection: Undue enlargement of abdomen with fullness at flanks, skin is tense and shiny, large striae.
Palpation: Height of the uterus is greater than period of amenorrhea, abdominal girth at the level of umbilicus is more than normal, fluid thrill may be elicited and fetal parts can not be felt definitely.
Auscultation: Fetal heart sound (FHS) is not clearly audible
Per vaginal (P/V): Cervix is taken up and high, os may be open
Investigation:
Ultrasonography (USG): Helpful for diagnosis of fetal anomalies and liquor pocket or amniotic fluid index (AFI) (In hydramnios liquor pocket is >8 cm and AFI is >25 cm) and also to diagnose multiple fetus, presentation of fetus, congenital defect of fetus.
Radiograph—can diagnose twin, congenital defect of fetus.

Blood group and Rh type, blood sugar, maternal serum alpha-fetoprotein (MSAFP) or amniotic fluid alphafeto protein [raised in fetal central nervous system (CNS) defect]

Amniotic fluid: Estimation of alpha fetoprotein which increases in open spina bifida.

> **Note**
>
> In USG, if AFI is 25–29.9 cm—mild hydramnios, moderate: AFI, 30–34.9 cm and severe: AFI ≥35 cm.

Q. What are the complications of hydramnios?

Ans. Maternal
   a. During pregnancy: Pre-eclampsia, malpresentation, preterm labor, premature rupture of membranes (PROM) and accidental hemorrhage following quick escape of large volume of liquor due to low artificial ruptue of membranes (ARM) and it is mainly due to decrease in the surface area of the uterus which leads to placental separation.
   b. During labor: Early rupture of membrane, cord prolapse, uterine inertia, difficult delivery due to mal presentation, retained placenta, postpartum hemorrhage (PPH).

Q. How do you manage hydramnios?

Ans. During pregnancy.

1. With no fetal anomalies

Expectant management if gestational age is <37 weeks:
   a. Bed rest, restriction of extra salt, treatment of PIH and diabetes if present.
   b. Amniocentesis: Slow decompression is done at the rate of 500 mL/hr (to avoid accidental hemorrhage) and total amount should not exceed 1-1.5 liter. The procedure of amnioreduction may need repetition weekly or semi-weekly.
   c. Pregnancy >37 weeks: Induction of labor.

2. With fetal anomalies

No expectant treatment

Termination of pregnancy by ARM. High rupture of membrane is beneficial but low rupture of membrane can be done with slow drainage of liquor by pressing the vulva with palms to avoid accidental hemorrhage and presenting part is pressed by first pelvic grip by assistant.

During labor

Chances of uterine inertia, cord prolapse, malpresentation.

After delivery: Care should be taken for management of PPH as the incidence of it is very high. So, active management of third stage of labor (AMTSL) is mandatory.

In acute case of hydramnios: Immediate relief by amniocentesis when USG and radiography shows no fetal anomalies, but chances of spontaneous abortion is high.

Q. What is the treatment of acute hydramnios?

Ans. a. Slow amnioreduction.
   b. Repeated abdominal amniocentesis after exclusion of fetal congenital malformation.
   c. Induction of labor by amniotomy and oxytocin drip.

> **Note**
> Chances of spontaneous abortion is high in early hydramnios.

> **Note**
> Role of indomethacin therapy in hydramnios: It is used in idiopathic hydramnios of gestational age of <37 weeks in a dose of 1.5–3 mg/kg/day for 2–11 weeks starting from 24–35 weeks. It decreases the fetal urine production, enhances the absorption of amniotic fluid.
> Side-effect: Premature closure of ductus arteriosus, necrotizing enterocolitis, intracranial hemorrhage and intrauterine fetal demise.

OLIGOHYDRAMNIOS OR OLIGOAMNIOS

Q. What is oligohydramnios?

Ans. Reduction of amniotic fluid volume to < 200 mL.

Q. Etiology of oligohydramnios?

Ans.
1. **Urinary tract anomalies of fetus**
   a. Impairment of production of urine: Renal agenesis (uni or bilateral), Horse shoe kidney, ectopic kidney and genetically inherited polycystic kidney.
   b. Impairment of passage of urine flow:
      High: At the level of uretero-pelvic junction (common in male baby)
      Median: At the level of distal ureter or U-V junction
      Low: Caused by urethral valve or agenesis.
2. **Feto-placental cause:** Intrauterine growth restriction (IUGR), Intrauterine fetal death (IUFD), Post-term pregnancy, PROM, monochorionic twin, twin-to-twin transfusion syndrome (TTTS), chorionic villi biopsy (CVS).
3. **Maternal causes:** Severe hypertension, anemia, diabetes, human immunodeficiency virus (HIV) antiphospholipid antibodies (APLAS), systemic lupus erythematosus (SLE), History of drugs like nonsteroidal anti-inflammatory drug (NSAID), angiotensin-converting enzyme (ACE) inhibitors.
4. **Amniotic nodosum:** Failure of secretion by the cells of amnion covering the placenta.
5. **Idiopathic:** 7.5–10%.

> **Note**
> Mnemonic: 'DRIPP'
> D–Demise of fetus; R–Renal anomalies; I–IUGR; P–PROM; P–Postmaturity.

Q. How do you diagnose oligohydramnios?

Ans. Clinical presentation:
   a. Uterus is small for date and full of fetus
   b. Fetus is in hyperflexed attitude
   c. Abnormal presentation—breech is common

d. History of less fetal movement
e. Mother may have hypertension, leaking p/v, and HIV infection.

Investigations:

USG is helpful
a. Liquor pocket (single pocket <2 cm and AFI <5 cm indicates oligohydramnios)
b. Can assess fetal growth
c. Identification of abnormal position of fetus
d. Detect congenital defect of fetus
e. USG Doppler diagnose placental insufficiency

MRI: Fetal urinary tract anomalies and pulmonary vasculature are better diagnosed.

Q. What are the complications of oligohydramnios?

Ans.
1. Abnormal presentation and attitude of fetus—hyperflexion of fetus and breech (common).
2. Pulmonary hypoplasia (lung size decreased and heart to lung ratio increased) due to less fluid intake by the fetal lung, which inhibits alveolar development.
3. Abnormal fetal development—due to compression of uterine wall, less space for fetal movement, adherent fetal parts, bands and adhesion between amnion and fetal parts may cause club foot, dislocated hip, finger amputation and Potter's face characterized by widely separated eyes, broad nasal bridge, low set ears and receding chin.
4. Fetal growth restriction.

During labor: Cord compression, meconium aspiration syndrome.

Q. How do you manage a case of oligohydramnios?

Ans. During pregnancy
a. Bed rest, nutritious diet
b. Hydration—oral/IV fluid may help to increase amniotic fluid
c. Offending drugs like NSAID should be avoided
d. Serial USG for fetal growth, amniotic fluid (AF) volume, assessment of fetal well-being and also to detect fetal anomalies
e. Treatment of underlying cause
f. Amino infusion—not very encouraging
g. Induction when maturity is achieved or fetal anomalies are detected.

Intranatal management
a. Proper counseling
b. Close fetal monitoring
c. Transcervical amino infusion—discussed in postdated pregnancy
d. In case of induction make everything ready for LSCS
e. Expert neonatologist for resuscitation of baby
f. Protection of vertical transmission of HIV.

> **Note**
> *Specific management by fetal surgery—vesicoamniotic shunt.*

PRETERM LABOR (PTL)

Q. What is preterm labor?
Ans. Onset of labor before 37 weeks of pregnancy. Early preterm occurs before 33 weeks, and late preterm between 34–36 completed weeks.

> **Note**
> Premature infant—born <37 weeks. Low-birth weight (LBW-BW) <2500 g, VLBW-BW <1500 g, extremely LBW body-BW <1000 g.

Q. What are the different causes of preterm labor?
Ans. Maternal:
   a. Diseases: Anemia, hypertension, heart disease, high fever.
   b. Other causes: Teen age, elderly women, cigarette smoking, and mental strain, low pre-pregnancy weight [body mass index (BMI) < 19.8 kg/m^2].
   c. Uterine causes: Incompetence of cervix, uterine fibroid and uterine anomalies.
   d. Fetal and placental causes: Multiple pregnancies, IUFD, congenital malformations, chrioamnionitis, PROM and antipartum hemorrhage (APH).
   e. Infection: Genitourinary infections like chlamydia, bacterial vaginosis, trichomoniasis, Group B streptococcus.
   f. Idiopathic.

Q. Criteria for diagnosis of preterm delivery (PTL)?
Ans.
   a. Uterine contraction—4 times/20 minute or 8 times/60 minutes plus progressive change in cervix.
   b. Cervical dilatation >1 cm in nulliparous and >3 cm in multipara.
   c. Cervical effacement >80%.

Q. Management.
Ans. 1. Prevention:
   a. Patient's education for signs and symptoms of PTL
   b. Cervicitis screening initially and again at 28–32 weeks
   c. Bed rest (doubtful value), use of progesterone is controversial
   d. Cerclage operation in patient with incompetent cervix.

2. Treatments:
Use of tocolytics: (Do not use tocolytic drugs for more than 48 hours) if:
   a. GA is < 37 weeks
   b. Cervix is less than 3 cm dilated on endovaginal sonography
   c. No chorioamnionitis, PIH, or active bleeding
   d. No fetal distress is noted

Confirm diagnosis of preterm labor by documenting cervical effacement over 2 hours.

If GA is < 34 weeks injection betamethasone 12 mg IM to mother, two doses at 24 hours apart or Dexamethasone 6 mg IM 4 doses 12 hours apart (weekly repeated doses are not indicated as IUGR and fetal brain

damage is shown by recent studies). Steroid is not recommended prior to 24 weeks of gestational age.
- Give tocolytic drugs and monitor the maternal and fetal conditions.
- If GA is <34 weeks and labor continues despite tocolysis or the woman is in advanced stage of labor (cervical dilatation >3 cm) allow delivery.

Treatment of infection like bacterial vaginosis by metronidazole 2 g orally for 2 consecutive days and intrapartum antimicrobial prophylaxis of Group B streptococcal (GBS) infection by ampicillin 2 g IV initial dose then 1 g IV 4 hourly or 2 g IV 6 hours or vancomycin 1 g IV every 12 hours until delivery.

> **Note**
> *Routine antibiotics use is not recommended for prolonging pregnancy in PTL.*

Labor: In induced or spontaneous labor continuous monitoring of fetal heart rate and uterine contractions are essential.

Delivery: In rigid perineum episiotomy is mandatory for delivery of preterm newborn. Routine forceps delivery is not essential. Resuscitation and preterm newborn care can improve the survival rate.

Q. What are the complications of PTL?
Ans.
a. Placental abruption
b. PROM
c. Intra-amniotic infection (chorioamnionitis): Subclinical infection may need maternal blood for leukocytes count and C-reactive protein estimation. If both are raised antibiotic may be needed for treatment.

Q. Name the tocolytic drugs used in obstetrics.
Ans. Isoxsuprine, ritodrine, salbutamol, indomethacin or other COX_2 inhibitors, Injection $MgSO_4$, nifedipine, hormone (progesterone), nitroglycerine, oxytocin receptor blocker—Atosiban.

> **Note**
> *When IV β-mimetic along with steroid are used chances of maternal pulmonary oedema is very high. Oral beta mimetics and subcutaneous (SC) administration of terbutaline include sudden death, pulmonary edema, cardiac arrhythmias, hepatitis, glucose intolerance and gestational diabetes mellitus (GDM).*
> - *Nifedipine 30 mg orally followed by 20 mg tds/day. Most practitioners do not recommend tocolytics after 33 weeks as after this time perinatal outcome is good in preterm neonates*
> - *Injection magnesium sulfate: The common clinical approach is 6 g IV bolus followed by 3 g/h (24 hours)*
> - *Indomethacin—orally, vaginally and rectally. Loading dose is 50–100 mg followed by 25 mg every 6–8 hours for 48–72 hours to avoid complications. Side effects: Nausea, gastrointestinal tract (GIT) upset, In fetus: Premature closure of fetal ductus arteriosus (at GA >32 weeks), pulmonary hypertension, oligohydramnios, IVH, and necrotizing enterocolitis with prolonged administration of the drug*

Contd...

Contd...

- Role of progesterone for prevention of PTL. It effectively decreases the incidence of recurrent preterm birth in subsequent pregnancy
  a. 17- hydroxy progesterone caproate: 250 g IM weekly at 16–20 weeks and continued till 37 weeks of GA.
  b. Micronized progesterone: 200 mg once per vagina per day.
- Atosiban—oxytocin receptor antagonist. Dosage: 6.75 mg IV bolus over 1 minute. Then an infusion of 18 mg/hr for 3 hours followed by 6 mg per hour for 45 hours. The total dose should be 330 mg.
- Side effects—these are fewer than other tocolytic agents. Nausea, vomiting, dyspnea, chest pain, palpitation, tachycardia and hypertension.

Q. What is the efficacy of oral tocolysis with β-mimetics?

Ans. Oral β-mimetic therapy is not very effective because:
   i. Drug should be taken at every 2–4 hours which may decrease compliance.
   ii. Long-term exposure of β-mimetic results in desensitization of the β-adrenergic receptors in the myometrium.
   iii. Development of tolerance is related to both duration of therapy and the total dose of β-mimetics.

> **Note**
> Tocolytics are used for short-term in modern obstetric practice for. (a) in utero transfer of fetus to higher centers in preterm labor, (b) for in utero fetal lung maturity by administration of steroids.

Q. What are the absolute contraindications of tocolytic therapy?

Ans. a. Severe PIH
   b. Severe abruptio placentae
   c. Severe bleeding per vagina
   d. Severe chorioamnionitis
   e. IUFD
   f. Severe fetal growth restriction (FGR) and fetal anomaly
   g. Mature lung of fetus
   h. Maternal cardiac arrhythmia.

Q. What are the maternal complications of beta-mimetics?

Ans. Nausea, vomiting, palpitation, hypotension, hyperglycemia, hyperinsulinemia, hypokalemia, pulmonary edema, arrhythmia, myocardial ischemia.

Q. What are the fetal complications of beta mimetics?

Ans. Tachycardia, increased cardiac output, myocardial ischemia, increased thickness of interventricular septum, hypoglycemia and intraventricular hemorrhage (IVH).

Q. When do you allow progression of labor?

Ans. Allow labor to progress if:
   a. GA > 37 weeks
   b. Cervix > 3 cm dilated

c. Active bleeding
d. Fetus is distressed, dead and has anomalies
e. Amnionitis or pre-eclampsia

Monitor the progress of labor by partograph

If labor continues and GA < 37 weeks

a. Give prophylactic antibiotics to prevent infection in neonates
b. Avoid vacuum as the risk of intracranial hemorrhage is high
c. Proper management of preterm and low birth weight (LBW) babies.

Q. What is fetal fibronectin (FFN) and what is its importance?

Ans. Fibronectin is an extracellular protein attached to the fetal membrane. It is found in cervicovaginal secretion at 20–22 weeks and again at the end of normal pregnancy as labor approaches. It is not normally present between 22 to 37 weeks. The presence of fibronectin after 22 weeks is a marker of disruption of the decidual-chorionic interface and is associated with preterm delivery and its absence is associated with low-risk of preterm delivery. Fetal fibronectin level is measured by ELISA and level >50 ng/mL is positive.

Q. What is the role of transvaginal sonography (TVS) in preterm delivery?

Ans. Transvaginal sonography (TVS) is performed at 18 to 20 weeks, if the cervical length is suspicious (2.0–2.9 cm), TVS is repeated at 1 to 2 weeks interval. Patient is advised for bed rest, and if cervical length is < 2.0 cm bed rest and cervical encirclage operation is advised.

> **Note**
> A short cervix is not a predictor of preterm delivery but funnelling and history of prior preterm birth is highly predictive.

Q. What is the role of newer marker PIGFBP-1 (phosphorylated insulin like growth factor binding protein-1)?

Ans. Progress of labor disrupts the choriodecidual interface releasing PIGFBP-1 in cervical secretion. Identification of PIGFBP-1 is thus indicative of labor process and predicts preterm labor. Commercial bed side kit test (ACTIM PARTUS) is available with detection limit of 10 µg/L. Positive result indicates preterm labor and negative test confirms that labor is remote.

Q. What is the role of other newer marker of PAMG-1 [human placental-alpha-microglobulin-1 (PAMG-1)]?

Ans. This is a protein released by the cells from the lining of the uterus into the amniotic cavity throughout pregnancy. The presence of PAMG-1 in cervicovaginal secretions indicates that preterm delivery is likely to occur within seven days and may be associated with an increased risk of intra-amniotic infection or inflammation. Its absence indicates no delivery within 7 days. The test uses monoclonal antibodies sufficiently sensitive to detect 4pg/µL of PAMG-1 in cervicovaginal discharge. The PartoSure test kit comprises immunochromatographic assay designed to identify the presence of PAMG-1.

Flying Questions

Q. Define lower uterine segment.

Ans.
1. It is the part of the uterus which is passive or noncontractile.
2. It is the part of the uterus lying between anatomical and histological internal os (isthmus of nonpregnant uterus).
3. The lower part of the uterus where peritoneum is loosely attached anteriorly, when fully formed it measures 7.5–10 cm from internal os.
4. It is limited superiorly by physiological retraction ring and inferiorly by fibromuscular junction of cervix and uterus.

> **Note**
> In pregnancy lower uterine segment forms as the isthmus elongates, hypertrophies and becomes infolded and part of the uterine cavity by 20th week of gestational age and disappears on the third day of puerperium.

Q. What is the clinical significance of lower uterine segment (LUS)?

Ans.
1. It passively dilates during normal labor.
2. It is poorly retractile, APH occurs when placenta is implanted on this area.
3. Chance of morbid adhesion of placenta for poor decidual reaction.
4. Lower segment cesarian section (LSCS) is performed through this area.
5. In obstructed labor it is very much stretched.

> **Note**
> History of one preterm labor, the risk increases to 17.2% in second pregnancy, while with history of 2 preterm labors, it increases to 28.4%. Complications of preterm baby: Respiratory distress syndrome (RDS), IVH, bronchopulmonary dysplasia (BPD), patent ductus arteriosus (PDA), sepsis, retinopathy, and necrotizing enterocolitis. It is now evidenced-based fact that delayed cord clamping of preterm neonates has several benefits like higher red cell volume, decreased need for blood transfusion, better circulatory stability and lower rate of intraventricular hemorrhage and necrotizing enterocolitis.

CHORIOAMNIONITIS

Q. What is chorioamnionitis?

Ans. It refers to inflammation and/or infection of the placenta and chorion and amnion (the fetal membrane).

Q. How do you diagnose chorioamnionitis?

Ans. Diagnosis is based on clinical examination.

Maternal features:
a. Maternal fever >100°F
b. Tachycardia—maternal and fetal
c. Uterine tenderness
d. Foul smelling amniotic fluid

Investigations:
a. Leukocytosis (count >15,000/cubic mm is suspicious for infection and left shift, i.e. increase in proportion of immature neutrophils)

b. Raised C-reactive protein (CRP > 2.5) and procalcitonin if sepsis
c. High vaginal swab for Gram stain and culture and sensitivity.

Fetal manifestations:
It includes tachycardia and non-reassuring fetal heart rate pattern.

Q. Describe management of chorioamnionitis.
Ans. a. Vaginal delivery is preferable with broad spectrum antibiotics. Injection of ampicillin, 2 g IV, 6 hourly after skin test and injection of gentamicin, 1.5 mg/kg body weight (BW), 8 hourly IV. Antibiotics should be started as early as possible with the diagnosis. Steroids should never be used for fear of flaring of infection of mother and neonates.
b. Expedition of delivery by vaginal route or LSCS according to the clinical situation.

Q. What are the maternal complications?
Ans. Early:
1. Preterm labor/PROM
2. Endometritis, wound sepsis, puerperal sepsis
3. Septic pelvic thrombophlebitis and septic shock
4. Sub-involution of uterus
5. Remote: Pelvic inflammatory disease (PID), ectopic pregnancy, infertility and chronic pelvic pain.

Q. What are the perinatal complications?
Ans.
1. No clinical effects
2. Preterm birth with risks of premature newborn especially intracranial hemorrhage and respiratory distress syndrome (RDS).
3. Infection of lungs, gut, meninges, brain and blood stream leading to septicemia.
4. Intrauterine fetal death.

SHOULDER DYSTOCIA

Q. What are the causes of shoulder dystocia?
Ans. DOPE—D-Diabetes, O-Obesity, P-Post-term, E-Excessive maternal weight gain.

Q. What is macrosomia?
Ans. Absolute birth weight of baby 4000 g or 9 lbs independent of GA and demographic variables. When AC value is > 90th percentile by USG, it correctly predicts macrosomia in 78% of cases antenatally.

Q. What is the important complication of macrosomia?
Ans. Shoulder dystocia as in macrosomia of uncontrolled diabetic mother.

Q. What is shoulder dystocia?
Ans. A prolonged head to body delivery time (>60 seconds or more) and/or the use of obstetric maneuver.

Q. How do you diagnose shoulder dystocia?

Ans.
a. The fetal head is delivered but remain tightly applied on the vulva
b. The chin retracts and depresses the perineum
c. Traction on the fetal head can not deliver the shoulder, which is caught behind the symphysis pubis.

Q. Management of shoulder dystocia.

Ans.
1. **McRobert's method** (commonly used): Patient overhangs at the lower edge of the table.
   Sharply flexion of maternal thighs over the maternal abdomen resulting in straightening of maternal sacrum relative to lumbar spine with consequent cephalic rotation of symphysis pubis. Suprapubic pressure should be given directed posteriorly by an assistant with episiotomy whenever necessary. [Do not give fundal pressure as it may cause (a) Impaction of anterior shoulder behind symphysis pubis, (b) Erb's palsy, (c) Thoracospinal cord injury of neonates]. If this method fails, follow the next method.

2. **Rubin's maneuver:** Fetal shoulders are rocked from side to side by applying force to the mother's abdomen. If it is not successful the most easily accessible fetal shoulder is pushed towards the anterior surface of fetus's chest. The shoulder to shoulder diameter is shown in Figure 11.1A by two small arrows. The most easily accessible shoulder [the anterior is shown here (Figure 11.1B)] is pushed towards the anterior chest wall of fetus. This most often causes adduction of both fetal shoulders, reducing shoulder to shoulder diameter and frees the impacted anterior shoulder from behind the symphysis pubis.
   If this maneuver fails, follow the next.

3. Delivery of posterior shoulder consists of sweeping of the posterior arm of the fetus across the chest followed by delivery of the arm. The shoulder girdle is rotated to one of the oblique diameter of the pelvis and subsequent delivery of anterior shoulder is accomplished.

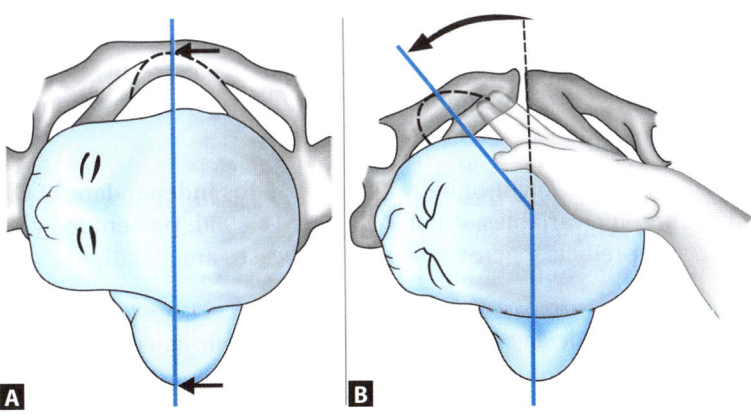

Figures 11.1A and B: Rubin's maneuver

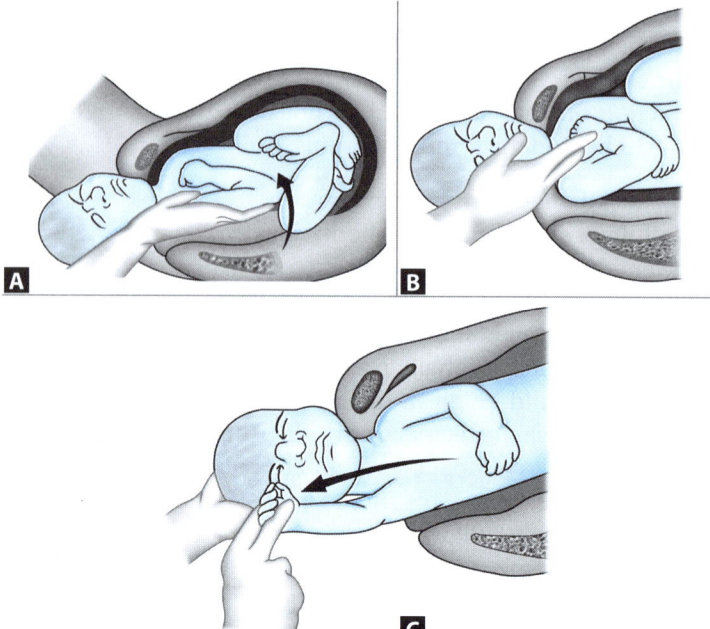

Figures 11.2 A to C: Delivery of posterior shoulder

Steps:
   a. The operator's hand is introduced in the vagina along the posterior surface of humerus and grasp it and the arm is swept across the chest keeping the arm flexed at elbow (Figure 11.2A) as this provide room for the shoulder that is anterior to move under the symphysis pubis.
   b. The fetal hand is grasped and the arm is extended along the side of face (Figure 11.2B).
   c. The posterior arm is delivered from the vagina (Figure 11.2C).
4. By applying pressure on the anterior surface of the posterior shoulder, the Wood's (corkscrew) maneuver attempt to push the posterior shoulder through a clockwise 180° arc, so that the impacted anterior shoulder is released (Figure 11.3).
5. If all the measures fail deliberate fracture of the clavicle by pressing the anterior clavicle against the ramus of the pubis which heals rapidly but less dangerous than brachial nerve injury, asphyxia and death of fetus.
6. In dead fetus cleidotomy (cutting of the clavicle by scissors) is usually used. In live fetus if cleidotomy is done, risk of injury of subclavian vessels is high and should never be tried.

Q. What are the complications of shoulder dystocia?

Ans. Maternal complications: Postpartum hemorrhage (PPH), cervico-vaginal lacerations, 3° perineal tear, bladder atony and uterine rupture.
Fetal complications:
1. Brachial plexus injury (nerve roots C 5–6, Erb's Duchene palsy) is more common in diabetic gravidas—90% resolve in 1 year.

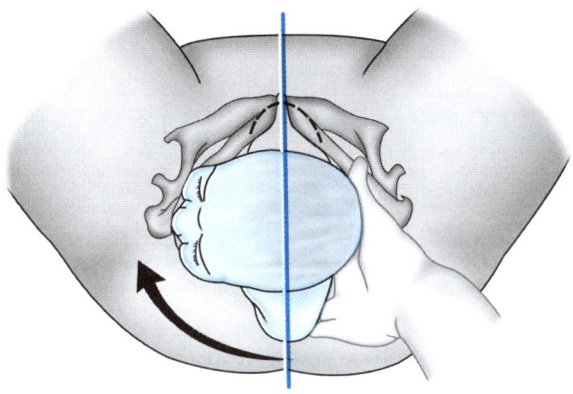

Figure 11.3: Wood's maneuver

The affected arm is held straight, internally rotated, the elbow is extended, the wrist and fingers are flexed, and finger function is usually retained.
2. Injury of C8-T1 nerve roots (Klumpke's palsy) in which hand is flaccid and resolved at one year.
3. Clavicular and humeral fracture may also occur.

INDUCTION OF LABOR

Q. What is induction of labor?

Ans. It is the process; by which quiescent uterus is stimulated to begin labor after 28 weeks (preferably after 37 weeks) of pregnancy by any methods like medical surgical or combined that aims to secure normal vaginal delivery.

Q. What is augmentation of labor?

Ans. Stimulation of the uterus during labor to increase the frequency, duration and strength of uterine contraction.

Q. Indications of induction of labor.

Ans.
a. Hypertensive disorder
b. Prolonged pregnancy
c. PROM > 37 weeks
d. Compromised fetus: PIH, eclampsia, intrauterine growth restriction (IUGR)
e. Maternal diabetes, Rh sensitization, SLE and renal disease
f. APH
g. Fetal anomalies and dead fetus
h. Marked polyhydramnios.

Q. How will you assess inducibility score?

Ans. Table 11.1.

Practical Manual of Obstetrics

Table 11.1: Bishop score

Examination	Points		
	1	2	3
Cervical dilatation (cm)	1–2	3–4	5–6
Cervical effacement (%)	40–50	60–70	80
Station of presenting part	–1, –2	0	+1, +2
Consistency of cervix	Medium	Soft	
Position of cervix	Middle	Anterior	

Total score =13; If score of greater than 6 is favorable, labor is successfully induced with oxytocin alone. If a score less than 5—unfavorable cervix—use PGs or Foley's catheter before induction.

Q. What are the contraindications of induction of labor?
Ans.
a. Cephalopelvic disproportion (CPD)
b. A floating or deflexed vertex or an unfavorable presentation including breech
c. Previous 2 cesarean section (CS), classical vesicovaginal fistula (VVF) repaired cases
d. Maternal cardiac diseases
e. Grand multipara (G4 or more)
f. Human immunodeficiency virus (HIV) or herpes genital infection.

Q. What are the different types of induction?
Ans.
a. Surgical
b. Medical
c. Combined.

Q. Surgical Induction.
Ans.
a. Stripping of membrane—half hearted method of induction
b. Artificial low rupture of membrane (ARM)—early amniotomy at 1-2 cm or late amniotomy at 5 cm of cervical dilatation
No anesthesia and analgesia is needed.

Techniques:
a. Aseptic precaution
b. Insert right index and middle fingers through the cervical os
c. The membrane is stripped off the lower uterine segment digitally and bag of membrane is ruptured by the tip of the Kocher's artery forceps holding by left hand
d. Color of the liquor is observed
e. Cord presentation (worm-like feeling) and cord prolapses should be excluded before or after the procedure
f. After ARM note the fetal heart sound (FHS) (if fetal heart rate (FHR) <100 bpm; or >180 bpm—fetal distress)
g. If delivery is not anticipated within 8 hours give prophylactic antibiotic (Injection ampicillin 2 g IV every 6 hours until delivery after skin test)
h. If good labor is not established after 1 hour of ARM begin oxytocin infusion.

Flying Questions

Q. Enumerate the absolute indication of ARM.

Ans. Pregnancy induced hypertension, eclampsia, APH (accidental hemorrhage and type-I and type-II anterior placenta previa), chronic hydramnios (slow release of liquor by pressing vulva to avoid placental separation and accidental hemorrhage and press the presenting part below by first pelvic grip or by multiple punctures of amniotic membrane by 16 gauge needle under direct visualization by vaginal speculum for slow gush of amniotic fluid), postmaturity, fetal growth restriction (FGR).

> **Note**
> Because of risk of cord prolapse and accidental hemorrhage, the fetal heart is assessed before and after amniotomy.

Q. What are the contraindications of ARM?

Ans.
a. IUFD for fear of infection
b. Very high floating head for fear of cord prolapse
c. Central placenta previa
d. HIV infected mother
e. Genital herpes infection.

Q. What are the complications of ARM?

Ans.
a. Failure to induce effective uterine contraction
b. Placenta separated in polyhydramnios
c. Bleeding—due to presence of vasa previa (fetal bleeding, not maternal bleeding)
d. Prolapse of the cord
e. Infection (chorioamnionitis is increased with early amniotomy)
f. Pulmonary embolism.

Q. What do you mean by ripe cervix?

Ans. A ripe cervix is ready for labor, when it is:
a. Soft
b. Taken up (cervix is <1.5 cm in length)
c. Dilated (admits 1 finger easily) or dilatable
d. Central on the presenting part.

Q. How do you induce labor in low cervical score?

Ans.
a. Prostaglandine E2 (PGE2) gel (0.5 mg) avalable as cerviprime gel is used intracervically. Two doses can be repeated every 6–12 hours, if needed.
b. 3 mg PGE2 as a vaginal pessary may also be introduced in high posterior fornix.
c. Introduction of Foley's catheter through the cervix appears to stimulate local production of prostaglandins (PGs) and may also ripe the cervix.
d. Extra-amniotic saline infusion (FASI) (30–40 mL/hr) by IV infusion pump through Foley's catheter. It released local prostaglandins and make cervix more favorable.

Q. What are the disadvantages of Foley's catheter?

Ans. a. Infection
b. Possibility of bleeding in choriodecidual space may lead to absorption of PGs causing uterus hypertonus.

> **Note**
> Monitoring of uterine contraction and FHR of all woman undergoing induction of labor.

Q. What is syntocinon?

Ans. It is a synthetic oxytocin.

Q. How will you induce by syntocinon?

Ans. It is better to start with a small dose of syntocinon in Ringer lactate (RL)/saline (salt solution) and should be infused slowly IV and the dose is to be increased steadily until the effective uterine contraction starts.

Q. How do you prepare 1 unit of syntocinon?

Ans. One ampoule of syntocinon contains 5 units of the drug. Take 5 mL of syringe and draw 5 unit of syntocinon (= 1 mL) and add 4 mL of normal saline to the same syringe and mix it up, now 5 mL contains 5 units of syntocinon and 1 mL of the mixture contain 1 unit of syntocinon and 2 mL of the solution contain 2 units of syntocinon.

Q. What is the approximate relation between drops/minute or milli unit (mU/minute)? (For example, If 1 unit of syntocinon is mixed in 500 mL of RL solution and start infusion at 15 drops/minute, then how much milli unit/minute will go?)

Ans. 1 unit = 1000 milli unit (mU)
500 mL contains 1 unit, i.e. 1,000 mU of syntocinon
1 mL contains 1,000/500 = 2 mU
So 1 mL contains 2 mU syntocinon
1 mL = 15 drops.
So if the solution of 1 unit is started at 15 drops/minute then 2 mU of syntocinon will be infused per minute.

Low dose regime (Table 11.2): Infuse oxytocin at 2 mU/min and increase it as needed every 15 minutes to 4, 8, 12, 16, 20, 25 and 30 mU/minute (Table 11.2).

Table 11.2: Relation between drops/minute

Units of oxytocin in 500 mL Ringer lactate (RL)	Drip speed (drops/minute)		
	15	30	60
1	2	4	8
2	4	8	16
8	16	32	64

Q. What is escalating dose of induction?

Ans. Table 11.3.

Flying Questions

Table 11.3: Escalating dose of induction		
Dose of oxytocin	Solution used	Escalating drops rate at 15 drops/minute
Start with 1 unit	500 mL	15–30–60
	Ringer lactate (RL)	
If no response —2 units	do	do
If still no response —5 units	do	do

In majority of cases 16 mU/min (2 units in 500 mL of RL with drip rate 60/minute) is sufficient to achieve 3 contractions in 10 minutes persisting for 40–60 seconds.

Q. What is high dose oxytocin regime for labor induction?

Ans. High dose oxytocin regime (see below).

Regimen	Starting dose (mU/min)	Incremental dose (mU/min)	Interval (min)
High dose	4	4	15
	4.5	4.5	15–30
	6	6	20–40*

*Tachysystole is more common with shorter interval

Q. What is hyperstimulation?

Ans. Any contraction lasting longer than 2 minutes (uterine hypertonus) or more than 6 contractions in 10 minutes, associated with fetal distress or nonreassuring fetal heart rate pattern is called hyperstimulation. The term hyperstimulation is now abandoned.

Q. What is tachysystole?

Ans. Increased contraction frequency and is defined by 6 or more uterine contractions within a 10 minute window for 2 consecutive windows. It is found in placental abruption or hyperstimulation of uterus with oxytocin.

> **Note**
> *Five contractions or less in 10 minutes, averaged over a 30 minutes window are normal uterine activity.*

Q. What is the line of management in hyperstimulation by oxytocin?

Ans. a. Stop syntocinon infusion
b. Terbutaline 250 mcg IV slowly over 5 minutes or Salbutamol 10 mg in 1L, IV fluid [normal saline (NS) or RL] at 10 drops/minute.

Q. What are the important observations during syntocinon induction?

Ans. a. Rate of flow of infusion
b. Response of uterine contraction—frequency, duration (place your right palm on uterus and feel contraction and note the time between appearance of contraction and disappearance of contraction, i.e. the duration and note how many contractions in 10 minutes occur, i.e. frequency).

c. FHR.
d. Maternal condition.
e. Progress of labor (POL).

Q. When do you stop syntocinon induction?
Ans.
a. Abnormal uterine contraction, i.e. hyperstimulation/tachysystole
b. Appearance of fetal distress
c. Appearance of maternal distress
d. Non-progress of labor.

Q. What is acceleration of labor?
Ans. The progress of labor can be speeded up by amniotomy and oxytocin infusion and by using this method most of the pregnant mother is delivered by 12 hours and avoid prolonged labor.

Q. What is the cause of failure of POL (progress of labor)?
Ans.
a. Patient not in labor
b. Malposition—occiput posterior
c. Cephalopelvic disproportion (CPD)—undiagnosed
d. Malpresentation
e. Cervical stenosis and pelvic tumor.

Q. What is dystocia?
Ans. Dystocia (= Difficult labor) is characterized by slow progress or eventual arrest of labor. Failure to progress means absence of cervical dilatation or progressive fetal descent. Failure to progress is recognized by true CPD (passenger or passage), ineffectual uterine activity or ineffective maternal expulsive force (power). Dystocia often involves combination of these factors. The cervix dilates 1 cm/hour in active phase of labor in primi mother and if cervical dilatation does not progress at this rate then the diagnosis of dystocia is made.

Q. What will you do if dystocia occurs after amniotomy?
Ans. After amniotomy oxytocin is infused to optimize coordinated uterine activity to manage the dystocia, where there is no evidence of malpresentation, malposition and CPD.

Q. What are the complications of dystocia?
Ans. *Maternal*
a. Intrapartum chorioamnionitis and postpartum pelvic infections in prolonged labor.
b. PPH occurs in prolonged and augmented labor.
c. Pathological retraction ring (Bandl's ring) followed by uterine rupture.
d. Fistula formation and pelvic floor injury
e. Injury of common fibular nerve due to pressure by inappropriate leg positioning in stirrups in prolonged second stage of labor.

Perinatal complications.
a. Sepsis, caput succedaneum and molding.
b. Mechanical trauma like nerve injury, fracture, and cephalhematoma.

Q. What are the complications of oxytocin or risk of induction?

Ans.
a. In-coordinate uterine contraction
b. Fetal distress
c. Hyperstimulation or tachysystole
d. Rupture of uterus
e. Water intoxication (if oxytocin used in large dosage and no salt solution is used) and convulsion
f. Failure of labor—if labor continues beyond 24 hours.

Q. What are the uses of oxytocin/syntocinon in obstetrics?

Ans.
a. Induction of labor
b. Augmentation of labor
c. Active management of 3rd stage of labor for prevention of PPH
d. In established cases of PPH
e. It stimulates the myoepithelial cells of breast and hence ejection of milk.

> **Note**
> Do not use oxytocin 10 units in 500 mL (i.e. 20 mU/minute) in multigravida or in post-CS pregnancy. If contraction is not adequate (<200 monte-video unit), fetal status is reassuring, and labor has arrested, use of oxytocin infusion at a rate of >48 mU/minute in nulliparous uterus has no risk.

Q. Name the other oxytocics used in obstetrics. Name the PGs used for induction of labor.

Ans. Ergometrine, methylergometrine
Prostaglandin
- Injection 15 methyl PGF2—always used by intramuscular route
- Tablet misoprostol (PGE1) use oral, PR/PV, primiprost (oral)—not available now.

Only misoprostol is used for induction of labor.

Q. Is methergine used for induction of labor?

Ans. No, as it causes retraction of uterus (retraction—permanent shortening of uterine muscle fibers).

Q. When do you discontinue PGs and begin oxytocin infusion?

Ans. Oxytocin infusion is generally used
a. If membrane is ruptured
b. Cervical ripening has been achieved
c. Good labor pain has not been established even after 8 hours of PG use.

Q. What are the indications of use of misoprostol in obstetrics?

Ans.
a. To ripen the cervix in highly selective cases
   1. Severe pre-eclampsia, when cervix is unfavorable or lower segment cesarean section (LSCS) is not immediately available or baby is too premature to survive
   2. IUFD
b. For prevention of PPH
c. For medical termination of pregnancy (MTP) in very early pregnancy (45–50 days) along with mifepristone (RU-486).

Q. How do you use misoprostol for induction of labor, for PPH, for MTP?

Ans. Per vagina: For labor
a. Misoprostol (25 µg) is used in posterior fornix of the vagina at 6 hours interval.
b. If no response is found after two doses of 25 µg increase to 50 µg every 6 hours.
c. Do not use > 50 µg dose at a time do not exceed four doses (200 µg).

Per oral:
a. 100 µg at 6 hour interval for 4 doses.

For PPH:
800 mcg (PR or oral)—oral: Onset of action is 12–15 minutes; duration of action is 20–40 minutes.

For MTP:
1st day—mifepristone—200 mg orally, on the third day—misoprostol (200 µg)—2 tablets orally or PV.

> **Note**
> Do not use oxytocin within 8 hours of using misoprostol. Misoprostol causes meconium stained liquor and incidence of meconium aspiration syndrome (MAS) is high in newborn babies.

Q. What are the advantages of misoprostol?

Ans. a. Tablet form.
b. Easy to use only sublingual (S/L), per vagina (PV), per rectum (PR) (not a good route).
c. Can be stored at room temperature.

Q. What are the disadvantages of misoprostol?

Ans. Cannot be withdrawn, when it is used.

Q. What are the disadvantages of syntocinon?

Ans. a. It reduces its potency, if it is kept at room temperature of above 30°C.
b. It cannot be used in high dose as a bolus IV may cause hypotension.

Q. What are the advantages of oxytocin?

Ans. a. Wider availability
b. Less systemic side effects
c. Less catastrophe
d. Infusion can be stopped immediately, if there is evidence of hyperstimulation or fetal distress.
e. The dose can be accurately titrated depending on the response.

Q. What is the management of prolonged latent phase?

Ans. Diagnosis of prolonged latent phase is subjective and Friedman's criteria are (>20 hours in nullipara and 14 hours in multipara) in between onset of labor and active phase.
If cervix >2 cm or 100% effaced offer admission with active management by oxytocin and amniotomy is usually best delayed until the cervix is > 2

cm dilated or station is > 2, especially if the vertex is not well applied to the cervix.

Q. How do you manage active phase disorder in labor?

Ans. a. Cervix must be at least 4 cm dilated to diagnose active phase of labor
b. Oxytocin infusion to achieve atleast three contractions in 10 minutes duration
c. Amniotomy should be performed if rupture of membrane has not already occurred
d. After 4 hours of abnormal progression, active labor (in a nullipara with no scarred uterus) can be continued up to 6 to 8 hours with good chances of vaginal delivery when fetal monitoring is reassuring having some evidence of progress.

Q. What are the intrapartum strategies to reduce the risks of dystocia?

Ans. a. Ambulation—neither helpful nor harmful
b. Maternal position in labor—comfortable position of mother
c. Continuous support—emotional and psychological support
d. Hydration—crystalloids 125-250 mL/hour
e. Judicious anesthesia—epidural.

Q. When will you ask the patient to bear down or pushing?

Ans. Pushing should start as soon as complete dilatation of cervix is achieved unless fetus is malpositioned (e.g. occiput posterior) or the epidural anesthesia is so dense that woman has no urge to push.

Q. What will happen in delayed bearing down pain in second stage of labor?

Ans. Delayed bearing down is associated with longer second stage of labor (normal in nulliparous: 3 hours with epidural and 2 hours without epidural; in multiparous: 2 hours with epidural and 1 hour without an epidural), with consequent increased risk of maternal and fetal-neonatal infection with lower neonatal pH.

Q. What is failed induction?

Ans. a. Cases where the cervix does not dilate beyond 4 cm, despite adequate oxytocic stimulation (maximum 40 mIU/min), over a reasonable period of time. In primigravida, 8–12 hours and in multigravida, 6–8 hours is considered as the reasonable period of time.
b. Adequate uterine contraction for 2 hours without cervical change.

Q. What is the onset and duration of action of syntocinon on puerperal uterus?

Ans. Onset of action is 1 minute and mean half-life of action is 3–5 minutes.

COMPLICATIONS OF THIRD STAGE OF LABOR

Q. What are the complications of IIIrd stage of labor?

Ans. 1. Postpartum hemorrhage, 2. Retained placenta, 3. Shock, 4. Sepsis of birth canal, 5. Acute inversion of uterus, 6. Embolism.

Q. What is PPH?

Ans.
1. WHO, 1990: Amount of blood loss in excess of 500 mL following birth of the baby.
2. Clinical definition: Any amount of bleeding from or into the genital tract following birth of the baby upto the end of puerperium which adversely affects the general condition of the patient evidenced by rise in pulse rate and falling BP is called PPH.
3. ACOG definition: A hematocrit change of 10% or the need for red cell transfusion after child birth.

> **Note**
> PPH can be minor (500–1000 mL) or major (>1000 mL); major causes can be divided into moderate (1000–2000 mL) or severe (>2000 mL).

Q. What is immediate (primary) PPH?

Ans. Bleeding within 24 hours of delivery due to (a) excessive bleeding during 3rd stage of labor (3rd stage hemorrhage) and (b) Bleeding due to uterine atonicity.

Q. What is delayed (secondary) PPH?

Ans. PPH occurring between 24 hours after delivery and 12 weeks postnatally.

Q. What are the causes of PPH?

Ans.
a. Atonic
b. Traumatic
c. Mixed
d. Disseminated intravascular coagulation (DIC)

> **Note**
> 4T's—Tone (poor uterine contraction after delivery), Tissue (retained products of conception and blood clots), Trauma (to genital tract), Thrombosis (coagulation abnormalities).

Q. How do you assess shock in PPH?

Ans. For the general management of PPH 'a rule of 30' has been proposed.
Patients
a. Systolic blood pressure (SBP) falls by <30 mm of Hg
b. Heart rate (HR) rise by 30 bpm
c. Respiratory rate (RR) increased to 30 breaths/minute

If the Hb/Hematocrit (Hct) drops by 30% and urinary output <30 mL/hour, then the patient is most likely to have lost at least 30% of her blood volume and is in moderate shock leading to severe shock.

Q. What is shock index (SI)?

Ans. HR/SBP = 0.5 to 0.7 normal, however with significant hemorrhage it increases to 0.9 to 1.1. SI correlates well in identifying easy blood loss than HR, SBP or diastolic blood pressure (DBP) used in isolation.

Q. How do you prevent PPH?

Ans.
a. Correct anemia antenatally as iron deficiency contributes to uterine atony due to deficiency of myoglobin level necessary for muscle action

b. Do active management of third stage of labor
c. Remain vigilant in immediate postpartum period.

Q. What is the active management of 3rd stage of labor for prevention of PPH?

Ans. a. Administration of oxytocin by IM route in the dose of 10 unit within 1 minute of delivery of baby vaginally. For women delivering by CS oxytocin (5 unit by slow IV injection) should be used as prophylaxis to encourage uterine contraction and to decrease blood loss.
b. Controlled cord traction (CCT)
c. Uterine massage (not mandatory in active management).

Q. How do you manage atonic PPH with retained placenta?

Ans. a. Start IV drip with RL with oxytocin infusion
b. Uterine massage
c. Expulsion of clots
d. Assess shock—if patient is in shock correct the shock, blood transfusion if necessary
e. Empty the bladder by catheterization
f. If there are signs of separation of placenta—CCT and placenta is delivered and examine the placenta after delivery
g. If there is no signs of separation of placenta—Manual removal of placenta (MROP) under general anesthesia and broad spectrum antibiotic should be started.

Q. How do you go for manual removal of placenta (steps)?

Ans. See the answer in obstetric intervention (Chapter—3).

Q. How do you manage a case of atonic PPH when placenta is delivered?

Ans. Atonic PPH means bleeding from placental site due to lack of tone of uterus and is responsible for 90% of PPH.
a. Call for help
b. Rub the fundus of uterus to expel the clot, bimanual uterine compression and emptying the bladder to stimulate uterine contraction represent the first line management of PPH. If massage is unsuccessful next measure is medical therapy (Table 11.4)
c. Give oxytocin 10 units IM
d. Start IV line and oxytocin infusion 40 unit in 500 mL of 0.9% of normal saline (NS) infused at a rate of 125 mL/minute. Oxytocin is the first line of drug. It is effective within 2–3 minutes of injection, other drugs mentioned in Table 11.4.
e. Blood grouping and cross matching [4 units, fresh frozen plasma (FFP), platelet (PLT), cryoprecipitate]
f. Continuous drainage of bladder should be maintained
g. If patient is in shock manage the problem of shock.

Resuscitation by: O_2 mask, fluid balance by wide bore needle (colloid 1.5 liters in 20 minutes, blood and blood component [packed red blood cells (pRBC), FFP, PLT, cryoprecipitate, factor VIII] therapy and monitoring by central arterial line, urine output (UOP) by Foley catheter, Hb%, coagulation profile and monitoring of other vital signs are also necessary.

> **Note**
>
> Management of primary PPH: **Tone**– See 'a–g' above.
> **Tissue**—Delivery of placenta by CCT/MROP according to condition and examination of placenta—if any placental beats is found inside, evacuation of uterus; **Trauma**—Assess episiotomy and tear of genital tract and repair; Thrombin-Coagulation profile studies and replacement by blood and specific component of blood (pRBC:FFP:platelet::2:1:1). If medical measures fail for management of atonic PPH, examination under anesthesia in OT and allow surgical management.

Table 11.4: Commonly used uterotonic drugs

Drug	Dose	Route of dose	Frequency	Contraindication
1. Oxytocin	10–40U 1000 mL NS/RL	IV infusion IM/umbilical cord vein	Continuous infusion	Nil In 20–30% of cases need another uterotonic agents
2. Methyl-ergometrine	0.2 mg	IM/IV	Every 2–4 hours	Increased blood pressure pre-eclampsia eclampsia and heart disease
3. 10-methyl PGF2α	0.25 mg	IM only	Every 15–90 minutes not exceeding 8 doses	Cardiac, pulmonary and liver diseases
4. Misoprostol	400–800 μg	Oral/PR/PV	Every 2 hours	Food and Drug Administration (FDA) approval is waiting for

Note: Inj tranexamic acid can be used in traumatic PPH.

Surgical Management:
a. Bimanual compression—effective for a short duration
b. Condom pressure pack
c. Uterine balloon tamponade
d. Aortic compression—adjunctive measure
e. Bilateral uterine artery and ovarian artery ligation on laparotomy
f. Uterine artery ligation by vaginal approach
g. Brace sutures—B-Lynch suture
h. Internal iliac artery ligation (complication—peripheral nerve ischemia)
i. Hysterectomy with or without adnexectomy—total or subtotal.

> **Note**
>
> Non-pneumatic antishock garments (NASG) is a temporary method to overcome shock and is not a treatment of PPH.

Q. What are the factors associated with uterine atony?

Ans.
a. Prolonged labor
b. Induction by oxytocin
c. General anesthesia (GA) (halothane)
d. Multiple gestations
e. Polyhydramnios

f. Big baby
g. Grand multiparity
h. Infection (chorioamnionitis).

> **Note**
> *If uterus is hard but PPH occurs, think of traumatic injury of genital tract (cervix and vagina) or coagulopathy.*

Q. What are the causes of sudden postpartum collapse?
Ans.
a. Amniotic fluid embolism
b. Massive pulmonary venous thromboembolism
c. Complications of regional anesthesia
d. Eclampsia
e. Myocardial infarction
f. Anaphylactic reaction due to drugs
g. Inversion of uterus.

Q. What are the causes of secondary PPH?
Ans. Any bleeding from genital tract after 24 hours postpartum and within 6 weeks of delivery is called secondary hemorrhage:
a. Uterine infection
b. Retained placental fragments
c. Abnormal involution of placental sites
d. Placental polyp
e. Coagulopathies.

Q. How do you manage a case of secondary PPH? USG: To see any retained beats of placenta.
Ans.
1. Medical (supportive): Oxytocics, PGs, antibiotics, tranexamic acids, and vasopressin. Hormones [oral contraceptive pills (OCP) and progestins] are of doubtful value. IV hydration and blood transfusion. For mild bleeding without retained bits conservative management is sufficient.
2. Surgical (Active management): Uterine evacuation—if products are noted inside the uterine cavity by USG, evacuation should be done under general anesthesia after 48 hours of injection antibiotic therapy and material should be sent for histopathological examination.

For excessive and continuous bleeding other surgical procedures are adopted like:
a. Uterine tamponade balloon
b. Uterine compression sutures
c. Pelvic artery ligation
d. Selective pelvic artery embolization
e. Relaparotomy and cesarean site may need hemostatic suture
f. Hysterectomy—when all measures fail.

Q. What is traumatic postpartum hemorrhage?
Ans. This is usually due to trauma of maternal soft tissues like, cervix, vagina and perineum in labor or by instrumental delivery. It should be suspected if uterine bleeding persists even after adequate uterine retraction.

Q. What is colporrhexis?

Ans. It is a condition where posterior vaginal fornix is torn and opens pouch of Douglas (POD). This is usually accompanied by cervical tear but can occur without any genital trauma. It usually requires hysterectomy with subsequent vaginal repair of the tear.

INVERSION OF UTERUS

Q. What is inversion of uterus?

Ans. It is the turning inside, out of the uterus.

Q. What are the degrees of inversion?

Ans. 1st degree: Depressed fundus of uterus reaches upto the internal os.
2nd degree: Body of the uterus is inverted upto the internal os and the fundus protrude through the external os into the vagina.
3rd degree: Uterus and cervix are completely inverted.

Q. What are the different types of uterine inversion?

Ans. **Acute inversion:** Detected within 24 hours of delivery
Subacute inversion: After 24 hours but within 4 weeks of delivery
Chronic inversion: After 4 weeks of delivery.

Q. What are the factors predisposing to uterine inversion?

Ans.
a. Short umbilical cord
b. Excessive traction of umbilical cord before separation of placenta
c. Vigorus fundal pressure
d. Fundal implantation of the placenta
e. Retained placenta or abnormal adherence of placenta
f. Rapid or prolonged labor
g. Previous uterine inversion
h. Drug promoting tocolysis (Injection $MgSO_4$).

Q. How do you diagnose a case of uterine inversion?

Ans. **History:**
a. Pulling of the umbilical cord in absence of uterine contraction.
b. Pulling of the cord in presence of placenta accreta
c. Excessive fundal pressure to deliver the baby and placenta.

On Examination:
a. Features of shock is out of proportion of blood loss
b. The fundus is absent on palpation of abdomen or cupping of the uterine fundal region
c. PV bleeding
d. Inverted uterus may be seen at vulva or felt in vagina.

Q. How do you prevent acute inversion?

Ans.
a. Do not pull the cord in relaxed uterus
b. Apply counter traction with other hand while using controlled cord traction (CCT)
c. Do not apply fundal pressure.

Flying Questions

Q. How do you manage the case of acute inversion?

Ans.
1. Evaluate woman's condition and call for help.
2. Examine the vital signs pulse/respirations/temperature/blood pressure (P/R/T/BP) and pallor to assess the features of shock—resuscitation and treatment of shock is mandatory.
3. Take written consent for operation.
4. Manual reposition of uterus under GA aseptically
   a. Insert the gloved hand in the vagina and try to feel the cervical rim
   b. Repose the uterus back starting with the part that comes out last (during inversion fundus comes out first and portion of the uterus just above the cervix comes out last)
   This part of the uterus just above the cervix is reposed first, then gradually going up
   c. If placenta is not delivered, manual removal of placenta (MRP) should be done after reposition of uterus to avoid severe hemorrhage.
   d. Give oxytocic drugs
   e. Monitor P/BP/fundal height at regular interval for 24 hours.

If fails hydrostatic pressure under GA:
1. Trendelenburg's position (low head 0.5 meter below the perineum)
2. Identify the posterior fornix (rogues vagina between the smooth vagina).
3. Place the nozzle of the douche (NS; 5L) in the posterior fornix and the douche can is placed at least 2 meters above the patient.
4. The douche fluid is prevented from escaping from the vagina by blocking the vaginal introitus by operator's wrist which holds the douche nozzle.
5. An assistant press the vulva around the doctor's forearm to prevent further leakage.
6. A large amount of fluid (5L) distends the vagina and gradually the inverted uterus will be corrected.

Combined abdomino-vaginal route:
   a. Opening of the abdomen
   b. Dilate the constricting cervical rim digitally
   c. Grasp the inverted fundus through the cervical rim by tenaculum or round ligament by Babcock/Allis tissue forceps
   d. Apply gentle traction to the fundus or round ligaments while assistant attempts manual correction vaginally.

Abdominal approach: If vaginal manipulation, or hydrostatic pressure fails to reposition uterus, laparotomy must be performed:
   1. Huntington's method: Allis forceps are placed at the dimple of the inverted fundus through abdominal route and gentle traction is applied. The forceps are further advanced till the fundus is repositioned.
   2. If traction fails incise the constriction ring posteriorly by longitudinal incission and fundus is repositioned by

operator's finger pressure and close the uterus in two layers (Haultain's operation).
3. Robinson's operation: Cut the anterior ring and reposition the fundus back. Risk of injury to the bladder is high in this case.
e. After correction close the abdomen
f. Postoperative IV fluid, blood, antibiotics and oxytocics is necessary.

ABORTION PROBLEM

(Early trimester bleeding in pregnancy: Abortion, ectopic pregnancy, hydatidiform mole, placental sign).

Q. Define spontaneous abortion or miscarriage?

Ans. Interruption of pregnancy with or without expulsion of products of conception before 20 weeks of gestation or below 500 g weighing fetus (WHO). This criteria is somewhat contradictory as the mean birth weight of a 20-week fetus is 320 g whereas 500 g is the mean for 22–23 weeks.

> **Note**
> *According to some 'age of viability is 22 weeks'.*

Q. What are the causes of spontaneous abortion in first and mid trimesters?

Ans. a. First trimester:
   i. Chromosomal defect (2/3rd)—autosomal trisomy (50%), polyploidy (20%), monosomy (25%)
   ii. Maternal defect (1/3rd)—luteal phase defect (LPD), progesterone hormonal deficiency, trauma (coitus, long travel and surgical trauma) and infection-viral [rubella, cytomegalovirus (CMV)], unknown.
b. Mid trimester:
   i. Cervical incompetence and anatomical defect of uterus like septate, bicornuate, low implantation of placenta.
   ii. Infection—syphilis, toxoplasmosis and malaria.
   iii. Endocrinal—hypo and hyperthyroidism and uncontrolled diabetes.

Q. What is threatened abortion? How do you diagnose it? Differential diagnosis (D/Ds), Management.

Ans. It is a type of abortion where products of conception are not expelled but continuation of pregnancy is possible.
Diagnosis:
a. Symptom: i. Period of amenorrhea, ii. Vaginal bleeding is minimal, iii. No abdominal pain but sometimes lower abdominal discomfort, iv. No expulsion of fleshy mass
b. Signs: Per speculum (P/S)-cervix is closed and per vaginal bleeding is mild, on bimanual examination uterus corresponds with the period of amenorrhea
c. USG—for detection of viability.

Differential diagnosis: Other stages of abortion, trophoblastic disease, ectopic pregnancy, cervical erosion, polyp, vaginal ulceration, cancer cervix.

Management:
a. Reassurance of continuation of pregnancy when bleeding settles
b. Avoid strenuous activity and restrict normal daily activity and coitus at least for 4 weeks
c. If bleeding continues rescan (USG) in about 7 day to confirm viability
d. Unfavorable outcome—lowering of β-hCG titer, sonographic evidence of decreasing fetus and embryo in size, a slow heart rate, and uterus not increasing in size on pelvic examination.

> **Note**
> Chances of fetal risks (prematurity, FGR, and perinatal death) and maternal risks like (APH, placenta previa, manual removal of placenta and incidence of cesarean delivery) are high in threatened abortion cases.

Q. What is inevitable miscarriage? Diagnosis.

Ans. It is the type of abortion when bleeding and cramping pain of lower abdomen is accompanied by dilatation of cervical canal.
Diagnosis is clinical. Vaginal bleeding with severe colicky pain. Cervical os is opened and product may be felt through os, no tissue is expelled.

Q. What is incomplete abortion? How do you diagnose it?

Ans. The miscarriage is incomplete when the products of conception are protruding through the external os or are in the vagina with persistent bleeding and cramping.
Diagnosis—Continuous vaginal bleeding which may be fatal sometime following amenorrhea, expulsion of fleshy mass and cervical os is opened through which the product hangs and uterus is smaller than period of amenorrhea.

Q. How do you treat inevitable and incomplete abortion?

Ans. a. Expectant—Wait for completion of miscarriage if the clinical condition permits and the patient wishes.
b. Uncontrolled bleeding or if the product hangs through the os—surgical evacuation under anaesthesia with IV infusion of normal saline (10–20 units of oxytocin)
c. Medical management with 800 μg of misoprostol (Four- 200 μg tablet) per vagina every 4 hours. Curettage is necessary in 28% of cases.
d. Counseling and support of the patient.

Q. What is complete miscarriage?

Ans. Type of miscarriage where product of conception is expelled enmass. Cervical os is closed; uterus remains smaller and per vaginal bleeding is scanty. USG shows empty uterine cavity without echo of placental tissue.

Q. What is missed abortion?

Ans. Retention of the product of conception in the uterus for a prolonged period which is uncertain. Symptoms of early pregnancy disappeared, uterus fails to grow, cessation of fetal movement, quantitative beta-human chorionic gonadotropin (β-hCG) level fall, no heart motion of fetus on USG. Laboratory estimation of blood for Hb%, bleeding time (BT), clotting time (CT), platelet and fibrinogen level is important.

Q. How do you treat missed abortion?

Ans. The uterus is emptied by dilatation and evacuation. In the second trimester—induction of labor with high titre oxytocin drip, intravaginal prostaglandin E_2 (PGE_2) gel or misoprostol. The cervix is first prepared by misoprostol or passively dilated with laminaria tent to avoid trauma before suction curettage. Medical management by misoprostol 200 mcg is placed high in the vagina 4 hourly until delivery of the fetus and placenta (maximum 5 doses), but possibility of retained placenta is not uncommon. If there is coagulation defect due to dead fetus fibrinogen replacement might be of help before induction.

Q. What is septic abortion?

Ans. Any abortion associated with fever and signs of pelvic and generalized sepsis are considered septic abortion. It may be due to unsafe abortion or sepsis following spontaneous or elective abortion.

Q. What are the different grades of septic abortion cases?

Ans. Grade 1: Infection is localized to the uterus
Grade 2: Infection spreads to the pelvic structures
Grade 3: Evidence of septic shock, generalized peritonitis, renal failure and coagulation failure.

Q. What is the bacteriology of sepsis?

Ans.
a. Endogenous—*E. coli*, anaerobic streptococci, *Cl. welchii*
b. Exogenous—Hemolytic streptococci, *Staph. pyogens*, Gonococci.

Q. How do you diagnose a septic abortion case?

Ans. History of interference for abortion

Symptoms
a. History of amenorrhea
b. Vaginal bleeding followed by foul smelling vaginal discharge
c. Lower abdominal pain
d. Product may or may not be expelled
e. Fever

Signs—High temperature, tachycardia, hypotension, jaundice, oliguria/anuria
P/A—Tender lower abdomen, rigid abdomen in peritonitis
P/V—Firm tender uterus, boggy mass in POD if pelvic abscess is present.

Investigations
a. Blood: Hemoglobin, hematocrit, complete blood count (CBC), electrolyte, creatinine, platelet count, blood urea nitrogen (BUN),

prothrombin time (PT-INR), activated partial thromboplastin time (aPTT), fibrinogen peripheral smear for toxic granules, blood culture and sensitivity test. C-reactive protein level is increased (CRP: normal value <5 mg/L), Procalcitonin—it is a peptide of calcitonin, which level is increased in sepsis of bacterial origin (normal value: <0.1 ng/mL)

b. Urine: Routine and microscopy and culture sensitivity
c. Abdominal X-ray: Identify the air and fluid levels in the bowel, gas may be seen in tissues in clostridia infection, gas under the diaphragm indicates bowel and uterine perforation.
d. USG: For any collection like blood, abscesses in the peritoneal cavity or for any retained products in the uterus.
e. CT scan: To differentiate gas in tissue spaces or to delineate the parametrial infections.

Q. What are the different steps of sepsis?

Ans.
a. Systemic inflammatory response syndrome (SIRS):
   i. Temperature >100.4°F/<96.8°F (>38°C or <32°C)
   ii. Pulse rate (PR) >90 per minute
   iii. Respiration rate (RR) >20 minute, $PaCO_2$ <32 mm of Hg.
   iv. WBC (>12000 per cubic mm or <4000 per cubic mm).
b. Sepsis
   i. 2SIRS + confirmed or suspected infection
c. Severe sepsis
   i. Sepsis + end organ damage
   ii. Hypotension (SBP <90 mm of Hg)
   iii. Lactate >4 mmol/L
d. Septic shock
   i. Severe sepsis
   ii. End-organ damage
   iii. Persistent hypotension
   iv. Lactate >4 mmol/L.

Q. How do you treat a septic abortion case?

Ans. First ensure vital signs (Pulse, Respiration, BP, Temperature, P/V bleeding, urine output)
a. High risk septic cases (high fever, evidence of shock), early goal directed therapy (EGDT): It is an approach consisting of fluid resuscitation, blood transfusion, and dobutamine administration to maintain MAP >65, CVP of 8–12 mm of Hg, mixed venous oxygen saturation ≥70% and urine output > 0.5 mL/kg/hr. EGDT performed in first 6 hours of severe sepsis or septic shock to standard therapy shows improved mortality, oxygen delivery, tissue perfusion and decreased hospital stay.
Management:
A–Ensure air way is open
B–Breathing support, oxygen (6–8 L/min) by mask when necessary
C–Maintenance of circulation by IV crystalloid fluids (saline, Ringer's solution-2-4 L in first hour) and subsequent fluid is given through

a large bore needle, measure urine output by Foley's catheter (at least 30 mL/hour) and blood for grouping and cross match for whole blood transfusion to maintain hematocrit between 30% to 35%. Watch for pulmonary edema secondary to fluid overload.

D–Drugs, IV antibiotics (give broad spectrum antibiotics like ampicillin 500 mg qid IV, gentamicin (1.5 mg/kg by slow IV every 8 hours), metronidazole 500 mg IV tid), tetanus toxoid, 250 U of tetanus immunoglobulin by deep IM. Vesopressors are used when fluid and blood cell replacement can not restore adequate organ perfusion

Dopamine drip when systolic BP is below 90 mm of Hg [low dose <5 µg/kg/min causes renal and mesenteric vasodilatation; at doses 5-10 µg/kg/min increases cardiac output and heart rate; when the dose is increased to >10 µg/kg/min it leads to arterial vasoconstriction and increase in blood pressure]. Tachycardia and arrhythmia are more common than norepinephrine. Norepinephrine: It increases blood pressure by vasoconstriction with a small increase in cardiac output and stroke volume. Attention should be paid that patients treated with norepinephrine are adequately volume resuscitated. Dose 0.01–3.3 µg/kg/min.

Steroid: use of steroid is controversial. It can be used in low dose in septic. Patients associated with adrenal insufficient.

Glycemic control by insulin to maintain blood sugar in 80–100 mg/dL as hyperglycemia is a common complication of sepsis and may also result from steroid use. Blood glucose level is frequently checked to prevent hypoglycemia.

E–Evaluation:
- Measuring central venous pressure (CVP) by inserting catheter in internal jugular vein- if lactate is greater than 4 mmol/L (36 mg/L)
- Measure central mixed venous oxygen saturation ($ScVO_2$), expect greater than 70% in sepsis
- Remeasure lactate if initial lactate is 4 mmol/L (36 mg/L)
- Urine output (UOP) [normal—0.5 mL/kg/hr].

Additional: Assess disseminated intravascular coagulation (DIC)

Note: Transfuse blood if Hb is <6 g/dL or Hct <15%

b. Low risk of septic cases—mild or moderate fever (temperature < 103°F, vital signs stable, a small uterus, localized infection only and no indication of shock)

Initial treatment:
  i. Monitor vital signs
  ii. IV fluid
  iii. IV antibiotics, injection tetanus toxoid and tetanus antitoxin by IM route
  iv. Control of pain
  v. Currettage should be done if needed.

> **Note**
> For management of sepsis follow Acronym 'ORDER': O—Oxygen; R—Replacement of fluid, D—Drugs; E—Evacuation of uterus; R—Re-evaluation of the condition. Additional—If bleeding disorder, assess DIC and laboratory test for CBC, BUN, serum urea, creatinine and electrolytes.

Operative intervention may be necessary:
1. Evacuation of uterus after 6-8 hours of antibiotic therapy when effective antibiotic level is achieved.
2. In gut injury by S/E or D/E, immediate laparotomy and repair of gut or intestinal anastomosis (small gut) or colostomy (large gut) should be done according to the condition.
3. Hysterectomy may be needed in complicated cases.

> **Note**
> DIC (blood does not clot and bleeding from multiple sites)—IV antibiotics and resuscitation by blood/plasma and blood component.

Q. What are the indications of hysterectomy in septic cases?
Ans.
a. Traumatic uterine perforation
b. *Clostridium welchii* infection
c. Peritonitis and septic shock not responding to medical treatment
d. Oliguria in normovolemic patient.

Q. What are the complications of septic abortion?
Ans. **Early:** Acute renal failure (ARF), DIC, acute lung injury (ALI), acute respiratory distress syndrome (ARDS), septic shock and maternal death
Late: Chronic pelvic pain, backache, dyspareunia, infertility, and ectopic pregnancy.

Q. What is medical termination of pregnancy (MTP)?
Ans. It is a safe hygienic and deliberate termination of pregnancy up to 20 weeks by a registered medical practitioners recognized by medical council of India.

> **Note**
> One licensed doctor can perform MTP upto 12 weeks but opinion of two medical practitioners is required beyond 12 weeks up to 20 weeks.

Q. Who can perform MTP?
Ans.
a. The registered doctor who has assisted 25 MTPs in a hospital or training center
b. The practitioner who has performed 6 months house job in gynecology and obstetrics
c. The doctor who has diploma and degree in the field of obstetrics and gynecology
d. One year practice in obstetrics and gynecology registered after 1971 Act or 3 years practice before 1971 Act.

Q. What are the indications of MTP?

Ans. MRCE: (M—Medical diseases, R—Rape, C—contraceptive failures, E—Eugenic).
   a. Medical diseases (heart disease leading to pulmonary hypertension) that deteriorate the maternal health
   b. Rape
   c. Contraceptive failure—not an important factor
   d. Eugenic—Fetal malformation, Down's syndrome.

> **Note**
> MTP first started from 1st April, 1972 following MTP Act passed by Indian Parliament in 1971 in a place approved by Director of Health Services or CMOH, or any Government hospitals.

Q. What are the different methods of termination of pregnancy in first trimester of pregnancy?

Ans. Manual vacuum aspiration (up to 8 weeks), suction evacuation from 6–12 weeks, dilatation and evacuation (6–12 weeks), medical agents up to 7 weeks [All are already discussed].

Q. Which investigations do you perform before MTP?

Ans. Determine the length of pregnancy by bimanual examination and recognition of other symptoms of pregnancy. Laboratory and USG testing to confirm pregnancy in doubt. Blood for hemoglobin, group and Rh, urine-for microscopy for pus cells and sugar and protein.

> **Note**
> Informed consent is necessary. Adult woman who is not mentally ill can undergo MTP with only her own consent.

Q. What are the complications of MTP?

Ans. a. **Early:** Incomplete abortion, failed abortion, hemorrhage, infection, uterine perforation and anesthesia-related complications.
   b. **Late:** Infection, sub-involution, infertility, bleeding per vagina and Hematoma.

Q. What are different methods of MTP in second trimester of pregnancy?

Ans. Intra-amniotic hypertonic saline infusion, extra-amniotic instillation of 0.1% ethacridine lactate (yellow dye with acridine derivative), IM, intra and extra-amniotic prostaglandin, abdominal hysterotomy in 13–20 weeks but vaginal insertion of 400 µg of misoprostol followed by D/E at 13–14 weeks is also practised.

> **Note**
> Hypertonic saline infusion causes hypernatremia, endotoxic shock, DIC, cerebral hemorrhage and hysterotomy causes scar endometriosis (1%). So both are not recommended nowaday routinely.

Flying Questions

Q. How do you insert ethacridine lactate for medical abortion?

Ans. A Foley catheter (16 size) is introduced transcervically into the extra-amniotic space above the internal os and the bulb is inflated with 10–20 mL distilled water to seal off the internal os. Ethacridine lactate (0.1%) is instilled through the catheter in dose of 10 mL per week (maximum 150 mL). Catheter is left in situ for 6 hours and then removed after deflating the bulb if not spontaneously expelled out. Uterine contraction starts by 12–18 hours. Oxytocin augmentation may be done. Induction-abortion interval is 24–36 hours, if no abortion occurs after 48 hours, reinstillation of the drug or some other technique may be adopted.

Complications:
a. Renal failure may occur in a very few percent of cases.
b. The prostaglandins and their analogue can be used as adjuncts to bring about safe abortion if the need arises.

Q. What is post-abortion care?

Ans.
a. Watch for vitals, per vaginal bleeding and treat by oral antibiotics, NSAID and injection anti-D globulin in RH negative mothers
b. Information regarding early detection of complications following surgical abortions and early report of post abortal traid [bleeding, lower abdominal pain (LAP) and low grade fever]
c. To counsel the woman regarding the choice of contraception available in India (tubectomy, COCPs IUCDs barrier methods)
d. A follow-up visit within 7 days of MTP
e. The patient should report if she misses her period beyond 6 weeks of termination of pregnancy.

> **Note**
> Routine use of antibiotics at the time of surgical procedure may reduce the risk of post-procedure infection.

GYNECOLOGICAL DISORDER IN PREGNANCY

A. Fibroid with Pregnancy

Q. What is the incidence?

Ans. The incidence of fibroid in pregnancy is 1 in 1,000.

Q. What are the symptoms of fibroid uterus related to pregnancy?

Ans.
a. Sub-fertility
b. Abortion and preterm labor
c. Malposition and malpresentation of fetus
d. Obstructed labor
e. Abnormal uterine action
f. When fibroid is impacted, pressure symptoms like retention of urine.

Q. What are the effects of fibroid on labor?

Ans. May be unaffected, uterine inertia, dystocia and PPH.

Q. What are the effects of fibroid on puerperium?

Ans. Sub-involution, sepsis, secondary PPH, lochiometra and pyometra.

Q. What are the effects of pregnancy on myoma?

Ans. a. Growth of the tumor in pregnancy increases due to congestion, edema and degeneration
b. Degeneration (red degeneration)
c. Torsion
d. Infection.

Red Degeneration

Q. When its incidence is common?

Ans. It is common during mid pregnancy and puerperium.

Q. What are the symptoms?

Ans. During mid-pregnancy the patient comes with the features of acute pain abdomen. Nausea, vomiting and pyrexia are also common.

Q. What is the pathogenesis?

Ans. Degeneration is due to sub-acute necrosis which is presumably caused by interference of blood supply. Arterial and venous thrombosis is also the contributory factors which cause infraction. RBCs and hemoglobin are lysed in the vessels before it escapes or after it has been extravasated and gives rise coloration.

Q. What are the differential diagnosis?

Ans. a. Torsion of the pedicle of fibroid and ovarian cyst
b. Abruption placentae
c. Acute pyelitis.

Q. Treatment of red degeneration.

Ans. Conservative treatment only: By rest, analgesic, sedation the acute symptoms subside within 3–10 days and pregnancy continues uneventfully.

Q. What is the treatment of fibroid uterus in pregnancy?

Ans. a. Uncomplicated—antenatal follow-up till delivery and vaginal examination at 36 weeks should be done to plan the mode of delivery
b. Complicated
  i. Cervical fibroid causing retention of urine—bladder is catheterized and manual reposition is attempted, if spontaneous correction does not happen due to impaction in early months.
  ii. Red degeneration—already mentioned (no operative treatment).
  iii. Tumor causing obstruction—cesarean section.
  iv. Proper management of PPH if occurs.

> **Note**
> *Scope of myomectomy during cesarean section (CS)—see the operation of myomectomy in gynecological part.*

B. Ovarian Tumor in Pregnancy

Q. What is the incidence?

Ans. Incidence is 1 in 2000.
[Incidence of dermoid increases two fold during pregnancy, serous cystadenoma is common, but malignant ovarian tumor is rare during pregnancy (3–5%)].

Q. Effects of tumor on pregnancy.

Ans. Malpresentation, nonengagement of the presenting part, mechanical distress in huge ovarian tumor and impaction leading to retention of urine.

Q. Effects of tumor on labor.

Ans. Obstructed labor may occur.

Q. What are the complications of tumor?

Ans. Torsion of pedicle, intracystic hemorrhage, rupture and hemorrhage.

Q. What is Hingorani sign?

Ans. When the pregnant mother with ovarian tumor is placed in head low down position the cystic tumor moves upward towards the epigastrium and a groove is felt in between the uterus and tumor on bimanual examination.

Q. How do you diagnose ovarian tumor?

Ans. Clinically by bimanual examination or by ancillary aid of USG and MRI.

Q. What is the treatment of benign ovarian tumor in pregnancy?

Ans. During pregnancy:
  a. Uncomplicated—Best time of removal is 14–18 weeks as chances of abortion is less and access to pedicle is easy.
  b. After 36 weeks—The operation is withheld till delivery and the tumor is removed in early puerperium.
  c. Complicated—The tumor is removed irrespective of period of gestation.

During labor:
  a. If the tumor is well above, a watchful expectancy of vaginal delivery.
  b. If impacted, LSCS with removal of tumor.

During puerperium:
Tumor is to be removed as early as possible otherwise there may be torsion of the pedicle due to involution of the uterus.

> **Note**
>
> **Ovarian cyst:** Management during pregnancy according to size;
> a. The cyst is more than 10 cm and asymptomatic: If it is detected in first trimester observe the growth and complication and if it is detected in second trimester remove by laparotomy to prevent complications.
> b. If the cyst size is between 5–10 cm: Follow-up and laparotomy may be urgent when the cyst increases in size or fails to regress.
> c. If the cyst size is <5 cm: It usually regresses and does not require any treatment.
> d. Germ cell tumor (common from birth to the age of 20 years) and gonadal stromal tumors are usually seen in the child bearing years.
> Both the tumors are more often unilateral.
> If findings at laparotomy are suggestive of malignancy the specimens is sent for histological examination and for management see the Chapter of flying questions, adenexal mass in gynecological part.

C. Cervical Cancer in Pregnancy

Pregnancy has no adverse effect on natural history and prognosis of cervical cancer.
a. If cervical cancer is detected at < 16 weeks of GA- Immediate treatment is recommended irrespective of its stage.
b. If cervical cancer is detected after 16 weeks of GA at an early stage (1A1-1B1):
   - Treatment can be delayed until fetal maturity
   - Antenatal steroid administration to promote fetal lung maturity with elective CS with and simple hysterectomy is to be performed for stage 1A2 cervical cancer
   - Wertheim's radical hysterectomy operation is performed for stage 1B1 cervical cancer
   - Patient with stage 1A1 cervical cancer is treated with laser loop excision of the transformation zone or cold knife conization 6 weeks postnatally.
c. If cervical cancer is detected after 16 weeks of GA at an advanced stage (1B2 or greater):
   - Consideration for delay up to 4 weeks must be based on the GA at the time of diagnosis
   - Classical CS is the recommended mode of delivery if the fetus is reached at the age of viability in order to damage to the cervix.

D. Genital Prolapse in Pregnancy

Q. What is the incidence of genital prolapse in pregnancy?

Ans. 1 in 250 pregnancies.

Q. What is the effect of genital prolapse in pregnancy, labor and puerperium?

Ans. *Pregnancy:*
   a. Increased incidence of abortion
   b. PROM
   c. Intrauterine infections

Labor:
Early rupture of membrane, cervical dystocia, prolonged labor and operative inference.
Puerperium:
Uterine sepsis and sub-involution of uterus.

Q. What are the symptoms and signs of genital prolapse in pregnancy?

Ans. *Symptoms:*
The symptoms are very much prominent in early months of pregnancy. The common symptoms are white discharge per vagina, backache, bladder symptoms—frequency of micturition, inability to complete evacuation of urine and stress incontinence, rectal symptoms like difficulty in defecation and constipation.
Signs:
Signs of pregnancy along with cystocele, rectocele, and uterine descent, the cervix may be ulcerated, edematous.

Q. What is the treatment?

Ans. Early pregnancy with uterine prolapse
- The cervix is replaced inside the vagina and is kept in situ by introducing ring pessary for 16–18 weeks. After this period the gravid uterus grows up out of the pelvis and pulls the cervix upwards.
- If the cervix remains out side the introitus even in later months of pregnancy the patient is to be admitted at 36 weeks.

During labor
a. The patient should be kept in bed to prevent early rupture of membrane.
b. In early labor the vagina should be packed with roller gauze soaked in glycerine and acriflavine solution to reduce the edema and also helps in dilatation of cervix.
c. Prophylactic antibiotic when the cervix remains outside the vagina or there is PROM.
d. For head coming low down with cervix becomes thin but undilated— delivery is done by Duhrssen's incision on the cervical lip at 2 and 10 o'clock position followed by application of ventouse or forceps.
e. If head is high up and cervix is edematous and undilated—LSCS.

Puerperium
a. Rest in bed
b. If the cervix is outside the vagina, cover it with gauze soaked in glycerine and acriflavine solution.
c. In sub-involution put the ring pessary until involution is completed. Proper pelvic floor operation should be done 6 months after delivery.

HYPEREMESIS GRAVIDARUM

Q. What is hyperemesis gravidarum (HG)?

Ans. This is characterized by excessive vomiting and inability of the woman to retain anything taken orally during pregnancy resulting in metabolic acidosis.

> **Note**
> Vomiting after 12 weeks of amenorrhea should not be regarded as HG. Other causes of vomiting like gastritis, cholecystitis, pancreatitis, peptic ulceration, hepatitis and UTI should be kept in mind.

Q. In which conditions hyperemesis gravidarum is common?

Ans. It is commonly seen in primigravida, multiple pregnancies, hydatidiform mole, and in women with pre-existing diabetes, hyperthyroidism and gastrointestinal disorders.

Q. What are the etiological factors of hyperemesis gravidarum?

Ans.
a. Hormones—high hCG concentration during early pregnancy
b. Cytokines—TNF-α and IL-4 also favors hCG production.
c. Genetics—i. Nausea and vomiting of pregnancy (NVP) is more common in monozygotic twin, ii. Siblings and mothers of patients affected with NVP are more likely to be affected than siblings of unaffected individuals, iii. NVP is more common in women with inherited glycoprotein hormone receptor defect.
d. Psychopathology.

Q. How do you diagnose hyperemesis gravidarum?

Ans. On examination the following signs are noted:
- Dehydration (dry tongue, loss of skin turgor, oliguria in severe cases)
- Tachycardia may be present
- Ketonuria may be present
- Laboratory abnormalities—the thyroid profile may be abnormal (TSH level is low in NVP), change in amylase, lipase and liver enzymes are transient, bilirubin level may also be high.

Q. How do you diagnose acetone in urine?

Ans.
a. **Rothera's test:** Take 5 mL of urine in a test tube. Ammonium sulfate is added to make it fully saturated. In this solution add 3–4 drops of freshly prepared sodium nitroprusside solution and then add 1 mL of concentrated ammonium hydroxide and wait for 1–2 minutes. Observation—a reddish-purple ring is found at the junction of two liquid. Inference—presence of acetone (if the ring is brown it has no significance).
b. **Ketostix test:** Dip the reagent impregnated strip in fresh specimen of urine and compare the color of the test with color chart supplied by manufacturer.

Q. What are the DDs?

Ans. Jaundice, meningitis, pancreatitis, gallstone, diabetic and uremic coma, peritonitis due to untreated septic abortion.

Q. What are the complications of HG?

Ans.
a. Mallory-Weiss tears of esophagus
b. Hematemesis
c. Muscle wasting and weakness

d. Vitamin B1 deficiency causing Wernicke's encephalopathy characterized by abnormal ocular movements, ataxia, confusion and death of fetus.

Q. How do you manage the condition?

Ans. a. Admit the patient in hospital.
b. Counsel the woman and family regarding the harmless nature of the condition.
c. Nutritious support—Start IV fluid, either Ringer's lactate (RL) or dextrose saline. Normal saline (NS) (0.9% with 20 mMol/L potassium chloride). Dextrose containing fluid should be avoided as this may cause central pontine myelinolysis and Wernicke's encephalopathy. (Dehydrated patient generally losses 6% of the fluid per kg of body weight, e.g. in 60 kg body weight the fluid loss is $6/100 \times 60 = 3.6$ L. So, total amount of fluid = 3.5–4 L/day. Drip rate/minute = Desired number of liters to be given/day × 12). 1 L should be given over 1–2 hours followed by second bottle in 2–4 hours.
d. Pulse, respiration, temperature and BP should be recorded on admission and every 2 hour during IV fluid treatment.

Pharmacology—Injectable antiemetics are used in acute case:
a. Metaclopramide 5–10 mg q8 h IV
b. Ondansetron 8 mg q8–12 h IV or PO
c. Additional MVI infusion daily.
Others are:
   i. Antihistamines (doxylamine, diphenhydramine, prométhazine, meclizine)
   ii. Phenothiazine (prochlorperazine, chlorpromazine)
   iii. Benzamides (metaclopramide)
   iv. $5\text{-}H_3$ antagonists (ondansetron, granisetron)
   v. Corticosteroids—Prednisolone, droperidol, methylprednisolone (16 mg tid for 3 days taper over 2 weeks to lowest effective dose and total duration of therapy 6 weeks)
d. Repeat urine examination every 4 hours till it becomes negative for ketone bodies
e. Once the vomiting stops and dehydration is corrected, discharge the patient
f. Advise the woman to take small, frequent carbohydrate meal, folic acid supplementation (5 mg once a day for 12 weeks), thiamine (50 mg tds/day) and oral antiemetics at home.

FOR POSTGRADUATES

NONIMMUNE HYDROPS FETALIS (NIH) AND FETAL ANEMIA

Q. What is NIH?

Ans. It is a disorder characterized by extensive accumulation of fluid in tissues or body cavities without any identifiable circulating antibody

against the red blood cell antigen. The sonographic diagnosis of hydrops is skin thickness of greater than 5.0 mm with 2 or more of the following:
1. Pleural effusion
2. Pericardial effusion
3. Ascites
4. Placental edema and enlargement.

Q. What is the basic pathophysiology of hydrops fetalis?

Ans. When the fetal hemoglobin concentration deficit exceeds 6 gm/dL hydrops develops. This is mainly due to extensive proliferation of the liver by erythropoietic tissues which give rise to parenchymal compression of portal vessels leading to portal hypertension. There is hypoproteinemia due to impaired protein synthesis and cardiac failure due to arrhythmias and structural cardiac defects. Fetal hydrops leads to fetal death in early pregnancy if uncorrected.

> **Note**
>
> *Pathophysiology*
> a. *Decreased osmotic pressure and hypoprotinemia*
> b. *Lymphatic abnormalities as seen in cystic hygroma, Turner's syndrome and skeletal dysplasia. Here umbilical venous pressure is normal*
> c. *Inadequate cardiac output (COP) due to obstructed outflow, inadequate ventricular filling and regurgitation may lead to cardiac failure and here umbilical venous pressure is increased.*

Q. What are the causes of NIH?

Ans. Maternal:
Anemia, preeclampsia, diabetes, indomethacin administration.
Fetal:
1. Anemia—thalassemia, fetomaternal hemorrhage, twin-to-twin transfusion syndrome (TTTS)
2. Cardiac—arrhythmia, cardiomyopathy, premature closure of ductus arteriosus
3. Chromosomal—Turner, trisomy 13 and 21
4. Infections—Parvovirus 19, herpes, toxoplasmosis, syphilis
5. Others—metabolic diseases, cystic hygroma, osteogenesis imperfecta, diaphragmatic hernia, congenital nephrosis.

Placental:
Chorioangioma of placenta.

Q. How do you investigate a case of NIH?

Ans. Noninvasive approach—Ultrasonography (USG), complete blood count (CBC), Kleihauer-Betke (K-B) analysis, toxoplasmosis, others—rubella, cytomegalovirus, herpes simplex (TORCH), echocardiography Invasive—amniocentesis, fetoscopy, cordocentesis, fetal karyotyping.
Maternal:
a. Full blood count
b. ABO/Rh
c. Hb electrophoresis

d. K-B test for fetomaternal hemorrhage
e. TORCH screen
f. Auto-antibody screen [systemic lupus erythematosus (SLE) and anti Ro and La] in cases of complete heart block
g. Oral glucose tolerance test (OGTT)
h. Liver function test (LFT) and renal function test (RFT).

Fetal:
a. Detailed anomaly scan
b. Fetal echocardiography
c. Amniotic fluid index (AFI)
d. Placental morphology and thickness
e. Doppler flow velocity studies
f. Cordocentesis at 18 weeks for CBC, blood group and Coomb test, thalassemia screen, blood gas analysis, karyotyping, glucose-6-phosphate dehydrogenase (G6PD) G6PD enzyme detection and TORCH.

Q. Why ultrasonography is important in NIH?

Ans. It is essential to detect:
1. Complete anatomical survey
2. Skin thickness > 5 mm
3. Placental thickness > 6 cm
4. Twins
5. AFI
6. Fetal Doppler
7. Fetal echo.

Q. How do you manage NIH?

Ans. Counselling regarding fetal prognosis, expensive investigations, shifting to tertiary center and early termination before 20 weeks is very important.

Treatment: 1. Medical 2. Surgery

1. **Medical:** Fetal therapy for anemia, arrhythmia, pulmonary condition and TTTS.
    a. *Transplacental drugs:*
    For the treatment of fetal dysrhythmias, particularly supra-ventricular tachycardia—drugs commonly used are digoxin, verapamil, amiodarone.
    b. *Direct fetal drug therapy:*
    As transplacental drug therapy is generally not effective in NIH, anemia can be treated by intrauterine fetal blood transfusion; digoxin and lasix can also be given to the fetus by intravenous route. Intrauterine transfusion of albumin can improve to some extent the idiopathic NIH.
2. **Surgery:**
Pleural effusion can be aspirated under USG guidance by pig-tail catheter or by pleuro-amniotic shunt. Diaphragmatic hernia can be treated by intrathecal balloon. Sacrococcygeal teratoma can be managed by radiofrequency ablation and TTTS is successfully managed

by laser photocoagulation of anastomotic placental vessels. Ascites can be treated by vesicoamniotic shunt or peritoneal- amniotic shunt.

Obstetric management:
1. Preterm delivery should be avoided
2. Some prefer routine LSCS to plan resuscitation with neonatologist
3. Vaginal delivery may be allowed
4. Active management of third stage of labor to prevent PPH.

Q. What is mirror syndrome?

Ans. In fetal hydrops the development of maternal edema in which fetus *mirrors* the mother is called mirror syndrome. It is also called triple edema because the fetus, mother and placenta, all are edematous. It is associated with Rhesus (Rh)-D alloimmunization, TTTS, chorioangioma of placenta, fetal cystic hygroma and sacrococcygeal teratoma, etc. It may be associated with hypertension, proteinuria, elevated liver enzyme and imbalance of angiogenic and antiangiogenic factors.

Treatment
a. Successful in utero treatment of fetal anemia, supraventricular tachycardia, hydrothorax and bladder outlet obstruction results in improvement of fetal hydrops and maternal mirror syndrome.
b. Prompt delivery may improve maternal edema within 9 days.

Fetal Anemia

Q. What is fetal anemia?

Ans. Fetal anemia is defined as hematocrit or hemoglobin concentration greater than 2SD below the mean of gestational age. Hemoglobin values should be expressed as multiples of the median (MoM) to adjust for the effects of gestational age.

Normal fetal hemoglobin values are ≥ 0.84 MoM (5th percentile)
Fetal anemia:
Mild—hemoglobin <0.84 MoM; Moderate—hemoglobin <0.65 MoM; Severe—hemoglobin <0.55 MoM.

Q. What are the different causes of fetal anemia?

Ans. Fetal anemia can be caused by alloimmune, non-immune, parvovirus B19 infection and idiopathic causes.

Q. What are the methods of diagnosis of fetal anemia in utero?

Ans. Noninvasive methods:
  A. Ultrasound imaging
   a. Middle cerebral artery peak systolic velocity (MCA-PSV) by Doppler-Fetal anemia is associated with increased arterial and venous blood flow velocities due to decreased viscosity and increased cardiac output. Fetal hemoglobin level is inversely related to MCA-PSV. If MCA peak systolic velocity is greater than 1.5 MoM (multiples of median) for the gestational age, 100 percent sensitivity in detection of moderate to severe anemia.

b. Liver length: Measured from the dome of the diaphragm to the tip of the right lobe on the right side of fetus.
c. Spleen perimeter: Spleen perimeter = (longitudinal diameter + transverse diameter) × 1.57 (values greater than 95th percentile are considered to be abnormal)
d. Doppler study of fetal descending aorta
e. Other findings:
  i. Prehydropic changes (early ascites and polyhydramnios)
  ii. Fetal hydrops—pleural effusion, pericardial effusion, scalp edema, subcutaneous edema
  iii. Placental thickness of more than 30 mm between 18 and 21 weeks of GA.

B. 2D Echocardiography
a. Increased biventricular outflow diameter during diastole and cardiothoracic ratio
b. Enlargement of fetal heart
c. Thickening of ventricular wall and interventricular septum
d. Hyperdensity of the myocardium
e. Tricuspid regurgitation

Invasive methods:
Fetal cordocentesis: It is reserved for patients when optical density (OD) 450 values and MCA-PSV are elevated. It is associated with 1–2% of fetal loss.
Amniocentesis: Amniotic fluid bilirubin measurement gives indirect estimation of hematological status, less invasive, but reliability before 27 weeks of gestation is questionable.

Q. Why diagnosis of fetal anemia is essential when the fetus is inside the uterus?

Ans.
1. To investigate the underlying cause
2. To ascertain the degree of fetal anemia
3. To diagnose before the development of hydrops fetalis as timely detection and early intervention may increase the survival rate of fetus to more than 90%.

Q. Why MCA –PSV is important?

Ans.
1. It responds quickly to hypoxemia
2. The incident angle between ultrasound beam and blood flow is maintained close to zero degrees and real velocity is determined
3. Middle cerebral artery is easy to locate
4. The results are highly accurate
5. Can detect fetal anemia due to:
   a. Parvovirus infection
   b. Fetomaternal hemorrhage (FMH)
   c. Fetal hydrops.

> **Note**
> *MCA-PSV can reduce the number of invasive tests in 70% of cases.*

Q. How MCA-PSV predicts moderate to severe fetal anemia?

Ans. MCA peak systolic velocity is expressed as multiples of median (MoM)
MoM = measured PSV/expected PSV
Expected MCA-PSV= $e^{(2.31 + 0.046\ GA)}$ where 'GA' is the gestational age
The relation between MoM for the peak systolic velocity and the MoMs for the hemoglobin concentration is evaluated by regression analysis. The optimum threshold values for peak systolic velocity in the MCA is kept at 1.29 times the median for mild anemia, 1.50 times the median for moderate anemia, and 1.55 times the median for severe anemia.

> **Note**
> The MCA-PSV can not diagnose all cases of fetal anemia. In mild anemic cases the velocity does not necessarily change. The correlation is more accurate as the severity of anemia increases.

Q. How do you manage fetal anemia?

Ans. A cut-off value of MCA-PSV of 1.5 MoM for the period of gestation is typically used to indicate anemia requiring treatment (fetal hematocrit <25%). Intrauterine transfusion at 18–24 weeks by aseptic precaution is helpful. Leukodepleted irradiated O-negative blood cross-matched to the mother's blood packed to a hematocrit of 75–85% is used.

The volume of blood transfused depends on the initial fetal hematocrit, size of the fetus, the donor hematocrit and the targeted hematocrit (Hct) to be achieved. The transfusion is given till a fetal Hct of 45–50% is achieved. The average neonatal survival rate is 80%. The loss rate from the procedure is 1–3%. The packed cells may be given intraperitoneally (IPT) or by intravascular route (IVT) through the umbilical vein either in the cord or intrahepatically. In fetal hydrops the intravascular route is preferred.

When fetal Hct is achieved by 45–50% serial 2 weekly follow-up is performed to decide the next transfusion, which will be typically 2–3 weeks after the first transfusion. The rate of drop of fetal hematocrit is around 0.8–1.1% per day. Combined with MCA Doppler this can be used as a guide to prefix the time the next transfusion. If fetus is well there is no need to deliver the baby preterm.

A special neonatal team is required during delivery of baby as previous IUT may need exchange transfusion or simple transfusion and management of hyperbilirubinemia.

Q. What are the complications of intrauterine transfusions?

Ans. Preterm labor, PROM, fetal bradycardia, and chorioamnionitis.

Q. What are the indications of intrauterine transfusion (IUT)?

Ans. Rh alloimmunization, fetal anemia caused by parvovirus B19 infection, chorioangiomas, twin anemia polycythemia sequences (TAPS).

Q. How do you follow-up fetal anemia by MCA-PSV?

Ans. In high-risk patients MCA-PSV can be done on weekly basis if values are below 1.5 MoM, if it becomes higher than 1.5 MoM, repeat the study in 2–3 days. If the value continues to rise, cordocentesis should be performed and IVT (intravascular transfusion should be given according to the fetal status).

MATERNAL DEATH

Q. What is maternal death?

Ans. The death of woman while pregnant or within 42 days of termination of pregnancy, irrespective of the duration and site of the pregnancy, from any cause related to or aggravated by the pregnancy or its management but not from accidental or incidental cause (WHO).

Q. What is maternal mortality ratio (MMR)?

Ans. The MMR is the number of maternal deaths per 100,000 live births per year (WHO).

$$MMR = \frac{\text{Total number of female death due to complications of pregnancy, child birth or within 42 days of a delivery in an area during given year}}{\text{Total number of live births in the same area and year}} \times 100,000$$

Maternal mortality ratio: Number of maternal deaths during a given time period for 100,000 live births during the same time period.
Maternal mortality rate: Number of maternal deaths in a given period per 100,000 women of reproductive age during the same time period.
Late maternal deaths: Complications of pregnancy and child birth can lead to death which was included in ICD-10 (the delayed death that occurs between 6 weeks and one year postpartum.
Pregnancy-related death: Death of women while pregnant or within 42 days of termination of pregnancy (TOP), irrespective of cause and death.

Q. What is the magnitude of the problem of MMR in India?

Ans. According to RGI-SRS report released in April, 2009 MMR in India has shown an appreciable decline from 398/100,000 live births in the year 1997–98 to 301/100,000 live births in the year 2001–03 to 254/100,000 live births in the year 2004–2006.
However, the National Rural Health Mission (NRHM) and Millennium Development Goal (MDG) is to reduce the MMR to less than 100/100,000 live births.
India:
In the year 2007–2009   MMR is 212 per lac
              2010–12   MMR is 178 per lac
A reduction of 34 points over a period of 3 years
              2013   MMR is 178 per 100,000 live births.

Q. What are the different causes of maternal death?

Ans.   *A. Direct Obstetric Causes:*
  I. Early pregnancy death (EPD) (first 20 weeks of pregnancy)
    i. Different kinds abortions
    ii. Ectopic pregnancy

iii. Molar pregnancy
iv. Induced abortions and sepsis.

II. Late pregnancy deaths (LPD)
   i. APH (after 20 weeks of pregnancy)
   ii. Obstructed labor/rupture uterus
   iii. PPH (primary or secondary)
   iv. Hypertensive disorder of pregnancy
   v. Sepsis related to pregnancy and child birth
   vi. Complications of anesthesia
   vii. Surgical complications
   viii. Transfusion reactions
   ix. Sudden deaths (pulmonary embolism, amniotic fluid embolism and sudden death due to undetermined cause)
   x. Other conditions (peripartum cardiomyopathy, suicide due to puerperal psychosis).

B. *Indirect Obstetric Causes:*
   i. Heart diseases complicating pregnancy
   ii. Anemia and its complications during pregnancy
   iii. Endocrine disorders (diabetes, thyroid and other endocrine problem)
   iv. Infectious diseases—(meningitis/encephalitis, maternal tetanus, HIV/AIDS, malaria, typhoid, TB)
   v. Liver disorder
   vi. Renal complications
   vii. Others (bronchial asthma, epilepsy, intracranial space occupying lesion, cancer, etc.).

Q. What are the different approaches of maternal death investigations?

Ans.
1. Community-based maternal death review (CBMDR) (verbal autopsy)
2. Facility based maternal death review (FBMDR)
3. Confidential enquiries into maternal deaths
4. Surveys of severe morbidity
5. Census
6. Household survey
7. Civil registration system—Routine registration of births and deaths
8. Sister head methods: Enquire the responders (representative sample) for survival of adult sisters and any death of sister during pregnancy, delivery or within 6 weeks of delivery
9. Clinical audit.

> **Note**
> *Government of India has taken up CBMDR and FBMDR to identify the gap in health care delivery systems to prioritize and plan for intervention strategies and to reconfigure health services.*

Q. What is community-based MDR?

Ans. Community-based reviews must be taken up for all deaths that occurred in the specified geographical area, irrespective of the place of death, be it at home, facility or in transit.

Flying Questions

Q. What is facility-based MDR?

Ans. Facility-based death reviews will be taken up for all government teaching hospitals, referral hospitals, and other hospitals [District, sub-district, community health centers (CHCs)] where more than 500 deliveries are conducted in a year.

Q. How do you prevent maternal mortality?

Ans.
a. Early registration of pregnancy
b. Minimum four antenatal check-up
c. Balanced diet including iron and folic acid prophylaxis for prevention of anemia
d. Treatment of medical complications like hypertension, diabetes, anemia, and renal disorders
e. Management of pregnancy complications like APH, PPH, infection, obstructed labor and ruptured uterus
f. Safe and clean delivery practice
g. Institutional delivery by different cash benefit scheme by Government of India
h. Institutional delivery of bad obstetric history (BOH) cases
i. Training of local dais in rural areas
j. Proper family planning services for proper birth spacing
k. Audit of each and every maternal death.

PERINATAL MORTALITY RATE

Q. What is perinatal mortality rate (PNMR)?

Ans. According to WHO

$$PNMR = \frac{\text{Late fetal death (> 28 weeks of GA) + early neonatal death (first week) in one year}}{\text{Live birth in the same year}} \times 1000$$

For international comparison (WHO expert committee on perinatal mortality and morbidity)

$$PNMR = \frac{\text{Late fetal and early neonatal death Weighing > 1000 g at birth}}{\text{Total birth weighing >1000 g at birth}} \times 1000$$

Q. What is the incidence of PNMR in India?

Ans. In India the PNMR is 38.7 per 1000 live births in urban areas and 43.3 in rural areas. National goal of PNMR was between 30 and 35 by the year 2000. Sample Registration System (SRS) estimation of perinatal mortality in India for the year 2010 was 32/1000 live births and stillbirths with 35 for rural area and 22 for urban area.

Q. Which risk factors are associated with high PNMR in India?

Ans. Low maternal age (<18 years), poor socioeconomic status, high parity, short maternal height, poor past obstetrical history, heavy smoking in rural areas, malnutrition and multiple pregnancies and lack of antenatal check-up.

Q. What are the different causes of PNM?

Ans. *a. Antenatal*
   i. Medical diseases associated with pregnancy: Anemia, hypertension, heart disease, diabetes, kidney disease, tuberculosis.
   ii. Complications in pregnancy: Pre-eclampsia, eclampsia, APH, jaundice.
   iii. Others: Advanced maternal age, congenital defects of uterus, pelvic diseases like pelvic inflammatory disease (PID), myoma, incompetent cervix.

b. Intranatal
   i. Obstetric complications
   ii. Birth injuries
   iii. Birth asphyxia

c. Postnatal causes
   i. Prematurity
   ii. Respiratory distress syndrome (RDS)
   iii. Respiratory tract infections and congenital anomalies.

Q. How do you prevent PNM?

Ans. a. Proper antenatal check-up
   b. Screening of high-risk pregnancies and early referral to higher centers for hospital delivery
   c. Improvement of nutrition by balanced diet and iron prophylaxis to prevent anemia during pregnancy
   d. Medical diseases should be treated properly till stable and then allow pregnancy
   e. Safe and clean delivery practice
   f. Essential newborn care and resuscitation when necessary
   g. Promote breastfeeding
   h. Good family planning services for birth spacing.

Note: See Figure 11.4

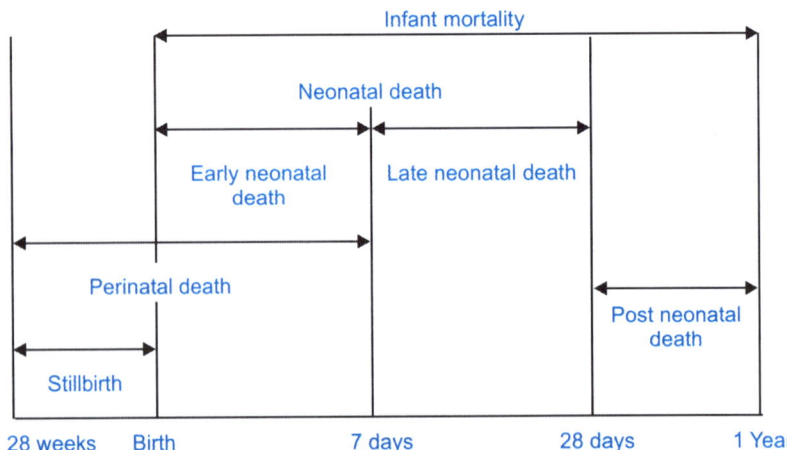

Figure 11.4: Time of stillbirths, perinatal and neonatal deaths

Appendices

APPENDIX 1: NUTRITION IN PREGNANCY

Q. What is the sample menu for pregnant mother?

Ans. Sample menu for pregnant mother is as follows:
   a. *Breakfast*: Tea/coffee/milk (1 cup = 225 mL), Biscuits = 2
   b. *Midmorning*:
      Non-vegetarians—two pieces of bread with butter or handmade bread (50 g), vegetables, eggs (duck or hen) = one (30 g), one cup of milk (150 mL).
      Vegetarians—all except egg.
   c. *Lunch*:
      Non-vegetarians—boiled rice (150 g)/four pieces of chapati, daal one cup (30 g), salad and tomato (150 g), potato (45 g), fish curry (25 g)/chicken curry (25 g), sour card (25 g), vegetables (30 g).
      Vegetarians—all except fish/chicken.
   d. *Afternoon*: Tea/coffee = one cup, biscuits = 2, fruits—guava, banana, cucumber, apple, orange in changing fashion (30 g)
   e. *Dinner*:
      Non-vegetarians—same as lunch
      Vegetarians—same except fish/chicken, dal (30 g)
   f. At bed time:
      Non-vegetarians—milk with sugar (200 mL)
      Vegetarians—milk with sugar (250 mL)
   g. Clean and boiled drinking water—10 glasses/day (normal 8 glasses/day).

Q. Prescribe a balanced diet for pregnant women doing sedentary work/24 hours.

Ans.
   1. For non-vegetarians/food stuffs in g:
      Cereals = 350, pulse = 45, green leafy vegetables = 150, other vegetables = 75, roots and tubers = 50, fruits = 30, milk = 225, fish and oils = 30, sugar and jaggery = 40, meat = 30, egg = 30.
   2. For vegetarians—food stuffs in g:
      All are same, except fish, meat and egg are not given. Also pulse = 60, milk = 325 (are in high amount).
   3. Calories 2,200, protein = 55 g, fat = 55 g.

Q. Relative protein value and protein energy (%) of some foods.

Ans. See Table 1.1

Table 1.1: Nutrition per 100 g

Food	Kcal	Protein (g)	Energy from protein	PE (%)
Fish	100	20.0	80	80
Milk (curd)	67	3.2	13	20
Pulse	350	21.0	84	24
Rice	350	7.0	28	8
Potato	100	1.6	6	6
Banana	100	1.0	4	4

Protein: Chapati = 11 g/100 g, vegetable = 2 g/100 g, fish = 21.8 g/100 g, chicken = 25.9 g/100 g, mutton muscle = 18.5 g/100 g, soyabean = 43.2 g/100 g.
Protein: Energy—4 kcal/g
Fat: Energy—9 kcal/g
Carbohydrate: Energy—4 kcal/g.

Q. What is PE (%)?

Ans. $PE (\%) = \dfrac{\text{Energy from protein}}{\text{Total energy in diet}} \times 100$

Q. How do you calculate kilocalories from the following diet chart?

Ans. See Table 1.2

Table 1.2: Calculation of kilocalories from diets

Cereals = 400 g	400 × 3.5	=	1400 kcal
Pulse = 30 g	30 × 3.5	=	105 kcal
Milk = 100 g	100 × 0.67	=	67 kcal
Egg = 30 g	30 × 2	=	60 kcal
Fish = 30 g	30 × 1	=	30 kcal
Oil = 10 g	10 × 9	=	90 kcal
Sugar = 10 g	10 × 4	=	40 kcal
Vegetables = 100 g	100 × 0.4	=	40 kcal
Potato = 100 g	100 × 1	=	100 kcal
Total		=	1,932 kcal

Q. What are the requirements of nutrients, minerals and vitamin in pregnancy and lactation?

Ans. N = normal, P = pregnancy, L = lactation
  a. Protein: N = 50 g (1 g/kg body weight), P = 50 + 10 = 60 g, L = 50 + 20 = 70 g.
  b. Fat: N = 50 g (1g/kg body weight), P = 50 g, L = 50 + 10 = 60 g.
  c. Carbohydrate: N=395 g, P = 460 g, L = 550 g.
  d. Minerals:
     i. Calcium: N = 400 mg, P = 1,000 mg, L = 1,000 mg
     ii. Phosphorus: N = 800 mg, P = 1,200 mg, L = 1,200 mg
     iii. Iron: N = 30 mg, P = 40 mg, L = 30 mg

Appendices

  iv. Zinc: N = 12 mg, P = 15 mg, L = 19 mg
  v. Iodine: N = 150 μg, P = 175 μg, L = 200 μg
  vi. Magnesium: N = 280 mg, P = 320 mg, L = 355 mg.
 e. Fat-soluble vitamins:
  i. Vitamin A: N = 5,000 IU, P = 6,000 IU, L = 8,000 IU
  ii. Vitamin D: N = 400 IU, P = 400 IU, L = 400 IU.
 f. Water-soluble vitamins:
 g. Folic acid: N = 0.5 mg, P = 1 mg
  i. Niacin: N = 15 mg, P = 17 mg, L = 20 mg
  ii. Riboflavin: N = 1.3 mg, P = 1.6 mg, L = 1.8 mg
  iii. Thiamine (B1): N = 1.1 mg, P = 1.5 mg, L = 1.6 mg
  iv. Pyridoxine (B6): N = 1.6 mg, P = 2.2 mg, L = 2.1 mg
  v. Cobalamin (B12): N = 2.0 μg, P = 2.2 μg, L = 2.6 μg
  vi. Vitamin C: N = 40 mg, P = 40 mg, L = 45 mg.

Q. What are the molecular functions of zinc?

Ans. a. Involved in nucleic acid and protein metabolism
 b. Zinc and zinc dependent enzymes are involved in the synthesis of deoxyribonucleic acid (DNA), ribonucleic acid (RNA) and ribosomes.
 c. Zinc is active in embryogenesis, cell differentiation and cell proliferation.
 d. In the immediate post-fertilization period, zinc deficiency can result in abnormal development of pre-implantation eggs.

Q. What is docosahexaenoic acid (DHA)?

Ans. DHA is a omega-3 fatty acids (Flowchart 1.1).

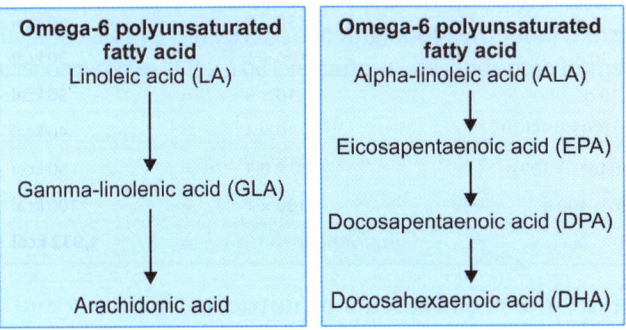

Flowchart 1.1: Conversion of essential fatty acids (EFA) to active metabolites in human body

> **Note**
> DHA is the predominant structural fatty acid in the human brain and retina.

Q. Why DHA supplementation is necessary during pregnancy and lactation?

Ans. 1. Due to low conversion of ALA to DHA, it is important to directly consume DHA especially during pregnancy and lactation.
 2. During pregnancy:
  a. Outcome of preterm delivery is less.

b. For fetus:
   i. Development of brain
   ii. Accretion in brain.
c. Postpartum depression of mother is high in DHA depletion.
d. DHA nutrition during lactation.

Advantages
i. Best psychomotor development of the baby
ii. Good mental and cognitive development of the baby
iii. Visual performance is also very good.

Q. What is the source of omega-3 fatty acids?

Ans. Fish and fish oils are rich in EPA and DHA. Alpha-linolenic acid is an omega-3 fatty acids present in seeds and oils, green leafy vegetables, nuts and beans.

Q. What is the source of omega-6 fatty acids?

Ans. It is present in grains, meats and the seeds of most plants.

Q. What are the recommendations of DHA intake?

Ans. According to British Nutrition and Foundation (BNF)—8 g EPA (Ecosapentaenoic acid) plus DHA per week, for women (1145 mg/day).

Glycemic index (GI) (Figure 1.1)

Some carbohydrate-containing food produces a rapid rise followed by a steep fall in blood glucose concentration, whereas others result in gradual rise followed by a slow decline—they differ in their glycemic response. These glycemic index quantitates these difference in the time course of postprandial glucose concentration.

So glycemic index is defined as area under the blood glucose curve seen after ingestion of meal with carbohydrate rich food, compared with area under the blood glucose curve after a meal consisting of same amount of carbohydrate as glucose (50 g). It is expressed as percentage:

$$GI = \frac{\text{Area under the blood glucose curve after test meal}}{\text{Area under the curve after ingestion of glucose}} \times 100$$

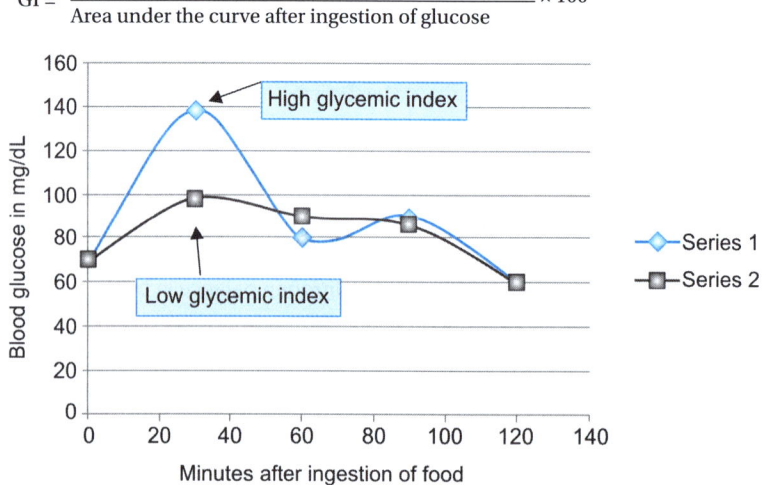

Figure 1.1: Blood glucose concentration of food with low or high glycemic index

Appendices

Glycemic Indices of different foodstuffs is shown in Table 1.3. GI of complex carbohydrate like starch is lower than glucose because of slower digestion and absorption of the former. Glycemic index of carbohydrate is also lower when it is associated with protein, fat and fibers. Foods with high fiber content have low glycemic index (e.g. whole grain, fruits, and vegetables) are preferable for consumption.

Table 1.3: Glycemic Indices of different foodgrains

Food grains	Glycemic index	Food grains	Glycemic index
Glucose	100	Potatoes, banana	60–70
Carrots*	90–95	Orange, apples	40–45

> **Note**
> How much a typical serving size of food raises blood glucose is referred to as the glycemic load (GL). Carrots* can have a high GI and low GL.

Generally foods are divided into three categories: see below

High glycemic index	70 or above
Medium glycemic index	50–69
Low glycemic index	49 or below

Foods with low glycemic index have some benefits which include low blood sugar levels, reduced appetite fluctuations, tend to create a sense of satiety over a longer period of time and may be helpful in limiting calorie intake.

Q. What is nitrogen balance?

Ans. A normal healthy adult is in a nitrogen(N) equilibrium as the daily dietary intake (I) is equal to the loss through urine(U), feces (F) and skin (S)[I = U+ F + S] Figure 1.2.

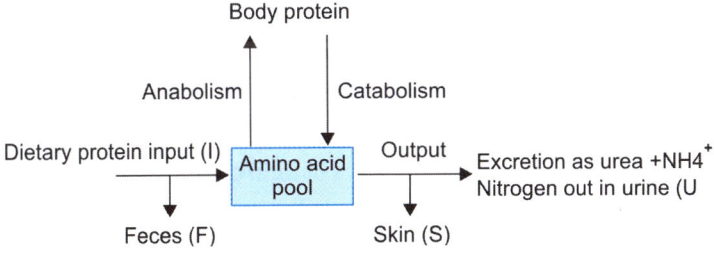

Figure 1.2: Nitrogen balance in body

Q. What is positive and negative nitrogen balance?

Ans. Positive nitrogen (N) balance: N input > N output; observed in pregnant woman, growing child.
Negative nitrogen (N) balance: N input < N output; child suffering from kwashiorkor or marasmus, trauma, burn, illness or surgery.

Q. What is biological value (BV) of protein?

Ans. BV is defined as percentage of absorbed nitrogen retained by the body.

$$BV = \frac{\text{Nitrogen retained}}{\text{Nitrogen absorbed}} \times 100$$

or, BV = N absorbed−N lost in metabolism/N absorbed × 100

It does not take into account the loss of nitrogen during the digestion process. If the ingested nitrogen is 100 mg, absorbed is 10 mg and retained is 6 mg, the BV = 6/10 × 100 = 60. This figure is erroneous as 90 mg of protein does not enter into body for utilization.

Q. What is net protein utilization (NPU)?

Ans.

$$NPU = \frac{\text{Nitrogen retained}}{\text{Nitrogen ingested}} \times 100$$

This index is better than BV as it takes into account the digestibility factor.

Q. What is Atkins diet?

Ans. Atkins diet is composed of fat and protein in high amount and carbohydrate in very low amount (<50 g/day; <10% of 2000 cal/day). It is utilized to lose weight in obese or overweight individual, but should never be used in pregnancy. High fat diet reduces appetite, reduces food intake, but long continued program is not favorable.

Q. What is RDA (recommended daily allowance)?

Ans. RDA represents the quantity of the nutrients to be provided in the diet daily for maintaining good health and efficiency of body, but not the minimum amount to meet the body needs.

Guideline for diet in diabetes

Energy: 25–30 kcal/kg body weight—reduce in obese and increase in underweight patient.

Carbohydrates (CHO): CHO contributes 60% of total calories. Complex carbohydrates like grains, cereals, pulses, beans vegetables and salads. Avoid simple carbohydrate, e.g. sugar, maida, honey, jaggery. Avoid bakery products and deep fired items.

Fats: 20–25% of total calories; saturated 6–7% of total calories; PUFA—6–7% of total calories; MUFA—10% of total calories; n6/n3 ratio =4:1.

Cooking oils should be as follows:

a. Groundnut oil, rice oil or sesame—have moderate quantity of linoleic acid
b. Use any of the above oils with alpha linolenic acid like mustard or soya bean oil—Intake of cholesterol is $\leq$ = 300 mg/day.

Proteins:

a. 15–20% of total calories
b. 1g/kg body weight + 14 g. Use of animal protein is important—fish, chicken, milk.

Fruits: Citrus fruits, oranges, guava, apple, papaya and water melon are helpful. These provide fiber and vitamins. Consumption of one fresh fruit per day.

Fiber diet: 30–40 g/day. Preferably from natural sources.

Avoid: Artificial sweeteners in pregnancy, alcohol, tobacco and smoking.

Others: Provide antioxidants, trace elements, minerals and omega-3 fatty acids.

APPENDIX 2: PHYSIOLOGICAL CHANGES IN PREGNANCY AND DIAGNOSIS OF PREGNANCY

PHYSIOLOGICAL CHANGES IN PREGNANCY

Q. Why physiological changes occur in pregnancy?

Ans.
- Suitable environment for nutrition, growth, and development of fetus
- Prepare the mother for the process of parturition and subsequent support for the newborn infant.

Q. What are the changes in genital organs?

Ans.

Vulva:	Edematous, pigmented, hypertrophied
Vagina:	Bluish or violet discoloration of mucosae—Jacquemier's sign, hypertrophied, vascular and edematous
Cervix:	Stroma: hypertrophy and hyperplasia, increased vascularity
	Marked softening of cervix—Goodell's sign
	Secretion—copious
Isthmus:	It becomes softer, hypertrophies, and 3-times its original length during the 1st trimester; but at 12 weeks it is incorporated in the uterine cavity.
Uterus:	It is enlarged, weight 900–1000 g, length = 35 cm

	Changes in muscles fibers.
	1. Hypertrophy (enlargement of muscle) and hyperplasia (increase in muscle number)
	2. Stretching of muscles fibers
	  • The fundus enlarges more than body
	  • Braxton-Hicks contraction
	  • Blood flow in UA increases from 50 mL at 10 weeks to 500–700 mL at term.

Breast:	• Size increased due to hypertrophy and proliferation of alveoli and ducts.
	• Vascularity increased
	• Nipple becomes large, erectile and deeply pigmented
	• Sebaceous gland hypertrophied—Montgomery's tubercle, in 2nd trimester—secondary areola colostrums can be expressed from the nipple after first few month (3–4 months) of pregnancy.

Appendices

Q. What are the cutaneous changes in pregnancy?

Ans.

Cutaneous change	Pigmentation
Face	Chloasma gravidarum, or pregnancy mask
Breast	As described before
Abdomen	Linea nigra, Striae gradivarum

Q. What is net weight gain in normal pregnancy?

Ans. Net weight gain in pregnancy is 24 lbs (11 kg): 1 kg in 1st trimester and 5 kg in 2nd and 3rd trimester.

Contribution of weight:
1. Reproductive—(a) Fetus, placenta, and liquor, (b) uterus, breasts
2. Net maternal weight gain—(a) increased in blood volume, (b) accumulation of fluid in the interstitial space, (c) deposition of fat and protein.

Q. What are the hematological changes?

Ans. The total blood volume increases by 30%, the increase in plasma volume is 30% and increase in total cell volume is 20%. This accounts hemodilution or physiological anemia in pregnancy (Table 2.1).

Table 2.1: Hematological changes

	Non-pregnant (NP)	Pregnancy (P) at term	Total increment	Change
Blood vol (mL)	4000	5500	1500	+30–40%
Plasma vol (mL)	2500	3750	1250	+40–50%
RBC vol (mL)	1400	1650	+250	+18–20%
Hb(g/dL)	12.5	11.5	Less	−12%
Hematocrit (whole body)	38%	32%		Diminished (-6%)
ESR	10 mm/hr	40 mm/hr		4 times increased

Leukocytes—10,000–15,000/cumm, labor 20,000/cumm (increased)
Total protein—Total plasma protein. Increases (from 180 g, non-pregnant to 230 g at term).
- Fall in albumin level (43–3 g%, 30% reduction)
- Slightly rise of globulin and normal A: G = 1.7:1 is diminished to 1:1

Blood coagulation factors change during pregnancy. Platelet count is reduced, but fibrinogen level becomes high (Table 2.2).

Table 2.2: Blood coagulation factors

	NP	P	Changes
Platelets (cumm)	2, 50,000	2, 10,000	15% reduction
Fibrinogen (mg %)	200–400	300–600	+50%
Fibrinolitic activity		Depressed	
Clotting time		Unaffected	

Different blood lipid levels become high during pregnancy (Table 2.3).

Table 2.3: Change of blood lipid levels during pregnancy

	NP	P	Changes
Total lipid (mg/100 mL)	650	1000	+50%
Cholesterol (mg/100 mL)	180	260	+40%
Phospholipid (mg/100 mL)	250	350	+40%

Q. What changes occur in cardiovascular system in normal pregnancy?

Ans
- The heart is pushed upward and outward
- The apex beat is shifted to the 4th IC space 2.5 cm outside the midclavicular line
- A continuous hissing murmur may be audible over the tricuspid area in left 2nd/3rd intercostal space—mammary murmur.
- X-rays shows enlarged cardiac shadow.
- ECG—left axis deviation
- Regional blood flow is increased
- Cardiac output (COP) is increased from early pregnancy (6 weeks) and peak at 32–34 weeks. COP is increased due to increase in pulse rate, stroke volume, fall in peripheral resistance (decrease in after load, increase in heart muscle contractility (positive ionotropic effect).

Q. What are the hemodynamic changes in pregnancy?

Ans. See Table 2.4.

Table 2.4: Hemodynamic changes in pregnancy

	NP	P	Changes
COP (L/min)	5	6.	increased (+40%)
Stroke vol (mL)	65	85	increased (+25%)
PR (per min)	70	85	increased (+15%)

Blood pressure: unaffected—may be mid-pregnancy drop of DBP
Peripheral resistance—markedly diminished
Blood viscosity—diminished
Supine hypotensive syndrome (10%) at term.

Q. What are the changes in respiratory system?

Ans. See Table 2.5.

Table 2.5: Changes in respiratory system

	NP	P	Changes
RR/min	15	15	Unaffected
Vital capacity (mL)	3200	3300	Almost unaltered
Tidal volume (mL)	500	700	+40%
Residual volume (mL)	1000	800	-20% (decreased)

Appendices

Q. What are the changes in acid-base balance in pregnancy?

Ans. There is variable changes in acid-base balance during pregnancy (Table 2.6).

Table 2.6: Changes in acid-base balance during pregnancy			
	NP	P	*Changes*
Arterial pCO_2 (mm of Hg)	38	32	Diminished
pH	7.40	7.44	Increased mild
Arterial pO_2 (mm of Hg)	95	105	Increased
Arterial oxygen saturation (%)	98.5	98	Slightly decreased

Q. What metabolic changes occur in normal pregnancy?

Ans. Protein: Pregnancy is a anabolic state with positive nitrogen balance. Conversion of amino acid to urea is suppressed, the blood urea level falls to 15–20 mg%.

Blood uric acid and creatinine levels are either normal or fall slightly.

Carbohydrate: Pregnancy is a diabetogenic state.
- Oral glucose tolerance test (OGTT) may show abnormal pattern
- Fasting blood glucose—low
- Slow rise of blood glucose level following ingestion of glucose due to decreased gastric empting and delayed absorption in pregnancy
- Blood glucose does not return to fasting level after 2 hours as in non-pregnant state due to peripheral resistance of insulin
- Transfer of glucose to fetus occurs due to high glucose level
- Glycosuria is found in 1/3 of cases
- Hyperinsulinemia in pregnancy due to hypertrophy and hyperplasia of β-cells of pancreas due to different diabetogenic hormones.

Fat metabolism:
- Carbohydrate is essential for oxidation
- Glycogen store is decreased in pregnancy
- Incomplete oxidation of fat produces ketone bodies.

Q. Effects of iron metabolism in pregnancy.

Ans. Additional iron (Fe) during pregnancy is 1,000 mg.
Daily requirement of Fe in pregnancy is 3.5 mg and in 2nd half 6 mg.

Q. What changes occur in other systems of body during pregnancy?

Ans. Urinary system: Renal plasma flow is increased (20–50%), GFR increases (50%), RFT—augmented
Ureter: Atonic, dilated, stasis is more marked at 20–24 weeks.
Bladder: Congestion and hypertrophy of muscles, frequency of micturition increases in 6–8 weeks, and again reappear in later month when presenting part descends in the pelvis.
Alimentary system: Gums spongy, muscle tone and motility of gastrointestinal tract (GIT) decreases.
Cardiac sphincter—relaxed leading to esophagitis and heart burn.
Nervous system: Psychosis, neuritis, carpal tunnel syndrome.

Calcium metabolism: Daily requirement 1,000 mg low calcium level causes low secretion of PTH, which leads to Ca++ resorption resulting osteomalacia and osteoporosis.

Q. Placental endocrinology.

Ans. Placental endocrinology
   a. Protein hormone:
      i. hCG: Luteotrophic, having two sub-units (α and β). α-subunit is structurally and immunologically similar to the LH, FSH and TSH. The hCG level is increased in multiple pregnancy, hydatidiform mole and Down syndrome but the level decreased in ectopic pregnancy and threatened abortion.
      ii. hPL (human placental lactogen): It promotes growth, insulin secretion, decreases insulin's peripheral effect, liberating maternal fatty acids and divert glucose to the fetus. It also stimulates mammary growth.
      iii. Human chorionic thyrotropin (hCT)
      iv. Pregnancy specific β-1 glycoprotein
      v. Pregnancy associated plasma protein (PAPP-A)
   b. Steroid hormone.
      i. Estrogen (estriol)—pregnancy is a hyperestrogenic state and most of the estriol is derived from fetal precursors. $DHEASO_4$ secreted by adrenals is hydroxylated in the fetal liver to 16-(OH) $DHEASO_4$ (as the placenta lacks the enzyme 16-hydroxylase), desulfated and aromatized in the placenta to produce estriol.
      ii. Progesterone: It sustains pregnancy.

Q. What changes occur in other maternal endocrine glands?

Ans.
- Thyroid—enlarged due to increased iodine uptake. Free T4 and T3 remain normal and serum TSH is lower in early pregnancy but remains normal throughout pregnancy.
- Pituitary—enlarged; PRL (increased), gonadotropin (decreased by placental steroids), GH (inhibited by placental lactogen) oxytocin markedly increases at term and labor.

DIAGNOSIS OF PREGNANCY

Q. How do you diagnose pregnancy in first trimester?

Ans. 1st trimester of pregnancy (first 12 weeks) can be diagnosed by the following ways:

Subjective symptoms
   a. Amenorrhea—cessation of menstruation
   b. Morning sickness—starts at 4–6 weeks and may continue till about 16 weeks
   c. Frequency of micturition—pressure exerted by growing fetus on bladder
   d. Breast discomfort
   e. Fatigue.

Objective tests

a. Chadwick sign—bluish discoloration of vagina due to congestion of blood vessels
b. Vaginal pulsation through lateral fornices—Osiander's sign (8th week)
c. Cervix become soft—Goodell's sign
d. Uterus—hen's egg 6th week
   - Cricket ball 8th week
   - Fetal head 12th week
e. Asymmetrical enlargement of uterus—Piskacek's sign
f. Hegar's sign—6-12 weeks due to softening and compressibility of isthmus

(The abdominal and vaginal fingers can be apposed below the body of the uterus).

g. Pregnancy test—immunological test, enzyme-linked immunosorbent assay (ELISA) test
h. Sonography by TVS
   - Gestational sac—5 week
   - Yolk sac—5-6 weeks
   - Fetal node—5½ weeks
   - Fetal heartbeat—by the end of 6th week
   - Crown rump length (CRL)—at 8-14 weeks gives accurate estimation of gestational age.

Q. How do you diagnose pregnancy in second trimester?

Ans. 2nd trimester (13-28 weeks)

Subjective symptoms:

a. Quickening (fluttering sensation felt by mother for active fetal movement for the first time),18 weeks in primi and 2 weeks earlier (at 16 weeks) in multigravida
b. Changes of the skin—pigmentation and striae on abdomen
c. Progressive enlargement of abdomen.

Sign:

a. Chloasma or melasma
b. Breast change—enlarged, secondary areola—20 weeks, montgomery's tubercle
c. Abdominal examination
   - Inspection—linea nigra, striae gravidarum (in multipara)
   - Palpation:
     – Uterine fundal height—
       - 16th week—5 cm above symphysis pubis
       - 20th week - 2.5 cm below umbilicus
       - 24th week—at the level of umbilicus
       - 28th week—lower 1/3rd of distance from umbilicus to ensiform cartilage
     – Uterus feels soft and elastic
     – Braxton-Hicks contraction (16th week) of uterus
     – Palpation of fetal parts (20th week)

- Active fetal movement (16–18 weeks)
- External ballottement (20th to 26th week)—can be elicited on dorsal position by two ways:
  - An outstretched left hand can grip the uterus and external ballottement can be felt by tossing the fetus
  - Tapping of fetus on one side can produce movement of fetus and the impulse can be felt on other side by palm of other hand.

  It is very difficult to elicit in thick and obese mother or in scanty liquor.
d. Auscultation: Fetal heart sound (18–20 weeks), uterine soufflé (a soft blowing sound synchronus with maternal pulse produced by passage of blood through dilated uterine artery), funic soufflé (15%) which is a sharp whizzing sound synchronous with fetal heart beat, heard due to passage of blood through the umbilical arteries
e. Vaginal examination:
   - Bluish discoloration
   - Internal ballottement (16th–28th weeks)—can be elicited on dorsal position of woman.

   Two fingers are placed on anterior vaginal fornix in front of cervix while other hand is placed firmly on the uterine fundus. The fetal head or buttocks may be felt by internal fingers. When internal fingers tap the fetal pole, it goes away and again settles on internal fingers.
f. Investigations:
   - Radiology (not very useful now for radiation hazards)
   - Sonography—BPD, head circumference (HC), abdominal circumference (AC), femur length (FL), etc.

Q. What are the different parameters for diagnosis of pregnancy in third trimester?

Ans. Last trimester (29–40 weeks)

Symptoms:
a. Amenorrhea
b. Frequency of micturition
c. Fetal movements
d. Enlargement of abdomen
e. Lightening (after 38th week)—feeling of emptiness at epigastrium due to engagement of presenting part and reduction of liquor amni.

Signs:
a. Cutaneous change
b. Fundal height:
   - At 28th week—uterine fundus reaches lower one-third distance between umbilicus and ensiform cartilage
   - At 32 weeks—fundus occupies lower two-third of the above space
   - At 36 weeks—fundus reaches near subcostal arch
   - At 38 weeks—fundus reaches the subcostal arch below ensiform cartilage
   - At 40 weeks fundus sinks below 36th week but above 32 weeks

c. McDonald's formula:

$$\frac{\text{Symphysio-fundal height (SFH)}}{3.5} = \text{Lunar months (Beyond 24 weeks)}$$

d. Uterine shape: cylindrical to spherical >36 weeks
e. Braxton-Hicks contraction—intermittent painless contraction felt per abdomen at irregular intervals of 10–20 minutes followed by relaxation. The women cannot feel such contraction. Absent in abdominal pregnancy
f. Fetal movement
g. Palpation of the fetal parts
h. Fetal heart sound—normal 110–160 bpm at 17th–20th week by stethoscope
i. Radiology— is not very useful now for hazards of radiation
j. USG is useful for assessment of fetal growth and fetal well-being.

> **Note**
> USG Doppler can detect FHS at 10 weeks; heart motion can be visualized by USG at 6 weeks.

Q. What are the absolute signs of pregnancy?
Ans.   a. Auscultation of fetal heart sounds.
b. Palpation of fetal parts and perception of fetal active movements
c. USG evidence of fetus in utero.

Q. What are the D/Ds of pregnancy?
Ans. Distended bladder, cystic ovarian tumor. Fibroid uterus, encysted peritonitis, pseudocyesis—false pregnancy due to obesity.

APPENDIX 3: FETAL CIRCULATION

FETAL CIRCULATION

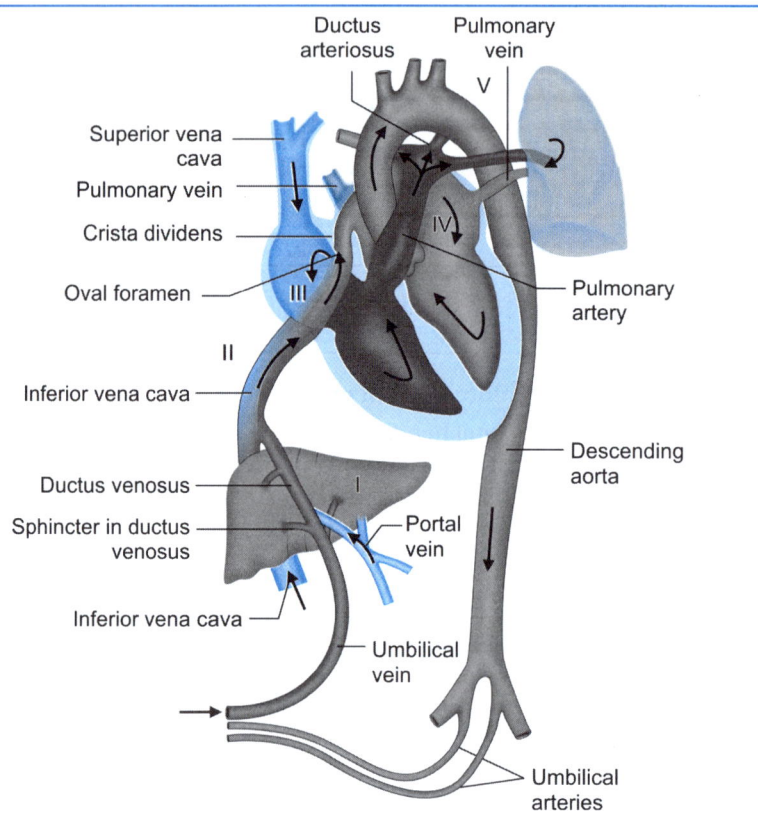

Figure 3.1: Fetal circulation before birth, arrows show direction of blood flow

Q. How does fetal circulation occur in utero?

Ans. Before birth, umbilical vein (UV) carries oxygenated (80%) blood from the placenta. On approaching the liver it gives off a branch ductus venosus, which carries the major part of the blood directly into the inferior vena cava (IVC) and then into the right atrium, short-circuiting the liver. A small amount enters the liver sinusoids and mixes the blood from the portal circulation. A sphincter mechanism in the ductus venosus, close to the entrance of umbilical vein regulates the flow of umbilical blood through the liver sinusoids. This sphincter closes when the uterine contraction renders venous return too high, preventing a sudden overloading of the heart. After a short course in the inferior vena cava, where placental blood (oxygenated) mixes with the de-oxygenated blood returning from lower limbs, it enters the right atrium. The well-oxygenated blood courses along the medial aspect of IVC and the less oxygenated blood along the lateral aspect. When this blood enters the right atrium, the well-oxygenated blood is shunted through the foramen ovale into the left atrium and a small amount is prevented from doing so by the lower edge of septum secundum, the crista dividens, and remains in the right atrium. Here it mixes with the desaturated blood from head and arms by way of superior vena cava.

From the left atrium where it mixes with a small amount of desaturated blood coming from the lungs, blood enters the left ventricle and ascending aorta. Since, the coronary artery and carotid arteries are the first branches of the ascending aorta, the heart musculature and the brain are supplied with well-oxygenated blood.

Desaturated blood coursing through the lateral aspect of IVC enters the right ventricle from the right atrium and then into the pulmonary trunk. During fetal life, resistance in the pulmonary vessels is high, so most of this blood passes directly through the ductus arteriosus into the descending aorta, where it mixes with the blood from proximal aorta.

The aorta divides into common iliacs, which further divide into internal and external iliacs. From the internal iliacs, the hypogastric arteries leave and ascending alongside the bladder flows towards the placenta by way of two umbilical arteries. The oxygen saturation in the umbilical arteries is approximately 58%.

During its course from the placenta to the organ of the fetus, blood in the umbilical vein gradually losses its oxygen content as it mixes with the desaturated blood (Figure 3.1).

Q. Mention the different places where mixing of oxygenated and deoxygenated blood may occur in fetal circulation?

Ans.   I. In the liver—by mixture with a small amount of blood returning from portal system.
II. In the IVC—which carries deoxygenated blood returning from the lower extremities, pelvis, and kidneys.
III. In the right atrium—by mixing the blood from head and limbs carried by SVC.
IV. In the left atrium—by mixture with blood returning from lungs.
V. At the entrance of ductus arteriosus into the descending aorta.

Q. What are the changes in fetal circulation at birth?

Ans. Fetal circulation changes after cord clamping due to:
1. Stoppage of placental circulation and massive venous return to the right heart.
2. Initiation of respiration.
   a. **Closure of the umbilical arteries:** Caused by smooth muscle contraction in their walls, due to thermal and mechanical stimuli and change in oxygen tension. Functionally the arteries close a few minutes after birth, though final closure is due to lumen obliteration by fibrous tissue taking 2–3 months.

Distal parts of the umbilical arteries from medial umbilical ligaments, and the *proximal part* remain open as superior vesical arteries.

b. **Closure of umbilical vein and ductus venosus:** Occurs shortly after umbilical arteries. So, blood from the placenta may enter the newborn for a few time after birth. After obliteration, the umbilical vein forms the ligamentum teres hepatis in the lower margin of the falciparum ligament. The ductus venosus constricts 12–96 hours after birth and closes anatomically by 2–3 weeks. The ductus venosus which courses from ligamentum teres to the IVC is also obliterated to form ligamentum venosum.

c. **Closure of the ductus arteriosus:** Closure occurs immediately after birth and bradykinin released from lungs during initial inflation causes contraction of muscular wall. Complete anatomical obliteration by proliferation of the intima is thought to take within 1–3 months. In the adult, the obliterated ductus arteriosus forms the ligamentum arteriosum.

d. **Closure of foramen ovale:** Caused by the increased pressure in the left atrium due to increase in pulmonary flow and increase in venous return, combined with decrease in pressure on the right side of heart due to clamping of umbilical cord. The first breath presses the septum primum against the septum secundum. During the first days of life, however this closure is reversible. Crying of the baby creates a shunt from right to left, which accounts for cyanotic periods in the newborn. Constant apposition causes fusion of the two septa in about 1 year. In 20% of individuals the perfect anatomical closure may not occur resulting probe patent foramen ovale.

Q. How does fetal circulation differ from adult circulation?

Ans. a. Fetal blood is not oxygenated in the lung.
  b. Major portion of right ventricular output bypasses the lungs.
  c. Chambers of fetal heart works in parallel, not in series as in adult.
  d. Well-oxygenated blood from left ventricle supplies heart and brain.
  e. Less oxygenated blood from the right ventricle supplies the rest of the body.

APPENDIX 4: DIFFERENT TYPES OF FEMALE PELVIS

Table 4.1: Different types of female pelvis

		Gynecoid	Anthropoid	Android	Platypelloid
Pelvic inlet	Widest transverse diameter of inlet	12 cm	< 12 cm	12 cm	12 cm
	Anteroposterior diameter of inlet	11 cm	> 12 cm	11 cm	10 cm
	Forepelvis	Wide	Divergent	Narrow	Straight
Pelvic midcavity	Side walls	Straight	Narrow	Convergent	Wide
	Sacrosciatic notch	Medium	Backward	Narrow	Forward
	Inclination of sacrum	Medium	Wide	Forward (lower third)	Narrow
	Ischial spines	Not prominent	Not prominent	Not prominent	Not prominent
Pelvic outlet	Subpubic arch	Wide	Medium	Narrow	Wide
	Transverse diameter of outlet	10 cm	10 cm	< 10 cm	10 cm

INDEX

Page numbers followed by *f* refer to figure and *t* refer to table

A

Abdomen 330, 339
   aortic compression per 102
   causes of pain 279
   flank of maternal 58
   progressive enlargement of 547
   X-ray of 9
Abdominopelvic method 308
Abortion 226
   causes of mid trimester 459
   complete 226
   first trimester 75
   incomplete 226, 513
   inevitable 226
   midtrimester 42
   missed 226, 227*f*, 229, 514
   problem 512
   recurrent mid-pregnancy 130
   second trimester 75
   surgical 131
   threatened 226, 512
   tubal 2
Abruptio placentae 78, 235, 359, 383, 428
Acardius acephalus 261
Acardius acormus 261
Acardius amorphous 261
Acardius anceps 261
Acardius fetus 261
Acetic acid 130
Acetone 524
Acetyl choline 65
Acid-base balance 545, 545*t*
Acquired immune deficiency syndrome 7, 398
Actinomycin 6
Adenexa, surgical extirpation of 20
Adenomyosis 48
Alanine aminotransferase 445
Alcohol 436
Alkali denaturation 364
Allis tissue
   forceps 39, 39*f*
      uses of 39
   pairs of 41

Amenorrhea 54, 476, 546
   lactational 335
   period of 18
   short period of 3, 4
Amniocentesis 139, 325
   indications of 139
Amnioinfusion 329
   benefit of 328
   intrapartum 328, 329
Amniotic fluid 213, 255, 484, 488
   bilirubin 63
   functions of 484
   index 56, 205, 235, 325, 328, 485, 527
   origin of 484
   volume 236, 326, 328, 484
Amniotic nodosum 487
Amniotic sacs, number of 312
Ampicillin 336
Anal canal, sphincters of 91
Analgesia 436
Ancillary tests 435
Anemia 270, 279, 336, 343, 344, 351, 436, 482
   causes of 344
   complications of 346
   correction of 23
   management of severe 349, 349*f*
   maternal 339
   prevent 346
   severe 85
   severity of 346, 346*t*
Anencephaly 256
   complications of 256
Anesthesia 88
   complications of local 130
   general 78, 99, 116, 508
   types of 78
Angiotensin converting enzyme 487
Anovulation, chronic 476
Antenatal card 324
Antenatal care 436
   general 400
Antenatal corticosteroid treatment 77
Antibiotic 332
   ointment 89

Antibody formation, types of 292
Anticardiolipin antibodies 266, 455
Anticoagulant
　role of 439
　　therapy 131
　　　monitor 440
Antidiuretic hormone 256
Antiepileptic drug 463
Antigen detection 399
Antihypertensive 458
Antinuclear antibody 458
Antiphospholipid antibody syndrome 264, 455
Antiretroviral
　classes of 408
　therapy, active 400
Antishock garments, non-pneumatic 508
Antithyroid drugs 473
Aorta, coarctation of 395, 441, 443
Aortic stenosis 444
　severe 442, 443
Apgar score 60
Arginine-vasopressin 57
Artery
　forceps, small 39
　ligation of 106
Asherman's syndrome 10, 42
Asphyxia 241
　causes of 59
　neonatorum 59
Aspirin, role of 392
Assisted reproductive technology 260, 476
Asthma 71
Atkins diet 540
Atonic uterus 84
Atrial septal defects 441
Autonomic nervous system 197, 198

B

Babcock's tissue forceps 39f
Baby friendly hospital initiative 340
Bacterial
　contamination 336
　endocarditis, subacute 435
　vaginosis 400
Bagel's sign 3
Bariatric surgery 477
Basal plate 26, 233
Battledore placenta 29, 29f
Bedside sickling test 482

Begin oxytocin infusion 503
Bell's sign 263
Beta adrenergic blocker 474
Betadine solution 91
Betamethasone, ampoule of 76f
Bile salt increased 445
Biliary cirrhosis, primary 445
Biophysical profile, modified 236, 326
Bioprosthetic valve 442
Biparietal diameter 157, 231, 255, 275
Bishop score 498t
Bladder 84, 545
　drainage, continuous 14
　dysfunction 79
　habit 269
　injury 42, 43, 64, 100, 358
　　repair of 43
　tenesmus 354
Bleeding
　in placenta previa 361
　per vagina 38, 49
　points 81
　reduction of 81
　severity of 362
　time 265, 514
Blood 333
　and blood products, transmission of 398
　borne diseases 481
　clot 91, 130
　coagulation factors 543t
　count, complete 4, 399, 514, 526
　dyscrasia 269
　fibrinogen in 266
　flow 242f
　　velocity 241
　glucose 264, 427
　　concentration of food 538f
　indices 345
　loss 84, 94, 336
　peritoneal collection of 3
　pressure 4, 90, 215, 270, 362, 427, 544
　smear, abnormal peripheral 447
　stained liquor 214
　sugar 486
　transfusion 84, 349, 482
　　indications of 349
　　requirement of 357
　urea nitrogen 22, 514
　vessels 88
　viscosity 544
　volume 348
Bluish discoloration 548

Index

Body
    mass index 280, 475, 489
    surface area 5
    weight 6, 494
Bolus dose, intravenous 68
Bone nibbling forceps 98, 98*f*
Bony pelvis 143*f*, 144*f*
Bowel injury 40
Brace suture 103
Bradycardia 57, 197*f*, 198
    mild 198, 208*f*
    severe 198, 208*f*
Brain tumor 388
Brandt-Andrews method 162
Brawny edema 338
Braxton Hicks contraction 9, 285
Breast 330, 542
    abscess 337, 338
    alveoli 342
    care 333
    complications 335
    engorged 330
    examination 339
    milk 333
    preparation of 342
Breastfeeding 333, 335, 340, 341, 430
    benefit of 340
    exclusive 406
Breathing spontaneous 60
Breech 248, 317
    delivery 134, 249
    habitual 248
    head of 110
    mobilization of 124
    presentation 247-251
        causes of 248
        type of 248
    uncomplicated 248, 250
British Nutrition and Foundation 538
Broad ligament hematoma 15
Bronchopulmonary dysplasia 493
Budin's cannula 96*f*

C

Calcium
    antagonists 394
    metabolism 546
    supplementation 393
Cancer cervix 43
Candidal vulvovaginitis 430
Cannula 49
    type of suction 55

Capillary
    blood glucose 429
    glucose 425
Carbimazole 474
Carbohydrate 333, 536, 540, 545
Carboprost 72
Carcinoma cervix 82, 356
Cardiac muscle 68
Cardiomyopathy 395, 434, 441
    hypertrophic 443
Cardiotocography 418
    external 194, 195
Cardiovascular system 238, 330, 433, 544
    dysfunction of 59
Catheter
    rubber 41
    simple rubber 41, 41*f*
    wall of 42
Cell injury, causes 65
Central nervous system 21, 202, 236, 423, 486
Central venous pressure 516
Cephalhematoma 152
    complications of 153
    treatment of 153
Cephalic
    curve 109
    index 232
    presentation 157, 250, 251, 329
    version, external 123, 124*f*, 253, 294
Cephalopelvic disproportion 12, 70, 78, 221, 286, 303, 498, 502
Cerclage operation 460
Cerebellum 237*f*
Cerebral
    artery, middle 245, 245*f*, 299, 300, 300*f*, 415, 528
    dysrhythmia 388
    edema 388
    hemorrhage 387
    malaria 388
    microcirculation 388
    palsy 357
Cerebrospinal fluid 44, 251
Cerebrovascular accident 388, 432
Cervical
    Canal
        ballooning of 11
        empty 10
    cancer 49, 522
    circlage, placement of 11
    dilatation, complications of 51
    dilators 49, 50, 93*f*

ectopic pregnancy 11
encirclage operation 64
incompetence 94, 239, 459
injury 47
insufficiency 240, 462
length 239, 240, 321
malignancy 360
orifice 252
pregnancy 10, 11
score 321
smear 399
spinal cord injury 249
stenosis 49, 51, 94
tear, repair of 44, 132, 133
Cervicitis 359
Cervix 49, 215, 542
amputation of 51, 52
anterior lip of 47
avulsion of 122
dilatation of 19
infection of 49
lip of 47
posterior aspect of 64
visualization of 44
Cesarean section 12, 57, 78, 294, 405, 498
indications of 85, 248, 391, 428
lower segment 13, 79, 80, 222, 253, 277, 493, 503
scar pregnancy 10
types of 353
Chemotherapy 20
course of 22
Chest circumference 334
Child immunization 340
Chlamydia trachomatis 336, 400
Cholelithiasis 445
Cholestasis 447
Cholestyramine 446
Chorioamnionitis 493
management of 494
Choriocarcinoma 16, 21, 23, 24
treatment of 23
uterus 53
Chorionic villi
biopsy 487
sampling 137, 239, 407
Chrioamnionitis 329
Circumvallate placenta 29*f*
Clot observation test 265
Clotting time 265, 514
Collagen vascular disease 395
Colostrum 332, 333
feeding, advantage of 333
Colpoperineorrhaphy, posterior 43, 45

Colporrhexis 510
Coma, stage of 388
Condom 340
Congenital heart disease 261, 434, 440, 441, 443
Contraception, permanent 334
Coomb's test 298
direct 302, 303
indirect 292, 295, 302
Cord
compression 365
entanglement 31, 123
prolapse 31, 38, 78, 253, 329
prevent recurrence of 65
traction 162
controlled 160, 507
Cordocentesis 140, 297, 299
Cornual pregnancy 8
fate of 8
Corticosteroids 76
Cranioclast 97*f*
Craniopagus 262
Craniotomy 12
indications of 95
operation 95, 98
Craniovertebral junction 237*f*
Creatinine level 382
Crown rump length 225, 547
Crystalloid hydration, intravenous 79
Culdocentesis 3, 4, 47
Cullen's sign 3
Cusco's speculum 46*f*
Cysteine aminopeptidase 27
Cystic ovarian tumor 549
Cysts 276
Cytomegalovirus 251
Cytotrophoblast 26, 27
trophoblastic proliferation of 16
Cytotrophoblastic shell 26

D

Dare's formula 281
Deaver's retractor 56*f*
use of 56
Deciduas basalis 26
Deferoxamine 481
Delivery
estimated time of 221
forceps 110
management 419, 419*f*
mode of 34, 330, 357, 381, 390, 402
normal 162

Index

preterm 259, 489
procedures, complications of 122
route of 258
timing and mode of 428
Deoxyribonucleic acid 7, 537
Depot medroxyprogesterone acetate 334, 340
Dexamethasone 475
Diabetes 395, 427, 485
    diet in 540
    in pregnancy 421, 425
    mellitus 205, 269, 432, 447
    uncontrolled 428
Diet chart 536
Dinoprostone 71
Disseminated intravascular coagulation 269, 506
Dizziness 131
Docosahexaenoic acid 537
Donald's method 308
Down's syndrome 238
Doyen's retractor 56f
    use of 55
Duchenne muscular dystrophy 137
Ductus arteriosus, closure of 552
Ductus venosus 238, 242, 246, 246f, 416f, 552
    abnormal 418
Dystocia 502, 505
    complications of 502

E

Eclampsia 385, 387-389
    bad signs of 388
    diagnosis of 388
Eclamptic seizure 195
Ecosapentaenoic acid 538
Ectopic
    mass 5
    pregnancy 1-4, 7, 47, 75, 130, 228, 229
        causes of 2
        chronic 3
        live 228f
        tubal 1, 2
        types of 3
        unruptured tubal 1, 1f
Edema 270
Eisenmenger's complex 435
Embryo, implantation of 10
Embryonic disc, development of 35
Embryotomy scissors 99, 101, 101f
    uses of 101

Endocarditis, infective 443
Endocrine disease 395
Endometrial
    ablation 52
    carcinoma 47, 52
    cavity, curetting of 53
    tissue 4
    tuberculosis 49
Endometriosis 2
Endometritis 357
Endovaginal sonography 3, 5, 223
Enzyme-linked immunosorbent assay 399
Epidural analgesia 110
Epidural block, disadvantages of 79
Epigastric pain 381
Epilepsy 388, 462, 464, 466
    in pregnancy 462
    on pregnancy, effect of 463
Epiphyseal bone centers 233
Episiotomy 86
    repair of 90f
    scissors 87f
    uses of 87
    steps of 88
    wound, repair of 90
Erythroblastosis 361
Erythropoiesis 343
Euglycemic goal 425
Eutocia 162
Exercise, abdominal 340
Extrauterine pregnancy 325

F

Fallopian tube 1, 2
Family planning 340, 430
Fascia 88
Fasting blood glucose 545
Fat 333, 536, 540
Fatigue 131
Fatty acid 537
    source of 538
Fatty liver
    acute 445
    of pregnancy, acute 445, 447, 451
    risk of 445
    treatment of acute 451
Feeding, exclusive replacement 405, 406
Female pelvis
    normal 149
    types of 553, 553t
Female urethra, length of 41

Femoral epiphysis, distal 233
Femur length 231, 233, 233*f*, 255, 548
Fern test 289
Ferric carboxy maltose 348
Fertilization 2
Fetal 264, 427
　acidemia 327
　anemia 299, 300, 525, 528-530
　　causes of 528
　　mild 298
　　moderate to severe 530
　aneuploidy 238
　anomalies 23, 230, 248, 460
　ascites 114
　baseline variability 209*f*
　bleeding disorders 123
　blood 57, 364, 552
　　cells 141
　　flow, rate of 27
　　sampling 206, 302
　　vessels 16
　bone 123
　capillaries, endothelium of 27
　cardiac activity 132
　circulation 550, 550*f*, 551
　coagulopathy 119
　complications 346, 387, 431, 443, 491
　compromise 418, 460
　condition 213, 309, 381, 382
　death 391, 457
　　antepartum 264
　　causes of recurrent 264
　　in eclampsia, causes of 391
　distress 31, 57, 78, 87, 119, 194, 195, 327, 328, 418, 428, 457
　　causes of 195
　　intrapartum 328
　　management of 207
　　signs of 57
　　treatment of 206
　echocardiogram 427
　electronic monitoring 211
　evaluation 382, 396
　fibronectin 321, 492
　foot 82
　gestational age 381
　growth 381, 457
　　failure 412
　　rate 231
　　restriction 69, 491, 499
　head 83, 155, 215, 310
　　attitude of 283*f*
　　hyperextension of 249
　　level of 65
　　position of 119, 156*f*
　heart rate 122, 124, 194, 199, 201, 202, 205, 209, 213, 217, 225*f*, 309, 326, 418, 427, 498
　　abnormal 207
　　causes of 196
　　classification of 196, 211*t*
　　monitoring 194
　　normal 56, 195
　　pattern 196
　　testing 396
　　traces 210, 210*t*
　heart sound 12, 56, 57, 80, 164, 195, 276, 314, 354, 485, 498
　hypoxia 241, 243
　intestinal cells 57
　kick chart, daily 427
　kidney, maturity of 255
　lung, maturity of 255
　macrosomia 429
　malpresentation 360
　maturity 254
　monitoring
　　electronic 194
　　intensive 436
　mortality, high 13
　movement 205, 549
　　active 548
　　count, daily 194, 212, 326, 381
　　excessive 57
　pole 224, 224*f*
　position 155, 155*f*
　scalp 65
　scalp blood
　　collect 57
　　sampling 211
　skin, mature 255
　skull 96, 97, 142, 149, 150*f*, 151, 151*f*, 154
　spinal cord transection 249
　status 396
　stomach 239*f*
　structure 141
　surface 30
　surveillance 417, 481
　　antepartum 194, 205
　tachycardia, persistent 57
　teratogenicity 436
　tissue 17, 93
　umbilical artery Doppler 212
　weight 231, 233, 363
　　estimated 327

Index

Fetomaternal hemorrhage 123, 293-295, 526, 529
Fetopelvic disproportion 248, 249
Fetoplacental hematoma 31
Fetus 44, 258*f*
   ankle of 83
   death of 13, 18
   delivery of 298
   demise of 487
   extraction of 12
   hyperextended neck of 248
   in utero, thalassemic 481
   loses blood 364
   papyraceus 318
   placenta, delivery of 78
   scalp of 64
Fever, puerperial 335
Fibroid uterus
   symptoms of 519
   treatment of 520
Fibromyoma 49
Figlu test 351
Fistula, rectovaginal 90
Foley's catheter 41, 42, 42*f*
   uses of 42
Folic acid 350, 351
   supplementation 482
   sources of 350
Foramen ovale 552
   closure of 552
Forceps
   Delivery
      complications of 113
      types of 110
   function of 118
   high 110
   low 110
   over ventouse, advantage of 122
   parts of 109
Fothergill's operation 53
Fresh frozen plasma 507
Frog faces 230*f*
Fundal grip 274, 274*f*
Fundus, height of 422
Fusion inhibitors 408

G

Gabapentin 464
Gallstone 445
Gamete intrafallopian transfer 2
Gardnerella vaginalis 336
Gas gangrene 266

Gastrointestinal tract 238, 490, 545
Genetic counseling 480
Genital
   organs 542
   prolapse 522
      in pregnancy 522
      signs of 523
      symptoms of 523
Genitofemoral nerve, branch of 88
Genitourinary system 423
Gentamicin 336
Gestational
   age, determination of 231
   diabetes mellitus 420, 490
   epilepsy 463
   sac 18, 223, 223*f*
      determination of 224
      number of 312
   trophoblastic disease 16, 21, 472
      persistent 24
Gestations, multiple 447
Ghost' cells 293
Glabella 150
Glaucoma 71
Glomerular filtration rate 447
Glucocorticoid 458
   regimes 76
Glucose tolerance test 77
Glycemic control 428
Glycemic index 425, 538, 539
   high 538*f*
   low 538*f*, 539
   medium 539
Grannum's classification 234
Graves disease 472
Green-Armytage hemostatic forceps 40, 40*f*
Growth retardation 429

H

Hawkin Ambler dilators 50, 51, 51*f*, 52
Hayman uterine compression suture 105*f*
Head
   circumference 231, 232, 334, 548
   deflexion of 173*f*
   delivery 83, 91
   double fixation of 100
   engagement of 282
   gripping of 116
   palpability measurement 287
   rotation of 116

Headache 65
   persistent 381
Health education 479
Heart 434
   disease 85, 110, 432, 436-438, 443
      contraception in woman with 439
      cyanotic 440, 442
      grading of 435
      types of 434
   failure 437, 438
   rate 59, 434, 506
Hegar's dilator 50f, 51
Hellin's rule 311
HELLP syndrome 384, 446-450
   management of 391, 449, 449f
Hematoma 448
Hematometra, drainage of 51, 52
Hematuria 359
Heme iron 344
Hemoglobin 422, 423, 483
Hemorrhage 13, 84, 360
   antepartum 28, 44, 79, 123, 215, 253, 277, 359, 414, 489
   intracerebral 290
   intracranial 62, 222
   intraventricular 491
   postpartum 28, 41, 42, 84, 69, 160, 315, 361, 486, 496
Hemorrhoidal nerve 88
Hepatic rupture 448
   diagnose 448
Hepatitis
   B
      surface antigen 276
      virus 452
      vaccine 400
      viral 445, 452
Herpes simplex virus 251
Hingorani sign 521
Hodge-Smith pessary 332
Holoprosencephaly, type of 36
Homan's sign 339
Hughes syndrome 455
Human
   brain 537
   chorionic
      gonadotropin 228
      thyrotropin 546
   immunodeficiency virus 7, 276, 397, 405, 487, 498
      exposed infants 406
      infection, course of 398
      infects body 398
      negative 411
      positive 399, 411
      status code 411
      subtype 409
      types of 397
   leukocyte antigen 409
   placenta, type of 25
Humeral epiphysis, proximal 233
Hydatidiform mole 16, 16f, 23, 48, 49, 55
   complete 17
   complications of 19
Hydralazine hydrochloride 68
Hydramnios 235, 256, 261, 304, 484, 485, 486
   acute 63
   chronic 485
   complications of 486
   treatment of acute 486
   types of 485
Hydrocephalic head 95
Hydrocephalus 33, 33f, 34, 237, 248, 250, 251, 261, 303
   cause of 33, 251
Hydrops fetalis 293, 526
Hyperemesis gravidarum 23, 445, 472, 523, 524
Hyperglycemia
   labor, effects of 430
   puerperium 430
Hypermetabolism 474
Hyperosmolar glucose 6
Hypersensitivity 71
Hyperstimulation 501
Hypertension 384, 447
   chronic 394
   duration of 395
   high-risk chronic 395
   persists 383
   treatment of 384
   uncontrolled 131
Hypertensive disorder 386, 392
Hyperthyroidism 23, 472, 473
   causes of 472
Hypocalcemia 431
Hypofibrinogenemia 265
Hypoglycemia, management of 327
Hypoproteinemia 270
Hypothalamic dysfunction 469
Hypothermia, prevention of 327
Hypothyroidism 468, 471
   causes of 469
   complications if 470
Hypoxemia 241

Index

Hypoxia 241
Hypoxic ischemic encephalopathy 419
Hysterectomy 14
    abdominal 37
    clamp 38
    indications of 7, 517
    subtotal 12*f*, 15
    total abdominal 8
Hysteroscopy 52
Hysterotomy 20

I

Iliac artery
    branches of internal 105
    division of internal 40
    internal 106
    ligation, internal 104, 105*f*
Ilioinguinal nerve 88
Immature immune system 409
Immunoglobulin G 292
In vitro fertilization 2
Incisions
    abdominal 80*f*
    types of 87
Infertility 53, 130
Injection magnesium sulphate, ampoule of 65*f*
Insulin 426, 427
    dependent diabetes mellitus 424
    resistance 454
    scale, supplemental rapid-acting 426
    schedule 424
    therapy 425
    zinc suspension 427
Interstitial laser 321
Intestine 84
Intrapartum
    fetal monitoring 207
    glycemic control 429
    insulin infusion, doses regimen of 429*t*
    stillbirth, causes of 266
Intrauterine
    adhesion 49
    fetal
        death 29, 215, 235, 249, 253, 263, 291, 487
        transfusion, types of 299
        growth restriction 29, 78, 196, 205, 233, 253, 315, 320, 412, 413, 487, 497
        asymmetrical 413
        types of 413
    intraperitoneal transfusion 299
    surgery, role of 252
    transfusion 299
        complications of 530
        indications of 530
    pregnancy 5, 11, 229
    contraceptive device 2, 46, 52, 334, 405
Iron 481
    deficiency
        anemia 345
        stages of 352, 352*t*
    dietary sources of 344
    sucrose 74
        injection, ampoule of 75*f*
Isoimmunization 293
Isthmus 542

J

Jaundice 85, 270, 444, 445
    in first trimester. 445
    in second trimester. 445
    in third trimester 445
Johnson's formula 281

K

Kaposi's sarcoma 403
Karman's cannula 55
Karyotype 17
    anomalies 318
Kernicterus 293
Kerr incision 85
Kilocalories, calculation of 536*t*
Kleihauer-Betke test 293, 294
Kocher's artery forceps 38, 39*f*
    uses of 38
Kronig incision 83
Kyphoscoliosis 149

L

Labor 286
    abnormalities, treatment of 167*t*
    acceleration of 502
    and delivery, care during 404
    arrest of progress of 418
    augmentation of 69, 497
    causes of preterm 489
    failed induction of 428

induction of 429, 497, 501, 503
management of 168
normal 162
obstructed 12, 221, 253
pain, true or false 285
preterm 123, 353, 430, 489
prevention of preterm 69
progress of 309, 382, 502
second stage of 86
stage of 14, 110, 163, 164
Lactate Ringer solution 429
Lambdoid suture 149
Laparoscopic surgery, procedure for 7
Laparotomy, indications of 53
Lecithin sphingomyelin 362, 418
Leopold's maneuvers 155
Lesithin 325
Leukocyte count 264, 336
    total 264, 336
Levator ani 88
Levetriacetum 394
Ligamentum arteriosum 552
Lignocain toxicity 135
Liley's chart 297
Lip of cervix, posterior 47
Liquor amnii 484
Litzmann's obliquity 159
Liver
    abdominal pain 519
    disease 446
    enzymes, elevated 447
    function test 446, 527
Lochia 329, 332, 333
    type of 339
Lochiometra, drainage of 52
Low birth weight 409, 492
Low-salt diet 436
Lumbar puncture
    needle 62
    uses of 62
Lung injury, acute 517
Lupus anticoagulant antibodies 455
Lupus erythematosus, systemic 487, 527
Luteal phase defect 53, 454, 512

M

Macrosomia 325, 428, 494
Magnesium sulfate 65, 394
    monitoring of 66
Malabsorption syndrome 414
Malaria parasite 336
Malformation, types of 466

Malnutrition 409
Marfan's syndrome 442
Martin classification 448
Mass screening 480
Massive perineal edema 43
Mastitis 337
Maternal age, extremes of 447
Maternal coagulopathy 79
Maternal complications 387, 476, 494
Maternal death 531
    causes of 531
    in eclampsia, causes of 391
    review 532
Maternal disease 264
    group C 413
Maternal endocrine glands 546
Maternal examination 382
Maternal factors 195
Maternal hypotension, refractory 79
Maternal monitoring 387
    continuous 14
Maternal mortality 13, 533
    ratio 531
Maternal pelvis 142, 155*f*
Maternal pulse, monitoring of 436
Maternal serum alpha-fetoprotein 361, 486
Maternal soft tissue 65
Maternal surface 25, 30
Maternal uterine artery Doppler 212
Maternal vital signs 309
McDonald stitch, steps of 461
McRobert's method 495
Meconium 325
    aspiration syndrome 73, 325, 327, 419
Medical abortion 131, 519
Medical termination of pregnancy 5, 72, 92, 503, 517
Mediolateral episiotomy 88
Megaloblastic anemia 351
Membrane
    bulging of 240
    premature rupture of 123, 249, 253, 288, 315, 486
    rupture of 44, 381
    thickness 312
Menstrual
    irregularities 94, 476
    period, last 223, 269, 323
Mentzer index 480
Mercury sphygmomanometer 270
Metal female catheter in obstetrics 43
Metastatic gestational trophoblastic disease 388

Methotrexate 6, 10
   act 7
   administration of 8
   place of 9
   systemic 6
      injection of 6
   therapy 7
Methylergometrine 70, 70f
Metronidazole 336
Metropathia hemorrhagica 48
Micturition, frequency of 546
Mifepristone 6
Milk, ejection of 342
Millennium development goal 531
Mirror syndrome 528
Miscarriage 353, 476, 512
   causes of recurrent 453
   complete 513
   inevitable 513
   recurrent 453, 456
Misoprostol 72, 73f, 160, 504
   advantages of 504
Mitral stenosis 438, 444
Mitral valve, normal 438
Mitral valvotomy, indications of 438
Molecular-weight heparin, low 440
Monoamniotic monochromic twin 322
Monochorionic diamniotic twins 318
Monochorionicity 312, 322
Monozygotic twins, types of 313
Morning sickness 546
Moro reflex 334
Morphine 437
Mucus membrane 411
Mucus sucker 58
Muller-Munro-Kerr method 308
Multicystic dysplastic kidneys 238
Multidrug resistant tuberculosis 341
Multiple pregnancies, antenatal management of 322
Muscle fibers, superficial 82
Muscular paresis 65
Myasthenia gravis 65
Mycoplasma 336
Myocardium, hypertrophic 438
Myoma 520
Myomectomy operation 42
Myometrial
   cells 71, 72
   contraction 69
   thickness 361
Myometrium
   invasion of 23
   trauma of 12
Myxedema coma 471

N

Naegele's formula 281
Naegele's obliquity 159
Naegele's pelvis 149
Nasal catheter 59
National Institute for Health and Care Excellence 271
Neisseria gonorrhoeae 400
Neonatal
   complications 443
   lupus erythematosus 458
   thyroid screening 470
   thyrotoxicosis 472
Nephritic syndrome 270
Nephritis, chronic 264
Nerve supply of vulva 88
Nervous system 545
Neural defects 350
   tube 32, 136, 261
Nevirapine 402
New York Heart Association 435
Nifedipine 68
Nipple, cracked 337
Nitabuch's membrane 27
Nitrazine test 289
Nitrogen 539
   balance 539, 539f
N-methyl-D aspartate 65
Nonimmune hydrops fetalis 525
Nonoligohydramniotic sac 321
Nonsteroidal anti-inflammatory drug 487
Non-stress test 194, 203, 205, 212, 326
Nontubal ectopic pregnancies 10
Normocardia 198
Nuchal cord 31
Nuchal translucency 238, 261
Nulligravida 278
Nullipara 278
Nulliparous gestations 447
Nutrition 340, 535

O

Obesity 339, 475, 476
Obstetric history, bad 428
Obstetrical pelvic axis 147f
Oldham's cranial perforator 95, 95f
Oligohydramnios 235, 248, 325, 328, 329, 384, 484, 487, 488
   complications of 488
Ophthalmoscopic examination 422
Opportunistic infection 400

Oral
  contraceptive pill 21, 405, 509
    combined 334, 432
  glucose
    challenge test 276, 420
    tolerance test 421, 527, 545
  hypoglycemic agents 431
  iron 348, 351
    absorption of 347
Ovarian artery 84
  ligation 103
Ovarian cystectomy operation 40
Ovarian ectopic pregnancy 8
Ovarian pregnancy 8, 10
  treatment of 8
  types of 8
Ovarian tumor 8, 230, 521
  treatment of benign 521
Ovary, position of 8
Overlapping of skull bones 263f
Ovum
  blighted 226
  forceps 37, 49, 54, 54f
Oxcarbazepine 464
Oxygen
  inhalation 327, 436
  partial pressures of 196
Oxytocin 214
  advantages of 504
  complications of 503
  infusion 74
  regime, high dose 501

P

Pain
  abdomen 18, 329, 353
  abdominal 3
  relief 167
Painful crisis 482
Paracervical block 133, 133f
Parametrial cellulitis 337
Parametrial phlegmon 337
Parenteral iron therapy, advantage of 348
Parietal bone 96
Parietal tissues 40
Partographic chart 213
Patellar reflex 385
Patent ductus arteriosus 441
Patwardhan's method 83
Pawlick's grip 275
Peak systolic velocity 300, 528

Pelvic
  abscess 337
  axis, anatomical 147f
  brim 142, 148, 154
  curve 109
    concavity of 83
  dimension 145, 146
    plane of least 146
  floor repair 269
  grip 274
    first 274, 275f
    second 275, 275f
  inflammatory disease 2, 94, 494, 534
  inlet 143, 553
    shape of 143
  outlet 145, 148, 553
  tumor 221
Pelvis 142, 146
  abnormalities of 149
  adequate 250
  axis of 110
  borderline 248
  contracted 221, 248, 303, 304, 357
  diameters of 146
  inclination of 143
  normal 308
  plane of 145
  shape of 160
  true 142
  type of 147, 310
Percutaneous umbilical blood sampling 140
Perinatal death 357
Perinatal mortality rate 533
Perinatal transmission, prevention of 407
Perineal injury 91
Perineal muscles 90f
Perineal tear
  degrees of 91
  repair of 134
    complete 45, 87
Perineal tissue, infiltration of 89f
Peripartum cardiomyopathy 442
Peripartum hysterectomy, indications of 85
Peripheral resistance 544
Peripheral vascular resistance, reduced 472
Peritonitis 13
Phagocytic cells 26
Phlebothrombosis 338, 339
Pinard's metal fetoscope 56

Index

Pinard's metal fetoscope 56
Pinch valve, releasing of 129*f*
Placenta 25*f*, 27, 31, 233
    abnormalities of 28
    accreta 85, 361, 365
        management of 365
    bipartia 28*f*
        or tripartia 28
    circumvallate 29*f*
    delivery of 37, 70
    diseases of 30
    duplex 28*f*
    functions of 27
    injury of 44
    lobules of 30
    manual removal of 14, 106, 298, 507
    maternal surface of 25*f*
    normal 27
    partial molar degeneration of 23
    previa 82, 85, 235, 248, 356, 359-363
        anterior 84
        causes of 359
        dangerous 364
    structures of 26
    succenturiata 28, 28*f*
Placental abruption 329
Placental alpha microglobulin-1 289
Placental dysfunction 413
Placental endocrinology 546
Placental infarction 361
Placental insufficiency 457
Placental masses, number of 312
Placental polyp 53
Placental site trophoblastic tumor 24
Plasma regain, rapid 276
Plasmapheresis 297
Plastic Karman's cannula 55*f*
Platelet 507
    concentrates 387
Platypelloid 149, 553
Pneumococcal vaccine 400
Pneumocystitis carinii pneumonia 400
Pneumocystitis jirovecii pneumonia 404
Podalic version, internal 125, 125*f*, 317
Polyglycolic suture material 82, 91
Polyhydramnios 248, 429, 430
Polymerase chain reaction 399
Ponderal index 413, 416
Post-term baby, complications of 325
Potassium chloride 6
Pouch of Douglas 3, 42
Pouch, opening of 47
Pre-eclampsia 445, 446, 457
    severe 382, 386

Pregnancy
    abdominal 10
    ascertain duration of 281
    associated plasma protein 27, 546
    blood volume 280
    causes of post-term 325
    cholestasis of 445
    continuation of 130
    early present 268
    fibroid with 519
    gynecological disorder in 519
    high-risk 213
    history of late 268
    hyperthyroidism in 469, 472
    induced hypertension 38, 234, 248, 270, 414
    induced hypotension 196
    interstitial 7, 9
    intrahepatic cholestasis of 451
    loss, recurrent 453, 454, 457
    molar 49
    morbidity 455
    multiple 248, 257, 261, 269, 311, 321-323, 329
    nausea and vomiting of 524
    on diabetes, effects of 424
    on epilepsy, effect of 462
    on thyroid function, effects of 467
    outcome, drugs to improve 456
    postdated 323, 326
    problems, first trimester 226
    secondary abdominal 9
    sickling disorder in 482
    termination of 131, 383, 418, 531
        indications of 435
    tubal 1,
    uncomplicated 356
    with epilepsy, antenatal care in 465
Pregnancy-induced hypertension, complications of 387
Pregnant mother with diabetes 421
Pregnant women 410*f*
    directly in labor 410*f*
Presteroid insulin doses, reduction of 77
Primigravida 87, 303, 362
Progesterone therapy 322
Progestogen-only pill 340
Propranolol 475
Propylthiouracil 473, 475
Prostaglandins 6, 383, 499
Prosthetic heart valve 443
Prosthetic valve 443
    types, benefit of 442

Prostodin ampoule 72f
Protamine sulphate 339
Protease inhibitors 401, 408
Protein 333, 536, 540, 545
   acetone 215
   biological value of 540
   C-reactive 460
   high 436
   hormone 546
Prothrombin time 446, 457
Pruritus
   character of 445
   prominent symptoms of 445
Pseudo sac, causes of 228
Pubic arch 147, 147f
Pudendal block 134
Pudendal nerve, branches of 88
Puerperal psychosis 335
Puerperal pyrexia, causes of 336
Puerperium 329, 331, 350, 390, 397, 430, 437, 476, 483
   complications of 335
Pulmonary edema 65, 84, 384, 387
   management of 437
Pulmonary embolism 435
Pulmonary hypertension
   effect of 442
   severe 442, 443
Pulse 59, 215, 536
   rate 3, 472, 515
Pyelonephritis 482
Pyometra, drainage of 51, 52
Pyopagus 262
Pyrexia, puerperal 335, 336

Q

Queenan chart 297
Quientero staging system 319

R

Rachitic pelvis 149
Radical hysterectomy 43
Red blood cells 292, 419
Red cell distribution width 347
Renal
   anomalies 487
   disease 351, 395
   failure 13, 387
      acute 517
   function 65
      test 422, 527
   glycosuria 424

Reproductive tract infection 436
Respiratory
   depression 65
   distress syndrome 62, 76, 315, 361, 431, 493, 494, 534
      acute 19, 517
      adult 84, 383
      rate 506
   system 544, 544t
   tract infections 336
Retention of urine 3, 42, 90
Retina 537
Retinopathy, proliferative 482
Retracted nipple 337
Rhesus 234
Rheumatic
   carditis, active 434
   fever 443
   valvular heart disease 434
Ribonucleic acid 397, 537
Ribs, crowding of 263
Ringer's lactate 4, 90, 168, 362, 500, 525
Robert's pelvis 149
Robert's sign 263
Rooting reflex 334
Roux-en-Y gastric bypass 477
Rubella 251
Rubin's criterion 11
Rubin's maneuver 495, 495f
Rudimentary horn 9
   tube of 8
Rupture
   of membrane, artificial 221, 257, 295, 407, 486
   tubal 2

S

Sacrocotyloid diameter 144
Sacrum 305
S-adenosylmethionine 446
Salpingectomy 1
   operation 5
Salt-restricted diet 437
Scalp blood pH measurement 207
Scalp hematoma 65
Scanzoni-Smellie maneuver 117
Scar dehiscence 354
Scar rupture 354, 355
Schilling test 351
Sepsis 332, 430, 515
   atonicity of 85
   bacteriology of 514
   puerperal 335, 336

Index

Septic abortion 514, 515, 517
Serum
    bile acid testing 445
    folate 351
    glutamic
        oxaloacetic transaminase 22
        pyruvic transaminase 22
    soluble transferrin receptor 345
Sexual intercourse 336, 398
Sexually transmitted diseases 398
Shirodkar's needle 63, 63f
Shock 4, 12, 15, 49
    correction of 15
    index 506
Shoulder
    delivery of posterior 496f
    dystocia 257, 494, 495
        causes of 494
        complications of 496
        management of 257, 495
    presentation, causes of 253
Sickle cell
    disease 479
    disorder 482
Sickling disorder 482
    diagnose 482
Silastic ventouse cup 123
Silent chorioamnionitis 336
Sim's anterior vaginal wall retractor 45f
Sim's double-bladed posterior vaginal speculum 44
Sim's position 46
    advantage of 46
Sim's speculum 44, 45f, 46
    disadvantages of 45
Sim's triad 46
Simpson's forceps 108f
Singleton pregnancy 329
Skeletal dysplasia 239
Skin 88
    cells 57
    incision 80
    infection 79
    integrity, altered 409
Small artery 90
Small gynecoid pelvis 149
Small menopausal uterus 49
Smythe catheter, drew 44, 44f
Snowstorm appearance 17, 18, 229f
Spalding's sign 263, 264, 264t
Spasmodic dysmenorrhea 52
Sphyngomyelin 325
Spiegelberg's criteria 8

Spina bifida 251
Spinal anesthesia 79
    complications of 79
Spinal blockade 79
    total 79
Spinal headache 79
Sponge holding forceps 37, 37f
Spontaneous abortion 430, 472, 482, 512
Staphylococcus aureus 336, 338
Status eclampticus 391
Steroids 446
Still birth, antepartum 357
Stress test, contraction 204, 212
Stress urinary incontinence 42
Stroke volume 438, 472
Stromal tissue 27
Stuck twin syndrome 321
Studdiford's criteria 9
Submucous fibroid 48
Subpubic angle 147
Suckling reflex 334
Sudden postpartum collapse, causes of 509
Supine hypotensive syndrome 195
Suprapubic pain 354
Symphysio-fundal height 331, 381, 549
    measurement 272f, 414
Symphysis pubis 305
Synclitism 159
Syncytiotrophoblast 26, 27
Syntocinon ampoule 69f
Systolic blood pressure 271, 506

T

Tachycardia 197f, 198
    mild 198
    severe 198, 208f
    unexplained 354
Tachysystole 501
Teeth vulsellum
    multiple 47, 47f
    parts of multiple 47
    uses of multiple 47
Temporal bones 150
Tennessee classification 448
Tenofovir 403
    disoproxil fumarate 408
Termination of pregnancy, methods of 518
Thalassemia 479, 526
    alpha 479
    beta 479

disease, E-beta 483
in population 479
major 479
minor 479
on child-bearing woman, effects of 479
Theca lutein cysts 20
Thoracic auscultation 435
Thoracopagus 35f
Thrombocytopenia 79, 448
Thromboembolism, high-risk of 443
Thrombophlebitis 338
   puerperal 338
Thromboplastin time
   activated partial 439, 440, 457
   partial 440
Thrombotic thrombocytopenic purpura 388
Thyroid 546
   disorder 467
   dysfunction 468
      primary 469
   hormones, exogenous 472
   storm 474, 475
   surgery 473, 474
Tibial epiphysis, proximal 233
Tissue forceps, type of 40
Tocolytic therapy 491
   role of 290
Tonic stage 388
Tooth
   disadvantages of single 47
   vulsellum, single 47f
Topiramate 464
Toxic adenomas 472
Toxic nodular goiter 472
Toxoplasmosis 251
Tranexamic acid 74
   injection, ampoule of 74f
Trans vaginal cervical length 322
Transcerebellar diameter 414
Transferrin saturation 352
Transient tachypnea 358
Transvaginal
   cervical length 321
   sonography 3, 492
      role of 492
Transverse arrest, deep 119, 172
Trauma 336
Traumatic postpartum hemorrhage 509
Trophoblast
   lysis of 6
   proliferative 18

Trophoblastic
   disease 229
   embolism 23
   hyperplasia 17
   neoplasia 17
   tumor, placental site 16, 24
Tubal pregnancy, rupture of 9
Tuberculosis 268
Tuberculous endometritis 53
Tumor, complications of 521
Twin
   anemia polycythemia sequence 320, 530
   cause of conjoined 35, 262
   conjoined 35, 261, 262, 313, 314
   deliver
      conjoined 36
      in second 318
   dizygotic 313
   fraternal 313
   head of second 119
   manage conjoined 262
   monozygotic 323
   peak sign 227f
   pregnancy 226, 258, 311, 314-316
      complications of 315
   pole 227
   type of 261, 311
   reversed arterial perfusion 315, 320
   syndrome, vanishing 259
   transfusion syndrome 258, 318
   types of 314f
      conjoined 262, 314
   vanishing 227
   with placenta, conjoined 35f
   X-ray of conjoined 262f
Twin-to-twin transfusion 243
   syndrome 315, 318, 487, 526

U

Umbilical artery 31, 241, 242f, 244, 414
   closure of 551
   Doppler, normal 244f
   single 31, 235, 261
Umbilical blood vessel 25f, 56
Umbilical cord 24, 30, 239f
   compression 328
   develops 31
   prolapse 123
   scissors 61, 61f
   vessel 25f
Umbilical grip 274

Index

Umbilical ligaments, medial 552
Umbilical vein 245, 550
   closure of 552
Umbilical vesicle, remnant of 31
Umbilicus, level of 273*f*
Uniovular twin pregnancy, placenta of 26*f*
United Nations Children's Fund 340
Ureter 545
Urethral damage 43
Urinary
   bladder, stone of 48
   system 545
   tract
      anomalies of fetus 487
      infection 43, 336, 405
Urine 336, 524, 539
   albumin 382
   output 382, 507, 516
   pregnancy test 355
Ursodeoxycholic acid 446
Uterine 84, 103
   anomalies 329
   artery 85, 244
      Doppler 242, 243*f*
      embolization 11
      waveform, abnormal 243*f*
      waveform, normal 243*f*
   atony, persistent 85
   bleeding, dysfunctional 53
   cavity 49, 53, 81, 93, 94, 94*f*
      length of 48
   compression, bimanual 101, 105*f*
   contraction 309, 460
      hyperactive 210*f*
   curette 52, 93, 93f, 94*f*
      uses of 53
   depth, measurement of 128*f*
   endometrium, status of 52
   fibroid 8, 48
   forceps 94, 94*f*
   hemorrhage, uncontrolled 85
   height of 58
   incision 81
      vertical 83
   infection 85
   inversion 510
      types of 510
   involution 331, 339
   isthmus, anterior part of 10
   length 48
   malformation 248
   muscle
      fibers, retraction of 70
      layer of deeper 82
      tone 248
   oxytocics 81
   polyp 54
   prolapse 48
   retraction 79
   rupture 85, 329
      causes of 12
      surgery of 43
   segment 82
      lower 15, 83, 85, 286, 493
   sepsis 49
   soufflé 284
   sound 48, 48*f*, 49
      uses of 48
   synechiae, treatment of 54
   tumors 230
   vessels 84
   wall 8, 44, 54, 84
      perforation, lateral 53
   waveform 243*f*
Uteroplacental
   fistula 9
   function 204
Uterotonic drug 160, 508*t*
Uterus 48, 49, 53, 55, 542
   acute infection of 49
   asymmetrical enlargement of 547
   atonicity of 85
   carcinoma of body of 53
   complications of ruptured 13
   degenerated fibroma of 229
   direction of 94
   emptying of 130
   evacuation of 130*f*
   fibroid 549
   fundus of 49
   hypertonicity of 329
   infection of 49
   inversion of 31, 48, 510
   involution of 331, 333
   irritable 307
   ligament of 80
   lower segment of 79, 83
   menopausal 48
   normal involution of 331
   packing of 11
   part of 8
   puerperal 49
   removal of 85
   rupture of 11, 12, 12*f*, 43, 123, 126
   sub-involution of 21, 48
   upper segment of 15
   walls of 54

V

Vagina 542
  ballooning of 46
Vaginal approach 134
Vaginal birth after cesarean section 355, 356
Vaginal bleeding 3, 18
  intractable 23
  mild 354, 357
Vaginal breech delivery 250
Vaginal delivery 85, 87, 258, 326, 387
  operative 404
  safe 249
  sign for successful 309
Vaginal discharge 329
Vaginal examination 14, 99, 222, 277
Vaginal ligation 47
Vaginal mucosa
  episiotomy in 90f
  posterior 88
Vaginal mucosae 89
Vaginal pessaries 462
Vaginal pulsation 547
Vaginal tissue 122
Vaginal wall
  anterior 45, 46
  posterior 45
Valproic acid 462
Valve syringe
  double 127f
  single 127f
Valvular stenosis 443
Vasa previa 364
Vascular disease 195, 395
Vasectomy, non-scalpel 405
Vein thrombosis, deep 335
Vena cava, inferior 550
Venereal disease research laboratory 276, 399
Ventilation, minute of 60
Ventouse delivery 119
Ventouse operation, indications of 119
Vesical artery, superior 552
Vesicles, discharge of 18
Vesicovaginal fistula 42, 45, 83, 222, 498
  repair of 269
Villi
  sampling, chrionic 483
  swelling of 17
  zone of terminal 27
Viral
  hepatitis 451
    types of 451, 451t
  illness 414
  isolation 399
Visual acoustic stimulation 204
Vital signs, supervision of 15
Vitamin
  A, supplementation of 400
  B_{12} deficiency anemia 351
  K 446
Vulsellum 47
Vulva 542
Vulval hematoma 90
  causes of 90

W

Weinberg's sign 9
White blood cell 22
Willets' scalp traction forceps 64, 64f
Wolf-Parkinson-White syndrome 473
World Health Organization 340, 407
Wound, episiotomy of 90f, 339
Wrigley's forceps 108f

X

Xylocain solution 136

Y

Yolk sac 224
  number of 312

Z

Zatuchni-Andros scores 249, 249t
Zidovudin 407
Zonisamide 464
Zygote, division of 35